A Clinical Guide to Skin Cancer

A Clinical Guide to Skin Cancer

Editor: Julio Casey

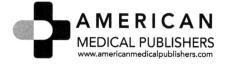

AMERICAN
MEDICAL PUBLISHERS
www.americanmedicalpublishers.com

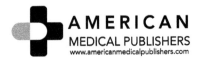

Cataloging-in-Publication Data

A clinical guide to skin cancer / edited by Julio Casey.
   p. cm.
Includes bibliographical references and index.
ISBN 978-1-63927-841-1
1. Skin--Cancer. 2. Skin--Cancer--Treatment. 3. Skin--Cancer--Prevention.
4. Skin--Cancer--Patients. 5. Skin--Cancer--Diagnosis. I. Casey, Julio.
RC280.S5 C55 2023
616.994 77--dc23

American Medical Publishers,
41 Flatbush Avenue,
1st Floor, New York,
NY 11217, USA

ISBN 978-1-63927-841-1 (Hardback)

Contents

Preface

The type of cancer that involves an abnormal growth of skin cells is called skin cancer. There are three prominent forms of this type of cancer named as basal cell carcinoma, squamous cell carcinoma, and melanoma. The main reason for development of skin cancer is exposure of skin to sun, and usually includes lips, ears, neck, face, and scalp. Basal cell carcinoma may appear like a pearly or waxy bump or as a flat, flesh colored scar-like lesion. Squamous cell carcinoma often affects people with darker skin tone and appears as a firm red nodule or as a flat lesion with a scaly crusted surface. The signs of melanoma include a large brownish spot with darker speckles, a painful lesion that itches or burns, or as a mole that changes in color and size. A weakened immune system, exposure to radiation, a personal history of skin cancer, fair skin, and excessive sun exposure are some factors that increase the risk of skin cancer. This book is a compilation of chapters that discuss the most vital concepts and emerging trends in the prevention and treatment of skin cancer. It aims to shed light on some of the unexplored aspects of this disease. The book will serve as a reference to a broad spectrum of readers.

This book has been the outcome of endless efforts put in by authors and researchers on various issues and topics within the field. The book is a comprehensive collection of significant researches that are addressed in a variety of chapters. It will surely enhance the knowledge of the field among readers across the globe.

It gives us an immense pleasure to thank our researchers and authors for their efforts to submit their piece of writing before the deadlines. Finally in the end, I would like to thank my family and colleagues who have been a great source of inspiration and support.

Editor

Skin Imaging Using Ultrasound Imaging, Optical Coherence Tomography, Confocal Microscopy and Two-Photon Microscopy in Cutaneous Oncology

Byung Ho Oh[1], Ki Hean Kim[2] and Kee Yang Chung[1]*

[1] Department of Dermatology and Cutaneous Biology Research Institute, Yonsei University College of Medicine, Seoul, South Korea, [2] Department of Mechanical Engineering, Pohang University of Science and Technology, Pohang-si, South Korea

*Correspondence:
Kee Yang Chung
kychung@yuhs.ac

With the recognition of dermoscopy as a new medical technology and its available fee assessment in Korea comes an increased interest in imaging-based dermatological diagnosis. For the dermatologist, who treats benign tumors and malignant skin cancers, imaging-based evaluations can assist with determining the surgical method and future follow-up plans. The identification of the tumor's location and the existence of blood vessels can guide safe treatment and enable the use of minimal incisions. The recent development of high-resolution microscopy based on laser reflection has enabled observation of the skin at the cellular level. Despite the limitation of a shallow imaging depth, non-invasive light-based histopathologic examinations are being investigated as a rapid and pain-free process that would be appreciated by patients and feature reduced time from consultation to treatment. In the United States, the current procedural terminology billing code was established for reflectance confocal microscopy in 2016 and has been used for the skin cancer diagnosis ever since. In this review, we introduce the basic concepts and images of ultrasound imaging, optical coherence tomography, confocal microscopy, and two-photon microscopy and discuss how they can be utilized in the field of dermatological oncology.

Keywords: skin imaging, skin cancer, benign skin tumor, ultrasound, optical coherence tomography, confocal microscopy, two-photon microscopy

INTRODUCTION

Efforts to diagnose skin cancer without skin biopsy are ongoing. The diagnoses of patients with suspected skin cancer are confirmed by punch biopsy followed by histopathological examination, which involve the collection of a small portion of the entire lesion to diagnose skin cancer (1). In this case, since only vertical information of a specific region is acquired, dermoscopy can supplement horizontal information of the entire lesion to identify the most suitable biopsy site. However, dermoscopy has an inherent depth limit confined to the upper dermis (**Table 1**).

TABLE 1 | Pros and cons of skin biopsy and dermoscopy.

	Skin biopsy	Dermoscopy
Advantages	1. Provide universal validity based on long-term accumulated histopathological criteria	1. Identify optimal biopsy sites 2. Reduce unnecessary biopsy 3. Determine horizontal extent of skin lesion 4. Continue to observe lesion treatment
Disadvantages	1. Limitation of evaluating whole lesion by vertical information of specific region 2. Limitations of repeated practice due to pain, bleeding, and infection risk	1. Inherent depth limitation (upper dermis) 2. Difficulty implementing 3D image 3. No reflection of functional and dynamic information (blood flow velocity, oxygen saturation, etc.) of the skin

TABLE 2 | Device resolution and imaging depths[1].

	Resolution	Penetration depth
Confocal microscopy	1 μm	~500 μm
Optical coherence tomography	2–10 μm	~2 mm
Ultrasonography	150 μm	~10 cm
High-resolution computed tomography	300 μm	Entire body
Magnetic resonance imaging	1 mm	Entire body

To observe lesions deep to the upper dermis, the maximum depth that can be observed with dermoscopy, non-invasive techniques, such as confocal microscopy, multiphoton microscopy, optical coherence tomography, and ultrasound must be used. Although each operation principle is different, they all use the reflection characteristic as if it is mirrored, and the skin's depth and resolution differ among device types (**Table 2**). Here we briefly discuss each available device and its clinical use in the dermatology field.

ULTRASOUND IMAGING

Ultrasound imaging uses high-frequency sound waves that cannot be heard by the human ear. When it is sent inside the human body, the degree of absorption and reflection is cut off depending on the constituents and the reflected sound waves are sensed and imaged (2). Therefore, the probe that sends and detects the sound waves forms the core equipment for ultrasound technology. Higher-frequency (MHz) sound waves enable high-resolution observation of the skin surface, but the observable depth decreases. In the field of dermatology, ultrasound is mainly used to identify benign tumor type and extent (**Table 3**). Before surgery, it can provide information about tumor type and size, locate the existence of surrounding vessels, identify the best location for the incision, and set the range while viewing the ultrasound screen in real time with the patient. It can also help the clinician evaluate whether the tumor was completely removed after surgery (**Figure 1**).

In the case of epidermoid cysts, one of the most common benign tumors, it is often seen as a well-defined ovoid-shaped heterogeneous hypoechoic lesion in the subcutaneous layer with strong posterior acoustic enhancement (**Figure 2**). Ultrasonographic findings corresponding to epidermal cyst rupture include pericystic changes, increased vascularity, deep abscess formation, and others (9). Trichilemmal cyst, a benign

appendage lesion derived from the outer root sheath of the hair follicle, is often seen as a well-defined hypoechoic lesion with internal calcification and posterior sound enhancement (**Figure 3**) (8). Identifying these sites just prior to surgery and optimizing the incision site and approach can improve the success rate and reduce recurrence rates.

Pilomatricoma, a benign superficial tumor of the hair follicle, is often seen as a well-defined mass with inner echogenic foci and a peripheral hypoechoic rim or a completely echogenic mass with strong posterior acoustic shadowing in the subcutaneous layer on ultrasonography (**Figure 4**) (7). Pilomatricoma often shows angiographic findings and may be difficult to differentiate from hemangioma.

A lipoma appears as a well-defined hypoechoic mass with multiple echogenic strands on ultrasound (**Figure 5**). If the encapsulation is well-formed, it is easier to remove. Ultrasonography is especially useful for diagnosing and treating lipoma in the forehead. A lipoma occurring in the forehead is often located under the frontalis muscles, and it is important to confirm its precise position using preoperative ultrasonography. It typically has a semispherical shape when located under the muscles and an ovoid shape when it is located in the subcutaneous fat layer (**Figure 6**) (11). However, this is not always the case, so a comprehensive judgment should be made by checking whether it is close to the periosteum or using a special technique that uses the angulation of the probe to point out the lateral borders of the lesion (12).

There are no obvious criteria that can diagnose malignant cutaneous tumors using ultrasound imaging. However, tumor size >5 cm, infiltrated margins, rapid clinical growth, moderate to severe intratumoral hypervascularity (**Figure 7**), and an absence of the typical features of benign tumors are highly suggestive of malignancy (13, 14). High-definition ultrasound with transducers up to 70 MHz, which can observe more detail, has been used to diagnose cutaneous angiosarcoma of the breast and is expected to be useful for the identification of malignant skin cancers (15).

OPTICAL COHERENCE TOMOGRAPHY

Optical coherence tomography (OCT), a three-dimensional (3D) imaging technique based on low coherence interferometry,

---

Abbreviations: OCT, optical coherence tomography; TPM, two-photon microscopy; EMPD, extramammary Paget's disease; SHG, second harmonic generation; MPM, multi-photon microscopy; BCC, basal cell carcinoma; SCC, squamous cell carcinoma; AK, actinic keratosis.

---

[1]Available online at: http://obel.ee.uwa.edu.au/research/fundamentals/introduction-oct/

TABLE 3 | Key articles comparing ultrasound imaging and histopathology.

Tumor type	Year	Main findings	Correlation with histopathological findings	Probe frequency	Sample size
Basal cell carcinoma (3)	2008	1. BCC tumor ultrasound shows an oval and hypoechoic lesion 2. Compare tumor thickness measurements between ultrasound and histology	Good thickness correlation with histology (intraclass correlation coefficient, 0.9)	7–15 MHz probe	25 patients
Basal cell carcinoma (4)	2007	Lesions that may have a higher aggressive potential may also appear as hyperechoic spots	Hypersonographic spots in BCCs seemed to correspond to calcification, horn cysts, or clusters of apoptotic cells in the centers of nests of basal cell carcinoma	15 or 30 MHz	29 basal cell carcinomas
Invasive squamous cell carcinoma (5)	2009	SCC metastasized to lymph node showed asymmetrical cortical area with high elasticity	Presence of metastatic tumor cells located asymmetrically in a small section of the cortical area	Not mentioned	1 patient
Merkel cell carcinoma (6)	2017	1. Hypoechoic pattern with variable vascularization 2. Useful in the diagnostic work-up of MCC and can help more precisely delimit the tumor prior to complete surgical resection	Not mentioned	18 MHz	7 patients
Pilomatricoma (7)	2005	Well-defined mass with inner echogenic foci and a peripheral hypoechoic rim or a completely echogenic mass with strong posterior acoustic shadowing	Inner echogenic foci may relate with calcification or ossification	7–12 MHz	20 pilomatricomas from 19 patients
Trichilemmal cyst (TC) (8)	2019	Well-defined hypoechoic lesions with internal calcification and posterior sound enhancement	TC contains homogeneous eosinophilic keratinous materials Calcified foci within this keratin can be found	3–12 MHz 6–18 MHz	54 TCs from 50 patients
Ruptured epidermal cyst (REC) (9)	2008	RECs were classified into three types: with lobulations showing echogenic inner contents (type I), with protrusions (type II), and with abscess pocket formations showing poorly defined pericystic changes and increased vascularity around the abscess formation (type III)	Histopathology of the excised RECs also showed similar morphology	5–10 MHz 5–12 MHz	13 patients
Lipoma in the forehead (10)	2016	1. Hyperechoic striated septae parallel to the skin suggestive of lipoma 2. Ultrasonographic findings were accurate in 9 of 14 cases (64.3%).	Unlike the preoperative ultrasonographic findings, 13 of 14 cases were confirmed as frontalis-associated lipomas intraoperatively	12 or 15 MHz	14 patients with lipomas in the forehead

creates an image by detecting the interference phenomena from light scattering or reflection as it passes through different layers of skin via the time domain or Fourier-domain method. OCT non-invasively provides skin images similar to the B mode of ultrasound to a depth of 1–2 mm and a resolution of 2–10 μm with high imaging speed. Functional OCT techniques that can provide additional information, such as polarization and vasculature were recently developed and applied for the detection of abnormal vasculature of a port-wine stain or skin cancer (16–18). Our research group developed a device that matches an OCT image with that obtained by dermoscopic imaging and provides more information than dermoscopy alone

(19). Through this, we expect to be able to assess the extent of scar treatment (**Figure 8**). It is expected that a stage of nevus flammeus will be established, and treatment feasibility and degree will be evaluated (**Figure 9**). The limitations of OCT are limited depth of examination and lack of resolution to observe cancer cell morphology. Line-field confocal OCT, which can reveal comprehensive structural mapping of the skin at the cellular level with an isotropic spatial resolution of ∼1 μm to a depth of ∼500 μm, was recently reported to correlate with conventional histopathological images of skin tumors (20). Key articles comparing OCT and histopathology are summarized in **Table 4**.

CONFOCAL MICROSCOPY

Confocal microscopy is based on the existence of one focal point when a laser, used as a light source, is reflected off a subject.

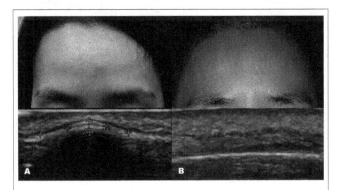

FIGURE 1 | Ultrasound images of forehead osteoma. **(A)** Before excision. **(B)** After excision performed through a remote incision above the hairline.

The "out of focus" signal is blocked by a pinhole, and contrast is generated by reflections at the interfaces of tissue and cellular structures due to variations of the index of refraction. Since image acquisition is not possible with a single signal point, imaging occurs by scanning across several pinholes. Imaging up to a depth of 100–200 μm at a 1-μm resolution is possible. Confocal microscopy is capable of providing rapid bedside pathological analysis by producing images with subcellular resolution without skin biopsy and physical sectioning (24–26). There are two ways to use this approach for Mohs surgery. One is used *in vivo* and can help the identification of the surgical margins in a perioperative setting (27). It is also possible to check the remaining lesion using intraoperative images *in vivo* after removing the main skin cancer mass (28). The other is for *ex vivo* use, in which the surgical margins are removed and confocal microscopy is used to confirm whether the tumor remains within it (29). However, when used for detection in Mohs surgery, the grayscale confocal image was difficult to interpret by the surgeons. To improve this, each frozen specimen was stained with acridine orange

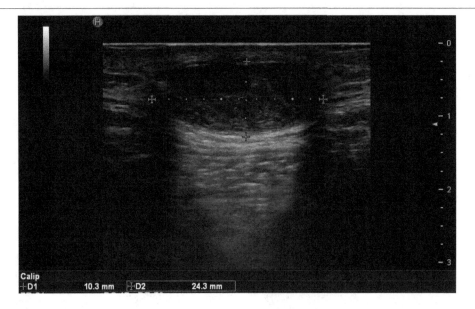

FIGURE 2 | Ultrasound image of epidermal cyst.

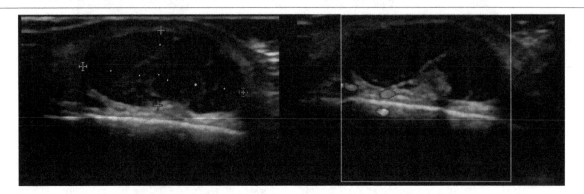

FIGURE 3 | Ultrasound image of trichilemmal cyst.

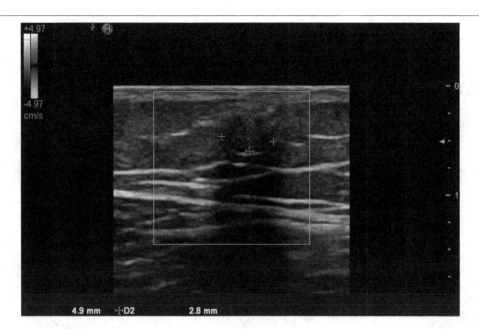

FIGURE 4 | Ultrasound image of pilomatricoma.

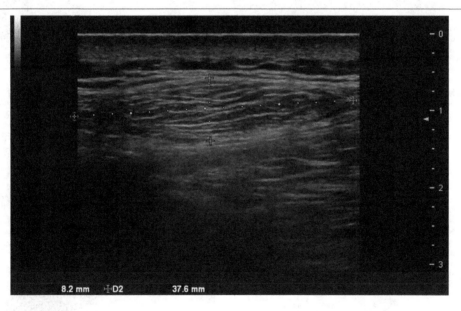

FIGURE 5 | Ultrasound image of lipoma.

(pH 6.0) and eosin (pH 6.0) and then scanned with confocal mosaicking microscopy to imitate hematoxylin and eosin-stained Mohs frozen sections. This approach and physician training can improve the accuracy of the non-melanoma skin cancer diagnosis (30). Key articles comparing confocal microscopy and histopathology are summarized in **Table 5**.

Confocal microscopy has also been applied to diagnose mammary and extramammary Paget's disease (EMPD) (37), frequently showing Paget cells predominantly within the epidermis (38). However, due to the limited depth of

imaging (100–200 μm) when applied non-invasively, the invasion site is difficult to determine. A major limitation of this technique is that it can only provide morphological information and does not reflect the tissue's internal structure or functional state.

TWO-PHOTON MICROSCOPY

Two-photon microscopy (TPM) is a technique that uses the fluorescence released after excitation from simultaneously

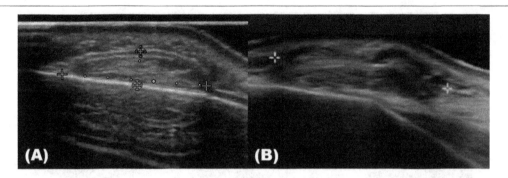

FIGURE 6 | Ultrasound image of forehead lipoma. **(A)** Submuscular layer. **(B)** Subcutaneous layer.

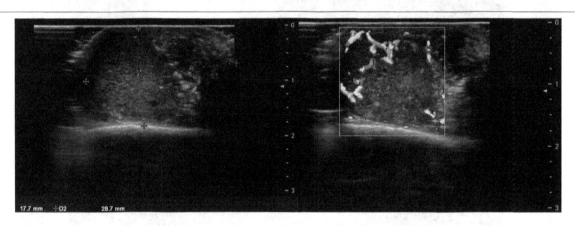

FIGURE 7 | Ultrasound image of malignant proliferating trichilemmal tumor.

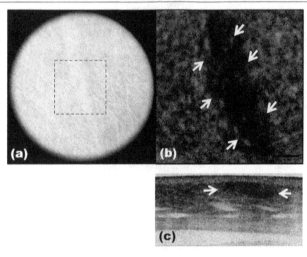

FIGURE 8 | Scar images by dermoscopy-guided multifunctional optical coherence tomography (OCT). **(a)** Dermoscopic image. **(b,c)** Intensity OCT showing a dark area and frequent banding pattern due to stronger light scattering and birefringence.

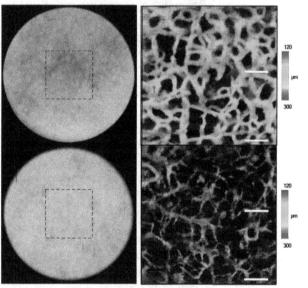

FIGURE 9 | Images of nevus flammeus and normal skin acquired by dermoscopy-guided angiographic optical coherence tomography.

absorbing two photons with long wavelengths and low energy. TPM allows observation of vital phenomena in cells and *in vivo* at the molecular level. In particular, it has the advantage of being able to identify the distribution of collagen within the dermis using the second harmonic generation (SHG) produced when two photons simultaneously interfere. Non-invasive *in vivo*

TABLE 4 | Key articles comparing optical coherence tomography and histopathology.

Tumor type	Year	Type	Main findings	Correlation with histopathology findings	Sample size
Basal cell carcinoma (BCC) (21)	2014	High-definition optical coherence tomography (HD-OCT)	Lobulated nodules, peripheral rimming, epidermal disarray	Peripheral rimming in HD-OCT correlates with peritumoral mucin deposition	25 cases of BCC
BCC (22)	2016	Dynamic OCT enables the detection of blood flow *in vivo* and visualization of the skin microvasculature	Blood vessels varied from dilated, larger-than normal vessels to the smallest detectable vessels	Loose and more vascularized dermis between tumor nests	1 patient with BCC on the cheek
BCC, Melanoma (20)	2018	Line-field confocal OCT	BCC: lobulated structures within the dermis, dark cleft due to mucin deposition; melanoma: general architectural disarrangement, disruption of the dermal-epidermal junction, pagetold spread of atypical melanocytes	BCC and melanoma approximate shapes observed in OCT appeared similar histopathologically	2 patients with BCC 2 patients with melanoma
Actinic keratosis (AK), Squamous cell carcinoma (SCC) (23)	2015	HD-OCT	Absence of an outlined dermo-epidermal junction on cross-sectional images allowed discriminating SCC from AK and normal skin	It related to irregular budding of the epidermis outstanding into the upper dermis and/or presence of periadenexal collars penetrating through the dermo-epidermal junction	37 cases of AK 16 cases of SCC

TABLE 5 | Key articles comparing confocal microscopy and histopathology.

Tumor type	Year	Type	Main findings	Correlation with histopathological findings	Sample size
Basal cell carcinoma (BCC) (31)	2002	Real-time, confocal reflectance microscopy (*in vivo*)	Confocal features correlated very well with hematoxylin and eosin (H&E)-stained sections of the biopsy specimen	Features that were readily identified by both *in vivo* confocal microscopy and standard microscopy of H&E-stained sections included parakeratosis, actinic changes overlying the BCC, relative monomorphism of BCC cells, BCC nuclei exhibiting characteristic elongated or oval appearance, high nucleocytoplasmic ratios, and the presence of prominent nucleoli, increased vascularity, and prominent predominantly mononuclear inflammatory cell infiltrate	8 BCC lesions
Actinic keratosis (AK), squamous cell carcinoma (SCC), keratoacanthoma (32)	2009	Reflectance confocal microscopy (*in vivo*)	All 38 cases displayed an atypical honeycomb and/or disarranged pattern of the spinous-granular layer of the epidermis; round nucleated cells were seen in 20 SCCs (65%) and 1 AK (14%) Round blood vessels were seen in the superficial dermis in 28 SCCs (90%) and 5 AKs (72%)	Round nucleated cells at the spinous-granular layer correspond to atypical keratinocytes or dyskeratotic cells	A total of 38 lesions in 24 patients with 7 AKs, 25 SCCs *in situ*, 3 invasive SCCs, and 3 keratoacanthomas
Bowen disease (BD) (33)	2012	Reflectance confocal microscopy (*in vivo*)	Two types of targetoid cells were seen: those presenting as large, homogeneous, bright cells with a dark halo; and round ones with a dark center, surrounding bright rim, and dark halo	Targetoid cells correlated dyskeratotic cells with condensed, eosinophilic cytoplasm and a retraction halo. Dyskeratotic cells were correlated with a dark central nucleus and a surrounding clear retraction halo	10 cases of BD
BCC (34)	2013	Comparison of reflectance confocal microscopy and multiphoton tomography findings (*in vivo*)	Elongated cells and palisading structures are easily recognized using both methods	Due to the higher resolution, changes in nucleus diameter or cytoplasm could be visualized using multiphoton tomography (MPT) Therefore, nucleus diameter, nucleus/cytoplasm ratio, and cell density are estimated for normal and BCC cells using MPT	9 patients with BCC

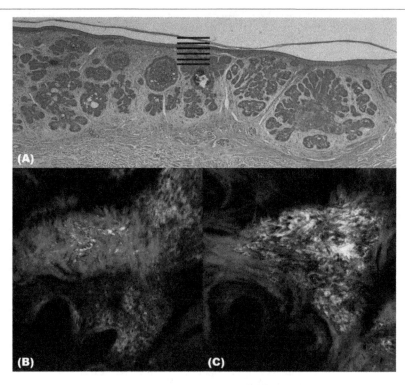

FIGURE 10 | Two-photon microscopy (TPM) images of basal cell carcinoma (BCC). **(A)** Histopathological finding. **(B,C)** TPM images showing parallel collagen fibers (blue) surrounding a BCC tumor nest.

TABLE 6 | Key articles comparing multiphoton microscopy and histopathology.

Tumor type	Year	Type	Main findings	Correlation with histopathological findings	Sample size
Basal cell carcinoma (BCC) (39)	2015	*In vivo* multiphoton microscopy (MPM)	1. Nests of basaloid cells palisading in the peripheral cell layer at the dermoepidermal junction and/or in the dermis 2. Parallel collagen and elastin bundles surrounding the tumors 3. Mucinous stroma adjacent to tumor was visualized using MPM	These features generally correlated well with histopathologic examination. However, histologic examination revealed palisading of peripheral layers in some of the tumor nests of the lesion, although this feature was not obvious in the nests imaged with MPM.	9 patients with a total of 10 BCC
Squamous cell carcinoma in situ (SCCIS), superfical BCC (SBCC) (40)	2008	*Ex vivo* MPM	The following findings were seen: SCCIS: bowenoid dysplasia, multinucleated cells, or hyperkeratosis SBCC: peripheral palisading of tumor cells	The morphologic features differed significantly between these lesions and perilesional skin.	5 specimens of SCCIS 6 specimens of SBCC
Actinic keratosis (AK), squamous cell carcinoma (SCC) (41)	2016	*In vivo* MPM	Changes in the morphology of the keratinocytes, such as broadened epidermis, large intercellular spaces, enlarged nucleus and a large variance in cell shape could easily be recognized.	AK: hyperparakeratosis and cell pleomorphism SCC: invasion of the dermis, keratin pearls and hyperchromatic nuclei	6 patients with AK 6 patients with SCC
Benign and malignant melanocytic nevi (BMMN) (42)	2014	*In vivo* MPM	They evaluate BMMN using 9-point scale showing different values according to two-photon excited fluorescence and second harmonic generation of nevi. Indices corresponding to common nevi (0–1), dysplastic nevi (1-4), and melanoma (5-8) were significantly different ($P < 0.05$).	Prominent qualitative correlations included the morphology of epidermal keratinocytes, the appearance of nests of nevus cells surrounded by collagen fibers, and the structure of the epidermal–dermal junction.	5 common nevi 5 dysplastic nevi 5 melanoma
BCC, SCC, dermatofibrosarcoma protuberans (DFSP) (43)	2019	*Ex vivo* moxifloxacin labeling-based MPM	Moxifloxacin MPM imaged both cells and collagen in the skin, similarly to label-free MPM, but with enhanced fluorescence intensities in cells and enhanced imaging speeds.	Moxifloxacin MPM could detect specific cellular features of various skin cancers in good correlation with histopathological images at the higher imaging speed than label-free MPM.	10 patients with BCC 1 patient with SCC 1 patient with DFSP

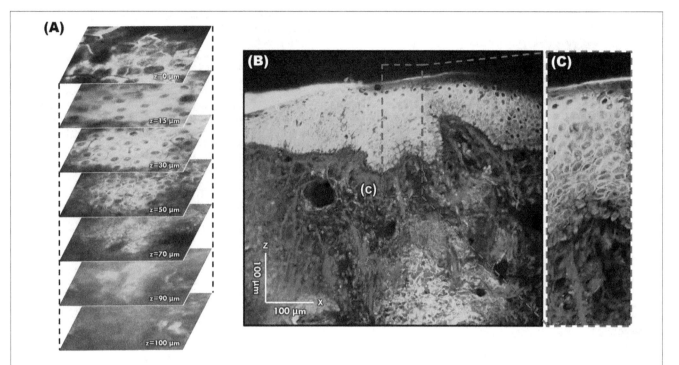

FIGURE 11 | Moxifloxacin-based multi-photon microscopy images of normal skin. **(A)** En face images at different depths. **(B,C)** Cross-sectional view of the epidermis and dermis.

multi-photon microscopy (MPM) imaging also reportedly provides label-free contrast and reveals several characteristic features of basal cell carcinoma lesions (39). This feature correlates well with histopathological examination, findings, and SHG in particular shows collagen and elastin bundles around the tumor (**Figure 10**) (**Table 6**).

However, since TPM and MPM utilize weak endogenous fluorescence in tissue, there is a need for high excitation laser power and extension of pixel duration (44, 45). To overcome this limitation and reduce photodamage, moxifloxacin, an FDA-approved antibiotic, has been reported as a cell-labeling agent for MPM (46). Moxifloxacin has bright intrinsic multi-photon fluorescence, good tissue penetration, and high intracellular concentration. In addition, moxifloxacin-based MPM imaging is 10 times faster than imaging based on endogenous fluorescence (**Figure 11**) (46).

Although imaging depth remains a limitation, various methods to achieve a clear and high-resolution image are being developed. It is also expected that the diagnosis rate can be increased by tumor marker labeling. A recent report stated that in patients with EMPD, a subclinical extension can be assessed by MPM using whole-mount immunostaining with anti-cytokeratin 7 antibody to label Paget cells (35). These trials will be used in the *ex vivo* skin tissue to find the tumor's margins, and it is anticipated that it may replace frozen sections in the future. For more generalized clinical applications, the cost of the equipment is the greatest hinderance. MPM equipment is expensive because it uses a femtosecond laser (36).

CONCLUSION

In addition to ultrasonic devices that can closely observe the skin and deep structures, the development of dermatological equipment that unites laser and optical technology has shown visible progress. The principle of these devices is to analyze signals reflected or scattered from the skin, and there is a fundamental limitation that it is evaluated by looking into the mirror. These limitations are expected to improve in the near future by the development of fluorescent probes targeting tumors or diseases and will be used more actively for the diagnosis and treatment of skin lesions.

For dermatologists, this is a good opportunity to strengthen the specialty of dermatology. We are already familiar with laser equipment and have demonstrated a correlation between clinical and histopathological findings. When we use imaging equipment to further investigate a patient's skin and present objectively explainable data by linking "clinical imaging–histopathological findings," a more robust doctor–patient relationship can be established.

AUTHOR CONTRIBUTIONS

BO conceived the concept and wrote the manuscript. KK co-conceived the concept and drafted the figures and tables. KC co-conceived the concept and edited and improved the manuscript.

REFERENCES

1. Elston DM, Stratman EJ, Miller SJ. Skin biopsy: biopsy issues in specific diseases. *J Am Acad Dermatol.* (2016) 74:1–16; quiz 7–8. doi: 10.1016/j.jaad.2015.06.033

2. Kleinerman R, Whang TB, Bard RL, Marmur ES. Ultrasound in dermatology: principles and applications. *J Am Acad Dermatol.* (2012) 67:478–87. doi: 10.1016/j.jaad.2011.12.016

3. Bobadilla F, Wortsman X, Munoz C, Segovia L, Espinoza M, Jemec GB. Pre-surgical high resolution ultrasound of facial basal cell carcinoma: correlation with histology. *Cancer Imaging.* (2008) 8:163–72. doi: 10.1102/1470-7330.2008.0026

4. Uhara H, Hayashi K, Koga H, Saida T. Multiple hypersonographic spots in basal cell carcinoma. *Dermatol Surg.* (2007) 33:1215–9. doi: 10.1097/00042728-200710000-00009

5. Aoyagi S, Izumi K, Hata H, Kawasaki H, Shimizu H. Usefulness of real-time tissue elastography for detecting lymph-node metastases in squamous cell carcinoma. *Clin Exp Dermatol.* (2009) 34:e744–7. doi: 10.1111/j.1365-2230.2009.03468.x

6. Hernandez-Aragues I, Vazquez-Osorio I, Alfageme F, Ciudad-Blanco C, Casas-Fernandez L, Rodriguez-Blanco MI, et al. Skin ultrasound features of Merkel cell carcinoma. *J Eur Acad Dermatol Venereol.* (2017) 31:e315–8. doi: 10.1111/jdv.14102

7. Hwang JY, Lee SW, Lee SM. The common ultrasonographic features of pilomatricoma. *J Ultrasound Med.* (2005) 24:1397–402. doi: 10.7863/jum.2005.24.10.1397

8. He P, Cui LG, Wang JR, Zhao B, Chen W, Xu Y. Trichilemmal Cyst: clinical and sonographic features. *J Ultrasound Med.* (2019) 38:91–6. doi: 10.1002/jum.14666

9. Jin W, Ryu KN, Kim GY, Kim HC, Lee JH, Park JS. Sonographic findings of ruptured epidermal inclusion cysts in superficial soft tissue: emphasis on shapes, pericystic changes, and pericystic vascularity. *J Ultrasound Med.* (2008) 27:171–6; quiz 7–8. doi: 10.7863/jum.2008.27.2.171

10. Huh JW, Kim MS, Choi KH, Park HJ, Jue MS. The accuracy of ultrasonography on the location of lipomas in the forehead. *Dermatol Surg.* (2016) 42:191–4. doi: 10.1097/DSS.0000000000000598

11. Oh BH, Seo J, Chung KY. Surgical treatment of 846 patients with benign skin tumors: experience of a dermatologic surgeon in Korea. *Korean J Dermatol.* (2015) 53:202–8. Available online at: https://www.koreamed.org/article/0048KJD/2015.53.3.202

12. Wortsman X. The accuracy of ultrasonography on location of lipomas in forehead. *Dermatol Surg.* (2017) 43:158–9. doi: 10.1097/DSS.0000000000000835

13. Chiou HJ, Chou YH, Chiu SY, Wang HK, Chen WM, Chen TH, et al. Differentiation of benign and malignant superficial soft-tissue masses using grayscale and color doppler ultrasonography. *J Chin Med Assoc.* (2009) 72:307–15. doi: 10.1016/S1726-4901(09)70377-6

14. Hung EH, Griffith JF, Ng AW, Lee RK, Lau DT, Leung JC. Ultrasound of musculoskeletal soft-tissue tumors superficial to the investing fascia. *AJR Am J Roentgenol.* (2014) 202:W532–40. doi: 10.2214/AJR.13.11457

15. Perrot JL, Habougit C, Biron Schneider AC, Couzan L, Tognetti L, Rubegni P, et al. Role of reflectance confocal microscopy and HD ultrasound in the diagnosis of cutaneous angiosarcoma of the breast. *Ann Dermatol Venereol.* (2019) 146:410–3. doi: 10.1016/j.annder.2018.12.008

16. Zhao S, Gu Y, Xue P, Guo J, Shen T, Wang T, et al. Imaging port wine stains by fiber optical coherence tomography. *J Biomed Opt.* (2010) 15:036020. doi: 10.1117/1.3445712

17. Mogensen M, Joergensen TM, Nurnberg BM, Morsy HA, Thomsen JB, Thrane L, et al. Assessment of optical coherence tomography imaging in the diagnosis of non-melanoma skin cancer and benign lesions versus normal skin: observer-blinded evaluation by dermatologists and pathologists. *Dermatol Surg.* (2009) 35:965–72. doi: 10.1111/j.1524-4725.2009.01164.x

18. Gambichler T, Plura I, Schmid-Wendtner M, Valavanis K, Kulichova D, Stucker M, et al. High-definition optical coherence tomography of melanocytic skin lesions. *J Biophotonics.* (2015) 8:681–6. doi: 10.1002/jbio.201400085

19. Kwon S, Yoon Y, Kim B, Jang WH, Oh B, Chung KY, et al. Dermoscopy guided dark-field multi-functional optical coherence tomography. *Biomed Opt Express.* (2017) 8:1372–81. doi: 10.1364/BOE.8.001372

20. Dubois A, Levecq O, Azimani H, Siret D, Barut A, Suppa M, et al. Line-field confocal optical coherence tomography for high-resolution noninvasive imaging of skin tumors. *J Biomed Opt.* (2018) 23:1–9. doi: 10.1117/1.JBO.23.10.106007

21. Gambichler T, Plura I, Kampilafkos P, Valavanis K, Sand M, Bechara FG, et al. Histopathological correlates of basal cell carcinoma in the slice and en face imaging modes of high-definition optical coherence tomography. *Br J Dermatol.* (2014) 170:1358–61. doi: 10.1111/bjd.12797

22. Ulrich M, Themstrup L, de Carvalho N, Manfredi M, Grana C, Ciardo S, et al. Dynamic optical coherence tomography in dermatology. *Dermatology.* (2016) 232:298–311. doi: 10.1159/000444706

23. Boone MA, Marneffe A, Suppa M, Miyamoto M, Alarcon I, Hofmann-Wellenhof R, et al. High-definition optical coherence tomography algorithm for the discrimination of actinic keratosis from normal skin and from squamous cell carcinoma. *J Eur Acad Dermatol Venereol.* (2015) 29:1606–15. doi: 10.1111/jdv.12954

24. Rajadhyaksha M, Grossman M, Esterowitz D, Webb RH, Anderson RR. *In vivo* confocal scanning laser microscopy of human skin: melanin provides strong contrast. *J Invest Dermatol.* (1995) 104:946–52. doi: 10.1111/1523-1747.ep12606215

25. Ulrich M, Lange-Asschenfeldt S. *In vivo* confocal microscopy in dermatology: from research to clinical application. *J Biomed Opt.* (2013) 18:061212. doi: 10.1117/1.JBO.18.6.061212

26. New K, Petroll WM, Boyde A, Martin L, Corcuff P, Leveque J, et al. *In vivo* imaging of human teeth and skin using real-time confocal microscopy. *J Scan Microsc.* (1991) 13:369–72. doi: 10.1002/sca.4950130507

27. Couty E, Tognetti L, Labeille B, Douchet C, Habougit C, Couzan C, et al. *In vivo* reflectance confocal microscopy combined with the 'spaghetti technique' for the identification of surgical margins of lentigo maligna: experience in 70 patients. *J Eur Acad Dermatol Venereol.* (2018) 32:e366–8. doi: 10.1111/jdv.14947

28. Flores ES, Cordova M, Kose K, Phillips W, Rossi A, Nehal K, et al. Intraoperative imaging during Mohs surgery with reflectance confocal microscopy: initial clinical experience. *J Biomed Opt.* (2015) 20:61103. doi: 10.1117/1.JBO.20.6.061103

29. Cinotti E, Perrot JL, Labeille B, Cambazard F, Rubegni P. *Ex vivo* confocal microscopy: an emerging technique in dermatology. *Dermatol Pract Concept.* (2018) 8:109–19. doi: 10.5826/dpc.0802a08

30. Mu EW, Lewin JM, Stevenson ML, Meehan SA, Carucci JA, Gareau DS. Use of digitally stained multimodal confocal mosaic images to screen for nonmelanoma skin cancer. *JAMA Dermatol.* (2016) 152:1335–41. doi: 10.1001/jamadermatol.2016.2997

31. Gonzalez S, Tannous Z. Real-time, *in vivo* confocal reflectance microscopy of basal cell carcinoma. *J Am Acad Dermatol.* (2002) 47:869–74. doi: 10.1067/mjd.2002.124690

32. Rishpon A, Kim N, Scope A, Porges L, Oliviero MC, Braun RP, et al. Reflectance confocal microscopy criteria for squamous cell carcinomas and actinic keratoses. *Arch Dermatol.* (2009) 145:766–72. doi: 10.1001/archdermatol.2009.134

33. Ulrich M, Kanitakis J, Gonzalez S, Lange-Asschenfeldt S, Stockfleth E, Roewert-Huber J. Evaluation of Bowen disease by *in vivo* reflectance confocal microscopy. *Br J Dermatol.* (2012) 166:451–3. doi: 10.1111/j.1365-2133.2011.10563.x

34. Ulrich M, Klemp M, Darvin ME, Konig K, Lademann J, Meinke MC. *In vivo* detection of basal cell carcinoma: comparison of a reflectance confocal microscope and a multiphoton tomograph. *J Biomed Opt.* (2013) 18:61229. doi: 10.1117/1.JBO.18.6.061229

35. Murata T, Honda T, Egawa G, Kitoh A, Dainichi T, Otsuka A, et al. Three-dimensional evaluation of subclinical extension of extramammary Paget disease: visualization of the histological border and its comparison to the clinical border. *Br J Dermatol.* (2017) 177:229–37. doi: 10.1111/bjd.15282

36. Tkaczyk E. Innovations and developments in dermatologic non-invasive optical imaging and potential clinical applications. *Acta Derm Venereol.* (2017) 218:5–13. doi: 10.2340/00015555-2717

37. Cinotti E, Galluccio D, Tognetti L, Habougit C, Manganoni AM, Venturini M, et al. Nipple and areola lesions: review of dermoscopy and reflectance confocal microscopy features. *J Eur Acad Dermatol Venereol.* (2019) 33:1837–46. doi: 10.1111/jdv.15727

38. Gonzalez S, Sanchez V, Gonzalez-Rodriguez A, Parrado C, Ullrich M. Confocal microscopy patterns in nonmelanoma skin cancer and clinical applications. *Actas Dermosifiliogr.* (2014) 105:446–58. doi: 10.1016/j.adengl.2014.04.007

39. Balu M, Zachary CB, Harris RM, Krasieva TB, Konig K, Tromberg BJ, et al. *In vivo* multiphoton microscopy of basal cell carcinoma. *JAMA Dermatol.* (2015) 151:1068–74. doi: 10.1001/jamadermatol.2015.0453

40. Paoli J, Smedh M, Wennberg AM, Ericson MB. Multiphoton laser scanning microscopy on non-melanoma skin cancer: morphologic features for future non-invasive diagnostics. *J Invest Dermatol.* (2008) 128:1248–55. doi: 10.1038/sj.jid.5701139

41. Klemp M, Meinke MC, Weinigel M, Rowert-Huber HJ, Konig K, Ulrich M, et al. Comparison of morphologic criteria for actinic keratosis and squamous cell carcinoma using *in vivo* multiphoton tomography. *Exp Dermatol.* (2016) 25:218–22. doi: 10.1111/exd.12912

42. Balu M, Kelly KM, Zachary CB, Harris RM, Krasieva TB, Konig K, et al. Distinguishing between benign and malignant melanocytic nevi by *in vivo* multiphoton microscopy. *Cancer Res.* (2014) 74:2688–97. doi: 10.1158/0008-5472.CAN-13-2582

43. Chang H, Jang WH, Lee S, Kim B, Kim MJ, Kim WO, et al. Moxifloxacin labeling-based multiphoton microscopy of skin cancers in Asians. *Lasers Surg Med.* (2019). doi: 10.1002/lsm.23138. [Epub ahead of print].

44. Thomas G, van Voskuilen J, Gerritsen HC, Sterenborg HJ. Advances and challenges in label-free nonlinear optical imaging using two-photon excitation fluorescence and second harmonic generation for cancer research. *J Photochem Photobiol B.* (2014) 141:128–38. doi: 10.1016/j.jphotobiol.2014.08.025

45. Dela Cruz JM, McMullen JD, Williams RM, Zipfel WR. Feasibility of using multiphoton excited tissue autofluorescence for *in vivo* human histopathology. *Biomed Opt Express.* (2010) 1:1320–30. doi: 10.1364/BOE.1.001320

46. Wang T, Jang WH, Lee S, Yoon CJ, Lee JH, Kim B, et al. Moxifloxacin: clinically compatible contrast agent for multiphoton imaging. *Sci Rep.* (2016) 6:27142. doi: 10.1038/srep27142

2

Strategies to Improve the Efficacy of Dendritic Cell-Based Immunotherapy for Melanoma

Kristian M. Hargadon*

Hargadon Laboratory, Department of Biology, Hampden-Sydney College, Hampden-Sydney, VA, United States

*Correspondence:
Kristian M. Hargadon
khargadon@hsc.edu

Melanoma is a highly aggressive form of skin cancer that frequently metastasizes to vital organs, where it is often difficult to treat with traditional therapies such as surgery and radiation. In such cases of metastatic disease, immunotherapy has emerged in recent years as an exciting treatment option for melanoma patients. Despite unprecedented successes with immune therapy in the clinic, many patients still experience disease relapse, and others fail to respond at all, thus highlighting the need to better understand factors that influence the efficacy of antitumor immune responses. At the heart of antitumor immunity are dendritic cells (DCs), an innate population of cells that function as critical regulators of immune tolerance and activation. As such, DCs have the potential to serve as important targets and delivery agents of cancer immunotherapies. Even immunotherapies that do not directly target or employ DCs, such as checkpoint blockade therapy and adoptive cell transfer therapy, are likely to rely on DCs that shape the quality of therapy-associated antitumor immunity. Therefore, understanding factors that regulate the function of tumor-associated DCs is critical for optimizing both current and future immunotherapeutic strategies for treating melanoma. To this end, this review focuses on advances in our understanding of DC function in the context of melanoma, with particular emphasis on (1) the role of immunogenic cell death in eliciting tumor-associated DC activation, (2) immunosuppression of DC function by melanoma-associated factors in the tumor microenvironment, (3) metabolic constraints on the activation of tumor-associated DCs, and (4) the role of the microbiome in shaping the immunogenicity of DCs and the overall quality of anti-melanoma immune responses they mediate. Additionally, this review highlights novel DC-based immunotherapies for melanoma that are emerging from recent progress in each of these areas of investigation, and it discusses current issues and questions that will need to be addressed in future studies aimed at optimizing the function of melanoma-associated DCs and the antitumor immune responses they direct against this cancer.

Keywords: dendritic cell, tumor, cancer immunotherapy, melanoma, immune suppression, immunogenic cell death, immunometabolism, microbiome

INTRODUCTION

Melanoma is responsible for ~10,000 deaths in the United States and ~55,000 deaths worldwide each year, making it the cause of over 75% of skin cancer-related deaths (1, 2). Importantly, data collected by the SEER Program show that melanoma incidence rates have continually risen the last 40 years (3), and a recent study projects melanoma incidence to continue increasing through at least 2022

(4). In the U.S. alone, annual costs for treatment and productivity losses associated with melanoma are near $3.3 billion (5). These numbers are even more staggering when considering the U.S. ranks only third in melanoma incidence worldwide (6), thus highlighting the need to address melanoma as a global public health concern.

Although it is the least common form of skin cancer, melanoma is by far the most lethal due to its propensity to metastasize to several vital organs, including the brain, lungs, liver, and other visceral organs (7). While surgical removal of primary melanomas is highly successful in eradicating disease prior to metastasis, many melanoma patients are not diagnosed until later stages of malignant disease. In these cases, surgery is often not possible or is largely ineffective (8). Moreover, traditional therapies such as chemotherapy and radiation also exhibit limited efficacy against malignant melanoma and are characterized by variable response rates, lack of durable responses, toxicity, and minimal impact on survival (9, 10). In recent years, important insights into the basic biology of melanoma progression have led to the development of several targeted therapies that have shown promise in the treatment of metastatic melanoma patients. In particular, vemurafenib, trametinib, dabrafenib, and other inhibitors of the BRAF–MEK signaling pathway that is hyperactive in melanoma patients bearing BRAF^{V600} mutations have proven superior to traditional chemotherapy in terms of both antitumor activity and clinical outcome (11–13). Unfortunately, drug resistance to BRAF or MEK inhibitors often develops within the first year of treatment and is accompanied by disease progression in many melanoma patients (14–16). While combination therapy with BRAF–MEK inhibitors delays melanoma progression and improves overall survival as compared to monotherapy, development of multi-drug resistance still leads to disease relapse in many patients (17, 18). A similar story has unfolded with regard to even the most promising immunotherapies for melanoma. Checkpoint blockade therapies with monoclonal antibodies targeting inhibitory receptors such as CTLA-4 and PD-1 on CD8$^+$ T lymphocytes have been developed to override cell intrinsic mechanisms that limit overstimulation of T cells and have dramatically improved both antitumor T cell function and clinical responses in melanoma patients. Both monotherapy and combinatorial approaches with nivolumab (anti-PD-1), pembrolizumab (anti-PD-1), and ipilimumab (anti-CTLA-4) have been promising, with reports of complete and objective responses in as high as 22 and 61% of melanoma patients, respectively (19–26). Despite these successes, though, many melanoma patients do not respond to these therapies, and others often experience disease relapse in as early as the first few months of treatment (27–29). Likewise, adoptive cell transfer (ACT) therapies that employ either naturally occurring tumor-infiltrating lymphocytes or genetically engineered T lymphocytes have produced complete tumor regression in as high as 25% of melanoma patients, though many other patients receive no clinical benefit from these regimens (30, 31). Therefore, while recent advances in the treatment of metastatic melanoma are encouraging, it is critical that we continue to explore strategies that will expand treatment options and optimize clinical outcome for patients with this disease.

Dendritic cells (DCs) have long been appreciated for their roles in the induction and maintenance of antitumor immune responses and are known to be critical regulators of both antitumor immune activation and immune tolerance. This dichotomy is highlighted by the variable outcomes of early trials employing DC-based therapies in melanoma patients. While tumor vaccines targeting host antigen (Ag)-presenting cells in situ or utilizing exogenous tumor Ag-loaded DC induced immunogenic responses that correlated with clinical benefits in a modest percentage of patients (32–35), many patients exhibited no clinical response to these therapies, and some immunization maneuvers even led to diminished tumor-specific T cell responses and the induction of immune tolerance, thereby potentially exacerbating disease progression (36, 37). Lessons learned from these first-generation cancer vaccines guided second-generation vaccination strategies that aimed to improve upon previous failures by (1) targeting tumor Ag to particular DC subsets in situ or (2) employing maturation cocktails to promote the immunostimulatory activity of exogenously generated monocyte-derived DCs. In addition to pulsing these latter DCs with recombinant synthetic peptides or tumor cell lysates, other approaches for tumor Ag loading onto exogenous DCs were also explored, including RNA/DNA electroporation and fusion of tumor cells to DCs. Details of these approaches have been described more extensively in recent reviews (38–40), and their translation to the clinic is highlighted in a recent Trial Watch (41). In brief, despite the improved immunogenicity of many of these approaches, they have unfortunately not been met with the success of checkpoint blockade and ACT therapies, and objective response rates have rarely exceeded 15%. Nevertheless, significant efforts in recent years have further improved our understanding of factors that regulate DC function in the context of cancer, and insights from this work have suggested novel strategies for improving the immunogenicity of both endogenous and exogenous DC. At the same time, advances in genetic engineering and other approaches that enable the manipulation of DC function are spearheading the translation of this basic research on DC immunobiology into novel clinical applications. Together, these findings have reinvigorated the pursuit of cutting-edge approaches that take advantage of the potential of DC as potent stimulators of robust, targeted antitumor immune responses, offering great promise for the future of DC-based cancer immunotherapies.

NEXT-GENERATION DC-BASED IMMUNOTHERAPY FOR MELANOMA

Although first- and second-generation DC vaccines, as well as other tumor Ag-based vaccines, have not yielded significant clinical benefit in a large percentage of melanoma patients to date, their relatively good safety profiles and ability to induce antitumor immune responses in some patients have encouraged the pursuit of next-generation melanoma vaccines that aim to improve upon the previous limitations of DC-based immunotherapy for this cancer. A major focus of one class of next-generation DC vaccines is the utilization of naturally occurring DC subsets, which differs from the artificial ex vivo generation of monocyte-derived and CD34$^+$ precursor-derived DC that predominated both first- and second-generation DC vaccination protocols. Though large clinical trials are needed to define which DC subsets provide optimal therapeutic efficacy in particular settings, early trials with plasmacytoid DC (pDC) and CD1c$^+$ myeloid DC (mDC) have both shown promise in melanoma patients. Intranodal injection of pDC that had been activated and pulsed with melanocyte differentiation Ag-derived peptides into tumor-free lymph nodes of patients with distant metastatic melanoma-induced Ag-specific CD8$^+$ T cell responses in nearly 50% of patients, and although the sample size was too small to make definitive assessments of clinical efficacy, a comparison of clinical outcomes for these patients versus matched control patients undergoing dacarbazine chemotherapy suggest vaccination benefits for both progression-free survival and overall survival (42). Likewise, immunization of stage IIIc/IV melanoma patients with autologous, peptide-pulsed CD1c$^+$ mDC promoted Ag-specific CD8$^+$ T cell responses in 33% of tested patients and induced long-term progression-free survival (12–35 months) in nearly 30% of patients (43). Other next-generation vaccination approaches currently being explored include immunization with tumor-specific neoantigens (either alone or loaded onto DC) that promote responses against mutated tumor-specific epitopes (44–46) as well as maneuvers that induce local or systemic activation of endogenous, tumor Ag-presenting DC (47, 48). These next-generation DC-based vaccines and the ways in which they might be incorporated as part of combinatorial regimens into the current cancer immunotherapy landscape that is being dominated by checkpoint blockade and ACT therapies have recently been reviewed more thoroughly elsewhere (49). Importantly, optimization of these next-generation approaches going forward will require careful consideration of the many factors that have emerged as regulators of DC function in the context of cancer. In this regard, this review highlights recent advances in our understanding of factors that influence DC function in melanoma immunity, including the immunogenicity of tumor cell death, immunosuppressive networks within the tumor microenvironment, tumor-altered immunometabolism, and microbiome-associated regulation of DC function and DC-mediated antitumor immunity. Additionally, particular focus is given to therapeutic strategies building on this knowledge that aim to improve the quality of next-generation DC-based immunotherapies for the treatment of melanoma.

INDUCTION OF IMMUNOGENIC CELL DEATH (ICD) AS A MEANS OF PROMOTING DC-MEDIATED ANTITUMOR IMMUNITY

ICD and DC Activation

As one of the primary mediators of immune surveillance, DC function as key sentinels that aim to maintain homeostasis within the body, invoking immune tolerance in the steady state and immune activation in times of stress, such as that which occurs during a pathogenic infection. In the steady state, DCs exist as immature, inactivated cells that are highly phagocytic but

tolerogenic in nature, expressing low levels of the costimulatory molecules and proinflammatory cytokines/chemokines necessary to invoke immune activation and effector cell recruitment to peripheral tissues. On the other hand, upregulation of these cell surface and soluble immunostimulatory molecules during DC maturation and activation promotes the induction of adaptive immunity capable of eliminating a particular source of Ag (50). While it was originally thought that DC maturation and activation status, and in turn the ability of DC to induce immune tolerance versus activation, was dictated solely by self/non-self discrimination (51), more recently, it has become appreciated that regardless of how self or foreign a source of Ag is, it is the microenvironmental cues within host tissues that are critical in driving the "friend or foe" decision made by DC upon Ag encounter (52). In this way, immature DC that encounter and phagocytose cells dying naturally from normal turnover can remove this cellular debris without risking aberrant autoimmune activation, while those that encounter cells dying from infection or other forms of stress (such as those ultimately imposed on at least some of the cancer cells within a growing tumor) receive "danger signals" that promote their maturation, activation, and ability to stimulate immune responses to combat the source of "danger." In the context of cancer, several of these "danger signals" have now been identified as damage-associated molecular patterns (DAMPs) (53). These include cell surface calreticulin and other endoplasmic reticulum (ER) chaperones exposed following the unfolded protein response, autophagy-mediated or conventional secretion of ATP, interleukin-1β (IL-1β) secretion as a result of inflammasome signaling, release of high-mobility group box 1 (HMGB1), and cell surface exposure/release of annexin A1, though this latter protein has been shown to promote both DC activation (54) and inhibition (55) in different settings, and its role as a DAMP is controversial. Nucleic acids released from dying tumor cells are another well-characterized DAMP that may signal through cytoplasmic sensors such as RIG-I or the TLR7/8/9-MyD88 pathway to stimulate DC. Additionally, their induction of type I IFN secretion by dying tumor cells can also lead to autocrine signals that trigger release of chemokines such as CXCL10 that promote recruitment of immune cell populations to the tumor (53, 56). Ultimately, it is the engagement of these types of DAMPs by pattern recognition receptors on DC that "alerts" these cells to an ICD and in turn promotes their stimulation of immune reactivity against "dangerous" immunogens (**Figure 1**). With this revised understanding of "danger/no danger" discrimination as the key regulator of immune activation, inducers of ICD in cancer have become a major area of investigation because of their potential to promote DC-mediated antitumor immunity.

Chemotherapy-Driven ICD and Its Potential for Activation of Endogenous Tumor-Associated DC

In recent years, a number of anticancer regimens have been investigated for their ability to induce ICD and enhance DC-based cancer immunotherapies (57–61). Interestingly, while it was once thought to be at odds with cancer immunotherapy

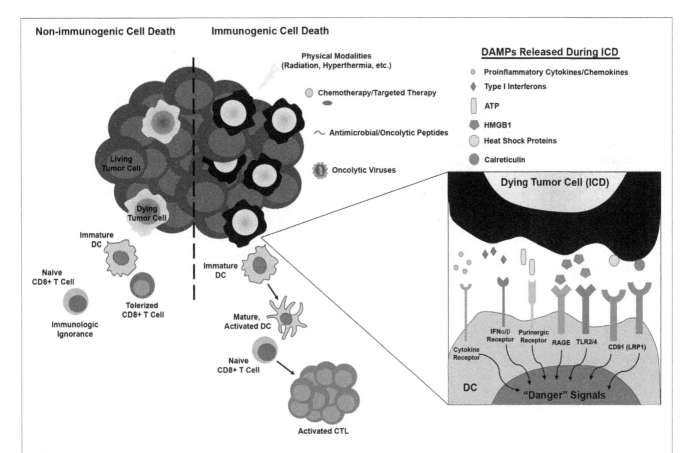

FIGURE 1 | The influence of immunogenic versus non-immunogenic tumor cell death on dendritic cell (DC) maturation/activation and DC-mediated antitumor immunity. Non-immunogenic tumor cell death does not elicit DC maturation or activation, leaving DC in an immature state in which they either (1) fail to "sense" tumor cell death and therefore do not acquire tumor antigen (Ag) for presentation to naïve T lymphocytes or (2) acquire tumor Ag through phagocytosis and induce T cell tolerance. On the other hand, immunogenic tumor cell death, which can be elicited by various physical, chemical, and biological modalities, results in the release of damage-associated molecular patterns (DAMPs) that are recognized by pattern recognition receptors on DC, resulting in the delivery of "danger" signals that promote the maturation and activation of DC capable of stimulating antitumor T cell activation.

because of its non-specific targeting of rapidly dividing cells (which could include not only tumor cells but also lymphocytes engaged in an antitumor immune response), chemotherapy has recently been revisited as a means of promoting ICD of tumor cells. Indeed, a number of chemotherapeutic agents approved for the treatment of various cancers, including doxorubicin, oxaliplatin, mitoxantrone, and others, are now known to induce ICD of some tumor cells (62). Dacarbazine is the only FDA-approved chemotherapeutic agent for the treatment of melanoma, and though its use in isolation has not produced clinical benefits of major significance (63), it has been shown to promote the efficacy of a peptide-based vaccine for melanoma patients by enhancing repertoire diversity of Melan-A-specific CTL (64, 65), suggesting that the benefit of dacarbazine as part of combinatorial therapy may be derived from its induction of melanoma ICD. Likewise, mitoxantrone has been implicated in ICD in an inducible murine model of *Braf*-driven melanoma, where the antitumor effects of this chemotherapeutic were both autophagy- and T lymphocyte-dependent (66). Studies with other chemotherapeutic agents have demonstrated either direct immunogenicity of killed melanoma cells or expression/

release of ICD biomarkers by melanoma cells exposed to a particular drug. In the B16-OVA model, the immunogenicity of doxorubicin-induced cell death was shown to be dependent on DC, as depletion of these cells by diphtheria toxin treatment of mice carrying the diphtheria toxin receptor transgene under control of the CD11c promoter prevented the accumulation of OVA$_{257}$-specific CD8$^+$ T cells that otherwise occurred in the lymph node draining the injection site. Although the OVA Ag in this model is more akin to a completely foreign oncoviral tumor Ag, this same study demonstrated in a humanized model of the B16-F10 murine melanoma cell line that tumor cells treated with doxorubicin and then injected into HLA-A2 transgenic hosts also conferred significant protection against a subsequent challenge with live tumor cells (67). Similarly, CD8$^+$ T cell responses were also elicited against endogenous gp100 Ag in mice immunized with oxaliplatin-treated, but not live, B16-F10 cells (68). Others have also shown that lysates from oxaliplatin-treated B16-F10 melanoma cells were found to be immunogenic, conferring partial protection against subsequent challenge with live tumor cells, and this chemotherapy-driven immunogenicity was associated with markers of ICD that include cell surface calreticulin and release of ATP and HMGB1 (69). Proinflammatory cytokines/chemokines and cell surface heat shock protein 90 (HSP90) are ICD biomarkers expressed by the human A375 melanoma cell line following treatment with melphalan, an alkylating agent whose toxicity against A375 cells promoted DC maturation *in vitro*. Similar effects in the murine B78 model were also associated with *bona fide* immunogenicity *in vivo*, as vaccination with melphalan-treated tumor cells conferred complete protection against re-challenge with live cells in 40% of mice. Interestingly, this vaccination effect was independent of HSP90 expression and could be augmented by coating of melphalan-treated tumor cells with recombinant calreticulin, which was not otherwise detectable on the cell surface (70). Together, these data highlight (1) the potential for artificial delivery of DAMPs to enhance the immunogenic nature of chemotherapy-killed tumor cells but also (2) a need to better understand the role of specific ICD markers in conferring antitumor immunogenicity. Importantly, it should also be emphasized that the immunogenic potential of many of these chemotherapeutic agents has been evaluated only in prophylactic settings, and in order to achieve clinical translatability it will be necessary going forward to determine whether the immunogenicity of these regimens confers any therapeutic benefit against established tumors.

Although the expression/release of ICD biomarkers often correlates with *bona fide* immunogenicity, as was shown to be the case in many of the aforementioned studies, detection of these markers alone is not sufficient to predict immunogenicity of dying tumor cells. For instance, although mafosfamide treatment induces HMGB1 release from both EG7 lymphoma cells and B16-F10 melanoma, this cyclophosphamide derivative promotes vaccine-verified ICD only in EG7 lymphoma (71). In fact, rather than simply failing to induce immunogenicity in melanoma, cyclophosphamide has actually been suggested to promote immune suppression. Studies in the Ret transgenic melanoma model show that although low-dose cyclophosphamide induced cell surface calreticulin on skin tumor-derived Ret cells and enhanced the *in vitro* maturation of co-cultured DC, this treatment alone did not produce any survival benefit in tumor-bearing animals and even led to an accumulation of myeloid-derived suppressor cells (MDSC) in primary tumors (72). This is in contrast to the adjuvant effect that cyclophosphamide has on a DC vaccine in the MC38 colon carcinoma model, where its contribution to tumor growth inhibition correlates with an increase in cytotoxic effector infiltration of tumors and a decrease in both regulatory T cells (Tregs) and MDSC (73). Such tumor-specific differences in responsiveness to chemotherapeutic agents remain poorly understood and underscore the need to gain new insights into factors that influence tumor cell sensitivity to chemotherapy-driven ICD. Moreover, discrepancies in ICD biomarker expression and genuine ICD following tumor cell exposure to chemotherapy drugs highlight both the importance of vaccination assays as a means of verifying *bona fide* ICD as well as the significance of future studies that are necessary to evaluate the immunologic effects of DAMPs, both individually and in combination, on DC and DC-mediated immune responses so that optimal strategies for promoting robust antitumor immunity can be realized.

Non-Chemotherapeutic Induction of ICD As a Means to Enhance Activation of Endogenous and Exogenous DC

While the aforementioned studies suggest potential utility for chemotherapy-driven ICD in promoting the immunogenicity of endogenous DC, whether this mode of ICD induction can be successful in enhancing the vaccination efficacy of exogenous DC is less clear. Combination therapy with cyclophosphamide and an autologous tumor Ag-pulsed DC vaccine has shown promise in a phase II study enrolling metastatic melanoma patients with progressive disease, but although cyclophosphamide's effect was shown not to be the result of Treg depletion, whether its adjuvant effect was the result of ICD induction is not clear (74). Another recent phase I study has demonstrated that intratumoral injection of IFNα-differentiated unloaded autologous DC 1 day following dacarbazine treatment is associated with induction of tumor-specific CD8+ T cell responses and stabilization of disease in a small cohort of stage IV melanoma patients (75). Despite these hints of success, though, there is concern by many investigators that multiple cycles of chemotherapy are incongruent with the potential immunologic benefits of DC vaccination due to the lymphoablative effects of such drugs. Moreover, chemotherapeutic induction of ICD in tumor cells prior to Ag loading of DC during the production of vaccines has the potential for cytotoxicity against DC and could lead to the unintended administration of residual chemotherapeutics to vaccinated patients (49).

A number of non-chemotherapeutic interventions that overcome these limitations have been investigated for their ability to induce ICD of melanoma. Various antimicrobial/oncolytic peptides have been shown to trigger DAMP release by killed melanoma cells and promote antitumor immune responses (76, 77). Oncolytic virus therapies that take advantage of the tumoricidal potential of measles virus, vaccinia virus, and reovirus have all been shown to induce melanoma ICD as well. Specifically, studies with these oncolytic viruses have shown that infected human melanoma cells or tumor-conditioned media from these cells promote the maturation of mDC *in vitro* (78–80), and Zhang et al. have shown in a murine model that an oncolytic adenovirus co-expressing IL-12 and GM-CSF enhances the immunogenicity and antitumor efficacy of a bone marrow-derived DC (BMDC) vaccine (81). Although ICD in the context of targeted therapy for melanoma has not been thoroughly investigated, one study has shown that vemurafenib can promote cell surface exposure of calreticulin and HSP90 on various human melanoma cell lines. This same study also demonstrated that MEK inhibition could trigger exposure of these ICD biomarkers on the surface of vemurafenib-resistant melanoma cells, and tumor cells pre-treated with these targeted drugs were able to promote the maturation of co-cultured DC (82). Based on these findings, it will be of interest going forward to assess how cancer immunization strategies might be coupled with targeted therapy to invoke anti-melanoma immune responses following drug-induced tumor cell death, an outcome that could result in immune-mediated eradication of tumor cells that might otherwise eventually acquire drug resistance. Finally, physical modalities that disrupt tumors, such as radiation, photodynamic therapy (PDT), high hydrostatic pressure, and hyperthermia, have been investigated for their ability to induce ICD-mediated activation of DC. Many of these approaches have been incorporated into DC vaccination setups and are currently being assessed in clinical trials for prostate cancer, ovarian cancer, and head and neck squamous cell carcinoma (83). However, melanoma resistance to many of these modalities has made their incorporation into combinatorial DC-based therapies a particular challenge. Melanoma's relative resistance to radiotherapy is well-documented (84), and many melanomas are also resistant to PDT as a result of optical interference by melanin in pigmented tumors, the antioxidant effect of melanin, sequestration of photosensitizers in melanosomes, and other mechanisms (85). Nevertheless, interest remains in (1) exploring strategies that might sensitize melanoma cells to these physical modalities and (2) identifying particular patient populations whose melanomas might be more susceptible to these types of physical disruptions. For instance, there is evidence that depigmented melanomas are more susceptible to PDT, meaning that at least a subset of melanoma patients might benefit from PDT/DC-based combination therapies, and interventions that result in even temporary depigmentation of melanomas have the potential to increase the percentage of patients who may benefit from such combinatorial regimens (86). Along with the diverse repertoire of ICD inducers known to be effective against melanoma (**Table 1**), ongoing efforts to refine the use of physical modalities for tumor destruction will increase the array of weapons that exhibit not only direct antitumor activity but also the ability to boost immune reactivity against living melanoma cells, thus doubling the impact of therapy. Importantly, further

optimization of therapeutic strategies with these and newly discovered ICD inducers in the future offers promise for enhancing not only naturally generated antitumor immune responses in melanoma patients but also DNA/RNA- and peptide/protein-based melanoma vaccines whose immunogenicity relies on endogenous DC to process and present Ag to tumor-specific T lymphocytes. Moreover, as is already being done with some of the aforementioned inducers of melanoma ICD, investigating how ICD inducers might maximize the immunogenicity of exogenous DC, either through *ex vivo* activation of these cells prior to immunization or through *in vivo* maintenance of their immunogenicity following infusion, will likely improve the quality and outcome of antitumor immune responses achieved by DC vaccines in future melanoma patients.

INTERFERING WITH IMMUNOSUPPRESSIVE NETWORKS THAT IMPAIR THE FUNCTION OF TUMOR-ASSOCIATED DC

Melanoma-Associated Suppression of DC Differentiation

A significant body of evidence now exists demonstrating that tumor cells as well as other immunosuppressive cell populations that accumulate within the tumor microenvironment produce a variety of factors that alter the function of DC (87). In the context of melanoma, such factors have been shown to interfere with the

TABLE 1 | Inducers of immunogenic cell death (ICD) in melanoma.

	Model system	ICD biomarker(s)	Bona fide ICD[a]	Reference
Chemotherapies				
Doxorubicin	B16-F10	Not determined	Yes	(67)
Oxilaplatin	B16-F10	Calreticulin, ATP, high-mobility group box 1 (HMGB1)	Yes	(68, 69)
Melphalan	A375	IL-8, CCL2, heat shock protein 90 (HSP90)	Not tested	(70)
	B78	HSP90	Yes	
Lidamycin	B16-F1	Calreticulin	Yes	(207)
R2016 heterocyclic quinone	B16-F10	Calreticulin, HMGB1, HSP60, HSP70, HSP90	Not tested	(208)
Ginsenoside Rg3	B16-F10	Calreticulin, HSP60, HSP70, HSP90	Not tested	(209)
Antimicrobial/oncolytic peptides				
LTX-315	B16-F1	HMGB1	Not tested	(76)
LTX-401	B16-F1	HMGB1, ATP, cytochrome c	Not tested	(77)
Oncolytic viruses				
Measles virus	Primary melanoma cells	IL-6, IL-8	Not tested	(78)
	Mel888, Mel624, MeWO, SkMel28	IL-6, IL-8, type I IFN, HMGB1		
Vaccinia virus	SK29-MEL	HMGB1, calreticulin (strain-dependent)	Not tested	(79)
Reovirus (type 3 Dearing strain)	Mel888, Mel624, MeWO, SkMel28	Proinflammatory cytokines (cell line-dependent)	Not tested	(80)
Targeted therapies				
Vemurafenib	A375, 451-LU, M1617	Calreticulin, HSP90	Not tested	(82)
U0126 (MEK inhibitor)	A375, 451-LU, M1617	Calreticulin, HSP90	Not tested	(82)
Bortezomib	A375, 451-LU, M1617	Calreticulin, HSP90	Not tested	(82)
Physical modalities				
Hyperthermia ± ionizing radiation	B16-F10	HMGB1, HSP70	Not tested	(210)

[a]Bona fide ICD can be verified only in murine tumor models, as it is determined by vaccination assays in which tumor cells killed by a particular agent in vitro are tested for their ability to invoke protective immunity against subsequent re-challenge with live tumor cells. ICD biomarkers are indicated only if detected in a context appropriate for ICD (i.e., cell surface calreticulin and heat shock proteins, secreted ATP and HMGB1, etc.).

development of DC from hematopoietic precursors, to suppress the maturation and activation of already-differentiated DC, and to induce the differentiation of regulatory DC with tumor-promoting functions. In terms of DC development, hyperactivation of the STAT3 and MAPK signaling pathways has been observed in progenitors that fail to differentiate into DC in the presence of melanoma-derived factors (88), and several groups have identified specific inhibitors contributing to melanoma-associated suppression of DC differentiation. Cyclooxygenase (COX)-derived prostanoids in primary melanoma-conditioned media have been shown to inhibit the differentiation of DC from both monocytes and CD34+ progenitors (89). Likewise, gangliosides from human melanoma tumors impair the differentiation of DC from monocytic precursors and promote the apoptosis of monocyte-derived DC (90). A similar apoptotic effect of melanoma-derived gangliosides has also been observed on epidermal Langerhans cells (91). In addition to inhibiting the generation and viable maintenance of distinct DC subtypes, melanoma-derived factors can also skew the differentiation of DC precursors toward other myeloid populations with immunosuppressive function. For instance, TGFβ1 in B16-F10 tumor-conditioned media is capable of preventing DC differentiation from bone marrow precursors and instead drives MDSC differentiation through upregulation of the Id1 transcriptional regulator (92). COX-2-driven prostaglandin E2 (PGE₂) in supernatants of cultured human melanoma cell lines can also promote MDSC differentiation from monocytes (93). Alternatively, macrophages capable of suppressing CD4+ and CD8+ T cell proliferation have been differentiated from monocytes cultured in conditioned media from both metastatic and non-metastatic human melanoma cell lines (94), and IL-10, which can be secreted at high levels by melanomas (95), has been shown to promote the trans-differentiation of monocyte-derived DC into tolerogenic CD14+ BDCA3+ macrophage-like cells similar to those known to be enriched in melanoma metastases (96). As immunosuppressive M2-like tumor-associated macrophages often accumulate in melanoma-bearing hosts (97–99), it is interesting to speculate that these cells may arise from an influence of tumor-derived factors on the differentiation of DC in vivo as well. Taken together, these influences of melanoma-derived factors on DC differentiation cannot only interfere with Ag presentation and the induction of anti-melanoma immune responses, but they can also lead to active suppression of such immune responses against melanoma.

Melanoma-Associated Suppression of DC Maturation and Activation

In addition to its influence on the differentiation of DC, melanoma has also been shown to modulate the maturation/activation of already-differentiated DC as well. Importantly, although the presence of mature DC within tumors and tumor-draining lymph nodes is a positive prognostic factor in melanoma patients, immature DC are often enriched in both melanoma lesions and tumor-draining lymph nodes of hosts with progressive disease (100–104), thus highlighting the significance of DC maturation status as a key determinant of the immunologic control of melanoma progression. Immune dysfunction stemming from melanoma-associated effects on DC maturation and activation

may result from defects in Ag processing and presentation (103, 105, 106) as well as diminished expression of costimulatory molecules and immunostimulatory cytokines, such as IL-12 (107–109). While an immature phenotype of tumor-associated DC may reflect a simple failure of tumor cells to support DC maturation and activation, active regulation of these processes by melanoma-derived factors has also been documented by several investigators. We have shown that tumor-conditioned media from murine melanoma cell lines suppresses costimulatory molecule expression and alters cytokine/chemokine expression profiles of multiple LPS-treated DC lines (110, 111), and our recent work has extended these observations to tissue-resident DC as well (99). This latter study has shown that the extent to which DC function is altered by melanoma-derived factors is tumor-dependent, such that LPS-induced costimulatory molecule expression on splenic DC-stimulated ex vivo as well as on lung tissue-resident DC in mice harboring melanoma lung metastases is suppressed by the rapidly progressing B16-F1 melanoma but not the poorly tumorigenic D5.1G4 melanoma. Moreover, we found that alterations to cytokine/chemokine expression profiles by DC in these systems also correlated with melanoma tumorigenicity and were partially driven by tumor-derived TGFβ1 and VEGF-A. Others have reported that immature tumor-infiltrating DC isolated from B16-F0 tumors are refractory to ex vivo stimulation with a cocktail of maturation stimuli but can be induced to undergo maturation following stimulation in the presence of an anti-IL-10R neutralizing antibody (112). Recently, Zelenay et al. employed CRISPR-Cas9 gene editing technology to demonstrate that COX-derived PGE₂ in a BRAF^V600E melanoma cell line also suppresses costimulatory molecule expression on CD103+ and CD103−, CD11b+ tumor-infiltrating DC as well as IL-12p40 expression by the CD103+ DC subset (113). In addition to these studies that have elucidated roles for extrinsic tumor-derived factors in the regulation of DC maturation and activation, studies from others have provided insights into dysregulated signaling pathways within tumor-associated DC that impact these processes as well. Upregulation of β-catenin, which has been reported in DC that mature but that fail to fully activate and secrete proinflammatory cytokines (114), has been observed both in DC from lymph nodes draining B16-F10 tumors and in splenic DC cultured with B16-F10-conditioned media, and its induction in tumor-associated DC suppresses their ability to cross-prime CD8+ T cells (115). Similarly, impaired DC activation as measured by IL-12 secretion has been associated with hyperactivation of both the STAT3 and MAPK signaling pathways in monocyte-derived DC exposed to conditioned media or tumor lysates from human melanomas (108, 116). Most recently, upregulation of the microRNA miR148-a in tumor-associated DC was shown to impair TLR-mediated maturation by suppressing expression of the DNA methyltransferase DNMT1, which in turn led to hypomethylation of the Socs1 gene and upregulation of the SOCS1 TLR signaling suppressor (117).

Melanoma-Associated Induction of Regulatory DC Function

Beyond limitations on the Ag processing/presentation and maturation/activation capacity of DC that can preclude induction of antitumor immunity and lead to tumor immune tolerance, respectively, melanoma-derived factors have also been shown to trigger development of regulatory DC with various tumor-promoting functions. Such DCs have been shown to contribute to tumor angiogenesis (118), the development and recruitment of immunosuppressive Tregs (119–121), and the direct suppression of CD4+ and CD8+ T cells (122, 123). Importantly, several studies have now provided mechanistic insights into both the induction of regulatory DC and the tumor-supporting activities mediated by these cells. One study has reported upregulation of the PD-L1 co-inhibitor that dampens CD8+ T cell effector function on tumor-infiltrating DC in the B16-F10 model (124). Another study has shown that melanoma-derived IL-10 and other unidentified factors contribute to an IL-12^{low}, IL-10^{high} phenotype in monocyte-derived DC capable of inducing CD4+ CD25+ FOXP3+ Treg development (125), and tumor-derived IL-6, VEGF, and TGFβ1 have all been implicated in the induction of IL-12^{low}, IL-10^{high} DC in the spontaneous Ret murine melanoma model (126). Differentiation of IL-10-producing regulatory DC has also been shown to be driven by autocrine IL-6/IL-10 signaling through STAT3 in DC, which is initiated by melanoma-derived factors that activate the TLR2 signaling pathway in these cells (127). Additionally, Treg expansion in melanoma can also be driven by TGFβ1-producing regulatory DC (128). Still others have found that regulatory DCs produce enzymes that diminish the availability of metabolites crucial for T cell activation, thereby inducing metabolic suppression of anti-melanoma immunity. In particular, mDC that were imprinted by ER stress in melanoma cells suppressed CD8+ T cell proliferation *via* secretion of the arginine-depleting enzyme arginase I (123), and melanoma-educated regulatory DCs have also been found to suppress CD4+ T cell proliferation in an arginase-dependent manner (122). Likewise, tryptophan catabolism by indoleamine 2,3-dioxygenase (IDO)-producing regulatory pDC recovered from melanoma-draining lymph nodes is associated both with suppression of CD8+ T cells (129) and with activation of CD4+ Tregs (130). In addition to this IDO-mediated regulation of anti-melanoma immunity, regulatory pDC have also been shown to drive T_H2 and Treg differentiation of CD4+ T cells through cell–cell interactions *via* OX40L and ICOSL, respectively (131).

Strategies to Overcome Melanoma-Associated Dysregulation of DC Function

While the previously described studies highlight diverse mechanisms by which melanoma may subvert DC-mediated antitumor immunity, insights into melanoma-altered DC function have suggested novel strategies for improving DC-based immunotherapies for this cancer (**Figure 2**). To overcome the paucity and poorly immunogenic nature of DC within melanoma lesions, strategies to increase tumor infiltration by DC and promote their activation *in situ* have shown promise in murine melanoma models. Salmon et al. recently demonstrated that systemic administration of Flt3L expanded and mobilized CD103+ DC progenitors from the bone marrow and led to the accumulation of immature CD103+ DC within tumor masses, and subsequent injection of polyI:C intratumorally induced local maturation of these cells and enhanced their ability to recruit and activate melanoma-specific

effector CD8+ T cells, leading to tumor regression (47). Similar findings were recently reported by Sánchez-Paulete et al., who demonstrated that Flt3L-mobilized Batf3-dependent DC activated by poly-ICLC synergized with anti-CD137 and anti-PD-1 monoclonal antibody therapy to promote Ag-specific CD8+ T cell cross-priming and tumor control (132). Likewise, Tzeng et al. found that administration of IFNα (as well as other DC maturation stimuli) after treatment of melanoma-bearing mice with a combination therapy that mediates tumor Ag release enhanced the cross-presentation and cross-priming activities of CD8α+ DC in tumor-draining lymph nodes (133). Importantly, although this maneuver led to complete regression of established tumors in a large percentage of mice, minimal benefit was observed when IFNα was administered either before or concomitantly with combination therapy, as the loss of phagocytic capacity that accompanied CD8α+ DC maturation at these early times limited the ability of these cells to acquire tumor Ag later released as a result of therapy. These data thus highlight the importance of treatment schedule and the temporal programming of DC maturation/activation in combinatorial approaches that rely on endogenous DC to trigger therapy-associated antitumor immune responses. Early clinical studies demonstrating that it is also possible to directly manipulate the frequency and maturation status of endogenous DC in melanoma patients have also reinforced the need for optimizing strategies to maximize the immunogenicity of these cells. For instance, local administration of a mix of CpG-B and GM-CSF at the site of primary melanoma excision resulted in the maturation of both pDC and conventional DC as well as an increase in the frequency of cross-presenting BDCA3+ CD141+ DC in sentinel lymph nodes, and this approach enhanced the frequency of melanoma Ag-specific CD8+ T cells in these nodes and reduced the frequency of lymph node metastasis (134, 135). At the same time, though, this approach also enhanced the suppressive activity of CD4+ Tregs in sentinel lymph nodes, suggesting that further optimization of this regimen may enable more robust antitumor immunity and even better clinical results. The identification of optimal DC stimulation cocktails and the implementation of combinatorial regimens that offset the deleterious activities of *in situ*-stimulated DC are therefore critical areas of investigation that may drive the development of more efficacious anti-melanoma immune therapies in the future. Moreover, advances in targeted delivery of therapeutics to endogenous DC, such as those that have already been achieved with IDO siRNA-encapsulated mannosed liposomes (136) and polypeptide micelle-based nanoparticles incorporating an miRNA148-a inhibitor (117), will enable selective reprogramming of melanoma-associated DC into potent stimulators of antitumor immune responses and likely improve the outcome of immunotherapy for melanoma patients going forward.

In contrast to strategies aimed at improving the immunogenicity of endogenous melanoma-associated DC, approaches to enhance the immunostimulatory capacity of exogenous DC have also improved the efficacy of many melanoma vaccines. For example, strategies that provide immune stimulating support for exogenous DC, such as the introduction of IL-6 or IL-21 transgenes into BMDC (137, 138) or the co-administration of oncolytic adenovirus engineered to express immune stimulators

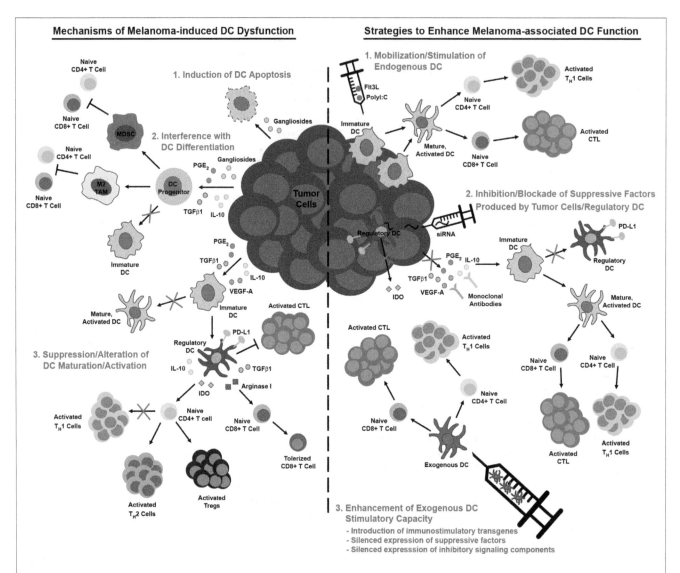

FIGURE 2 | Melanoma-associated dendritic cell (DC) dysfunction and therapeutic interventions to enhance DC-mediated anti-melanoma immune responses. Melanoma interferes with the function of DC by numerous mechanisms, including induction of DC apoptosis, blocking/altering DC development from hematopoietic precursors, suppressing DC maturation/activation, and driving the differentiation of tumor-promoting regulatory DC (left). Insights into these mechanisms of melanoma-altered DC dysfunction have informed strategies to augment DC-mediated anti-melanoma immune responses. These strategies include approaches that mobilize and stimulate endogenous DC, interventions that impede the production or action of immunosuppressive factors released by melanoma and associated cells in the tumor microenvironment, and regimens that employ exogenous DC that have been manipulated to resist suppressive elements and stimulate robust antitumor immunity (right).

such as IL-12 and GM-CSF (64, 119), have been shown to significantly improve vaccine efficacy, resulting in complete regression of established melanomas in some cases. Combinatorial approaches that aim to neutralize the effects of tumor-derived factors on exogenously administered DC, such as local siRNA-mediated silencing of TGFβ1 at the tumor site (139), have also been effective. Alternatively, manipulation of exogenous DC prior to immunization by gene-silencing approaches can promote the immunostimulatory capacity of these cells in two ways. First, silencing the expression of genes involved in signaling pathways that limit the immunostimulatory function of melanoma-associated DC can prevent their immunosuppression by tumor-derived

factors. In this regard, vaccines employing SOCS1-silenced DC improve the control of established B16 melanoma (140, 141), a finding that offers exciting proof-of-principle for this approach and that suggests the silencing of other immunosuppressive signaling molecules often dysregulated in melanoma-altered DC, such as STAT3 and β-catenin, may also improve the antitumor efficacy of DC vaccines for melanoma. Second, silencing the expression of suppressive factors known to be released by melanoma-induced regulatory DC can prevent conversion of exogenous DC from immune activating cells to immunosuppressive ones. Indeed, vaccination of mice with IDO-silenced DC confers partial protection against B16 melanoma (142), and a recent case report has revealed immunologic and clinical benefits of an IDO-silenced DC vaccine in a melanoma patient (143). Similarly, *in vitro* studies have shown that IL-10-silenced human mDC are better able to elicit CTL activation against an antigenic epitope of MART-1 (144), suggesting that immunization with such DCs might improve antitumor immunity in melanoma patients as well. Altogether, these and related strategies for improving the function of DCs in the context of melanoma offer exciting promise for DC-based immunotherapies designed to overcome melanoma-imposed limitations on these cells and the antitumor immune responses they mediate.

OVERCOMING METABOLIC CONSTRAINTS ON DC FUNCTION WITHIN THE TUMOR MICROENVIRONMENT

Metabolic Reprogramming of DC and Tumor Cells

The emerging role of immunometabolism in the regulation of DC function in recent years has revealed new mechanisms by which tumors may subvert DC-mediated antitumor immunity. Indeed, beyond the aforementioned mechanisms of tumor-associated immunosuppression of DC, metabolic suppression of DC in the tumor microenvironment is now recognized as a significant barrier to DC function, which is controlled by key metabolic pathways regulating the bioenergetic and biosynthetic needs of these cells. While immature DC in the steady state rely on fatty acid oxidation and oxidative phosphorylation (OXPHOS) as their primary modes of metabolism, TLR-stimulated DC undergo a metabolic switch to aerobic glycolysis within minutes of the maturation and activation process (145). This early switch to glycolytic metabolism provides a source of carbon for the pentose phosphate pathway and tricarboxylic acid (TCA) cycle, both of which produce intermediates for fatty acid synthesis needed to support the expansion of membrane mass for the ER and Golgi apparatus, thus allowing DC to meet the demands of protein synthesis, transport, and secretion that are associated with maturation/activation (146). Long-term commitment to glycolytic metabolism in activated DC then fuels ATP production and survival in the face of decreasing mitochondrial metabolism, which results from OXPHOS inhibition by nitric oxide in inflammatory DC (147) and from autocrine type I IFN induction of the HIF1α transcription factor that blocks mitochondrial respiration in conventional DC (148). Interestingly, metabolic suppression of tumor-associated DC is often a consequence of metabolic reprogramming in tumor cells themselves, which are driven by the activation/deactivation of oncogenes/tumor suppressor genes and harsh environmental conditions (such as hypoxia) to switch from OXPHOS to glycolysis as the primary mode of metabolism, in this case to support the energy and biosynthetic demands of rapidly proliferating cells. Indeed, even under normoxic conditions, tumor cells are reprogrammed for a primarily glycolytic-based mode of energy production (aerobic glycolysis, otherwise known as the "Warburg effect" in tumor cells), thus allowing intermediates of the glycolytic pathway to function as important metabolites for macromolecule biosynthesis by mitochondria no

longer relied as heavily upon for OXPHOS (149–151). Therefore, as metabolically reprogrammed tumors grow, their increasing demand for glucose consumption contributes to an environment that is metabolically hostile to infiltrating DC and other immune cell populations, with competition for limiting nutrients and accumulation of toxic metabolic byproducts released by tumor cells into the extracellular space both impairing immune system function.

Metabolic Suppression of DC in the Context of Melanoma

In melanoma, metabolic rewiring for glycolysis may be driven by multiple signaling pathways, including BRAF-driven MAPK hyperactivation that negatively regulates OXPHOS (152) and PI3K/AKT/mTOR/HIF1α signaling that positively regulates glycolysis (153). These signaling pathways induce expression of glucose transporters as well as enzymes that favor glycolytic metabolism, such as lactate dehydrogenase A (LDHA) that converts the glycolysis end-product pyruvate into lactic acid, thus diverting pyruvate from utilization in the TCA cycle as fuel for OXPHOS (154). Importantly, depletion of glucose in the tumor microenvironment by melanomas exhibiting high glycolytic activity may impair glycolysis, and in turn ATP production, in tumor-infiltrating DC. Such effects may alter the AMP:ATP ratio in DC and lead to AMP-mediated activation of the nutrient/energy sensor AMPK (155), which is known to promote OXPHOS and suppress mTOR and HIF1α signaling (156–158), thus further contributing to the negative regulation of glycolysis in these cells. Beyond the effects of glucose deprivation in the tumor microenvironment on DC function, buildup of lactic acid in the extracellular space of glycolytically active melanomas can also suppress DC. In this regard, melanoma-derived lactic acid inhibits the differentiation of monocyte-derived DC and suppresses IL-12 production by previously differentiated monocyte-derived DC stimulated with LPS *in vitro* (159). Although the mechanism by which lactic acid influences tumor-associated DC function has yet to be elucidated, there is speculation that altered membrane transport in the lactate-rich tumor microenvironment might contribute to its suppressive effect (160, 161). Because lactate is transported passively by facilitated diffusion through monocarboxylate transporters, high levels of extracellular lactate within the tumor microenvironment might promote import of melanoma-derived lactic acid into DC while at the same time precluding export of lactic acid produced within DC also undergoing aerobic glycolysis, leading to a buildup of lactate within DC that impairs the glycolytic flux necessary to maintain an activated phenotype. Alternatively, lactate was recently shown to inhibit macrophage activation by binding to the GPR81 lactate receptor and suppressing TLR signaling (162), and it is possible that this pathway might also contribute to lactate-associated suppression of DC stimulated by tumor-derived DAMPs. Finally, evidence is emerging that suppression of glycolysis in DC is not merely a consequence of the metabolic limitations imposed by glycolytically active tumor cells, as tumor-derived immunosuppressive cytokines have also been shown to alter DC metabolism. For instance, IL-10 was found to suppress the metabolic switch to aerobic glycolysis in LPS-stimulated DC by antagonizing TLR ligand-mediated hypophosphorylation of AMPK (145). Similarly, IL-10 is known to promote *Socs3* gene expression (163), and melanoma-associated DC have been found to exhibit SOCS3-mediated inhibition of the M2 pyruvate kinase (PKM2) that catalyzes conversion of phosphoenolpyruvate into pyruvate in the final step of glycolysis (164).

In addition to the key role played by glycolytic metabolism in the activation of DC, the metabolism of fatty acids has also been shown to be an important regulator of DC function. Although lipid synthesis is important for ER and Golgi biogenesis during DC activation, the accumulation of lipids in DC in the context of cancer is often associated with immune dysfunction. In particular, Herber et al. demonstrated that several species of triglycerides accumulate in DC cultured with various tumor explant supernatants, including that of B16-F10 melanoma, and that high lipid content in tumor-associated DC impaired tumor Ag processing and cross-presentation (165). Interestingly, DC cultured with tumor-derived supernatant also exhibited increased expression of the scavenger receptor MSR1, suggesting that the accumulation of lipids in these DCs might arise from tumor-derived factors that promote DC uptake of fatty acids in the form of lipoproteins, as triglycerides are typically not taken up by DC but can be synthesized from lipoprotein precursors within cells. Subsequent studies revealed that lipid accumulation in tumor-associated DC defective in cross-presentation resulted from an increase in polyunsaturated fatty acids, particularly linoleic acid and to a lesser extent arachidonic acid, and that DC isolated from tumor-bearing mice or exposed to tumor explant supernatants *in vitro* exhibited significantly higher levels of oxidized free fatty acids and oxidatively truncated triglycerides (166). Of note, these DC did not exhibit oxidation of phospholipids that would be a major component of ER and Golgi membranes. These data may therefore explain the apparent discrepancy between the need for DC to undergo *de novo* lipogenesis to support ER and Golgi biogenesis during activation and the dysfunction that results from lipid accumulation in the context of tumors, suggesting that it is the nature and oxidation status of the fatty acids accumulating in tumor-associated DC that is detrimental to their function. Indeed, oxidized fatty acids have been shown to inhibit DC maturation through binding and activation of the peroxisome proliferator-activated receptor PPARγ, which promotes fatty acid synthesis and storage (167). Additionally, others have reported that lipid peroxidation by reactive oxygen species within tumor-associated DC yields byproducts that upregulate the ER stress sensor XBP1, which activates genes involved in the biosynthesis and accumulation of triglycerides known to be linked with DC dysfunction (168). Altogether, these studies reveal the complex regulation of lipid metabolism that controls DC function, and they highlight how factors in the tumor microenvironment can alter this process to ultimately promote tumor immune escape.

While alterations to glycolysis and lipid metabolism impair tumor-associated DC function by influencing how major macromolecules necessary for cell survival and activation are utilized, other metabolites that frequently accumulate in the tumor microenvironment are also known to compromise the function

of DC and DC-mediated immune responses. Adenosine is a particularly well-characterized metabolite that accumulates in the extracellular space of many tumors, including melanoma (169). Although ATP released from tumor cells may serve as a DAMP to promote DC activation (see Induction of Immunogenic Cell Death (ICD) as a Means of Promoting DC-Mediated Antitumor Immunity), melanoma cells often express on their surface the CD39 and CD73 ectonucleotidases that hydrolyze ATP into adenosine (170–172), thereby leading to its buildup in the tumor microenvironment. In addition to its role in the suppression of T cell signaling (173) and immunosuppressive activity of Tregs (174), adenosine has also been shown to impair DC function. *In vitro* studies with LPS-stimulated human monocyte-derived DCs have shown that adenosine promotes IL-10 secretion while suppressing IL-12 and TNFα secretion as well as the capacity of DC to promote T_H1 differentiation (175). Others have shown that DC differentiated from monocytic precursors in the presence of adenosine acquire several tumor-promoting functions that are dependent on signaling through the A_{2B} adenosine receptor. These pro-tumor functions include increased expression of angiogenic factors, immunosuppressive cytokines, and proteins that disrupt immunometabolism such VEGF, TGFβ, IDO, and arginase 2, among others (176). In the context of melanoma, *in vivo* studies in B16-F10 tumor-bearing mice have shown that adenosine signaling through the A_{2A} adenosine receptor on DC is associated with a slight decrease in MHC II and IL-12 expression and a significant increase in the expression of IL-10 (177). Interestingly, recent studies have shown that adenosine receptor signaling in DC also promotes accumulation of intracellular cAMP (178), suggesting that adenosine may ultimately suppress DC activation by influencing AMPK activity and decreasing glycolytic metabolism in these cells. Finally, whereas melanoma cells are one of the major sources of adenosine in the tumor microenvironment, immunoregulatory metabolites that compromise DC function may also be produced by other cell types known to infiltrate tumors. For instance, arginase I-producing cells such as MDSC produce ornithine as a byproduct of arginine metabolism, and ornithine decarboxylation yields polyamines that enhance IDO-1 expression in DC, thus conditioning these cells for immunosuppressive activity (179). Even melanoma-associated DC themselves can contribute immunosuppressive metabolites to the extracellular milieu of progressive tumors. Specifically, melanoma-induced activation of β-catenin signaling in DC from tumor-draining lymph nodes promotes expression of enzymes involved in vitamin A metabolism, leading to DC secretion of the vitamin A metabolite retinoic acid that in turn promotes differentiation of immunosuppressive Tregs (120). Collectively, these studies highlight the metabolically hostile nature of the tumor microenvironment that must be overcome in order for DC to elicit and maintain effective antitumor immune responses.

Metabolic Interventions to Promote DC Function in the Context of Melanoma

Just as insights into melanoma-associated immune suppression of DC have informed therapeutic strategies to enhance the immunogenicity of these cells, so too have insights into the

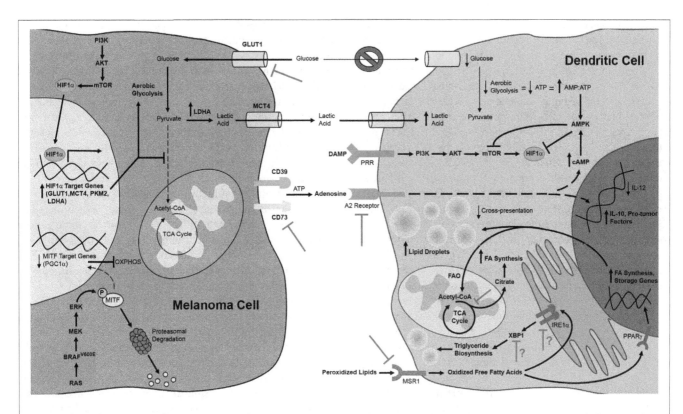

FIGURE 3 | Alterations to tumor cell and dendritic cell (DC) metabolism in the context of melanoma and therapeutic strategies to overcome metabolic suppression of melanoma-associated DC. DC function in the context of melanoma is compromised by constraints on metabolic pathways essential to DC maturation and activation. Metabolic suppression of DC in the tumor microenvironment arises from nutrient depletion and the buildup of toxic waste that results from metabolic rewiring of melanoma cells for aerobic glycolysis. Uptake of peroxidized lipids within the tumor microenvironment also promotes DC dysfunction, leading to an accumulation of oxidized lipids in DC that impairs cross-presentation of tumor antigen. Additionally, tumor cell release of immunosuppressive metabolites such as adenosine that signal through DC inhibit the antitumor function of these cells. Mechanistic insights into these phenomena have identified novel targets for therapies designed to interfere with metabolic pathways in melanoma cells or to prevent tumor-altered metabolism of melanoma-associated DC. Pharmacologic interventions or tissue-specific gene-silencing approaches that target factors upregulated by melanoma cells have direct antitumor effects and are also likely to improve DC function indirectly by creating a more hospitable metabolic microenvironment. Similarly, DC-targeted delivery of therapeutics that prevent uptake of suppressive metabolites or that block metabolic pathways associated with tolerogenicity can improve the immunostimulatory function of endogenous DC, and manipulation of exogenous DC to resist the induction of metabolic suppression can improve the efficacy of DC vaccines. Bold arrows and type designate metabolic pathways, metabolites, intermediates, and processes that are elevated in melanoma cells and tumor-altered DC. Arrows and type not in bold represent those that are downregulated in these cells. Red inhibition symbols highlight proteins and metabolic pathways that have been successfully targeted in melanoma cells and DC in preclinical studies, as described in the text. Red inhibition symbols with red question marks indicate targets that have been associated with both immune activating and immune suppressing functions in different models and whose inhibition may therefore be appropriate only in certain contexts, as is discussed in more detail in the text.

metabolic suppression of melanoma-associated DC (**Figure 3**). To overcome the immune dampening effects of retinoic acid signaling, a retinoic acid receptor α antagonist has been used to enhance the efficacy of a peptide-pulsed DC vaccine against B16 melanoma. In addition to enhancing DC production of IL-12 and lowering DC production of TGFβ and IL-10, this antagonist reduced the number of FOXP3⁺ IL-10⁺ Tregs that infiltrated tumors (180). Pharmacologic inhibition of the β-catenin/TCF pathway that promotes melanoma-associated DC production of retinoic acid has also been shown to reduce the expression of vitamin A-metabolizing genes in DC isolated from tumor-draining lymph nodes, and the antitumor activity associated with this inhibition correlated with reduced Treg and increased effector CD8⁺ T cell infiltration of subcutaneous melanomas (120). Likewise, inhibition of adenosine in the tumor microenvironment

may be approached in a number of ways to prevent its deleterious effects on DC function. Pharmacological antagonists of the A₂B receptor block the effects of adenosine on DC differentiation *in vitro*, and DC from both A₂A and A₂B receptor knockout mice are resistant to the suppressive effects of adenosine (176, 177). Therefore, neutralization of adenosine signaling in DC *via* pharmacologic agents or gene-silencing approaches that knock down expression of adenosine receptors on either endogenous or exogenous DC might improve the antitumor immunogenicity of these cells. Alternatively, strategies that interfere with the CD73 ectonucleotidase on melanoma cells have already been shown to improve antitumor immunity in preclinical models (169, 181), and this outcome is likely due to a reduction in the immunoregulatory effects of adenosine on multiple immune cell populations, including DC.

In addition to overcoming the suppressive effects of extracellular metabolites on DC in the tumor microenvironment, maneuvers that interfere with the metabolism of macromolecules in melanoma cells and/or DC may also restore metabolic and immune function in tumor-associated DC. Pharmacologic regulation of lipid levels in DC using an inhibitor of acetyl-CoA carboxylase that blocks fatty acid synthesis improved the antitumor efficacy of a peptide vaccine against B16-F10 melanoma (165). It is also possible to regulate lipid levels in DC by targeting the MSR1 scavenger receptor that promotes lipid uptake or the IRE1α/XBP1 pathway that triggers triglyceride synthesis in tumor-associated DC. To this point, immunization of tumor-bearing mice with MSR1 gene-silenced BMDC improved vaccine-induced CD8$^+$ T cell responses against multiple melanoma antigens and enhanced immunologic control of established B16 melanomas in both subcutaneous and lung metastasis models (182). Likewise, targeted delivery of nanoparticles encapsulating siRNA has been used to silence in tumor-associated DC the expression of either XBP1 or the IRE1α endoribonuclease that cleaves *Xbp1* mRNA into a form that encodes functional protein during ER stress. In a murine model of ovarian cancer, this approach reduced triglyceride levels in tumor-associated DC, augmented the activation of tumor Ag-specific T cells, and improved tumor immune control and overall survival of tumor-bearing mice (168). As triglycerides are also known to accumulate in dysfunctional melanoma-associated DC (165), silencing of IRE1α or XBP1 expression in these cells might also improve DC-mediated immune responses against this cancer in certain contexts. It is worth noting, however, that overexpression of XBP1 in BMDC actually improves DC survival, activation, and T cell stimulatory capacity, leading to enhanced immune control of established B16 melanoma following vaccination (183). Additionally, in an inducible BRAF^{V600E}/PTEN-driven melanoma model, a DNA vaccine that promotes XBP1 expression in endogenous DC conferred CD8$^+$ T cell-mediated immune control of small established tumors (184). While tumor microenvironment-specific differences in these ovarian cancer and melanoma models may explain differences in the impact of XBP1 on DC function, it is also possible that these discrepancies are due to differences in the particular DC under study, including the endogenous/exogenous nature of these cells and the extent of ER stress in the DC in which XBP1 is active. It is interesting to speculate that in DC which have not previously been exposed to the hostile tumor microenvironment (i.e., exogenous BMDC) or which are found in the context of early stage tumors and have not yet accumulated the types of fatty acids associated with immune dysfunction, XBP1 promotes DC immunogenicity by protecting these cells against ER stress as they increase protein synthesis during their activation. On the other hand, in endogenous DC that have incorporated significant polyunsaturated fatty acids within the microenvironment of late-stage tumors, XBP1 activation may lead to the generation of oxidized triglycerides that impair DC function. Future studies will be necessary to test this hypothesis and define the parameters under which XBP1 activation versus inactivation in DC is appropriate for optimizing the antitumor activity of these cells.

Finally, glycolytic metabolism in both melanoma cells and DC can be targeted to enhance the immunostimulatory capacity of DC. Recent studies have demonstrated that silencing of the GLUT1 glucose transporter or the CD147 gene product that regulates its expression in melanoma cell lines impairs the growth and metastasis of transplanted tumors (185, 186). In addition to having direct antitumor effects, interfering with glycolysis in melanoma cells may have pro-immune consequences as well, resulting in enhanced DC-mediated antitumor immune responses by increasing glucose availability and decreasing lactic acid concentration in the tumor microenvironment. Therefore, targeting glucose transporters and other enzymes (such as LDHA) that are involved in glycolytic metabolism in melanoma cells is a potentially attractive therapeutic option for the treatment of melanoma. While selective targeting of such therapies specifically to tumor cells might be difficult for some cancer types and could lead to compromised function of DC and other immune cell populations that also rely on glycolysis for induction and maintenance of an activated phenotype, the identification of tissue-specific genes in melanoma (such as those involved in the melanin deposition pathway) opens up the possibility of DNA-based therapies in which siRNA/shRNA expression is driven off of tissue-specific promoters active only in melanoma cells. Such a strategy would overcome issues with selective *delivery* of siRNA/shRNA to tumor cells and instead would rely on selective *activation* of a gene-silencing therapeutic specifically in melanoma cells. Alternatively, it is also possible to minimize the reliance of DC on glycolysis as the sole bioenergetic mode of metabolism during activation. Although signaling through mTOR is associated with a metabolic switch to aerobic glycolysis during DC activation as described above, this switch results less from a preference for glycolytic metabolism and more from a requirement for glycolysis as a means of generating ATP in the face of mitochondrial suppression by reactive oxygen species. Interestingly, it has been reported that inhibition of mTOR in DC does not preclude ATP synthesis in these cells and instead extends the lifespan of activated DC by reducing reactive oxygen species and preserving mitochondrial function, thus allowing flexibility in the metabolic pathways utilized by DC for bioenergetic purposes (187). Indeed, multiple groups have shown that interfering with mTOR function in BMDC enhances vaccine-induced CD8$^+$ T cell responses and immunologic control of established B16 melanomas (188, 189). Together, these data highlight how metabolic interventions may shift the profile of tumor-associated DC from tolerogenic to immunogenic, and they suggest great promise for metabolism-based therapies, either alone or in combination with immunotherapies, in the treatment of melanoma.

MODULATING THE MICROBIOME TO AUGMENT DC-MEDIATED ANTITUMOR IMMUNITY

Gut Microbiome Influences on Natural Antitumor Immunity to Melanoma

As data have emerged demonstrating that the microbiota and dysbiosis play significant roles in both cancer progression and the efficacy of anticancer therapies (190), there has been considerable interest in understanding how the microbiome regulates the quality of antitumor immune responses. In the context of melanoma, altering the composition of the gut microbiota has been shown to impact both natural and therapy-associated antitumor immunity, and in many cases, regulation of these responses has been associated with microbial influences on DC activation. Antibiotic treatment with a mixture of ampicillin, vancomycin, and neomycin sulfate (which leads to a decreased frequency of gut bacteria belonging to the Bacteroidetes phylum and an increased frequency of gut bacteria belonging to the Firmicutes phylum) prior to B16-F10 challenge enhances tumor outgrowth and is associated with defects in natural antitumor immunity that include a decrease in the frequency of DC among tumor-infiltrating leukocytes and a reduced expression of genes associated with DC maturation and immune activation within tumor tissue (191). Addition of metronidazole to the aforementioned cocktail of antibiotics yields a different type of gut dysbiosis in treated mice (decreased frequency of both Firmicutes and Bacteroidetes phyla members and increased frequency of members of the Proteobacteria phylum), and this alteration also leads to impaired immune control of B16-F10 lung metastases (192). This latter effect results from an antibiotic-associated decrease in IL-17$^+$ $\gamma\delta$T cells in the lungs of treated mice. Although the mechanism by which microbial dysbiosis influences $\gamma\delta$T cell function remains to be elucidated in this model, the authors speculated that a lack of DC stimulation by PAMPs in antibiotic-treated mice could contribute to the observed decrease in gene expression in the lungs of IL-6 and IL-23, cytokines known to activate IL-17 production by $\gamma\delta$T cells.

Gut Microbiome Influences on Therapy-Associated Immunity to Melanoma

The first study to report microbial influences on the outcome of immune therapy for cancer demonstrated that the therapeutic benefit of total body irradiation prior to adoptive T cell transfer arises in part from activation of the innate immune system following radiation-induced damage to the GI tract and subsequent translocation of gut microbiota (*Enterobacter cloacae, Escherichia coli, Lactobacillus,* and *Bifidobacterium*) to mesenteric lymph nodes (193). In addition to mobilizing the gut microbiome, total body irradiation also led to elevated serum LPS levels and an increase in the absolute number of CD86^{hi} DC in the spleen and lymph nodes, which in turn correlated with enhanced activation of adoptively transferred gp100-specific CD8$^+$ T cells and improved control of established B16-F10 tumors. Interestingly, when mice were administered the broad-spectrum antibiotic ciprofloxacin beginning two days prior to irradiation, microbial translocation to lymph nodes was not observed, nor was any elevation in serum LPS levels. Likewise, the immunologic and antitumor benefits of DC and CD8$^+$ T cell activation were also abrogated following ciprofloxacin depletion of gut microbiota. Additional experiments with the LPS-blocking antibiotic polymyxin B as well as TLR4$^{-/-}$ mice revealed that the therapeutic effect of gut microbiota translocation following total body irradiation resulted from LPS stimulation of innate immune cells that support the activation of adoptively transferred CD8$^+$ T cells. In related work, Iida et al. showed that treating mice with a cocktail of antibiotics (vancomycin, imipenem, and neomycin) abrogated the antitumor effects of combination immunotherapy with anti-IL-10 receptor antibody and intratumoral CpG-oligodeoxynucleotides (ODN) in B16-F10 tumor-bearing mice (194). Though the mechanistic basis for these findings was not further studied in the B16 melanoma model, the authors reported analogous findings in the MC38 colon adenocarcinoma model, where antibiotic treatment decreased both the frequency of TNF-producing tumor-infiltrating DC (and other leukocytes) as well as CD86 expression and IL-12p40 production by tumor-associated DC. Similar results were also observed following combination immunotherapy of germ-free MC38-bearing mice, suggesting that commensal microbes are necessary to prime DC and other myeloid cell populations for inflammatory cytokine production in response to this immune therapy.

More recently, the microbiome has been shown to influence DC function and antitumor immunity in the context of checkpoint blockade therapies for melanoma as well. In the B16-SIY melanoma model, the success of α-PD-L1 Ab therapy was shown to rely on the presence within the intestinal microbiota of *Bifidobacterium* species that enhance the antitumor effects of therapy (195). Specifically, the presence of natural *Bifidobacterium* species in C57Bl/6 mice from The Jackson Laboratory (JAX) or the introduction of *Bifidobacterium* species by oral gavage into C57Bl/6 mice from Taconic (TAC), which do not naturally harbor these bacteria, correlated with tumor-specific CD8$^+$ T cell responsiveness to α-PD-L1 Ab therapy and tumor control. Of note, the presence of intestinal *Bifidobacterium* species in these mice was also associated with an increase in the frequency of intratumoral DC expressing high levels of MHC class II, and genome-wide transcriptional profiling of these cells revealed elevated expression of several genes known to play roles in DC maturation, Ag processing and presentation, costimulation, and chemokine-mediated recruitment of immune effectors. Moreover, DC isolated from lymphoid tissues of JAX mice and *Bifidobacterium*-fed TAC mice induced higher levels of IFNγ production by CD8$^+$ T cells than did DC from untreated TAC mice that had not been exposed to *Bifidobacterium* species. In other work investigating microbial influences on checkpoint blockade therapy, pretreatment of mice with a cocktail of broad-spectrum antibiotics blocked the efficacy of α-CTLA-4 Ab therapy for established Ret murine melanomas (196). Interestingly, in mice not treated with antibiotics, CTLA-4 blockade promoted T cell-mediated destruction of intestinal epithelial cells and was associated in general with a decrease in Bacteroidales and Burkholderiales member species and an increase in Clostridiales member species in the feces, suggesting that induction of immunity to members of the Bacteroidales and Burkholderiales orders may be linked to the induction of antitumor T cell responses. In this regard, antibiotic-treated or germ-free mice that otherwise failed to exhibit any antitumor effects following α-CTLA Ab therapy were able to control tumors when fed with *Bacteroides thetaiotaomicron, Bacteroides fragilis, Burkholderia cepacia,* or a combination of *B. fragilis* and *B. cepacia* shortly after therapy, and this response was associated with enhanced maturation of intratumoral DC and T$_H$1 immune responses in tumor-draining lymph nodes. Moreover, fecal transplantation studies in which feces from ipilimumab-treated

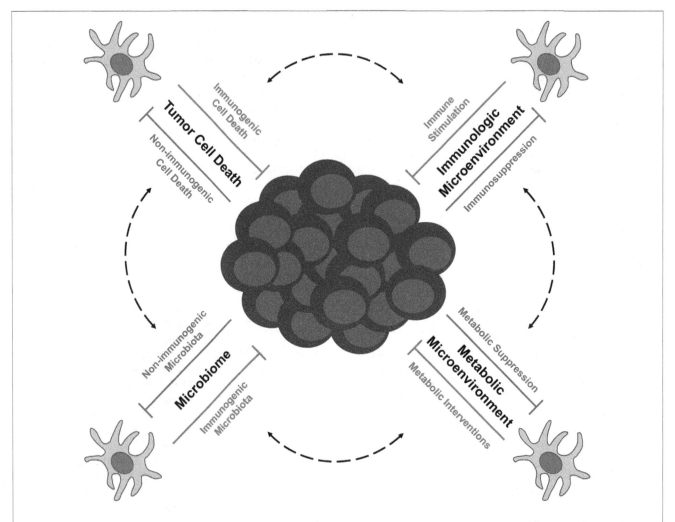

FIGURE 4 | Multifactorial influences on the function of melanoma-associated dendritic cells (DC). A variety of complex factors contribute to the immunoregulation of DC in the context of melanoma. Elements that control the immunogenicity of tumor cell death, the balance of immunostimulatory versus immunosuppressive signals in the tumor microenvironment, metabolic influences on DC function, and the microbiome all interact to dictate the immune stimulatory capacity of melanoma-associated DC. Mechanistic insights into each of these layers of DC immune regulation provide opportunities for therapeutic interventions to enhance the immunogenicity and antitumor function of melanoma-associated DC as described in more detail in the text.

metastatic melanoma patients clustered by stool microbial composition were transferred to germ-free mice two weeks prior to tumor challenge and α-CTLA-4 Ab therapy supported a role for *Bacteroides* species in promoting responsiveness to therapy. In these studies, feces from only one cluster of melanoma patients promoted colonization of immunogenic *B. thetaiotaomicron* and *B. fragilis* in mice, and these animals were the only fecal transplant recipients to mount effective antitumor responses following α-CTLA-4 Ab treatment. While these data suggest that the presence of commensal *Bacteroides* species in the gut may be a useful prognostic indicator for identifying patients most likely to benefit from checkpoint blockade therapy, it should be noted that confounding data on the influence of *Bacteroides* species on therapeutic efficacy in metastatic melanoma patients have emerged from recent clinical studies. Indeed, in a prospective study of metastatic melanoma patients receiving ipilimumab therapy, a high proportion of baseline gut *Bacteroides* actually correlated

with poor clinical benefit, whereas long-term benefit (progression-free and overall survival) was associated with enrichment of *Faecalibacterium* species and other Firmicutes phylum members (unclassified *Ruminococcaceae*, *Clostridium* XIVa, and *Blautia*) (197). Similarly, Bacteroidales family members were found to be enriched in the gut microbiome of metastatic melanoma patients classified as non-responders to α-PD-1 therapy, while responders were found to exhibit greater microbial diversity in the gut and enrichment of members belonging to the Clostridiales order (198). It is possible that the differences reported in these clinical studies versus the study by Vetizou et al. (196) are due either to species-specific differences between mouse and man or to biased reconstitution of gut microbiota following fecal transplantation from humans to mice. However, it is worth noting that another clinical study comparing the baseline gut microbiota of responders versus non-responders to various checkpoint blockade regimens reported data from melanoma patients similar to that described by Vetizou et al.—that is, that enrichment of *Bacteroides* species correlated positively with patient response to therapy (199). In this most recent study, gut microbiome diversity was not significantly different in responders versus non-responders, but metagenomic shotgun sequencing analysis of pretreatment fecal samples identified enrichment of particular species in responding patients that was unique for each therapeutic regimen under study. When comparing responders versus non-responders to all checkpoint blockade regimens under study, both *Bacteroides caccae* and *Streptococcus parasanguinis* were enriched in the gut microbiomes of responders. When analyzing patients responding to ipilimumab/nivolumab combination therapy, Firmicutes phylum members (*Faecalibacterium prausnitzii* and *Holdemania filiformis*) and the Bacteroidetes phylum member *B. thetaiotaomicron* were enriched in responders. Finally, the Firmicutes phylum member *Dorea formicigenerans* was enriched in responders to therapy with pembrolizumab. Based on these collective data, it is clear that additional studies with larger cohorts of patients are necessary to resolve these early discrepant findings and determine how particular gut microbiota regulate both natural antitumor immune responses as well as responsiveness to various tumor immunotherapies. Additionally, as evidence is accumulating that the gut microbiome also influences immunometabolism (200) as well as the metabolism and antitumor activity of chemotherapeutic drugs (201), future studies are needed to investigate how particular microbial species and their metabolites regulate chemotherapy-driven ICD and the function of DC and other immune cell populations in the context of melanoma. Together, these insights will be important for the optimization of strategies to manipulate the gut microbiome in ways that enhance antitumor immune reactivity while also minimizing adverse events such as therapy-associated colitis (202).

The Role of the Skin Microbiome in Immunity to Melanoma?

While a number of studies have been initiated to gain insights into the gut microbiome's influence on the progression of melanoma and other cancers, little is currently known about how the skin microbiome might impact immunologic protection from either the development of primary melanomas or the recurrence of melanoma in the skin or surrounding/distant tissues. To date, only one study has compared the skin microbiome of cutaneous melanomas and benign melanocytic nevi (203). While the cutaneous microbial diversity of melanomas was found to be slightly lower than that of melanocytic nevi, these differences did not reach statistical significance, and no differences were found in the relative abundance of bacterial genera between patients from these groups. However, the limited sample size of this study (15 cutaneous melanoma cases versus 17 melanocytic nevi cases) precludes any strong conclusions that the skin microbiome has no impact on melanoma progression or anti-melanoma immunity in the skin. With regard to microbial influences on cutaneous immunity, others have reported associations between the skin microbiome and patient susceptibility to inflammatory skin conditions such as atopic dermatitis (204), and dysbiosis of the skin microflora has recently been linked to autoimmune vitiligo

as well (205, 206). As vitiligo results from immune-mediated destruction of melanocytes, microbial species that influence this process may be of particular relevance to melanoma. In this light, a recent study comparing bacterial communities in lesional versus non-lesional skin of vitiligo patients revealed a decrease in microbial diversity in vitiliginous lesions, and intra-community network analyses showed that Actinobacterial species predominate the microbial interaction network of non-lesional skin, while members of the Firmicutes phylum exhibit the highest degree of interactions in lesional skin (205). Future studies will be necessary to determine the cause–effect relationship of these alterations in cutaneous microbial communities during cases of vitiligo and whether such alterations might also impact immune reactivity against melanoma cells. Answers to these questions and others that address how the cutaneous microbiota might influence the maturation/activation of Langerhans cells and other skin-resident DC populations may suggest microbial interventions that support the promotion of robust, DC-mediated anti-melanoma immune responses. Coupled with an improved understanding of the gut microbiome's influence on DC-mediated immune responses against melanoma, these findings may identify appropriate dietary modifications, prebiotic/probiotic supplements, antibiotic regimens, and/or fecal transplantation strategies that can be implemented to support DC-based and other immune therapies for the treatment of melanoma.

CONCLUSION AND FUTURE DIRECTIONS

As highlighted throughout this review, DC function at the center of antitumor immunity and play major roles in determining immune activation versus tolerance against cancer. Regulation of immunity to melanoma by DC is controlled by a variety of intrinsic and extrinsic factors, and it is the collective interplay between these factors that ultimately shape the quality of DC-mediated antitumor immune responses (**Figure 4**). Advances in our understanding of the ways in which DC function is influenced by ICD, immunosuppressive networks within the tumor microenvironment, tumor-altered immunometabolism, and the microbiome have provided crucial insights into the immunoregulation of tumor-associated DC, and these insights have informed novel strategies for improving the immunogenicity of DC in the context of melanoma and other cancers. Some of these strategies have already reached patients and have improved the immunologic control of melanoma, and many others have shown great promise in murine models and in preclinical settings. It will therefore be exciting to follow the translation of these and related strategies for enhancing the immunostimulatory function of melanoma-associated DC into the clinic in the future. As we continue to build on these findings, the challenge going forward will be to dissect the complex interplay between the regulatory mechanisms discussed herein and discern how these diverse factors act in concert to control DC function. In this regard, in what ways does the microbiome impact the induction of ICD in melanoma cells? Can particular microbes provide metabolic support for DC by removing toxic byproducts from the tumor microenvironment, and how do microbe-derived metabolites themselves contribute to the metabolic milieu and its influence on DC in the tumor microenvironment? To what extent do immunosuppressive factors in the tumor microenvironment blunt DC function through regulation of metabolic pathways in these cells, and how might altering the balance of these factors impact the abundance and diversity of the microbiota and its contribution to tumor-associated DC function? Collectively, how do these factors influence the ability of DC to maintain the immune reactivity of T cells supported by checkpoint blockade therapy, and how might DC-based therapies best be utilized in combinatorial approaches to induce antitumor T cell responses in patients who have not mounted natural responses to melanoma and are therefore currently poor candidates for treatment by checkpoint blockade? These additional insights into DC immunoregulation in the context of melanoma, coupled with ongoing technological advances that enable fine-tuned manipulation of DC function,

will arm scientists with the tools necessary to devise multifaceted approaches to overcome melanoma-imposed limitations on DC immunogenicity. Based on the advances that have already been seen in recent years, there is great optimism within the field that these novel approaches will significantly improve the antitumor efficacy and clinical outcome of DC-based immunotherapies for melanoma patients in the future.

AUTHOR CONTRIBUTIONS

KH was solely responsible for the conception and writing of this review article.

REFERENCES

1. American Cancer Society. *Cancer Facts & Figures 2016*. Atlanta: American Cancer Society (2016). p. 1–9.
2. Ferlay J, Soerjomataram I, Dikshit R, Eser S, Mathers C, Rebelo M, et al. Cancer incidence and mortality worldwide: sources, methods and major patterns in GLOBOCAN 2012. *Int J Cancer* (2015) 136:E359–86. doi:10.1002/ijc.29210
3. Howlader N, Noone AM, Krapcho M, Miller D, Bishop K, Altekruse SF, et al., editors. *SEER Cancer Statistics Review 1975–2013 National Cancer Institute SEER Cancer Statistics Review 1975–2013 National Cancer Institute. SEER Cancer Stat Rev 1975–2013*. Bethesda, MD: Natl Cancer Institute (2016). Available from: http://seer.cancer.gov/csr/1975_2013/
4. Whiteman DC, Green AC, Olsen CM. The growing burden of invasive melanoma: projections of incidence rates and numbers of new cases in six susceptible populations through 2031. *J Invest Dermatol* (2016) 136:1161–71. doi:10.1016/j.jid.2016.01.035
5. Guy GP, Machlin SR, Ekwueme DU, Yabroff KR. Prevalence and costs of skin cancer treatment in the U.S., 2002-2006 and 2007-2011. *Am J Prev Med* (2015) 48:183–7. doi:10.1016/j.amepre.2014.08.036
6. Erdmann F, Lortet-Tieulent J, Schüz J, Zeeb H, Greinert R, Breitbart EW, et al. International trends in the incidence of malignant melanoma 1953-2008-are recent generations at higher or lower risk? *Int J Cancer* (2013) 132:385–400. doi:10.1002/ijc.27616
7. Leung AM, Hari DM, Morton DL. Surgery for distant melanoma metastasis. *Cancer J* (2012) 18:176–84. doi:10.1097/PPO.0b013e31824bc981
8. Lejeune FJ. The impact of surgery on the course of melanoma. *Recent Results Cancer Res* (2002) 160:151–7. doi:10.1007/978-3-642-59410-6_18
9. Atkins MB, Sosman JA, Agarwala S, Logan T, Clark JI, Ernstoff MS, et al. Temozolomide, thalidomide, and whole brain radiation therapy for patients with brain metastasis from metastatic melanoma: a phase II Cytokine Working Group study. *Cancer* (2008) 113:2139–45. doi:10.1002/cncr.23805
10. Atkins MB, Hsu J, Lee S, Cohen GI, Flaherty LE, Sosman JA, et al. Phase III trial comparing concurrent biochemotherapy with cisplatin, vinblastine, dacarbazine, interleukin-2, and interferon alfa-2b with cisplatin, vinblastine, and dacarbazine alone in patients with metastatic malignant melanoma (E3695): a trial coordinated by the Eastern Cooperative Oncology Group. *J Clin Oncol* (2008) 26:5748–54. doi:10.1200/JCO.2008.17.5448
11. McArthur GA, Chapman PB, Robert C, Larkin J, Haanen JB, Dummer R, et al. Safety and efficacy of vemurafenib in BRAFV600E and BRAFV600K mutation-positive melanoma (BRIM-3): extended follow-up of a phase 3, randomised, open-label study. *Lancet Oncol* (2014) 15:323–32. doi:10.1016/S1470-2045(14)70012-9
12. Hauschild A, Grob J-J, Demidov LV, Jouary T, Gutzmer R, Millward M, et al. Dabrafenib in BRAF-mutated metastatic melanoma: a multicentre, open-label, phase 3 randomised controlled trial. *Lancet* (2012) 380:358–65. doi:10.1016/S0140-6736(12)60868-X
13. Flaherty KT, Robert C, Hersey P, Nathan P, Garbe C, Milhem M, et al. Improved survival with MEK inhibition in BRAF-mutated melanoma. *N Engl J Med* (2012) 367:107–14. doi:10.1056/NEJMoa1203421
14. Van Allen EM, Wagle N, Sucker A, Treacy DJ, Johannessen CM, Goetz EM, et al. The genetic landscape of clinical resistance to RAF inhibition in metastatic melanoma. *Cancer Discov* (2014) 4:94–109. doi:10.1158/2159-8290. CD-13-0617
15. Rizos H, Menzies AM, Pupo GM, Carlino MS, Fung C, Hyman J, et al. BRAF inhibitor resistance mechanisms in metastatic melanoma: spectrum and clinical impact. *Clin Cancer Res* (2014) 20:1965–77. doi:10.1158/1078-0432. CCR-13-3122
16. Kim KB, Kefford R, Pavlick AC, Infante JR, Ribas A, Sosman JA, et al. Phase II study of the MEK1/MEK2 inhibitor trametinib in patients with metastatic *BRAF*-mutant cutaneous melanoma previously treated with or without a BRAF inhibitor. *J Clin Oncol* (2013) 31:482–9. doi:10.1200/JCO.2012. 43.5966
17. Long GV, Flaherty KT, Stroyakovskiy D, Gogas H, Levchenko E, de Braud F, et al. Dabrafenib plus trametinib versus dabrafenib monotherapy in patients with metastatic BRAF V600E/K-mutant melanoma: long-term survival and safety analysis of a phase 3 study. *Ann Oncol* (2017) 28:1631–9. doi:10.1093/annonc/mdx176
18. Long GV, Weber JS, Infante JR, Kim KB, Daud A, Gonzalez R, et al. Overall survival and durable responses in patients with BRAF V600-mutant metastatic melanoma receiving dabrafenib combined with trametinib. *J Clin Oncol* (2016) 34:871–8. doi:10.1200/JCO.2015.62.9345
19. Postow MA, Chesney J, Pavlick AC, Robert C, Grossmann K, McDermott D, et al. Nivolumab and ipilimumab versus ipilimumab in untreated melanoma. *N Engl J Med* (2015) 372:2006–17. doi:10.1056/NEJMoa1414428
20. Weber JS, D'Angelo SP, Minor D, Hodi FS, Gutzmer R, Neyns B, et al. Nivolumab versus chemotherapy in patients with advanced melanoma who progressed after anti-CTLA-4 treatment (CheckMate 037): a randomised, controlled, open-label, phase 3 trial. *Lancet Oncol* (2015) 16:375–84. doi:10.1016/S1470-2045(15)70076-8
21. Felix J, Lambert J, Roelens M, Maubec E, Guermouche H, Pages C, et al. Ipilimumab reshapes T cell memory subsets in melanoma patients with clinical response. *Oncoimmunology* (2016) 5:1136045. doi:10.1080/2162402X.2015.1136045
22. Yun S, Vincelette ND, Green MR, Wahner Hendrickson AE, Abraham I. Targeting immune checkpoints in unresectable metastatic cutaneous melanoma: a systematic review and meta-analysis of anti-CTLA-4 and anti-PD-1 agents trials. *Cancer Med* (2016) 5:1481–91. doi:10.1002/cam4.732
23. Robert C, Schachter J, Long GV, Arance A, Grob JJ, Mortier L, et al. Pembrolizumab versus ipilimumab in advanced melanoma. *N Engl J Med* (2015) 372:2521–32. doi:10.1056/NEJMoa1503093
24. Daud AI, Wolchok JD, Robert C, Hwu W-J, Weber JS, Ribas A, et al. Programmed death-ligand 1 expression and response to the anti-programmed

death 1 antibody pembrolizumab in melanoma. *J Clin Oncol* (2016) 34:4102–9. doi:10.1200/JCO.2016.67.2477

25. Zimmer L, Apuri S, Eroglu Z, Kottschade LA, Forschner A, Gutzmer R, et al. Ipilimumab alone or in combination with nivolumab after progression on anti-PD-1 therapy in advanced melanoma. *Eur J Cancer* (2017) 75:47–55. doi:10.1016/j.ejca.2017.01.009

26. Chuk MK, Chang JT, Theoret MR, Sampene E, He K, Weis SL, et al. FDA approval summary: accelerated approval of pembrolizumab for second-line treatment of metastatic melanoma. *Clin Cancer Res* (2017) 23:5666–70. doi:10.1158/1078-0432.CCR-16-0663

27. Gibney GT, Kudchadkar RR, DeConti RC, Thebeau MS, Czupryn MP, Tetteh L, et al. Safety, correlative markers, and clinical results of adjuvant nivolumab in combination with vaccine in resected high-risk metastatic melanoma. *Clin Cancer Res* (2015) 21:712–20. doi:10.1158/1078-0432.CCR-14-2468

28. Coens C, Suciu S, Chiarion-Sileni V, Grob J-J, Dummer R, Wolchok JD, et al. Health-related quality of life with adjuvant ipilimumab versus placebo after complete resection of high-risk stage III melanoma (EORTC 18071): secondary outcomes of a multinational, randomised, double-blind, phase 3 trial. *Lancet Oncol* (2017) 18:393–403. doi:10.1016/S1470-2045(17)30015-3

29. Kim JM, Chen DS. Immune escape to PD-L1/PD-1 blockade: seven steps to success (or failure). *Ann Oncol* (2016) 27:1492–504. doi:10.1093/annonc/mdw217

30. Rosenberg SA, Yang JC, Sherry RM, Kammula US, Hughes MS, Phan GQ, et al. Durable complete responses in heavily pretreated patients with metastatic melanoma using T-cell transfer immunotherapy. *Clin Cancer Res* (2011) 17:4550–7. doi:10.1158/1078-0432.CCR-11-0116

31. Robbins PF, Kassim SH, Tran TLN, Crystal JS, Morgan RA, Feldman SA, et al. A pilot trial using lymphocytes genetically engineered with an NY-ESO-1-reactive T-cell receptor: long-term follow-up and correlates with response. *Clin Cancer Res* (2015) 21:1019–27. doi:10.1158/1078-0432.CCR-14-2708

32. Slingluff CL, Petroni GR, Yamshchikov GV, Barnd DL, Eastham S, Galavotti H, et al. Clinical and immunologic results of a randomized phase II trial of vaccination using four melanoma peptides either administered in granulocyte-macrophage colony-stimulating factor in adjuvant or pulsed on dendritic cells. *J Clin Oncol* (2003) 21:4016–26. doi:10.1200/JCO.2003.10.005

33. Slingluff CL, Petroni GR, Yamshchikov GV, Hibbitts S, Grosh WW, Chianese-Bullock KA, et al. Immunologic and clinical outcomes of vaccination with a multiepitope melanoma peptide vaccine plus low-dose interleukin-2 administered either concurrently or on a delayed schedule. *J Clin Oncol* (2004) 22:4474–85. doi:10.1200/JCO.2004.10.212

34. Banchereau J, Palucka AK, Dhodapkar M, Burkeholder S, Taquet N, Rolland A, et al. Immune and clinical responses in patients with metastatic melanoma to CD34(+) progenitor-derived dendritic cell vaccine. *Cancer Res* (2001) 61:6451–8.

35. Nestle FO, Alijagic S, Gilliet M, Sun Y, Grabbe S, Dummer R, et al. Vaccination of melanoma patients with peptide- or tumor lysate-pulsed dendritic cells. *Nat Med* (1998) 4:328–32. doi:10.1038/nm0398-328

36. Slingluff CL, Petroni GR, Olson WC, Smolkin ME, Ross MI, Haas NB, et al. Effect of granulocyte/macrophage colony-stimulating factor on circulating CD8+ and CD4+ T-cell responses to a multipeptide melanoma vaccine: outcome of a multicenter randomized trial. *Clin Cancer Res* (2009) 15:7036–44. doi:10.1158/1078-0432.CCR-09-1544

37. Slingluff CL, Petroni GR, Chianese-Bullock KA, Smolkin ME, Ross MI, Haas NB, et al. Randomized multicenter trial of the effects of melanoma-associated helper peptides and cyclophosphamide on the immunogenicity of a multipeptide melanoma vaccine. *J Clin Oncol* (2011) 29:2924–32. doi:10.1200/JCO.2010.33.8053

38. Palucka K, Banchereau J. Dendritic-cell-based therapeutic cancer vaccines. *Immunity* (2013) 39:38–48. doi:10.1016/j.immuni.2013.07.004

39. Anguille S, Smits EL, Lion E, van Tendeloo VF, Berneman ZN. Clinical use of dendritic cells for cancer therapy. *Lancet Oncol* (2014) 15:e257–67. doi:10.1016/S1470-2045(13)70585-0

40. Rodríguez-Cerdeira C, Gregorio MC, López-Barcenas A, Sánchez-Blanco E, Sánchez-Blanco B, Fabbrocini G, et al. Advances in immunotherapy for melanoma: a comprehensive review. *Mediators Inflamm* (2017) 2017:1–14. doi:10.1155/2017/3264217

41. Garg AD, Vara Pérez M, Schaaf M, Agostinis P, Zitvogel L, Kroemer G, et al. Trial watch: dendritic cell-based anticancer immunotherapy. *Oncoimmunology* (2017) 6:e1328341. doi:10.1080/2162402X.2017.1328341

42. Tel J, Aarntzen EHJG, Baba T, Schreibelt G, Schulte BM, Benitez-Ribas D, et al. Natural human plasmacytoid dendritic cells induce antigen-specific T-cell responses in melanoma patients. *Cancer Res* (2013) 73:1063–75. doi:10.1158/0008-5472.CAN-12-2583

43. Schreibelt G, Bol KF, Westdorp H, Wimmers F, Aarntzen EHJG, Duiveman-de Boer T, et al. Effective clinical responses in metastatic melanoma patients after vaccination with primary myeloid dendritic cells. *Clin Cancer Res* (2016) 22:2155–66. doi:10.1158/1078-0432.CCR-15-2205

44. Carreno BM, Magrini V, Becker-Hapak M, Kaabinejadian S, Hundal J, Petti AA, et al. Cancer immunotherapy. A dendritic cell vaccine increases the breadth and diversity of melanoma neoantigen-specific T cells. *Science* (2015) 348:803–8. doi:10.1126/science.aaa3828

45. Ott PA, Hu Z, Keskin DB, Shukla SA, Sun J, Bozym DJ, et al. An immunogenic personal neoantigen vaccine for patients with melanoma. *Nature* (2017) 547:217–21. doi:10.1038/nature22991

46. Sahin U, Derhovanessian E, Miller M, Kloke BP, Simon P, Löwer M, et al. Personalized RNA mutanome vaccines mobilize poly-specific therapeutic immunity against cancer. *Nature* (2017) 547:222–6. doi:10.1038/nature23003

47. Salmon H, Idoyaga J, Rahman A, Leboeuf M, Remark R, Jordan S, et al. Expansion and activation of CD103 + dendritic cell progenitors at the tumor site enhances tumor responses to therapeutic PD-L1 and BRAF inhibition. *Immunity* (2016) 44:924–38. doi:10.1016/j.immuni.2016.03.012

48. Kranz LM, Diken M, Haas H, Kreiter S, Loquai C, Reuter KC, et al. Systemic RNA delivery to dendritic cells exploits antiviral defence for cancer immunotherapy. *Nature* (2016) 534:396–401. doi:10.1038/nature18300

49. Garg AD, Coulie PG, Van den Eynde BJ, Agostinis P. Integrating next-generation dendritic cell vaccines into the current cancer immunotherapy landscape. *Trends Immunol* (2017) 38:577–93. doi:10.1016/j.it.2017.05.006

50. Joffre O, Nolte MA, Spörri R, Reis e Sousa C. Inflammatory signals in dendritic cell activation and the induction of adaptive immunity. *Immunol Rev* (2009) 227:234–47. doi:10.1111/j.1600-065X.2008.00718.x

51. Janeway CA. The immune system evolved to discriminate infectious nonself from noninfectious self. *Immunol Today* (1992) 13:11–6. doi:10.1016/0167-5699(92)90198-G

52. Matzinger P. Tolerance, danger, and the extended family. *Annu Rev Immunol* (1994) 12:991–1045. doi:10.1146/annurev.iy.12.040194.005015

53. Galluzzi L, Buqué A, Kepp O, Zitvogel L, Kroemer G. Immunogenic cell death in cancer and infectious disease. *Nat Rev Immunol* (2017) 17:97–111. doi:10.1038/nri.2016.107

54. Vacchelli E, Ma Y, Baracco EE, Sistigu A, Enot DP, Pietrocola F, et al. Chemotherapy-induced antitumor immunity requires formyl peptide receptor 1. *Science* (2015) 350:972–8. doi:10.1126/science.aad0779

55. Weyd H, Abeler-Dörner L, Linke B, Mahr A, Jahndel V, Pfrang S, et al. Annexin A1 on the surface of early apoptotic cells suppresses CD8+ T cell immunity. *PLoS One* (2013) 8:e62449. doi:10.1371/journal.pone.0062449

56. Sistigu A, Yamazaki T, Vacchelli E, Chaba K, Enot DP, Adam J, et al. Cancer cell-autonomous contribution of type I interferon signaling to the efficacy of chemotherapy. *Nat Med* (2014) 20:1301–9. doi:10.1038/nm.3708

57. Spisek R, Charalambous A, Mazumder A, Vesole DH, Jagannath S, Dhodapkar MV. Bortezomib enhances dendritic cell (DC)-mediated induction of immunity to human myeloma via exposure of cell surface heat shock protein 90 on dying tumor cells: therapeutic implications. *Blood* (2007) 109:4839–45. doi:10.1182/blood-2006-10-054221

58. Tsang YW, Huang CC, Yang KL, Chi MS, Chiang HC, Wang YS, et al. Improving immunological tumor microenvironment using electro-hyperthermia followed by dendritic cell immunotherapy. *BMC Cancer* (2015) 15:708. doi:10.1186/s12885-015-1690-2

59. Ji J, Fan Z, Zhou F, Wang X, Shi L, Zhang H, et al. Improvement of DC vaccine with ALA-PDT induced immunogenic apoptotic cells for skin squamous cell carcinoma. *Oncotarget* (2015) 6:17135–46. doi:10.18632/oncotarget.3529

60. Garg AD, Vandenberk L, Koks C, Verschuere T, Boon L, Van Gool SW, et al. Dendritic cell vaccines based on immunogenic cell death elicit danger signals and T cell-driven rejection of high-grade glioma. *Sci Transl Med* (2016) 8:328ra27. doi:10.1126/scitranslmed.aae0105

61. Mikyšková R, Štěpánek I, Indrová M, Bieblová J, Šímová J, Truxová I, et al. Dendritic cells pulsed with tumor cells killed by high hydrostatic pressure induce strong immune responses and display therapeutic effects both in murine TC-1 and TRAMP-C2 tumors when combined with docetaxel chemotherapy. *Int J Oncol* (2016) 48:953–64. doi:10.3892/ijo.2015.3314

62. Pol J, Vacchelli E, Aranda F, Castoldi F, Eggermont A, Cremer I, et al. Trial Watch: immunogenic cell death inducers for anticancer chemotherapy. *Oncoimmunology* (2015) 4:e1008866. doi:10.1080/2162402X.2015.1008866

63. Lui P, Cashin R, Machado M, Hemels M, Corey-Lisle PK, Einarson TR. Treatments for metastatic melanoma: synthesis of evidence from randomized trials. *Cancer Treat Rev* (2007) 33:665–80. doi:10.1016/j.ctrv.2007.06.004

64. Nisticò P, Capone I, Palermo B, Del Bello D, Ferraresi V, Moschella F, et al. Chemotherapy enhances vaccine-induced antitumor immunity in melanoma patients. *Int J Cancer* (2009) 124:130–9. doi:10.1002/ijc.23886

65. Palermo B, Del Bello D, Sottini A, Serana F, Ghidini C, Gualtieri N, et al. Dacarbazine treatment before peptide vaccination enlarges T-cell repertoire diversity of melan-A-specific, tumor-reactive CTL in melanoma patients. *Cancer Res* (2010) 70:7084–92. doi:10.1158/0008-5472.CAN-10-1326

66. Michaud M, Xie X, Bravo-San Pedro JM, Zitvogel L, White E, Kroemer G. An autophagy-dependent anticancer immune response determines the efficacy of melanoma chemotherapy. *Oncoimmunology* (2014) 3:e944047. doi:10.4161/21624011.2014.944047

67. Casares N, Pequignot MO, Tesniere A, Ghiringhelli F, Roux S, Chaput N, et al. Caspase-dependent immunogenicity of doxorubicin-induced tumor cell death. *J Exp Med* (2005) 202:1691–701. doi:10.1084/jem.20050915

68. Ghiringhelli F, Apetoh L, Tesniere A, Aymeric L, Ma Y, Ortiz C, et al. Activation of the NLRP3 inflammasome in dendritic cells induces IL-1β–dependent adaptive immunity against tumors. *Nat Med* (2009) 15:1170–8. doi:10.1038/nm.2028

69. Rodríguez-Salazar MDC, Franco-Molina MA, Mendoza-Gamboa E, Martínez-Torres AC, Zapata-Benavides P, López-González JS, et al. The novel immunomodulator IMMUNEPOTENT CRP combined with chemotherapy agent increased the rate of immunogenic cell death and prevented melanoma growth. *Oncol Lett* (2017) 14:844–52. doi:10.3892/ol.2017.6202

70. Dudek-Perić AM, Ferreira GB, Muchowicz A, Wouters J, Prada N, Martin S, et al. Antitumor immunity triggered by melphalan is potentiated by melanoma cell surface-associated calreticulin. *Cancer Res* (2015) 75:1603–14. doi:10.1158/0008-5472.CAN-14-2089

71. Schiavoni G, Sistigu A, Valentini M, Mattei F, Sestili P, Spadaro F, et al. Cyclophosphamide synergizes with type I interferons through systemic dendritic cell reactivation and induction of immunogenic tumor apoptosis. *Cancer Res* (2011) 71:768–78. doi:10.1158/0008-5472.CAN-10-2788

72. Sevko A, Sade-Feldman M, Kanterman J, Michels T, Falk CS, Umansky L, et al. Cyclophosphamide promotes chronic inflammation-dependent immunosuppression and prevents antitumor response in melanoma. *J Invest Dermatol* (2013) 133:1610–9. doi:10.1038/jid.2012.444

73. Rossowska J, Pajtasz-Piasecka E, Anger N, Wojas-Turek J, Kicielińska J, Piasecki E, et al. Cyclophosphamide and IL-12-transduced DCs enhance the antitumor activity of tumor antigen-stimulated DCs and reduce Tregs and MDSCs number. *J Immunother* (2014) 37:427–39. doi:10.1097/CJI.0000000000000054

74. Ellebaek E, Engell-Noerregaard L, Iversen TZ, Froesig TM, Munir S, Hadrup SR, et al. Metastatic melanoma patients treated with dendritic cell vaccination, interleukin-2 and metronomic cyclophosphamide: results from a phase II trial. *Cancer Immunol Immunother* (2012) 61:1791–804. doi:10.1007/s00262-012-1242-4

75. Rozera C, Cappellini GA, D'Agostino G, Santodonato L, Castiello L, Urbani F, et al. Intratumoral injection of IFN-alpha dendritic cells after dacarbazine activates anti-tumor immunity: results from a phase I trial in advanced melanoma. *J Transl Med* (2015) 13:139. doi:10.1186/s12967-015-0473-5

76. Camilio KA, Berge G, Ravuri CS, Rekdal O, Sveinbjørnsson B. Complete regression and systemic protective immune responses obtained in B16 melanomas after treatment with LTX-315. *Cancer Immunol Immunother* (2014) 63:601–13. doi:10.1007/s00262-014-1540-0

77. Eike LM, Mauseth B, Camilio KA, Rekdal Ø, Sveinbjørnsson B. The Cytolytic amphipathic β(2,2)-amino acid LTX-401 induces DAMP release in melanoma cells and causes complete regression of B16 melanoma. *PLoS One* (2016) 11:e0148980. doi:10.1371/journal.pone.0148980

78. Donnelly OG, Errington-Mais F, Steele L, Hadac E, Jennings V, Scott K, et al. Measles virus causes immunogenic cell death in human melanoma. *Gene Ther* (2013) 20:7–15. doi:10.1038/gt.2011.205

79. Heinrich B, Klein J, Delic M, Goepfert K, Engel V, Geberzahn L, et al. Immunogenicity of oncolytic vaccinia viruses JX-GFP and TG6002 in a human melanoma in vitro model: studying immunogenic cell death, dendritic cell maturation and interaction with cytotoxic T lymphocytes. *Onco Targets Ther* (2017) 10:2389–401. doi:10.2147/OTT.S126320

80. Errington F, White CL, Twigger KR, Rose A, Scott K, Steele L, et al. Inflammatory tumour cell killing by oncolytic reovirus for the treatment of melanoma. *Gene Ther* (2008) 15:1257–70. doi:10.1038/gt.2008.58

81. Zhang SN, Choi IK, Huang JH, Yoo JY, Choi KJ, Yun CO. Optimizing DC vaccination by combination with oncolytic adenovirus coexpressing IL-12 and GM-CSF. *Mol Ther* (2011) 19:1558–68. doi:10.1038/mt.2011.29

82. Martin S, Dudek-Perić AM, Maes H, Garg AD, Gabrysiak M, Demirsoy S, et al. Concurrent MEK and autophagy inhibition is required to restore cell death associated danger-signalling in Vemurafenib-resistant melanoma cells. *Biochem Pharmacol* (2015) 93:290–304. doi:10.1016/j.bcp.2014.12.003

83. Adkins I, Fucikova J, Garg AD, Agostinis P, Špíšek R. Physical modalities inducing immunogenic tumor cell death for cancer immunotherapy. *Oncoimmunology* (2015) 3:e968434. doi:10.4161/21624011.2014.968434

84. Khan M, Almasan N, Almasan A, Macklis R. Future of radiation therapy for malignant melanoma in an era of newer, more effective biological agents. *Onco Targets Ther* (2011) 4:137. doi:10.2147/OTT.S20257

85. Huang YY, Vecchio D, Avci P, Yin R, Garcia-Diaz M, Hamblin MR. Melanoma resistance to photodynamic therapy: new insights. *Biol Chem* (2013) 394:239–50. doi:10.1515/hsz-2012-0228

86. Sharma KV, Davids LM. Depigmentation in melanomas increases the efficacy of hypericin-mediated photodynamic-induced cell death. *Photodiagnosis Photodyn Ther* (2012) 9:156–63. doi:10.1016/j.pdpdt.2011.09.003

87. Hargadon KM. Tumor-altered dendritic cell function: implications for anti-tumor immunity. *Front Immunol* (2013) 4:192. doi:10.3389/fimmu.2013.00192

88. Oosterhoff D, Lougheed S, van de Ven R, Lindenberg J, van Cruijsen H, Hiddingh L, et al. Tumor-mediated inhibition of human dendritic cell differentiation and function is consistently counteracted by combined p38 MAPK and STAT3 inhibition. *Oncoimmunology* (2012) 1:649–58. doi:10.4161/onci.20365

89. Sombroek CC, Stam AGM, Masterson AJ, Lougheed SM, Schakel MJAG, Meijer CJLM, et al. Prostanoids play a major role in the primary tumor-induced inhibition of dendritic cell differentiation. *J Immunol* (2002) 168:4333–43. doi:10.4049/jimmunol.168.9.4333

90. Péguet-Navarro J, Sportouch M, Popa I, Berthier O, Schmitt D, Portoukalian J. Gangliosides from human melanoma tumors impair dendritic cell differentiation from monocytes and induce their apoptosis. *J Immunol* (2003) 170:3488–94. doi:10.4049/jimmunol.170.7.3488

91. Bennaceur K, Popa I, Portoukalian J, Berthier-Vergnes O, Péguet-Navarro J. Melanoma-derived gangliosides impair migratory and antigen-presenting function of human epidermal Langerhans cells and induce their apoptosis. *Int Immunol* (2006) 18:879–86. doi:10.1093/intimm/dxl024

92. Papaspyridonos M, Matei I, Huang Y, do Rosario Andre M, Brazier-Mitouart H, Waite JC, et al. Id1 suppresses anti-tumour immune responses and promotes tumour progression by impairing myeloid cell maturation. *Nat Commun* (2015) 6:6840. doi:10.1038/ncomms7840

93. Mao Y, Poschke I, Wennerberg E, Pico de Coaña Y, Egyhazi Brage S, Schultz I, et al. Melanoma-educated CD14 + cells acquire a myeloid-derived suppressor cell phenotype through COX-2-dependent mechanisms. *Cancer Res* (2013) 73:3877–87. doi:10.1158/0008-5472.CAN-12-4115

94. Wang T, Ge Y, Xiao M, Lopez-Coral A, Azuma R, Somasundaram R, et al. Melanoma-derived conditioned media efficiently induce the differentiation of monocytes to macrophages that display a highly invasive gene signature. *Pigment Cell Melanoma Res* (2012) 25:493–505. doi:10.1111/j.1755-148X.2012.01005.x

95. Gerlini G, Tun-Kyi A, Dudli C, Burg G, Pimpinelli N, Nestle FO. Metastatic melanoma secreted IL-10 down-regulates CD1 molecules on dendritic cells in metastatic tumor lesions. *Am J Pathol* (2004) 165:1853–63. doi:10.1016/S0002-9440(10)63238-5

96. Lindenberg JJ, van de Ven R, Lougheed SM, Zomer A, Santegoets SJ, Griffioen AW, et al. Functional characterization of a STAT3-dependent dendritic cell-derived CD14 + cell population arising upon IL-10-driven maturation. *Oncoimmunology* (2013) 2:e23837. doi:10.4161/onci.23837

97. Chen P, Huang Y, Bong R, Ding Y, Song N, Wang X, et al. Tumor-associated macrophages promote angiogenesis and melanoma growth via adrenomedullin in a paracrine and autocrine manner. *Clin Cancer Res* (2011) 17:7230–9. doi:10.1158/1078-0432.CCR-11-1354

98. Tham M, Wai Tan K, Keeble J, Wang X, Hubert S, Barron L, et al. Melanoma-initiating cells exploit M2 macrophage TGFβ and arginase pathway for survival and proliferation. *Oncotarget* (2014) 5:12027–42. doi:10.18632/oncotarget.2482

99. Hargadon KM, Bishop JD, Brandt JP, Hand ZC, Ararso YT, Forrest OA. Melanoma-derived factors alter the maturation and activation of differentiated tissue-resident dendritic cells. *Immunol Cell Biol* (2016) 94:24–38. doi:10.1038/icb.2015.58

100. Ladányi A, Kiss J, Somlai B, Gilde K, Fejős Z, Mohos A, et al. Density of DC-LAMP+ mature dendritic cells in combination with activated T lymphocytes infiltrating primary cutaneous melanoma is a strong independent prognostic factor. *Cancer Immunol Immunother* (2007) 56:1459–69. doi:10.1007/s00262-007-0286-3

101. Movassagh M, Spatz A, Davoust J, Lebecque S, Romero P, Pittet M, et al. Selective accumulation of mature DC-lamp+ dendritic cells in tumor sites is associated with efficient T-cell-mediated antitumor response and control of metastatic dissemination in melanoma. *Cancer Res* (2004) 64:2192–8. doi:10.1158/0008-5472.CAN-03-2969

102. Elliott B, Scolyer RA, Suciu S, Lebecque S, Rimoldi D, Gugerli O, et al. Long-term protective effect of mature DC-LAMP+ dendritic cell accumulation in tumors in sentinel lymph nodes containing micrometastatic melanoma. *Clin Cancer Res* (2007) 13:3825–30. doi:10.1158/1078-0432.CCR-07-0358

103. Stoitzner P, Green LK, Jung JY, Price KM, Atarea H, Kivell B, et al. Inefficient presentation of tumor-derived antigen by tumor-infiltrating dendritic cells. *Cancer Immunol Immunother* (2008) 57:1665–73. doi:10.1007/s00262-008-0487-4

104. Vermi W, Bonecchi R, Facchetti F, Bianchi D, Sozzani S, Festa S, et al. Recruitment of immature plasmacytoid dendritic cells (plasmacytoid monocytes) and myeloid dendritic cells in primary cutaneous melanomas. *J Pathol* (2003) 200:255–68. doi:10.1002/path.1344

105. Gerner MY, Mescher MF. Antigen processing and MHC-II presentation by dermal and tumor-infiltrating dendritic cells. *J Immunol* (2009) 182:2726–37. doi:10.4049/jimmunol.0803479

106. Ataera H, Hyde E, Price KM, Stoitzner P, Ronchese F. Murine melanoma-infiltrating dendritic cells are defective in antigen presenting function regardless of the presence of CD4+CD25+ regulatory T cells. *PLoS One* (2011) 6:e17515. doi:10.1371/journal.pone.0017515

107. Ott PA, Henry T, Baranda SJ, Frleta D, Manches O, Bogunovic D, et al. Inhibition of both BRAF and MEK in BRAFV600E mutant melanoma restores compromised dendritic cell (DC) function while having differential direct effects on DC properties. *Cancer Immunol Immunother* (2013) 62:811–22. doi:10.1007/s00262-012-1389-z

108. Jackson AM, Mulcahy LA, Zhu XW, O'Donnell D, Patel PM. Tumour-mediated disruption of dendritic cell function: inhibiting the MEK1/2-p44/42 axis restores IL-12 production and Th1-generation. *Int J Cancer* (2008) 123:623–32. doi:10.1002/ijc.23530

109. Enk AH, Jonuleit H, Saloga J, Knop J. Dendritic cells as mediators of tumor-induced tolerance in metastatic melanoma. *Int J Cancer* (1997) 73:309–16. doi:10.1002/(SICI)1097-0215(19971104)73:3<309::AID-IJC1>3.0.CO;2-3

110. Hargadon KM, Forrest OA, Reddy PR. Suppression of the maturation and activation of the dendritic cell line DC2.4 by melanoma-derived factors. *Cell Immunol* (2012) 272:275–82. doi:10.1016/j.cellimm.2011.10.003

111. Hargadon KM, Ararso YT, Forrest OA, Harte CM. Melanoma-associated suppression of the dendritic cell lines DC2.4 and JAWSII. *Am J Immunol* (2012) 8:179–90. doi:10.3844/ajisp.2012.179.190

112. Vicari AP, Chiodoni C, Vaure C, Ait-Yahia S, Dercamp C, Matsos F, et al. Reversal of tumor-induced dendritic cell paralysis by CpG immunostimulatory oligonucleotide and anti-interleukin 10 receptor antibody. *J Exp Med* (2002) 196:541–9. doi:10.1084/jem.20020732

113. Zelenay S, van der Veen AG, Böttcher JP, Snelgrove KJ, Rogers N, Acton SE, et al. Cyclooxygenase-dependent tumor growth through evasion of immunity. *Cell* (2015) 162:1257–70. doi:10.1016/j.cell.2015.08.015

114. Jiang A, Bloom O, Ono S, Cui W, Unternaehrer J, Jiang S, et al. Disruption of E-cadherin-mediated adhesion induces a functionally distinct pathway of dendritic cell maturation. *Immunity* (2007) 27:610–24. doi:10.1016/j.immuni.2007.08.015

115. Liang X, Fu C, Cui W, Ober-Blobaum JL, Zahner SP, Shrikant PA, et al. β-Catenin mediates tumor-induced immunosuppression by inhibiting

116. Iwata-Kajihara T, Sumimoto H, Kawamura N, Ueda R, Takahashi T, Mizuguchi H, et al. Enhanced cancer immunotherapy using STAT3-depleted dendritic cells with high Th1-inducing ability and resistance to cancer cell-derived inhibitory factors. *J Immunol* (2011) 187:27–36. doi:10.4049/jimmunol.1002067

117. Liu L, Yi H, Wang C, He H, Li P, Pan H, et al. Integrated nanovaccine with microRNA-148a inhibition reprograms tumor-associated dendritic cells by modulating miR-148a/DNMT1/SOCS1 axis. *J Immunol* (2016) 197:1231–41. doi:10.4049/jimmunol.1600182

118. Fainaru O, Almog N, Yung CW, Nakai K, Montoya-Zavala M, Abdollahi A, et al. Tumor growth and angiogenesis are dependent on the presence of immature dendritic cells. *FASEB J* (2010) 24:1411–8. doi:10.1096/fj.09-147025

119. Xia S, Wei J, Wang J, Sun H, Zheng W, Li Y, et al. A requirement of dendritic cell-derived interleukin-27 for the tumor infiltration of regulatory T cells. *J Leukoc Biol* (2014) 95:733–42. doi:10.1189/jlb.0713371

120. Hong Y, Manoharan I, Suryawanshi A, Majumdar T, Angus-Hill ML, Koni PA, et al. β-catenin promotes regulatory T-cell responses in tumors by inducing vitamin A metabolism in dendritic cells. *Cancer Res* (2015) 75:656–65. doi:10.1158/0008-5472.CAN-14-2377

121. Holtzhausen A, Zhao F, Evans KS, Tsutsui M, Orabona C, Tyler DS, et al. Melanoma-derived Wnt5a promotes local dendritic-cell expression of IDO and immunotolerance: opportunities for pharmacologic enhancement of immunotherapy. *Cancer Immunol Res* (2015) 3:1082–95. doi:10.1158/2326-6066.CIR-14-0167

122. Liu Q, Zhang C, Sun A, Zheng Y, Wang L, Cao X. Tumor-educated CD11b^{high} Ia^{low} regulatory dendritic cells suppress T cell response through arginase I. *J Immunol* (2009) 182:6207–16. doi:10.4049/jimmunol.0803926

123. Mahadevan NR, Anufreichik V, Rodvold JJ, Chiu KT, Sepulveda H, Zanetti M. Cell-extrinsic effects of tumor ER stress imprint myeloid dendritic cells and impair CD8+ T cell priming. *PLoS One* (2012) 7:e51845. doi:10.1371/journal.pone.0051845

124. Nakahara T, Oba J, Shimomura C, Kido-Nakahara M, Furue M. Early tumor-infiltrating dendritic cells change their characteristics drastically in association with murine melanoma progression. *J Invest Dermatol* (2016) 136:146–53. doi:10.1038/JID.2015.359

125. Yaguchi T, Goto Y, Kido K, Mochimaru H, Sakurai T, Tsukamoto N, et al. Immune suppression and resistance mediated by constitutive activation of Wnt/β-catenin signaling in human melanoma cells. *J Immunol* (2012) 189:2110–7. doi:10.4049/jimmunol.1102282

126. Zhao F, Falk C, Osen W, Kato M, Schadendorf D, Umansky V. Activation of p38 mitogen-activated protein kinase drives dendritic cells to become tolerogenic in ret transgenic mice spontaneously developing melanoma. *Clin Cancer Res* (2009) 15:4382–90. doi:10.1158/1078-0432.CCR-09-0399

127. Tang M, Diao J, Gu H, Khatri I, Zhao J, Cattral MS. Toll-like receptor 2 activation promotes tumor dendritic cell dysfunction by regulating IL-6 and IL-10 receptor signaling. *Cell Rep* (2015) 13:2851–64. doi:10.1016/j.celrep.2015.11.053

128. Ghiringhelli F, Puig PE, Roux S, Parcellier A, Schmitt E, Solary E, et al. Tumor cells convert immature myeloid dendritic cells into TGF-beta-secreting cells inducing CD4+CD25+ regulatory T cell proliferation. *J Exp Med* (2005) 202:919–29. doi:10.1084/jem.20050463

129. Munn DH, Sharma MD, Hou D, Baban B, Lee JR, Antonia SJ, et al. Expression of indoleamine 2,3-dioxygenase by plasmacytoid dendritic cells in tumor-draining lymph nodes. *J Clin Invest* (2004) 114:280–90. doi:10.1172/JCI21583

130. Sharma MD, Hou DY, Liu Y, Koni PA, Metz R, Chandler P, et al. Indoleamine 2,3-dioxygenase controls conversion of Foxp3+ Tregs to TH17-like cells in tumor-draining lymph nodes. *Blood* (2009) 113:6102–11. doi:10.1182/blood-2008-12-195354

131. Aspord C, Leccia MT, Charles J, Plumas J. Plasmacytoid dendritic cells support melanoma progression by promoting Th2 and regulatory immunity through OX40L and ICOSL. *Cancer Immunol Res* (2013) 1:402–15. doi:10.1158/2326-6066.CIR-13-0114-T

132. Sánchez-Paulete AR, Cueto FJ, Martínez-López M, Labiano S, Morales-Kastresana A, Rodríguez-Ruiz ME, et al. Cancer immunotherapy with immunomodulatory anti-CD137 and anti-PD-1 monoclonal antibodies

cross-priming of CD8+ T cells. *J Leukoc Biol* (2014) 95:179–90. doi:10.1189/jlb.0613330 requires BATF3-dependent dendritic cells. *Cancer Discov* (2016) 6:71–9. doi:10.1158/2159-8290.CD-15-0510

133. Tzeng A, Kauke MJ, Zhu EF, Moynihan KD, Opel CF, Yang NJ, et al. Temporally programmed CD8α(+) DC activation enhances combination cancer immunotherapy. *Cell Rep* (2016) 17:2503–11. doi:10.1016/j.celrep.2016.11.020

134. Sluijter BJR, van den Hout MFCM, Koster BD, van Leeuwen PAM, Schneiders FL, van de Ven R, et al. Arming the melanoma sentinel lymph node through local administration of CpG-B and GM-CSF: recruitment and activation of BDCA3/CD141+ dendritic cells and enhanced cross-presentation. *Cancer Immunol Res* (2015) 3:495–505. doi:10.1158/2326-6066.CIR-14-0165

135. van den Hout MFCM, Sluijter BJR, Santegoets SJAM, van Leeuwen PAM, van den Tol MP, van den Eertwegh AJM, et al. Local delivery of CpG-B and GM-CSF induces concerted activation of effector and regulatory T cells in the human melanoma sentinel lymph node. *Cancer Immunol Immunother* (2016) 65:405–15. doi:10.1007/s00262-016-1811-z

136. Chen D, Koropatnick J, Jiang N, Zheng X, Zhang X, Wang H, et al. Targeted siRNA silencing of indoleamine 2, 3-dioxygenase in antigen-presenting cells using mannose-conjugated liposomes. *J Immunother* (2014) 37:123–34. doi:10.1097/CJI.0000000000000022

137. Bhanumathy K, Zhang B, Ahmed K, Qureshi M, Xie Y, Tao M, et al. Transgene IL-6 enhances DC-stimulated CTL responses by counteracting CD4+25+Foxp3+ regulatory t cell suppression via IL-6-induced Foxp3 downregulation. *Int J Mol Sci* (2014) 15:5508–21. doi:10.3390/ijms15045508

138. Aravindaram K, Wang PH, Yin SY, Yang NS. Tumor-associated antigen/IL-21-transduced dendritic cell vaccines enhance immunity and inhibit immunosuppressive cells in metastatic melanoma. *Gene Ther* (2014) 21:457–67. doi:10.1038/gt.2014.12

139. Conroy H, Galvin KC, Higgins SC, Mills KHG. Gene silencing of TGF-β1 enhances antitumor immunity induced with a dendritic cell vaccine by reducing tumor-associated regulatory T cells. *Cancer Immunol Immunother* (2012) 61:425–31. doi:10.1007/s00262-011-1188-y

140. Shen L, Evel-Kabler K, Strube R, Chen SY. Silencing of SOCS1 enhances antigen presentation by dendritic cells and antigen-specific anti-tumor immunity. *Nat Biotechnol* (2004) 22:1546–53. doi:10.1038/nbt1035

141. Evel-Kabler K, Song XT, Aldrich M, Huang XF, Chen SY. SOCS1 restricts dendritic cells' ability to break self tolerance and induce antitumor immunity by regulating IL-12 production and signaling. *J Clin Invest* (2005) 116:90–100. doi:10.1172/JCI26169

142. Zheng X, Zhang X, Vladau C, Li M, Suzuki M, Chen D, et al. A novel immune-based cancer therapy using gene-silenced dendritic cells (48.8). *J Immunol* (2007) 178(1 Suppl):S76.

143. Sioud M, Nyakas M, Sæbøe-Larssen S, Mobergslien A, Aamdal S, Kvalheim G. Diversification of antitumour immunity in a patient with metastatic melanoma treated with ipilimumab and an IDO-silenced dendritic cell vaccine. *Case Rep Med* (2016) 2016:1–7. doi:10.1155/2016/9639585

144. Chhabra A, Chakraborty NG, Mukherji B. Silencing of endogenous IL-10 in human dendritic cells leads to the generation of an improved CTL response against human melanoma associated antigenic epitope, MART-1 27-35. *Clin Immunol* (2008) 126:251–9. doi:10.1016/j.clim.2007.11.011

145. Krawczyk CM, Holowka T, Sun J, Blagih J, Amiel E, DeBerardinis RJ, et al. Toll-like receptor-induced changes in glycolytic metabolism regulate dendritic cell activation. *Blood* (2010) 115:4742–9. doi:10.1182/blood-2009-10-249540

146. Everts B, Amiel E, Huang SC, Smith AM, Chang CH, Lam WY, et al. TLR-driven early glycolytic reprogramming via the kinases TBK1-IKK? supports the anabolic demands of dendritic cell activation. *Nat Immunol* (2014) 15:323–32. doi:10.1038/ni.2833

147. Everts B, Amiel E, van der Windt GJW, Freitas TC, Chott R, Yarasheski KE, et al. Commitment to glycolysis sustains survival of NO-producing inflammatory dendritic cells. *Blood* (2012) 120:1422–31. doi:10.1182/blood-2012-03-419747

148. Pantel A, Teixeira A, Haddad E, Wood EG, Steinman RM, Longhi MP. Direct type I IFN but not MDA5/TLR3 activation of dendritic cells is required for maturation and metabolic shift to glycolysis after poly IC stimulation. *PLoS Biol* (2014) 12:e1001759. doi:10.1371/journal.pbio.1001759

149. DeBerardinis RJ, Chandel NS. Fundamentals of cancer metabolism. *Sci Adv* (2016) 2:e1600200. doi:10.1126/sciadv.1600200

150. Pavlova NN, Thompson CB. The emerging hallmarks of cancer metabolism. *Cell Metab* (2016) 23:27–47. doi:10.1016/j.cmet.2015.12.006

151. Renner K, Singer K, Koehl GE, Geissler EK, Peter K, Siska PJ, et al. Metabolic hallmarks of tumor and immune cells in the tumor microenvironment. *Front Immunol* (2017) 8:248. doi:10.3389/fimmu.2017.00248

152. Haq R, Shoag J, Andreu-Perez P, Yokoyama S, Edelman H, Rowe GC, et al. Oncogenic BRAF regulates oxidative metabolism via PGC1α and MITF. *Cancer Cell* (2013) 23:302–15. doi:10.1016/j.ccr.2013.02.003

153. Laurenzana A, Chillà A, Luciani C, Peppicelli S, Biagioni A, Bianchini F, et al. uPA/uPAR system activation drives a glycolytic phenotype in melanoma cells. *Int J Cancer* (2017) 141:1190–200. doi:10.1002/ijc.30817

154. Ratnikov BI, Scott DA, Osterman AL, Smith JW, Ronai ZA. Metabolic rewiring in melanoma. *Oncogene* (2017) 36:147–57. doi:10.1038/onc.2016.198

155. Auciello FR, Ross FA, Ikematsu N, Hardie DG. Oxidative stress activates AMPK in cultured cells primarily by increasing cellular AMP and/or ADP. *FEBS Lett* (2014) 588:3361–6. doi:10.1016/j.febslet.2014.07.025

156. Hardie DG, Ross FA, Hawley SA. AMPK: a nutrient and energy sensor that maintains energy homeostasis. *Nat Rev Mol Cell Biol* (2012) 13:251–62. doi:10.1038/nrm3311

157. Shaw RJ, Bardeesy N, Manning BD, Lopez L, Kosmatka M, DePinho RA, et al. The LKB1 tumor suppressor negatively regulates mTOR signaling. *Cancer Cell* (2004) 6:91–9. doi:10.1016/j.ccr.2004.06.007

158. Shackelford DB, Vasquez DS, Corbeil J, Wu S, Leblanc M, Wu CL, et al. mTOR and HIF-1alpha-mediated tumor metabolism in an LKB1 mouse model of Peutz-Jeghers syndrome. *Proc Natl Acad Sci U S A* (2009) 106:11137–42. doi:10.1073/pnas.0900465106

159. Gottfried E, Kunz-Schughart LA, Ebner S, Mueller-Klieser W, Hoves S, Andreesen R, et al. Tumor-derived lactic acid modulates dendritic cell activation and antigen expression. *Blood* (2006) 107:2013–21. doi:10.1182/blood-2005-05-1795

160. Dong H, Bullock TNJ. Metabolic influences that regulate dendritic cell function in tumors. *Front Immunol* (2014) 5:24. doi:10.3389/fimmu.2014.00024

161. Huber V, Camisaschi C, Berzi A, Ferro S, Lugini L, Triulzi T, et al. Cancer acidity: an ultimate frontier of tumor immune escape and a novel target of immunomodulation. *Semin Cancer Biol* (2017) 43:74–89. doi:10.1016/j.semcancer.2017.03.001

162. Hoque R, Farooq A, Ghani A, Gorelick F, Mehal WZ. Lactate reduces liver and pancreatic injury in toll-like receptor – and inflammasome-mediated inflammation via GPR81-mediated suppression of innate immunity. *Gastroenterology* (2014) 146:1763–74. doi:10.1053/j.gastro.2014.03.014

163. Cassatella MA, Gasperini S, Bovolenta C, Calzetti F, Vollebregt M, Scapini P, et al. Interleukin-10 (IL-10) selectively enhances CIS3/SOCS3 mRNA expression in human neutrophils: evidence for an IL-10-induced pathway that is independent of STAT protein activation. *Blood* (1999) 94:2880–9.

164. Zhang Z, Liu Q, Che Y, Yuan X, Dai L, Zeng B, et al. Antigen presentation by dendritic cells in tumors is disrupted by altered metabolism that involves pyruvate kinase M2 and its interaction with SOCS3. *Cancer Res* (2010) 70:89–98. doi:10.1158/0008-5472.CAN-09-2970

165. Herber DL, Cao W, Nefedova Y, Novitskiy SV, Nagaraj S, Tyurin VA, et al. Lipid accumulation and dendritic cell dysfunction in cancer. *Nat Med* (2010) 16:880–6. doi:10.1038/nm.2172

166. Ramakrishnan R, Tyurin VA, Veglia F, Condamine T, Amoscato A, Mohammadyani D, et al. Oxidized lipids block antigen cross-presentation by dendritic cells in cancer. *J Immunol* (2014) 192:2920–31. doi:10.4049/jimmunol.1302801

167. Coutant F, Agaugué S, Perrin-Cocon L, André P, Lotteau V. Sensing environmental lipids by dendritic cell modulates its function. *J Immunol* (2004) 172:54–60. doi:10.4049/jimmunol.172.1.54

168. Cubillos-Ruiz JR, Silberman PC, Rutkowski MR, Chopra S, Perales-Puchalt A, Song M, et al. ER stress sensor XBP1 controls anti-tumor immunity by disrupting dendritic cell homeostasis. *Cell* (2015) 161:1527–38. doi:10.1016/j.cell.2015.05.025

169. Young A, Ngiow SF, Madore J, Reinhardt J, Landsberg J, Chitsazan A, et al. Targeting adenosine in BRAF-mutant melanoma reduces tumor growth and metastasis. *Cancer Res* (2017) 77:4684–96. doi:10.1158/0008-5472.CAN-17-0393

170. Bastid J, Regairaz A, Bonnefoy N, Déjou C, Giustiniani J, Laheurte C, et al. Inhibition of CD39 enzymatic function at the surface of tumor cells alleviates

their immunosuppressive activity. *Cancer Immunol Res* (2015) 3:254–65. doi:10.1158/2326-6066.CIR-14-0018

171. Sadej R, Spychala J, Skladanowski AC. Expression of ecto-5'-nucleotidase (eN, CD73) in cell lines from various stages of human melanoma. *Melanoma Res* (2006) 16:213–22. doi:10.1097/01.cmr.0000215030.69823.11

172. Wang H, Lee S, Nigro CL, Lattanzio L, Merlano M, Monteverde M, et al. NT5E (CD73) is epigenetically regulated in malignant melanoma and associated with metastatic site specificity. *Br J Cancer* (2012) 106:1446–52. doi:10.1038/bjc.2012.95

173. Linnemann C, Schildberg FA, Schurich A, Diehl L, Hegenbarth SI, Endl E, et al. Adenosine regulates CD8 T-cell priming by inhibition of membrane-proximal T-cell receptor signalling. *Immunology* (2009) 128:e728–37. doi:10.1111/j.1365-2567.2009.03075.x

174. Ohta A, Sitkovsky M. Extracellular adenosine-mediated modulation of regulatory T cells. *Front Immunol* (2014) 5:304. doi:10.3389/fimmu.2014.00304

175. Panther E, Corinti S, Idzko M, Herouy Y, Napp M, la Sala A, et al. Adenosine affects expression of membrane molecules, cytokine and chemokine release, and the T-cell stimulatory capacity of human dendritic cells. *Blood* (2003) 101:3985–90. doi:10.1182/blood-2002-07-2113

176. Novitskiy SV, Ryzhov S, Zaynagetdinov R, Goldstein AE, Huang Y, Tikhomirov OY, et al. Adenosine receptors in regulation of dendritic cell differentiation and function. *Blood* (2008) 112:1822–31. doi:10.1182/blood-2008-02-136325

177. Cekic C, Day YJ, Sag D, Linden J. Myeloid expression of adenosine A2A receptor suppresses T and NK cell responses in the solid tumor microenvironment. *Cancer Res* (2014) 74:7250–9. doi:10.1158/0008-5472.CAN-13-3583

178. Cekic C, Kayhan M, Koyas A, Akdemir I, Savas AC. Molecular mechanism for adenosine regulation of dendritic cells. *J Immunol* (2017) 198(1 Suppl):67.8.

179. Mondanelli G, Bianchi R, Pallotta MT, Orabona C, Albini E, Iacono A, et al. A relay pathway between arginine and tryptophan metabolism confers immunosuppressive properties on dendritic cells. *Immunity* (2017) 46: 233–44. doi:10.1016/j.immuni.2017.01.005

180. Galvin KC, Dyck L, Marshall NA, Stefanska AM, Walsh KP, Moran B, et al. Blocking retinoic acid receptor-α enhances the efficacy of a dendritic cell vaccine against tumours by suppressing the induction of regulatory T cells. *Cancer Immunol Immunother* (2013) 62:1273–82. doi:10.1007/s00262-013-1432-8

181. Young A, Ngiow SF, Barkauskas DS, Sult E, Hay C, Blake SJ, et al. Co-inhibition of CD73 and A2AR adenosine signaling improves anti-tumor immune responses. *Cancer Cell* (2016) 30:391–403. doi:10.1016/j.ccell.2016.06.025

182. Yi H, Guo C, Yu X, Gao P, Qian J, Zuo D, et al. Targeting the immunoregulator SRA/CD204 potentiates specific dendritic cell vaccine-induced T-cell response and antitumor immunity. *Cancer Res* (2011) 71:6611–20. doi:10.1158/0008-5472.CAN-11-1801

183. Tian S, Liu Z, Donahue C, Falo LD, You Z. Genetic targeting of the active transcription factor XBP1s to dendritic cells potentiates vaccine-induced prophylactic and therapeutic antitumor immunity. *Mol Ther* (2012) 20:432–42. doi:10.1038/mt.2011.183

184. Zhang Y, Chen G, Liu Z, Tian S, Zhang J, Carey CD, et al. Genetic vaccines to potentiate the effective CD103 + dendritic cell-mediated cross-priming of antitumor immunity. *J Immunol* (2015) 194:5937–47. doi:10.4049/jimmunol.1500089

185. Su J, Gao T, Jiang M, Wu L, Zeng W, Zhao S, et al. CD147 silencing inhibits tumor growth by suppressing glucose transport in melanoma. *Oncotarget* (2016) 7:64778–84. doi:10.18632/oncotarget.11415

186. Koch A, Lang SA, Wild PJ, Gantner S, Mahli A, Spanier G, et al. Glucose transporter isoform 1 expression enhances metastasis of malignant melanoma cells. *Oncotarget* (2015) 6:32748–60. doi:10.18632/oncotarget.4977

187. Amiel E, Everts B, Fritz D, Beauchamp S, Ge B, Pearce EL, et al. Mechanistic target of rapamycin inhibition extends cellular lifespan in dendritic cells by preserving mitochondrial function. *J Immunol* (2014) 193:2821–30. doi:10.4049/jimmunol.1302498

188. Amiel E, Everts B, Freitas TC, King IL, Curtis JD, Pearce EL, et al. Inhibition of mechanistic target of rapamycin promotes dendritic cell activation and enhances therapeutic autologous vaccination in mice. *J Immunol* (2012) 189:2151–8. doi:10.4049/jimmunol.1103741

189. Raïch-Regué D, Fabian KP, Watson AR, Fecek RJ, Storkus WJ, Thomson AW. Intratumoral delivery of mTORC2-deficient dendritic cells inhibits B16 melanoma growth by promoting CD8(+) effector T cell responses. *Oncoimmunology* (2016) 5:e1146841. doi:10.1080/2162402X.2016.1146841

190. Bhatt AP, Redinbo MR, Bultman SJ. The role of the microbiome in cancer development and therapy. *CA Cancer J Clin* (2017) 67:326–44. doi:10.3322/caac.21398

191. Xu C, Ruan B, Jiang Y, Xue T, Wang Z, Lu H, et al. Antibiotics-induced gut microbiota dysbiosis promotes tumor initiation via affecting APC-Th1 development in mice. *Biochem Biophys Res Commun* (2017) 488:418–24. doi:10.1016/j.bbrc.2017.05.071

192. Cheng M, Qian L, Shen G, Bian G, Xu T, Xu W, et al. Microbiota modulate tumoral immune surveillance in lung through a T17 immune cell-dependent mechanism. *Cancer Res* (2014) 74:4030–41. doi:10.1158/0008-5472.CAN-13-2462

193. Paulos CM, Wrzesinski C, Kaiser A, Hinrichs CS, Chieppa M, Cassard L, et al. Microbial translocation augments the function of adoptively transferred self/tumor-specific CD8+ T cells via TLR4 signaling. *J Clin Invest* (2007) 117:2197–204. doi:10.1172/JCI32205

194. Iida N, Dzutsev A, Stewart CA, Smith L, Bouladoux N, Weingarten RA, et al. Commensal bacteria control cancer response to therapy by modulating the tumor microenvironment. *Science* (2013) 342:967–70. doi:10.1126/science.1240527

195. Sivan A, Corrales L, Hubert N, Williams JB, Aquino-Michaels K, Earley ZM, et al. Commensal *Bifidobacterium* promotes antitumor immunity and facilitates anti-PD-L1 efficacy. *Science* (2015) 350:1084–9. doi:10.1126/science.aac4255

196. Vetizou M, Pitt JM, Daillere R, Lepage P, Waldschmitt N, Flament C, et al. Anticancer immunotherapy by CTLA-4 blockade relies on the gut microbiota. *Science* (2015) 350:1079–84. doi:10.1126/science.aad1329

197. Chaput N, Lepage P, Coutzac C, Soularue E, Le Roux K, Monot C, et al. Baseline gut microbiota predicts clinical response and colitis in metastatic melanoma patients treated with ipilimumab. *Ann Oncol* (2017) 28:1368–79. doi:10.1093/annonc/mdx108

198. Wargo JA, Gopalakrishnan V, Spencer C, Karpinets T, Reuben A, Andrews MC, et al. Association of the diversity and composition of the gut microbiome with responses and survival (PFS) in metastatic melanoma (MM) patients (pts) on anti-PD-1 therapy. *J Clin Oncol* (2017) 35(15 Suppl): 3008–3008. doi:10.1200/JCO.2017.35.15_suppl.3008

199. Frankel AE, Coughlin LA, Kim J, Froehlich TW, Xie Y, Frenkel EP, et al. Metagenomic shotgun sequencing and unbiased metabolomic profiling identify specific human gut microbiota and metabolites associated with immune checkpoint therapy efficacy in melanoma patients. *Neoplasia* (2017) 19:848–55. doi:10.1016/j.neo.2017.08.004

200. Rooks MG, Garrett WS. Gut microbiota, metabolites and host immunity. *Nat Rev Immunol* (2016) 16:341–52. doi:10.1038/nri.2016.42

201. Roy S, Trinchieri G. Microbiota: a key orchestrator of cancer therapy. *Nat Rev Cancer* (2017) 17:271–85. doi:10.1038/nrc.2017.13

202. Dubin K, Callahan MK, Ren B, Khanin R, Viale A, Ling L, et al. Intestinal microbiome analyses identify melanoma patients at risk for checkpoint-blockade-induced colitis. *Nat Commun* (2016) 7:10391. doi:10.1038/ncomms10391

203. Salava A, Aho V, Pereira P, Koskinen K, Paulin L, Auvinen P, et al. Skin microbiome in melanomas and melanocytic nevi. *Eur J Dermatol* (2016) 26:49–55. doi:10.1684/ejd.2015.2696

204. Chng KR, Tay ASL, Li C, Ng AHQ, Wang J, Suri BK, et al. Whole metagenome profiling reveals skin microbiome-dependent susceptibility to atopic dermatitis flare. *Nat Microbiol* (2016) 1:16106. doi:10.1038/nmicrobiol.2016.106

205. Ganju P, Nagpal S, Mohammed MH, Nishal Kumar P, Pandey R, Natarajan VT, et al. Microbial community profiling shows dysbiosis in the lesional skin of Vitiligo subjects. *Sci Rep* (2016) 6:18761. doi:10.1038/srep18761

206. Vujkovic-Cvijin I, Wei M, Restifo NP, Belkaid Y. Role for skin-associated microbiota in development of endogenous anti-melanocyte immunity in vitiligo. *J Immunol* (2017) 198(1 Suppl):58.14.

207. Yang J, Qin Y, Li L, Cao C, Wang Q, Li Q, et al. Apoptotic melanoma B16-F1 cells induced by lidamycin could initiate the antitumor immune response in BABL/c mice. *Oncol Res* (2016) 23:79–06. doi:10.3727/096504015X14478843952942

208. Son KJ, Choi KR, Ryu CK, Lee SJ, Kim HJ, Lee H. Induction of immunogenic cell death of tumors by newly synthesized heterocyclic quinone derivative. *PLoS One* (2017) 12:e0173121. doi:10.1371/journal.pone.0173121

209. Son K, Choi KR, Lee SJ, Lee H. Immunogenic cell death induced by ginsenoside Rg3: significance in dendritic cell-based anti-tumor immunotherapy. *Immune Netw* (2016) 16:75. doi:10.4110/in.2016.16.1.75

210. Werthmöller N, Frey B, Rückert M, Lotter M, Fietkau R, Gaipl US. Combination of ionising radiation with hyperthermia increases the immunogenic potential of B16-F10 melanoma cells *in vitro* and *in vivo*. *Int J Hyperth* (2016) 32:23–30. doi:10.3109/02656736.2015.1106011

3

The Role and Necessity of Sentinel Lymph Node Biopsy for Invasive Melanoma

Yasuhiro Nakamura*

Department of Skin Oncology/Dermatology, Saitama Medical University International Medical Center, Saitama, Japan

*Correspondence:
Yasuhiro Nakamura
ynakamur@saitama-med.ac.jp

Sentinel lymph node biopsy (SLNB) is a widely accepted procedure for melanoma staging and treatment. The development of lymphatic mapping and SLNB, which was first introduced in 1992, has enabled surgeons to detect microscopic nodal metastases and stage-negative regional nodal basins with low morbidity. SLNB has also facilitated the selective application of regional lymph node dissection for patients with microscopic nodal metastases, enabling unnecessary lymph node dissection. In contrast, recent major randomized phase III trials (DeCOG-SLT and MSLT–II trial) compared the clinical benefit of early completion lymph node dissection with observation after detecting microscopic nodal disease. The results of those studies indicated that there was no significant difference in the survival between the two groups, although regional control was superior after early completion lymph node dissection compared to that obtained after observation. Thus, the role and value of early completion lymph node dissection worldwide are currently very limited for patients with microscopic nodal disease. However, the use of SLNB is still controversial. In addition, the recent approval of adjuvant therapy using novel agents, such as anti-programmed death-1 antibodies, and molecular targeted therapeutics may influence the skipping of complete lymph node dissection in patients with micrometastatic nodal disease in a real-world setting. Furthermore, modern neoadjuvant therapy, which is now under investigation, may have the potential to change the surgical procedure used for nodal disease. Herein, we describe the current role and value of SLNB and completion lymph node dissection and discuss the major controversies as well as the favorable future outlook.

Keywords: melanoma, lymphatic metastasis, sentinel lymph node biopsy, completion lymph node dissection, observation, adjuvant therapy

INTRODUCTION

Malignant melanoma is among the most common types of cancer, with an increasing incidence rate of 7.9 per 100,000 people in 1975 to 25.8 per 100,000 people in 2015 (1). Approximately 7% of patients are diagnosed with stage III disease, who have a 5 year survival rate was 60.8% (2). The treatment approach for stage III patients is crucial because cutaneous melanoma often metastasizes first to the regional lymph nodes and the sentinel lymph node (SLN) is the first lymph node to receive lymphatic drainage from the primary site.

The surgical approach for treating regional lymph node metastasis has continued to develop, particularly considering sentinel lymph node biopsy (SLNB). Although most patients with melanoma have no clinical nodal disease at the first visit, some patients have clinically undetectable micrometastasis in the regional lymph node. The main controversy is whether completion lymph node dissection (CLND) improves the overall or disease-specific survival of patients with SLN micrometastasis. Furthermore, the advent of promising systemic therapies, confirmed in recent clinical trials, and the results of several trials, confirming the efficacy of SLNB and immediate CLND in patients with positive SLN, may drastically change the conventional methods used for surgical control of the regional lymph nodes by using CLND for all patients with a positive SLNB.

APPLICATION OF SLNB

SLNB is the most appropriate technique for accurate staging of clinical stage I and II disease. The main risk variables associated with higher SLN metastasis are Breslow thickness (BT), ulceration, and a number of mitoses. Per the 8th edition cancer staging guidelines recommended by the American Joint Committee on Cancer (AJCC) (3), SLNB is generally not recommended for melanoma patients with a BT of <0.8 mm without ulceration because the probability of a positive SLN is <5%. However, SLNB should generally be considered for melanoma patients with clinical stage IB or II disease, with the following considerations:

1. T1b (BT of <0.8 mm with ulceration or BT of 0.8 mm^{-1} mm with or without ulceration) or T1a lesions with BT < 0.8 mm with other adverse features [e.g., very high mitotic index ≤2/mm^2 (particularly in young patients), lymphovascular invasion, or a combination of these factors], because the probability of a positive SLN is 5–10%. SLNB should be considered for these patients after discussion.
2. Stage IB (T2a) or II (BT of >1 mm with any feature), because the probability of a positive SLN is >10%. SLNB should be offered SLNB for these patients after discussion.

No globally accepted protocols are available for processing SLNs. However, small metastases are overlooked in conventional processing, which involves the examination of a single routine hematoxylin-eosin (HE)-stained section obtained by bivalving the SLN along the long axis (4, 5). In another procedure, the SLN is sectioned serially along the short axis (breadloaf technique) to increase the amount of subcapsular tissue in the HE-stained sections (6). When routine H&E staining does not reveal SLN metastases, immunohistochemistry (IHC) for S100, HMB-45, and MART-1/Melan-A is useful for detecting additional SLN-positive patients (7, 8). Reverse transcription-polymerase chain reaction (RT-PCR) and cell culture can increase the detection rates of positive SLN even when there are only a few metastatic melanoma cells in the SLN (9); however, these molecular biology techniques are not widely used in most institutions.

MANAGEMENT OF PATIENTS WITH POSITIVE SLN: RESULTS OF RECENT STUDIES AND THE ROLE OF SLNB

When patients show positive results for SLN metastasis, CLND has traditionally been indicated. However, the findings of recent studies regarding the therapeutic value of SLNB and immediate CLND after positive SLNB have resulted in a change in this traditional strategy.

DERMATOLOGIC COOPERATIVE ONCOLOGY GROUP-SENTINEL LYMPH NODE TRIAL (DECOG-SLT)

The Dermatologic Cooperative Oncology Group-Sentinel Lymph node Trial (DeCOG-SLT), conducted in Germany, was the first phase III randomized clinical trial to evaluate the efficacy of immediate CLND in patients with melanoma on the trunk and limbs with BT of ≥1.0 mm and positive SLN (10). The patients were randomly assigned to the immediate CLND group (n = 240) or the observation group (n = 233; patients underwent delayed CLND only if regional metastasis was suspected on ultrasonography performed every 3 months). There were no significant differences in the distant metastasis-free survival, recurrence-free survival, and overall survival (OS) between the two groups. In this study, most patients (n = 311) had SLN tumor burdens of ≤1.0 mm. This high proportion of SLN micrometastasis leads to the high probability of negative non-SLN in both groups. There was no significant difference in distant metastasis-free survival between the two groups in this cohort. Therefore, distant metastasis-free survival in the cohort with SLN tumor burdens of >1.0 mm was also analyzed. There was no significant difference in the distant metastasis-free survival between the two groups, but the sample size was small in each group (n = 62 in the CLND group and n = 59 in the observation group). The authors concluded that immediate CLND was not associated with improved distant metastasis-free survival, recurrence-free survival, and OS after a median follow-up of 72 months, and no longer recommend CLND for patients with micrometastases.

MULTICENTER SELECTIVE LYMPHADENECTOMY TRIAL (MSLT-II)

MSLT–II enrolled a large number of patients with positive SLN (9). This was also a multicenter, phase III randomized trial that compared the immediate CLND group (n = 824) with the observation group (n = 931; patients underwent CLND only when regional metastasis was suspected on ultrasonography performed every 4 months). The mean 3 year melanoma-specific survival rate was statistically insignificant between the two groups after a median follow-up of 43 months. The disease-free survival (DFS) was slightly significantly better in the CLND group than in the observation group ($P = 0.05$). A positive non-SLN status was a reliable, independent prognostic factor for recurrence [hazard ratio (HR), 1.78; $P = 0.005$]. The occurrence of post-operative lymphedema was higher in the CLND group (24.1%) than in the observation group (6.3%). Likewise, the authors concluded that immediate CLND was not associated with improved melanoma-specific survival, but improved the regional recurrence rate and provided prognostic information.

HOW ARE PATIENTS HARBORING POSITIVE SLN MANAGED?

The above-mentioned two randomized trials demonstrated no survival benefit even if patients received immediate CLND after positive SLNB, although the nodal recurrence rate decreased in the immediate CLND group. The results of these trials do not recommend routine CLND in most patients after positive SLNB. However, their conclusions are still limited, as most patients in these studies had lower tumor burdens in the SLN (>60%). Those populations have a low probability of positive non-SLN in both groups. The true efficacy of immediate CLND after positive SLNB in patients with a higher risk, with SLN tumor burdens of >1 mm, is still unknown because of the small sample size in these trials. Therefore, current NCCN guidelines still recommend CLND, along with careful observation in patients with positive SLN after appropriate risk stratification (11). Accordingly, some guides, such as nomograms, should be utilized for accurate prediction of non-SLN status, regional control, and prognosis. This will enable us to conduct clinical trials for confirming the survival advantage of CLND in a more homogenous cohort with positive non-SLNs. Previously published predictive models for positive non-SLNs (12–18) are shown in **Table 1**. Although several studies have suggested similar clinicopathological characteristics as predictive parameters, a recent study by Bertolli et al. proposes BT, the number of positive SLNs, and large tumor diameter as significant predictive parameters, using their nomogram (18). This model shows the best discriminatory power (AUC 0.752) and Brier score (0.085) among all published predictive models (18) (**Table 1**).

The racial difference in the proportion of clinical type is also crucial for considering the role of SLNB and immediate CLND. For example, acral melanoma (AM) shows drastic differences from other clinical types considering the biological, genetic, and clinicopathological aspects, although SLNB is also widely applied in clinical practice. The actual role of SLNB in this cohort remains unclear, as limited number of AM patients were included in the large trials of SLNB (i.e., DeCOG-SLT and MSLT-II) that mainly investigated Caucasian people (9, 10, 19). Ito et al. retrospectively investigated Japanese AM patients ($n = 116$) who received SLNB (20). Positive SLN was associated with significantly shorter melanoma-specific survival and DFS. The impact of positive SLNs on melanoma-specific survival was increased in AM patients with >1 mm thickness (5 year survival, 22.7 vs. 80.8%; $P = 0.0005$). Although the sample size was small in these studies, the trends of positive SLN status in association with more frequent recurrence and worsened survival in AM patients were similar to those trends in larger prospective randomized trials; however, there are no data regarding the efficacy of immediate CLND compared with observation.

ROLE OF ADJUVANT THERAPY FOR POSITIVE SLN PATIENTS WITHOUT IMMEDIATE CLND

The recent development of novel agents, including immune checkpoint inhibitors (ICIs) and molecular target agents, and their approval in many countries worldwide changed the treatment strategy for not only disease in the advanced stage but also treatment in the post-operative adjuvant setting. All these clinical trials mainly included stage III patients who underwent CLND and no patients skipped CLND after positive SLNB.

ANTI-CTLA-4 ANTIBODIES

A phase III randomized controlled trial (EORTC 18071) comparing ipilimumab with placebo for stage III melanoma patients indicated a significant improvement in the 3 year relapse-free survival (RFS), distant metastasis-free survival, and OS in the ipilimumab group (21). However, severe immune-related adverse events were observed in 41.6% of patients in the ipilimumab group, leading to discontinuation of ipilimumab in half of the patients.

ANTI-PD-1 ANTIBODIES

The clinical benefits of two anti-PD-1 agents as adjuvant therapy were reported recently. A phase III randomized controlled trial (Checkmate 238) comparing nivolumab with ipilimumab for stage IIIB to IV melanoma patients (22) demonstrated better 1 year RFS with lower toxicity in the nivolumab group than in the ipilimumab group. Likewise, a phase III randomized trial (KEYNOTE-054) comparing pembrolizumab with placebo for stage III patients, except for <1 mm of tumor burden in the SLN, also demonstrated improvement in the recurrence-free survival of patients receiving pembrolizumab compared to those receiving placebo after a median follow-up of 15 months (HR, 0.57; $P < 0.001$) (23).

BRAF INHIBITOR/MEK INHIBITOR

A phase III randomized trial (COMBI-AD) comparing dabrafenib plus trametinib with placebo for patients with stage III BRAF mutant melanoma, except for <1 mm of tumor burdens in the SLN, showed improved RFS in the dabrafenib/trametinib group after a median follow-up of 44 months in the dabrafenib/trametinib group and 42 months in the placebo group (24). There also was a trend of improvement in the OS [the 3-year OS rate was 86% in the dabrafenib/trametinib group and 77% in the placebo group (HR, 0.57; $P = 0.0006$)], although the data obtained on statistical analysis did not fulfill the pre-specified interim analysis boundary ($P = 0.000019$) (25).

Based on the above-mentioned clinical trials, the latest NCCN guidelines recommend adjuvant nivolumab for stage IIIB/C

TABLE 1 | The performance of published prediction models for non-sentinel lymph node positivity.

References	Patient no. for research	Significant clinicopathological parameters	Discrimination AUC (95% CI)	Calibration brier score (95% CI)
Lee et al. (12)	191	Breslow thickness SLN tumor burden diameter	0.65 (0.60–0.70)	0.19 (0.18–0.20)
Sabel et al. (13)	221	Sex Breslow thickness Extranodal extension in SLN No. of positive SLNs	0.67 (0.63–0.74)	0.18 (0.16–0.20)
Gershenwald et al. (14)	343	SLN tumor burden diameter Breslow thickness No. of SLNs harvested	0.65 (0.60–0.70)	0.18 (0.17–0.20)
Murali et al. (15)	309	Sex Primary tumor regression No. of positive SLNs SLN tumor burden diameter SLN metastasis site	0.65 (0.60–0.70)	0.18 (0.17–0.19)
Kibrite et al. (16)	171	Breslow thickness SLN tumor burden diameter	0.65 (0.60–0.70)	0.19 (0.18–0.20)
Rossi et al. (17)	1220	Breslow thickness Primary tumor site SLN tumor burden diameter SLN metastasis site No. of SLNs harvested No. of positive SLNs	0.74 (0.70–0.79)	0.16 (0.15–0.17)
Bertolli et al. (18)	1213	Breslow thickness No. of positive SLNs SLN tumor burden diameter	0.86 (0.73–0.99)	0.085 (N.A.)

SLN, sentinel lymph node; AUC, area under the curve; CI, confidence interval; N.A., not available.

and IV melanoma patients after complete tumor removal. Pembrolizumab was recommended for stage III melanoma patients with ≥1 mm tumor burden in the SLN. In patients with BRAF mutations, dabrafenib plus trametinib can also be alternatively recommended for stage III disease with ≥1 mm tumor burden in the SLN.

The result of SLNB can be used to classify patients without clinical nodal disease for undergoing adjuvant therapy. However, all the above-mentioned clinical trials required CLND before initiating adjuvant therapy. Conversely, in the real-world setting, patients who have positive SLN and do not undergo CLND will increase considering the results of the DeCOG-SLT and MSLT-II trials, even if the patients' tumor burdens exceed 1 mm. Currently, there are no data about the survival benefit of adjuvant therapy with the novel agents in patients who skipped CLND after positive SLNB. Therefore, further research is required to investigate the survival differences between the clinical trial populations and the more heterogeneous real-world population.

POSSIBLE ROLE OF NEOADJUVANT THERAPY

The reports of modern neoadjuvant clinical trials using ICIs or molecular targeted agents demonstrate promising efficacy, mainly for clinical stage III disease. All agents for neoadjuvant use have not yet been approved worldwide.

ANTI-PD-1 ANTIBODIES AND ANTI-PD-1/ANTI-CTLA-4 ANTIBODY

Huang et al. conducted a phase Ib trial investigating the safety of neoadjuvant/adjuvant pembrolizumab for resectable clinical stage III and IV melanoma (26). Enrolled patients received neoadjuvant/adjuvant pembrolizumab (1 cycle of neoadjuvant pembrolizumab 3 weeks before surgery and 17 cycles of adjuvant pembrolizumab). Eight of 27 patients (30%) achieved complete or major pathological response, and they remain free of disease.

Amaria et al. reported a randomized phase II trial comparing the efficacy and safety of neoadjuvant nivolumab (four cycles of neoadjuvant and 13 cycles of adjuvant nivolumab) to neoadjuvant nivolumab/ipilimumab (three cycles of neoadjuvant nivolumab/ipilimumab and 13 cycles of adjuvant nivolumab) for resectable clinical stage III and IV melanoma (27). Neoadjuvant nivolumab/ipilimumab demonstrated higher response rates (RRs) [objective RR, 73 vs. 25%; pathological complete response (pCR), 45 vs. 25%] but also showed higher toxicity (grade 3 treatment-related adverse events, 73 vs. 8%).

Blank et al. also reported a randomized phase II trial (OpACIN) comparing neoadjuvant nivolumab/ipilimumab (two cycles of neoadjuvant nivolumab/ipilimumab and two cycles of adjuvant nivolumab/ipilimumab) with adjuvant nivolumab/ipilimumab (four cycles of adjuvant nivolumab/ipilimumab) in patients with palpable stage III melanoma (28). The neoadjuvant arm achieved high pathological responses (78%), and no patients showing response developed recurrence during the median follow-up or 25.6 months. However, 9 of 10 patients experienced grade 3/4 adverse events in both treatment arms.

Rozeman et al. conducted a phase II randomized trial (OpACIN-neo) comparing three different doses and cycles of neoadjuvant nivolumab/ipilimumab for resectable clinical stage III melanoma (29). The following were three protocols: group A, two cycles of nivolumab (1 mg/kg) and ipilimumab (3 mg/kg); group B, two cycles of nivolumab (3 mg/kg) and ipilimumab (1 mg/kg); and group C, two cycles of ipilimumab (3 mg/kg) followed by two cycles of nivolumab (3 mg/kg). The objective radiological and pathological RRs were 63% (19/30) and 80% (24/30) in group A, 57% (17/30) and 77% (23/30) in group B, and 35% (9/26) and 65% (17/26) in group C, respectively. The rate of grade 3/4 immune-related adverse events was lower in group B than in groups A and C (group A, 40% [12/30]; group B, 20% [6/30]; group C, 50% [13/26]). One group A patient died of encephalitis.

BRAF INHIBITOR/MEK INHIBITOR

Amaria et al. reported a randomized phase II trial for patients with resectable clinical stage III or oligometastatic stage IV melanoma harboring BRAFV600E/K mutation (30). The patients were randomly assigned to either undergo surgery followed by adjuvant therapy without ICIs or targeted agents or to receive neoadjuvant/adjuvant dabrafenib/trametinib (8 weeks of neoadjuvant and 44 weeks of adjuvant dabrafenib/trametinib). The neoadjuvant group showed significantly long event-free survival (median event-free survival: 19.7 vs. 2.9 months; HR 0.016; $P < 0.0001$).

Long et al. also reported a single-arm phase II trial (NeoCombi) for patients with resectable clinical stage IIIB-C (AJCC 7th edition) melanoma harboring BRAFV600 mutation (31). The patients received neoadjuvant/adjuvant dabrafenib/trametinib (12 weeks of neoadjuvant and 40 weeks of adjuvant dabrafenib/trametinib). Thirty of 35 patients (86%) achieved a response (46%, complete response; 40%, partial response). All patients achieved pathological response, including 17 patients (49%) with pCR.

These novel neoadjuvant therapies, involving active regimens mainly for clinical stage III melanoma, showed high pathological RRs. Remarkably, no patients achieving pCR after treatment with ICIs developed recurrence during the follow-up periods. However, these esults must be interpreted with caution as these trials did not report OS after long-term follow-up.

IMMUNOLOGY OF SLNs

Immunohistological and molecular characteristics of SLNs may be useful in predicting the development of regional or distant metastasis, because the SLN represents the immunological site at which anti-tumor immune dysfunction is established and where potential prognostic immunologic markers can be found. Considering the immunologic microenvironment, the number of CD3+, CD4+, and CD8+ tumor-infiltrating lymphocytes in positive SLN is associated with better recurrence-free survival and OS (32). Elevated levels of regulatory T cell markers, such as FOXP3 and indoleamine 2,3-dioxygenase, correlate with increasing rates of local, regional, and distant metastases (33, 34). A study focused on regression of the primary tumor indicated that a regression of more than 10% was a reliable cutoff to divide different risk categories (35). Only a small number of CD4+/CD25+, FOXP3+/CD4+, or PD1+/CD4+ lymphocytes infiltrated the regressed areas. These lymphocytes were correlated with anergy and lower CD8+ lymphocyte immune response to melanoma cells. Thus, these findings may help in developing novel therapeutic strategies for selecting SLNB and immediate CLND for patients with stage III melanoma. As for molecular characteristics, Vallacchi et al. reported a pilot study involving integrated analysis of genome-wide transcriptional profiles and *in vitro* assessment of immune cells present in positive SLNs. This analysis identified microRNA, involved in the regulation of the TNF receptor superfamily member 8 gene that encodes the CD30 receptor, as a marker in the lymphocytes of melanoma patients with progressive disease. These findings demonstrate that microRNA is associated with the regulation of immune dysfunction in SLNs, providing a valuable prognostic molecular marker for identifying stage III melanoma patients at risk of recurrence.

CONCLUSIONS

SLNB has contributed to the selection of earlier CLND in patients without nodal disease by detecting microscopic positive SLN. Conversely, it is questionable whether CLND is required if SLN itself was therapeutic in patients with microscopic positive SLN alone. The results of two recent randomized clinical trials suggested that immediate CLND for positive SLN patients was not associated with DFS, OS, and metastasis-free survival, despite an increased risk of delayed non-SLN recurrence. Currently, SLNB provides prognostic information and has a therapeutic role in patients with a low tumor burden with intermediate-thickness melanoma. SLNB is also useful to select patients with the appropriate stage for undergoing post-operative adjuvant therapy. Immediate CLND is no longer routinely recommended for all patients with positive SLNB, particularly for patients without suspected non-SLN metastasis. At present, immediate CLND is ideal for patients at low risk of distant metastasis but at high risk of delayed regional metastasis.

The future of SLNB and CLND will depend on the development of promising neoadjuvant/adjuvant therapies and excellent biomarkers, which may drastically change the treatment strategies for stage III melanoma patients as well as the current TNM classification. This may lead to the advent of a new era in which surgical procedures would not be required for high-risk patients, including those with stage III disease.

AUTHOR CONTRIBUTIONS

YN had full access to all of the data in the study and take responsibility for study concept and design, acquisition, analysis, interpretation of data, drafting of the manuscript, and critical revision of the manuscript for important intellectual content.

REFERENCES

1. Siegel RL, Miller KD, Jemal A. Cancer statistics, 2018. *CA Cancer J Clin.* (2018) 68:7–30. doi: 10.3322/caac.21442
2. Cronin KA, Lake AJ, Scott S, Sherman RL, Noone AM, Howlader N, et al. Annual report to the nation on the status of cancer, part I: National Cancer Statistics. *Cancer.* (2018) 124:2785–800. doi: 10.1002/cncr.31551
3. Gershenwald JE, Scolyer RA, Hess KR, Sondak VK, Long GV, Ross MI, et al. Melanoma staging: evidence-based changes in the American Joint Committee on Cancer eighth edition cancer staging manual. *CA Cancer J Clin.* (2017) 67:472–92. doi: 10.3322/caac.21409
4. Prieto VG. Use of frozen sections in the examination of sentinel lymph nodes in patients with melanoma. *Semin Diagn Pathol.* (2008) 25:112–5. doi: 10.1053/j.semdp.2008.04.001
5. Gershenwald JE, Colome MI, Lee JE, Mansfield PF, Tseng C, Lee JJ, et al. Patterns of recurrence following a negative sentinel lymph node biopsy in 243 patients with stage I or II melanoma. *J Clin Oncol.* (1998) 16:2253–60. doi: 10.1200/JCO.1998.16.6.2253
6. Prieto VG, Clark SH. Processing of sentinel lymph nodes for detection of metastatic melanoma. *Ann Diagn Pathol.* (2002) 6:257–64. doi: 10.1053/adpa.2002.35400
7. Abrahamsen HN, Hamilton-Dutoit SJ, Larsen J, Steiniche T. Sentinel lymph nodes in malignant melanoma: extended histopathologic evaluation improves diagnostic precision. *Cancer.* (2004) 100:1683–91. doi: 10.1002/cncr.20179
8. Yu LL, Flotte TJ, Tanabe KK, Gadd MA, Cosimi AB, Sober AJ, et al. Detection of microscopic melanoma metastases in sentinel lymph nodes. *Cancer.* (1999) 86:617–27. doi: 10.1002/(SICI)1097-0142(19990815)86:4<617::AID-CNCR10>3.3.CO;2-J
9. Faries MB, Thompson JF, Cochran AJ, Aracena CJ, Lotti T. Completion Dissection or Observation for Sentinel-Node Metastasis in Melanoma. *N Engl J Med.* (2017) 376:2211–22. doi: 10.1111/dth.12544
10. Leiter UM, Stadler R, Mauch C, Hohenberger W, Brockmeyer N, Berking C, et al. Final analysis of DECOG-SLT trial: survival outcomes of complete lymph node dissection in melanoma patients with positive sentinel node. *J Clin Oncol.* 36(15_suppl):9501. doi: 10.1200/JCO.2018.36.15_suppl.9501
11. Fiddian-Green RG, Silen W. *NCCN Clinical Practice Guidelines in Oncology (NCCN Guidelines²) Melanoma Version 2.2019.* (2019). Available online at: https://www.nccn.org/professionals/physician_gls/pdf/cutaneous_melanoma.pdf (accessed March 12, 2019).
12. Lee JH, Essner R, Torisu-Itakura H, Wanek L, Wang H, Morton DL. Factors predictive of tumor-positive nonsentinel lymph nodes after tumor-positive sentinel lymph node dissection for melanoma. *J Clin Oncol.* (2004) 22:3677–84. doi: 10.1200/JCO.2004.01.012
13. Sabel MS, Griffith K, Sondak VK, Lowe L, Schwartz JL, Cimmino VM, et al. Predictors of nonsentinel lymph node positivity in patients with a positive sentinel node for melanoma. *J Am Coll Surg.* (2005) 201:37–47. doi: 10.1016/j.jamcollsurg.2005.03.029
14. Gershenwald JE, Andtbacka RH, Prieto VG, Johnson MM, Diwan AH, Lee JE, et al. Microscopic tumor burden in sentinel lymph nodes predicts synchronous nonsentinel lymph node involvement in patients with melanoma. *J Clin Oncol.* (2008) 26:4296–303. doi: 10.1200/JCO.2007.15.4179
15. Murali R, Desilva C, Thompson JF, Scolyer RA. Non-Sentinel Node Risk Score (N-SNORE): a scoring system for accurately stratifying risk of non-sentinel node positivity in patients with cutaneous melanoma with positive sentinel lymph nodes. *J Clin Oncol.* (2010) 28:4441–9. doi: 10.1200/JCO.2010.30.9567
16. Kibrité A, Milot H, Douville P, Gagné ÉJ, Labonté S, Friede J, et al. Predictive factors for sentinel lymph nodes and non-sentinel lymph nodes metastatic involvement: a database study of 1,041 melanoma patients. *Am J Surg.* (2016) 211:89–94. doi: 10.1016/j.amjsurg.2015.05.016
17. Rossi CR, Mocellin S, Campana LG, Borgognoni L, Sestini S, Giudice G, et al. Prediction of non-sentinel node status in patients with melanoma and positive sentinel node biopsy: an Italian Melanoma Intergroup (IMI) study. *Ann Surg Oncol.* (2018) 25:271–9. doi: 10.1245/s10434-017-6143-5
18. Bertolli E, Franke V, Calsavara VF, de Macedo MP, Pinto CAL, van Houdt WJ, et al. Validation of a nomogram for non-sentinel node positivity in melanoma patients, and its clinical implications: a Brazilian-Dutch study. *Ann Surg Oncol.* (2019) 26:395–405. doi: 10.1245/s10434-018-7038-9
19. Morton DL, Thompson JF, Cochran AJ, Mozzillo N, Nieweg OE, Roses DF, et al. Final trial report of sentinel-node biopsy versus nodal observation in melanoma. *N Engl J Med.* (2014) 370:599–609. doi: 10.1056/NEJMoa1310460
20. Ito T, Wada M, Nagae K, Nakano-Nakamura M, Nakahara T, Hagihara A, et al. Acral lentiginous melanoma: who benefits from sentinel lymph node biopsy? *J Am Acad Dermatol.* (2015) 72:71–7. doi: 10.1016/j.jaad.2014.10.008
21. Eggermont AM, Chiarion-Sileni V, Grob JJ, Dummer R, Wolchok JD, Schmidt H, et al. Prolonged survival in stage III melanoma with ipilimumab adjuvant therapy. *N Engl J Med.* (2016) 375:1845–55. doi: 10.1056/NEJMoa1611299
22. Weber J, Mandala M, Del Vecchio M, Gogas HJ, Arance AM, Cowey CL, et al. Adjuvant nivolumab versus ipilimumab in resected stage III or IV melanoma. *N Engl J Med.* (2017) 377:1824–35. doi: 10.1056/NEJMoa1709030
23. Eggermont AMM, Blank CU, Mandala M, Long GV, Atkinson V, Dalle S, et al. Adjuvant pembrolizumab versus placebo in resected stage III melanoma. *N Engl J Med.* (2018) 378:1789–801. doi: 10.1056/NEJMoa1802357
24. Hauschild A, Dummer R, Schadendorf D, Santinami M, Atkinson V, Mandalà M, et al. Longer follow-up confirms relapse-free survival benefit with adjuvant dabrafenib plus trametinib in patients with resected BRAF V600-mutant stage III melanoma. *J Clin Oncol.* (2018) 2018:JCO1801219. doi: 10.1200/JCO.18.01219
25. Long GV, Hauschild A, Santinami M, Atkinson V, Mandalà M, Chiarion-Sileni V, et al. Adjuvant dabrafenib plus trametinib in stage III BRAF-mutated melanoma. *N Engl J Med.* (2017) 377:1813–23. doi: 10.1056/NEJMoa1708539
26. Huang AC, Orlowski RJ, Xu X, Mick R, George SM, Yan PK, et al. A single dose of neoadjuvant PD-1 blockade predicts clinical outcomes in resectable melanoma. *Nat Med.* (2019) 25:454–61. doi: 10.1038/s41591-019-0357-y
27. Amaria RN, Reddy SM, Tawbi HA, Davies MA, Ross MI, Glitza IC, et al. Neoadjuvant immune checkpoint blockade in high-risk resectable melanoma. *Nat Med.* (2018) 24:1649–54. doi: 10.1038/s41591-018-0197-1
28. Blank CU, Rozeman EA, Fanchi LF, Sikorska K, van de Wiel B, Kvistborg P, et al. Neoadjuvant versus adjuvant ipilimumab plus nivolumab in macroscopic stage III melanoma. *Nat Med.* (2018) 24:1655–61. doi: 10.1038/s41591-018-0198-0
29. Rozeman EA, Menzies AM, van Akkooi ACJ, Adhikari C, Bierman C, van de Wiel BA, et al. Identification of the optimal combination dosing schedule of neoadjuvant ipilimumab plus nivolumab in macroscopic stage III melanoma (OpACIN-neo): a multicentre, phase 2, randomised, controlled trial. *Lancet Oncol.* (2019) 20:948–60. doi: 10.1016/S1470-2045(19)30151-2

30. Amaria RN, Prieto PA, Tetzlaff MT, Reuben A, Andrews MC, Ross MI, et al. Neoadjuvant plus adjuvant dabrafenib and trametinib versus standard of care in patients with high-risk, surgically resectable melanoma: a single-centre, open-label, randomised, phase 2 trial. *Lancet Oncol.* (2018) 19:181–93. doi: 10.1016/S1470-2045(18)30015-9

31. Long GV, Saw RPM, Lo S, Nieweg OE, Shannon KF, Gonzalez M, et al. Neoadjuvant dabrafenib combined with trametinib for resectable, stage IIIB-C, BRAF(V600) mutation-positive melanoma (NeoCombi): a single-arm, open-label, single-centre, phase 2 trial. *Lancet Oncol.* (2019) 20:961–71. doi: 10.1016/S1470-2045(19)30331-6

32. Kakavand H, Vilain RE, Wilmott JS, Burke H, Yearley JH, Thompson JF, et al. Tumor PD-L1 expression, immune cell correlates and PD-1+ lymphocytes in sentinel lymph node melanoma metastases. *Mod Pathol.* (2015) 28:1535–44. doi: 10.1038/modpathol.2015.110

33. Speeckaert R, Vermaelen K, van Geel N, Autier P, Lambert J, Haspeslagh M, et al. Indoleamine 2,3-dioxygenase, a new prognostic marker in sentinel lymph nodes of melanoma patients. *Eur J Cancer.* (2012) 48:2004–11. doi: 10.1016/j.ejca.2011.09.007

34. Ryan M, Crow J, Kahmke R, Fisher SR, Su Z, Lee WT. FoxP3 and indoleamine 2,3-dioxygenase immunoreactivity in sentinel nodes from melanoma patients. *Am J Otolaryngol.* (2014) 35:689–94. doi: 10.1016/j.amjoto.2014.08.009

35. Osella-Abate S, Conti L, Annaratone L, Senetta R, Bertero L, Licciardello M, et al. Phenotypic characterisation of immune cells associated with histological regression in cutaneous melanoma. *Pathology.* 2019. doi: 10.1016/j.pathol.2019.04.001

4

Recent Successes and Future Directions in Immunotherapy of Cutaneous Melanoma

Hassan Sadozai[1†], Thomas Gruber[1†], Robert Emil Hunger[2] and Mirjam Schenk[1*]

[1] Institute of Pathology, Experimental Pathology, University of Bern, Bern, Switzerland, [2] Department of Dermatology, University Hospital Bern, Bern, Switzerland

*Correspondence:
Mirjam Schenk
mirjam.schenk@pathology.unibe.ch

[†] These authors have contributed equally to this work.

The global health burden associated with melanoma continues to increase while treatment options for metastatic melanoma are limited. Nevertheless, in the past decade, the field of cancer immunotherapy has witnessed remarkable advances for the treatment of a number of malignancies including metastatic melanoma. Although the earliest observations of an immunological antitumor response were made nearly a century ago, it was only in the past 30 years, that immunotherapy emerged as a viable therapeutic option, in particular for cutaneous melanoma. As such, melanoma remains the focus of various preclinical and clinical studies to understand the immunobiology of cancer and to test various tumor immunotherapies. Here, we review key recent developments in the field of immune-mediated therapy of melanoma. Our primary focus is on therapies that have received regulatory approval. Thus, a brief overview of the pathophysiology of melanoma is provided. The purported functions of various tumor-infiltrating immune cell subsets are described, in particular the recently described roles of intratumoral dendritic cells. The section on immunotherapies focuses on strategies that have proved to be the most clinically successful such as immune checkpoint blockade. Prospects for novel therapeutics and the potential for combinatorial approaches are delineated. Finally, we briefly discuss nanotechnology-based platforms which can in theory, activate multiple arms of immune system to fight cancer. The promising advances in the field of immunotherapy signal the dawn of a new era in cancer treatment and warrant further investigation to understand the opportunities and barriers for future progress.

Keywords: melanoma, immunotherapy, immune checkpoint blockade, tumor microenvironment, adoptive T cell transfer, programmed cell death protein 1, tumor-infiltrating lymphocyte, tumor-infiltrating dendritic cell

METASTATIC MELANOMA

Malignant melanoma is a highly aggressive cancer and accounts for the majority (60–80%) of deaths from skin cancer (1, 2). Non-melanoma skin cancers, including basal cell carcinomas and squamous cell carcinomas, have much lower metastatic potential and associated mortality than melanoma (3). Melanoma arises from pigment-producing cells called melanocytes that are found primarily in the skin and the eyes and to a lesser extent, in a wide range of body tissues (2, 4, 5). Melanocytes originate from the embryonic neural crest and migrate to the epidermis where they mature and produce melanin that is subsequently transferred to neighboring keratinocytes (6, 7). Melanin plays a crucial role in protecting the skin from ultraviolet (UV) solar radiation (6, 8). Neoplasia of melanocytes varies from benign melanocytic naevi to malignant melanomas (4, 5).

Malignancies can arise from any of the tissues where melanocytes are present but by far the most common type is cutaneous melanoma, comprising over 90% of all melanoma cases (5, 9). Hence, the central focus of this review will be on cutaneous melanoma. Due to the recent advances in tumor immunotherapy, a number of novel cancer treatment strategies have emerged. As such, this review will discuss the development of cancer immunotherapy in the context of melanoma and highlight potential avenues for further research.

Epidemiology

Melanoma is a fairly common cancer with an estimated global incidence rate of 3 per 100,000 (9–11). In 2015, it was reported that there were approximately 352,000 new cases of melanoma worldwide with an age-standardized incidence rate of 5 cases per 100,000 persons (12). There were nearly 60,000 deaths worldwide due to melanoma (12). The incidence rate is observed to be higher in males than in females and is associated with a younger median age (~57 years) at diagnosis than other solid tumors (~65 years) (9, 10, 12). The three regions with the highest incidence of melanoma were found to be Australasia (54%), North America (21%), and Western Europe (16%) (12). Furthermore, it is particularly concerning that the global incidence rates of melanoma continue to rise. In 2005, there were roughly 225,000 new cases of melanoma but in 2015, that number climbed to roughly 352,000 cases, representing a 56% increase (13). A large-scale cohort study from 39 countries showed that while incidence rates for melanoma are beginning to stabilize in North America and Australia, they are continuing to rise in Southern and Eastern Europe (11). Therefore, melanoma constitutes a significant burden of disease worldwide and warrants both novel treatments and prevention strategies.

Pathophysiology and Clinical Subtypes

The exact etiology of melanoma development is not well understood (4). However, there has been tremendous study on the histological and molecular profiles of the various subtypes of melanoma (14–16). Overall, it has been observed that melanomas which arise from skin that is chronically sun-damaged (CSD) occur in anatomical locations such as the head and neck. By contrast, non-CSD melanomas are found in anatomical regions that suffer only limited sun exposure such as the trunk and extremities (4). Overall, non-CSD melanomas also have lower mutational loads than CSD melanomas (4, 16). A significant number of melanomas are usually associated with benign neoplasms of melanocytes. These lesions are termed naevi (commonly called moles), and an increased presence of naevi is deemed a risk factor for melanoma (2, 4). These lesions include benign naevi, dysplastic naevi, which display atypical cellular characteristics, and non-invasive melanoma *in situ* (4, 17). Melanoma *in situ* is by definition confined to the epidermis and if resected entirely, has a 100% survival rate (17). The current staging system for melanoma is the one used by the American Joint Committee on Cancer (AJCC) and relies upon analysis of the tumor (T), the number of metastatic nodes (N), and the presence of distant metastases

(M) (18, 19). These are then grouped to provide clinical stages of the cancer, ranging from 0 to stage IV (19). Stage IV melanoma is classified as metastatic melanoma due to the presence of distant metastases, while stage III is only marked by metastases in regional lymph nodes (LN) (20).

Historically, malignant melanoma was divided into four major histological subtypes but due to the complexity of the disease, a fraction of melanomas cannot be completely classified into either subtype (15, 21, 22). Moreover, as this classification system is reliant on clinical and morphological features, it yields little prognostic value but serves as a useful strategy in identifying the various histological forms of the disease (22). The four primary subtypes of melanoma are as follows: (i) superficial spreading melanoma (SSM), (ii) nodular melanoma (NM), (iii) lentigo maligna melanoma (LMM), and (iv) acral lentiginous melanoma (ALM) (14, 22). However, in recent years, a number of novel clinical subtypes have also been defined. These include desmoplastic melanoma (DM), melanoma arising from a blue naevus and persistent melanoma (22). The five common histogenic subtypes of melanoma warrant further description here. A pictorial overview of the clinical manifestation and histopathology of melanoma is presented in **Figure 1**.

Superficial Spreading Melanoma

Superficial spreading melanomas are the most common subtype representing between 50 and 70% of all cases (14, 23). They occur in relatively younger patients (~50 s) and present on anatomical regions such as the trunk, back, and extremities (22). SSM presents as a flat or a slightly elevated lesion with varying pigmentation (24). Histologically, SSM is marked by atypical melanocytes with nested or single cell upward migration (22). Malignant melanocytes display lateral spreading throughout the epidermis, poor circumscription, and increased melanization in the cytoplasm (14, 22).

Nodular Melanoma

Nodular melanomas are a fairly common subtype of melanoma (15–35%) that can present most commonly on the head and neck as a growing nodule that shows ulceration (22–24). Histologically, NMs show similarities to SSMs but differ in that they show distinct circumscription. They do not display radial growth but aggressive vertical growth evidenced by large dermal nests and sheets of atypical melanocytes (14, 22).

Lentigo Maligna Melanoma

Lentigo maligna melanomas present almost exclusively on the sun-exposed upper extremities or head and neck of elderly people (mostly octogenarians) (22). It is relatively uncommon (5–15%), and topically can be seen as patch of discolored skin showing variegated coloring (23, 24). Lentigo maligna (Hutchinson's freckle) is the term for the *in situ* melanoma phase, and a small percentage of these patients progress to invasive LMM (23). Histologically, the skin exhibits extensive solar damage resulting in an atrophic epidermis and lentiginous (back-to-back) proliferation of melanocytes, which are hyperchromatic (22). Multinucleated (starburst form)

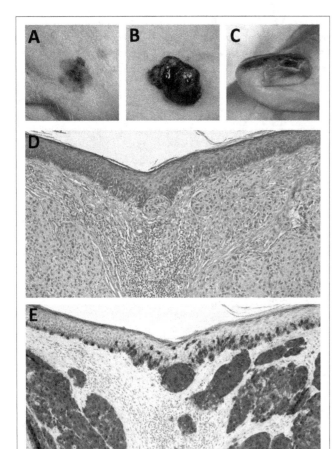

FIGURE 1 | Clinical and histological presentation of melanoma.
(A) Superficial spreading melanoma (SSM), **(B)** nodular melanoma (NM),
(C) acrolentiginous melanoma (ALM), **(D)** H&E stain of NM depicting
asymmetrical nodular tumor infiltrates in the upper dermis. Nests of
atypical cells are visible in the dermis and at the dermoepidermal junction.
(E) Immunohistochemical staining for Melan-A reveals red stained atypical
tumor cells in the dermis and epidermis (Images courtesy of RH).

melanocyte cells and solar elastosis are also hallmarks of this
type of melanoma (14).

Acral Lentiginous Melanoma

Acral lentiginous melanomas are a fairly uncommon subtype
(5–10%) and occur primarily in non-Caucasian populations
such as people of African or Japanese descent (23). They present on acral sites such as palms, soles of the feet, or under
the nails. On the skin they present as slow growing patches
with variegated pigmentation (22). Histologically, this subtype
displays single cells or nests of melanocytes along the dermal–epidermal junction, and the association of lymphocyte
infiltrates can be used as a diagnostic marker for this subtype
of melanomas (14, 22).

Desmoplastic Melanoma

Desmoplastic melanoma is a rare form of melanoma comprising 4% of primary melanomas and defined by the histological
features observed in its dermal component (22, 25). It occurs

primarily on the head and neck region in elderly individuals
and is associated with higher probability of recurrence but a
lower incidence of metastasis (25). Histologically, it is characterized by spindle-shaped melanocytes and a desmoplastic
stroma, i.e., new collagen formation, and usually appears to be
amelanotic (22, 25).

Risk Factors and Driver Mutations

Melanoma occurs via a complex interplay of genetic and environmental risk factors. The primary environmental risk factor of
concern is UV solar radiation as well as, UV rays from tanning
beds (26, 27). Individual risk factors include the increased
presence of melanocytic naevi, skin complexion, and in certain
cases, family history of melanoma (26, 28). Melanomas display
one of the highest mutational burdens among solid tumors
(25). Thus, the molecular profiles that are associated with various subtypes of melanoma are the subject of current studies.
In particular, it is crucial to distinguish "driver" mutations, or
mutations that confer a survival advantage, from "passenger"
mutations, which have negligible or no contribution to tumor
growth (29). Understanding the mutational landscapes of
a cancer allows for the development of targeted therapies
that can significantly improve clinical outcomes. A massive
study conducted by researchers of The Cancer Genome Atlas
Network, was reported in 2015, and determined the first-ever
comprehensive genomic classification system for cutaneous
melanomas (30). These four distinct subtypes were based on
the pattern of the major significantly mutated genes, i.e., BRAF,
RAS, neurofibromin 1 (NF1), and triple wild type (WT), which
denotes a lack of mutations in the three aforementioned genes
but is associated with higher copy number and structural rearrangement abnormalities. These subtypes do not correlate with
outcome but may help delineate the genomic changes associated
with melanoma thereby providing potential molecular targets
(30). Of further interest was the observation that immune gene
expression, and immune cellular infiltrates did correlate with
patient survival (30). As the studies of the major genomic aberrations in melanoma have been extensively reviewed elsewhere,
this section will describe a number of the most common driver
mutations seen in cutaneous melanoma [BRAF, NRAS, NF1,
microphthalmia-associated transcription factor (MITF), and
PTEN] (4, 15, 25, 28, 31).

BRAF

Nearly 60% of melanoma cases have mutations in BRAF (v-raf
murine sarcoma viral oncogene homolog B) (25, 32). Thus, a
brief overview of BRAF signaling is warranted. *BRAF* codes for
a serine/threonine protein kinase constituting part of the RAS–
rapidly accelerated fibrosarcoma (RAF)–mitogen-activated protein kinase kinase (MEK)–extracellular signal-regulated kinase
(ERK) [mitogen-activated protein kinase (MAPK)] pathway,
which is activated by the binding of extracellular growth factors to receptor tyrosine kinases (32). This binding leads to the
activation of RAS (named for *Rat sarcoma*) family of GTPases
(proteins that bind and hydrolyze guanosine triphosphate to
guanosine diphosphate, i.e., GTP to GDP), which recruit and
activate RAF serine/threonine protein kinases, which in turn

activate MEK resulting finally in the phosphorylation of ERK (32–35). The activation of ERK leads to downstream signaling and activation of transcription factors that mediate cell differentiation, growth, and inhibit cell death (33, 36).

BRAF is one of three mammalian RAF isoforms, and one that has the highest basal kinase activity and thus is the most common isoform mutated in human cancers that include melanoma but also hairy cell leukemia, papillary thyroid cancer and colorectal cancer (CRC) (33, 36). The missense mutation, V600E, results in a substitution from valine to glutamic acid at the 600th amino acid position and represents the majority (80%) of all BRAF activating mutations in melanoma (25, 28). Other BRAF mutations include V600K (valine–lysine) and V600R (valine–arginine). BRAF-activating mutations result in constitutively active MEK signaling leading to tumor progression. *In vitro*, the V600E mutation confers 500-fold higher activity in BRAF than normal and promotes the transformation of melanocytes to melanoma (37). BRAF^{V600E} mutations are also found in benign naevi indicating that alone, these mutations may not be sufficient for tumor progression (38). The presence of these mutations has led to the development and approval of two BRAF inhibitors (BRAFi) for melanoma treatment, namely, vemurafenib (Genentech/Plexxikon) and dabrafenib (GlaxoSmithKline) as well as, a MEK inhibitor trametinib (GSK) (33, 39).

NRAS

The second most common type of driver mutations in melanomas occur in NRAS (neuroblastoma RAS viral v-ras oncogene) and are found in 15–20% of melanoma patients (28). The most common mutation in NRAS occurs at codon 61 resulting in the replacement of glutamine by lysine or arginine, thereby resulting in a constitutively active RAS (38). This leads to upregulation of both the MAPK and phosphatidylinositol 3′ kinase (PI3K) pathways and results in increased cell proliferation and invasiveness (25). NRAS mutant melanomas have increased thickness and display high rates of mitosis (25). NRAS mutations are also found in benign congenital nevi (28). NRAS and BRAF activations rarely occur in the same melanoma, albeit NRAS mutations being observed in patients with advanced BRAF tumors who had failed BRAFi therapy and which therefore may mechanistically contribute to resistance to BRAFi treatment (28). Efforts to target NRAS have focused on downstream inhibitors for the MAPK pathway and include the MEK inhibitor binimetinib, which is undergoing clinical trials (25).

Neurofibromin 1

Neurofibromin 1 encodes a large protein of more than 2,800 amino acids with multiple functional domains (40). It contains several functional domains with one domain bearing resemblance to the catalytic region of GTPase-activating protein. This is the most well-characterized domain of NF1 and acts as a negative regulator for RAS by converting the active RAS-GTP to the inactive RAS-GDP, thus playing the role of a tumor suppressor gene (40, 41). Germline mutations in NF1 lead to a genetic syndrome called neurofibromatosis type 1 (NF1), a

relatively frequent genetic condition with an incidence of 1 in 3,000, resulting in a higher predisposition to multiple tumors arising from various cell types (40). The incidence of melanoma in patients with neurofibromatosis type 1 is very low. However, NF1 somatic mutations are found in a range of cancers, and it is the third common driver mutation in melanoma found in nearly 14% of tumors (25, 41). Mutations in NF1 are more commonly observed on skin with chronic UV exposure and in elderly patients (40). NF1 inactivating mutations were found in 48% of a cohort of wild-type BRAF and NRAS melanomas and are often associated with mutations in other RAS-related genes such as RAS p21 protein activator 2 (RASA2), PTPN11, and SPRED1 (25, 40). Recent studies have also shown that NF1 may be a unique driver mutation in DMs as NF1 loss-of-function in DM is more common than for other histogenic subtypes (25). Due to the crucial role of NF1 upstream of RAS/MAPK and PI3K/mTOR pathways, NF1 mutant tumors have been targeted with tyrosine kinase inhibitors (e.g., imatinib), MEK inhibitors (trametinib), and mTOR inhibitors (sirolimus), but to date, none of these agents have been reported in treatment of NF1 mutant melanomas (40).

Microphthalmia-Associated Transcription Factor

Microphthalmia-associated transcription factor is a helix-loop-helix leucine zipper transcription factor required for differentiation, proliferation, and survival of melanocytes and thus, its expression is also necessary for melanoma survival (42, 43). MITF also plays an important antiapoptotic function in melanoma cells by activating the expression of genes such as *BLC2A1*, *BCL2*, and *BIRC7* (43). MITF is observed to be amplified in 20% of metastatic melanomas and is associated with poor survival (25). MITF is regulated by the MAPK pathway and in particular, BRAF^{V600E} causes induction of MITF through the transcription factor BRN2 (N-Oct-3) (25). Alternately, increased ERK signaling can also target MITF for degradation (44). Finally, MITF is also purported to contribute to BRAFi resistance through the regulation of the *BCL2A1* antiapoptotic gene (44). Although targeting of MITF directly may not be viable, the use of histone deacetylase (HDAC) inhibitors can reduce MITF expression. Hence, the HDAC inhibitor panobinostat in combination with decitabine and chemotherapy is being studied in clinical trials for metastatic melanoma treatment (25).

PTEN

Phosphatase and tensin homolog (*PTEN*) is a commonly mutated gene in melanoma and PTEN mutations were found in 14% of all melanoma samples from the TCGA genome classification study mentioned above (25, 30). *PTEN* codes for a phosphatase which targets phosphatidylinositol (3,4,5)-triphosphate and thus plays a crucial role in the aforementioned PI3K–Akt pathway (45). PTEN silencing therefore results in dysregulated apoptosis, cell cycle progression and migration, contributing to tumorigenesis (25, 45). It has been observed that *PTEN* mutations are more frequent in metastatic melanomas as opposed to early stage primary tumors (25). The loss of PTEN also interferes with genetic stability, thus sensitizing PTEN-deficient cells to polyadenosine diphosphate ribose polymerase (PARP) inhibitors (46). Currently, there are no PARP inhibitor trials underway for the treatment of metastatic melanoma (46).

Current Treatments for Malignant Melanoma

The multiple clinical approaches to the treatment of early and advanced melanoma are reviewed elsewhere (18, 20, 47). As previously mentioned, the median survival associated with metastatic melanoma (stage IV) remains very poor, and the 10-year survival for all patients is under 10% (47). Melanoma treatments involve the use of surgery, radiation or systemic therapy (which includes immunotherapy) (18, 20). For most primary melanomas, surgical excision of the tumor remains the standard-of-care therapy. Biopsy and histological examination of the sentinel LN is an important component of melanoma staging and has been found to be a strong prognostic measure (18, 20). When surgical excision is not an option, primary lentigo maligna may also be treated with radiation or cryotherapy (20). The treatment modalities for metastatic melanoma are more complex as most single or even combination therapies are only successful in a subset of patients (18, 48). For patients with oligometastatic disease, surgery remains a primary treatment (18, 48). Melanoma is considered a relatively radiation-resistant cancer type, but radiation therapy continues to be utilized for patients with brain metastases (47, 48). Systemic therapy includes chemotherapy, targeted therapy, and immunotherapy (18, 47). Studies with various agents, including combination chemotherapy approaches, have shown that it has limited efficacy in melanoma (18, 47). The major chemotherapy drugs that have been used to treat melanoma including the alkylating agents dacarbazine, temozolomide, and nitrosoureas such as fotemustine and carmustine (47). Platinum analogs (e.g., cisplatin) and antimicrotubular agents such as vinblastine and paclitaxel have also shown modest efficacies in patients with metastatic melanoma (47). Recently, clinical studies have been performed using biochemotherapy, which combines cytotoxic drugs with immunotherapies such as interleukin-2 (IL-2) and IFNα (interferon alpha), and despite showing increased response rates these patients did not experience prolonged overall survival (OS) (18). In patients with recurrent metastatic melanoma in the limb, high doses of the cytotoxic drug melphalan and recently, tumor necrosis factor (TNF) and IFNγ are given to the patient via isolated limb perfusion to reduce systemic toxicity (48). A significant improvement in melanoma treatment was observed using targeted therapies, which pharmacologically inhibit key mutations in melanoma. These include the BRAFi drugs vemurafenib and dabrafenib, and the MEK inhibitor trametinib (39). Targeted therapies for melanoma have been expertly reviewed elsewhere (39, 49). The major clinically approved immunotherapies for melanoma include adjuvant treatments such as IL-2 and interferon alfa (18, 48). A few clinical groups have had success with adoptive T cell therapy in a subset of patients (50). Finally, immune checkpoint blockade (ICB) with antibodies targeted to cytotoxic T lymphocyte antigen-4 (CTLA-4) (ipilimumab) and programmed cell death protein 1 (PD-1) (nivolumab and pembrolizumab) has resulted in significant improvements in clinical outcomes for a proportion of melanoma patients (39). Targeting the ligand for PD-1 (i.e. PD-L1) is also being studied in clinical trials (51, 52). This review will summarize the evolution of immunotherapies in the context of melanoma and discuss novel opportunities to significantly enhance tumor immunotherapy. To assess the results of clinical studies, it is pertinent to mention some of the key measures used in clinical trials and criteria defined within the RECIST (Response Evaluation Criteria in Solid Tumors) (53). OS is defined as the time from randomization of the treatment subject to time of death due to any cause, while the more utilized progression-free survival (PFS) metric, denotes time from randomization until tumor progression or death (54). The overall objective response rate (ORR) is a measure of the percentage of patients who have had either a partial response (PR) or complete response (CR) to treatment (54). PR is defined as a decrease of at least 30% in the sum of the diameters of the target tumor lesions while CR indicates the disappearance of all target lesions (53). Finally, progressive disease (PD) is defined as at least a 20% increase in the sum of the target lesions' diameters while stable disease (SD) denotes a state where the lesions do not shrink enough to signal PR or increase sufficiently to indicate PD (53). Thus, these parameters provide an objective methodology to measure the results of a treatment (53, 54).

IMMUNOBIOLOGY OF MELANOMA

Cancer Immunoediting

Over the past decade, cancer immunotherapy has emerged as a vital new approach to cancer treatment (55, 56). The earliest evidence of the involvement of the immune response in fighting cancer was observed over a century ago. In 1893, William Coley, a surgeon in New York published a report describing tumor regression in a number of patients treated with cultures of the bacterium *Streptococcus pyogenes* (57, 58). However, the immunological basis of these results was not yet known and the approach did not gain wide acceptance in the medical field. Nevertheless, subsequent observations in murine models led to the formulation of the "cancer immunosurveillance" hypothesis by Macfarlane Burnet and Lewis Thomas in the middle of the century (59, 60). The hypothesis posited that lymphocytes played a protective role by continuous recognition and elimination of malignant cells (61). Currently, the concept of "cancer immunoediting" is forwarded as a comprehensive depiction of the continuous interplay between tumors and the immune system (62, 63). Cancer immunoediting posits the existence of three distinct phases, namely, elimination, equilibrium, and escape (63, 64). In the *elimination* phase, innate and adaptive immune mechanisms eradicate neoplastic cells before they become clinically detectable cancers (64). This phase has not been directly observed *in vivo* but the increased susceptibility to developing cancer in immunodeficient mouse models provides evidence of the existence of this stage of immunoediting (64). Further observations in humans such as the increased risks of cancers in patients with immunodeficiencies or undergoing immunosuppression for organ transplantation, as well as cases of spontaneous tumor regression lend further proof to this paradigm (64, 65). During the *equilibrium* stage, rare cancerous cells that were not destroyed during the elimination phase, are kept in check by the immune system while influencing the immunogenicity of the tumor (62). This state results in a form of tumor dormancy and is considered to last a long time, potentially lasting the lifetime of an individual. Furthermore, this phase enacts a selective pressure on the tumor cells, allowing those with the potential to evade the immune system to escape immune control and manifest as clinical disease (62, 64). A landmark study in 2007 demonstrated the existence of the equilibrium phase *in vivo*. Using a carcinogenic compound (3′-methylcholanthrene -MCA), the authors were able to study stable tumor masses at the site of MCA injection (66). When treated with a cocktail of antibodies targeting CD4, CD8, and IFNγ, 60% of the mice developed rapidly growing tumors. Furthermore, the authors demonstrated that these rapidly growing tumors resembled "unedited" tumors from MCA-injected RAG$^{-/-}$ mice (mice lacking recombination activation gene RAG1) (66). Finally, it was shown that this equilibrium state required components of adaptive immunity (IL-12, IFNγ, CD4$^+$, and CD8$^+$ cells) but not key components of innate immunity such as NK cell recognition and effector functions (66). Thus, while the immune system is capable of controlling cancerous cells during the equilibrium phase, it also drives the selection of cells that are able to evade immune attack and develop into a progressively growing tumor. This stage is known as the *escape* phase of immunoediting. This escape is made possible due to a number of potential mechanisms which have been reviewed in detail (61, 63, 65). Briefly, the cells can evade immune detection by reducing the expression of immunogenic tumor antigens or by reducing major histocompatibility complex class I (MHC I) (62, 64). Another route of escape involves decreased susceptibility to immune-mediated cytotoxicity through upregulation of oncogenes and anti-apoptotic mediators (64). Finally, tumor cells harbor the potential to modulate the immune system by producing immunosuppressive cytokines such as transforming growth factor beta (TGFβ) and vascular endothelial growth factor (VEGF). Moreover, tumor cells can recruit regulatory immune cells [e.g., regulatory T cells (Treg)] or engage in adaptive immune resistance via the expression of immune checkpoint ligands such as programmed death-ligand 1 (PD-L1) (64). Finally, the notion of "reverse immunoediting" has been proposed as some cancers can cause the selective depletion of specific high-avidity cytotoxic T cell (CTL) clones via hitherto unknown mechanisms and thus actively shape the immune repertoire of the host (67). The pathways used by tumor cells to escape the immune system are therefore studied extensively to devise immunotherapeutic approaches for cancer treatment.

Immune Response to Melanoma

The immune response to tumor cells is currently one of the major areas of research in biomedical science. An overview of antitumor immune response is provided by the concept of the cancer-immunity cycle as described by Chen and Mellman (68).

It commences with the release of tumor antigens that are presented by antigen-presenting cells (APC), primarily dendritic cells (DC), to T cells in the LN (**Figure 2**). This is followed by the trafficking of T cells including CD8$^+$ cytotoxic T lymphocytes (CTL), to the tumor where they can recognize and kill malignant cells, thereby releasing more cancer antigens (68). However, at each step, there are negative regulators that can disrupt the cancer-immunity cycle and allow progression of the tumor (68). One of the primary aims of cancer immunotherapy is therefore to ensure a sustained T cell response against the tumor (55). The complex biology of the interactions between tumor cells and the innate and adaptive immune system has been extensively reviewed elsewhere (68–72). Thus, the primary focus of this section will be to provide a basic primer to cancer immunology and in particular, to the biological and therapeutic significance of the major types of immune cells in the tumor microenvironment (TME) in melanomas. For the purposes of this review, the populations of interest are tumor-infiltrating lymphocytes (TIL), tumor-infiltrating dendritic cells (TIDC), and tumor-infiltrating natural killer (NK) cells. The cancer-specific roles of tumor-associated macrophages (TAM), NKT cells, the more recently described myeloid-derived suppressor cells (MDSC), and non-NK innate lymphoid cell subsets (ILC) have been thoroughly reviewed elsewhere (73–77).

Tumor Antigens

As tumors arise from a host's own tissue, immune recognition of these cells is hindered by the fact that a majority of potentially autoimmune cells are deleted during central (thymic) and peripheral mechanisms of self-tolerance (78). However, as early as 1943, it was observed that mice could immunologically reject chemically induced tumors (79). In the late 1970s, the ability to grow CTL cultures using IL-2 allowed for screening of tumor-derived DNA libraries to characterize tumor antigens (79). In 1988, the gene coding for a murine tumor antigen (P91A) was cloned (80). Shortly afterward, the first human tumor antigen gene was identified in melanoma, namely, *MAGEA1* (melanoma antigen family A, 1) and was found to be expressed in various types of tumors (81). Interestingly, the gene was not observed to be expressed in normal tissue except for trophoblastic cells and male germline cells (79). Since then, several tumor antigens have been discovered, and their underlying biology has been the subject of much study (82, 83). There are several types of tumor antigens, but they have been broadly classified into three major categories. The first category includes antigens that are caused by non-synonymous mutations, or are encoded by viral genes in tumors of viral etiology (83). These are labeled tumor-specific antigens (TSA) or "neoantigens" (83, 84). Alternately, tumor-associated antigens (TSA) are usually expressed at low levels in normal tissues but are found to be overexpressed in cancer cells such the surface receptor, human epidermal growth factor 2 (HER2 or ERBB2) in breast cancer, and other malignancies (85). Finally, cancer/testis antigens (CTA) such as the aforementioned MAGE family of proteins are expressed in several tumor types and only in normal germline cells such as trophoblasts, ovaries and the testes (82, 83). The advent of high-throughput next-generation sequencing technology has

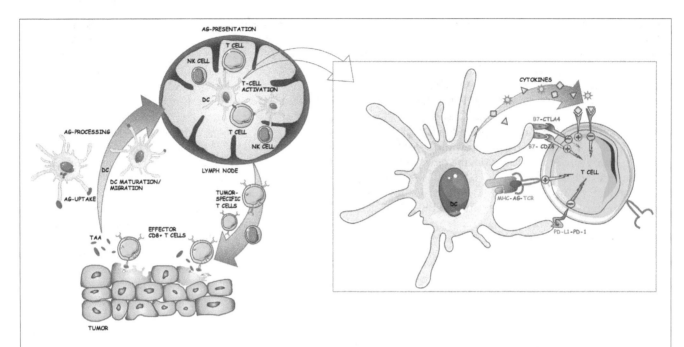

FIGURE 2 | Schematic of the roles dendritic cells (DC) play in antitumor immune response. DC take up and process tumor-associated/tumor-specific antigens (TAA/TSA) from dying tumor cells, undergo maturation, and migrate to tumor draining lymph nodes (LN) where they can present antigen to lymphocytes. Tumor-specific T cells then egress from the LN and infiltrate the tumor. Effector CD8+ cytotoxic T lymphocytes play a major role in killing tumor cells, leading to further release of TAA/TSA for DC uptake and subsequent presentation. Inset panel: Costimulatory and inhibitory interactions at the antigen-presenting cell (APC)–T cell immunological synapse. The activation of T cells by APC is tightly regulated by multiple ligand–receptor interactions. TCR binds to cognate antigen (AG) in the context of their specific MHC. Costimulatory molecules such as CD80 (B7.1) and CD86 (B7.2) on APC can either bind to CD28 on T cells resulting in downstream activation of T cell effector genes or to cytotoxic T lymphocyte antigen-4 (CTLA-4) resulting in inhibition. Further T cell activation is achieved through cytokines. Programmed cell death protein 1 (PD-1) is another immune checkpoint receptor and is expressed on activated T cells. The primary ligand for PD-1 (PD-L1) is expressed on APC and on some tumor cells, and upon binding to PD-1 acts to inhibit T cell activation.

allowed for relatively low-cost detection of somatic mutations in tumor cells. There are currently several approaches being formulated to tailor individualized immunotherapies for patients on the basis of their expression of tumor neoantigens (83). Although currently personalized approaches are highly expensive, it is posited that with the continuing reduction of sequencing costs and using combinatorial treatments, it may be possible to even target tumors that are non-responsive to immunotherapy (83). Since their discovery, tumor antigens have been used for multiple purposes in cancer treatment. They have been used as diagnostic markers, cancer vaccines, and as targets for adoptive T cell therapy (82, 86, 87). In general, most tumor antigens elicit a weak immune response against cancer and have been tested clinically in combination with adjuvants or additional treatments (87). To date, cancer vaccination or adoptive transfer targeting specific tumor antigens has not shown major survival advantages in melanoma (48, 88). The three major types of tumor antigens that have been described and used in melanoma immunotherapy are discussed below. A majority of described melanoma antigens are restricted to human leukocyte antigen A2 (HLA-A2) (89).

MAGE Family
The MAGE (melanoma antigen) family is divided into two major groups type I MAGEs and type II MAGEs. The type I MAGE

subfamily consists of 25 functional genes located on the X chromosome in the regions *MAGEA*, *MAGEB*, and *MAGEC* (82, 90). These genes are classified as CTAs and are expressed in melanoma as well as other cancer types such as colon cancer, non-small cell lung cancer (NSCLC), and breast cancers (90). Conversely, type II MAGE genes are expressed in several types of normal tissue and are not X chromosome restricted. Both type I and type II MAGEs contain the MAGE homology domain (90). Due to the extensive homology between the MAGE proteins, there is a lack of antibodies that recognize specific MAGE antigens. In several cancer types, nuclear and cytoplasmic staining using widely reactive anti-MAGE antibodies have been performed and although the functions of MAGE proteins are not known, there is some evidence that they play a role in cell cycle progression and apoptosis (91). The MAGE family of proteins may serve as useful targets for immunotherapy. After encouraging results from Phase I/II studies, the DERMA phase III clinical trial aimed to assess a vaccine using MAGE-A3 protein in combination with an immunostimulant, in melanoma patients following tumor resection (92). However, in 2016 the trial was ended as it failed to show efficacy (NCT 00796445). Nevertheless, the lack of MAGE family gene expression in normal tissue and their overexpression in cancer cells is one of the key reasons they remain attractive targets for future immunotherapy treatments. Other CTAs observed in melanoma include the B-M antigen-1 (BAGE) and

G antigen (GAGE) family of proteins, and their functions are currently being studied (86).

NY-ESO-1

NY-ESO-1 (New York esophageal squamous cell carcinoma-1) is a CTA that is also located on chromosome X and is expressed in a wide range of malignancies (93). In normal cells, this antigen is primarily expressed on spermatogonia and at very low levels in pancreas, liver, and placenta (93). A homolog of NY-ESO-1, LAGE-1 has also been reported and is expressed in a wide variety of human cancer types. The biological functions of both proteins are unknown (93). NY-ESO-1 is a highly immunogenic tumor antigen and is able to elicit a detectable antibody response. In human melanoma, it is observed in a large frequency of melanoma patients (46%) and some studies indicate that its expression may be higher in metastatic lesions (93, 94). Due to its expression in a large fraction of melanomas, immunotherapy trials continue to be conducted using the NY-ESO-1 antigen as part of a tumor vaccine, or more recently using adoptively transferred lymphocytes with recombinant TCRs specific for NY-ESO-1 (95, 96). The adoptive transfer trial resulted in objective responses in 55% of treated melanoma patients but the most efficacious strategy for targeting NY-ESO-1 in melanoma immunotherapy remains to be determined.

Melanoma Differentiation Antigens

A number of TAA in melanoma that are recognized by both CD4+ and CD8+ T lymphocytes are on proteins specifically expressed on melanocytes and involved in melanocyte-specific functions (86, 97). These TAA are located in melanosomes, the organelles in which melanin is synthesized. Moreover, their role in oncogenesis is not known (86). These antigens include *tyrosinase, tyrosinase-related proteins 1 and 2 (TRP-1 and TRP-2), Melan-A (MART-1), and gp100 (pmel17)* (82, 97). *Tyrosinase* and *TRP-1/-2* are copper and zinc containing metalloenzymes with homology at several sequences and they play crucial roles in melanin synthesis (98). *Tyrosinase* is the key enzyme in melanin synthesis and is located on the membrane of melanosomes. It is observed in over 80% of primary and metastatic melanomas (86). The exact function of *TRP-1* (gp75) remains unclear, but it is purported to play a role in stabilizing tyrosinase (98). *TRP-2* is a DOPAchrome tautomerase and its overexpression is believed to contribute to the chemoresistance and radiotherapy resistance of metastatic melanoma (86, 97). *Melan-A* (melanoma antigen recognized by T cells-1 or MART-1) is a single domain transmembrane protein of 118 amino acids found primarily in melanosomes, endoplasmic reticulum, and trans-Golgi network (86, 99). MART-1 is crucial for the expression, trafficking, and stability of the protein gp100 (pmel17) (99). It is expressed in all melanocytic naevi, and a majority of primary and metastatic melanomas (86). It has been observed that significantly higher frequencies (100- to 1,000-fold) of naive CTL are found against a specific MART-1 peptide (Melan-A$_{26-35}$) compared to other antigens in normal (non-cancerous) individuals who express HLA-A2 (79). However, T cell recognition of MART-1 does not necessarily result in improved clinical outcomes (97). Finally, the protein gp100 (premelanosomal protein-pmel17), is a transmembrane protein that has a role in melanosome biogenesis and melanin polymerization (86). The gp100 gene was found to be widely expressed in malignant melanoma at all stages but was significantly reduced in normal melanocytes (100). HMB-45, a mouse monoclonal antibody (mAb) to gp100, is used for diagnostic purposes to distinguish non-melanocytic from melanocytic tumors (99). All of the aforementioned differentiation antigens are recognized by CD4+ and CD8+ T cells, while TRP-1, TRP-2, tyrosinase, and gp100 can also elicit antibody responses (97). Thus, these antigens are considered to be useful targets for melanoma immunotherapy (86). The B16 syngeneic transplant model, obtained initially from C57BL/6 mice, is one of the most widely utilized models in melanoma research (101). The most obvious advantage of this model is that it expresses murine homologs of the melanoma differentiation antigens (tyrosinase, gp100, MART-1, TRP-1, and TRP-2) (102). Melanocyte differentiation antigens continue to be used in a number of clinical studies in combination with various adjuvants and immunostimulants such as granulocyte-macrophage colony-stimulating factor (GM-CSF), but none of the studies have to date shown significant improvements in OS in melanoma patients (87, 103, 104). Due to the multiple mechanisms of tumor immune escape, it remains particularly difficult to sustain a prolonged response to cancer antigens. However, recently the use of nanoparticles (NP) containing mRNA encoding the melanoma antigens, NY-ESO-1, tyrosinase, MAGE-A3, and a novel CTA TPTE (a transmembrane phosphatase), has shown early clinical promise in a pilot study of three patients (105). To be successful, future immunotherapy trials will need to not only consider the tumor antigens to be used but also the delivery vector, the format (RNA, DNA or protein), and the appropriate adjuvants.

Tumor-Infiltrating Lymphocytes

A cardinal feature of cancer is the immunosuppressive TME (106, 107). As the disease progresses, T cells in the TME exhibit a phenotype analogous to that seen in chronic viral infection known as T cell exhaustion (108). T cell exhaustion denotes a state of hyporesponsiveness to antigen with reduced cytokine secretion and cytotoxic function (108, 109). Nevertheless, the overwhelming majority of studies in human patients have demonstrated a correlation between TIL and better disease outcomes in cancers (110, 111). An exception to this observation is that FOXP3 expression, a marker of Treg that has been shown to correlate to poor prognosis in various types of human cancer (112, 113). The term TIL was first described by Wallace Clark, who was instrumental in developing the first histological classifications for melanoma as mentioned above (114, 115). TIL have been described in primary tumors, tumor-bearing LN, and in metastases of melanoma and various other cancer types (114). The range of immune cells that infiltrate a tumor, i.e., the "immune contexture" of a tumor is heterogeneous and consists of various types of T lymphocytes, B cells, NK cells, macrophages, and DC (111, 114). In 1989, Clark published a classification of the three major patterns of lymphocyte infiltration that are commonly used today (115). The *brisk* pattern is indicated by interposed lymphocytes between tumor cells that may be diffusely present throughout the tumor nodule or along the advancing (basal) periphery of the nodule (114, 115). The *non-brisk* pattern delineates a scattered multifocal presence of lymphocytes throughout the vertical growth phase of the nodule. Finally, an *absent* pattern is associated with a lack of lymphocytes in the tumor, or if they are present, their lack of interaction with melanoma cells (115). In recent years, various groups have attempted to further classify TIL or propose novel grading schemes, but the Clark model remains widely accepted and highly reproducible (114). In a recently published report, it was shown that melanoma tumors with *brisk* TIL patterns in primary melanoma H&E tissue, even in the absence of immunohistochemistry for specific markers, was associated with increased OS in patients versus tumors with *non-brisk* and *absent* patterns (116). The importance of TIL has been used to establish a novel classification system for cancer based on an "Immunoscore," which relies upon the quantitation of CD3 and CD8 lymphocytes with the additional marker CD45RO used to mark memory T cells. The "Immunoscore" was found to be superior to the conventional AJCC TNM system for prognosis of stage I–III colorectal cancer (CRC) (117). Similar approaches are now being tested for immunoscoring of melanoma but have not been tested in large patient cohorts (118).

An additional feature observed in cancer, and other situations of chronic inflammation is the formation of tertiary lymphoid structures (TLS—also called tertiary lymphoid organs) (119, 120). These TLS can range from loose aggregates of various immune cells to complex structures that resemble secondary lymphoid organs such as LN. They consist of T cell-rich regions containing mature DC expressing DC-LAMP (lysosomal associated membrane protein), B cells, and high endothelial venules, which play a role in immune cell extravasation and production of key chemokines (120). In 2012, Messina et al. reported that a gene expression profile consisting of 12 chemokines could accurately predict the histological presence of LN-like TLS in stage IV melanoma (primary tumors and metastases), and the TLS correlated strongly with improved overall patient survival (121). Other studies have shown that the presence of TLS is a positive prognostic indicator in melanoma and a range of other cancer types including breast carcinoma, CRC, and pancreatic cancer (120). Thus, these results suggest that lymphocyte infiltration mediates a protective immune response to cancer.

However, many tumors are not T cell inflamed, and the mechanisms underlying T cell infiltration into the tumor are poorly understood (89, 122). In the context of melanoma, a recent study compared all major classes of melanoma tumor antigens between T cell inflamed and non-T cell inflamed tumors and found that there were no differences between both groups in terms of antigen load (123). Rather it was shown that non-T cell inflamed melanomas displayed reduced gene expression associated with Batf3-dependent, CD141$^+$ DC (123). Furthermore, studies have pointed to the ability of tumors to interfere with chemokines that recruit leukocytes to tumors. Finally, the abnormal tumor vasculature may express reduced adhesion molecules required for homing and directly or indirectly suppress T cells by expression of molecules such as PD-L1, PD-L2, VEGF, and TGFβ (122). Once T cells infiltrate the TME, they are acted upon by a range of immunoregulatory mechanisms that prevent complete eradication of the tumor (72). These can be tumor-specific escape mechanisms or the recruitment of suppressive immune cells. For instance, mutations in BRAF or PTEN loss are associated with increased T cell inhibition by production of IL-1 and VEGF (72). Furthermore, conserved immunoregulatory mechanisms are also at play within the TME the production of immunosuppressive mediators [TGFβ and indoleamine 2,3 dioxygenase (IDO)], and the recruitment of regulatory myeloid and lymphoid cell populations (72). Another important consideration is that although, CD8$^+$ T cells are canonically considered the primary cytotoxic cells involved in tumor eradication, CD4$^+$ T cells can also kill tumor cells (89). However, the precise mechanisms of CD4$^+$ antitumor immunity are not well described, and the role of CD4$^+$ T cell infiltration in the TME has not been explored significantly with the exception of FOXP3$^+$CD4$^+$ Treg (72, 89). A recently concluded meta-analysis demonstrated that FOXP3$^+$ Treg infiltrates were predominantly associated with worse OS in a review of over 17 types of cancer (124). In most tumors, such as cervical, renal, breast cancers, and melanoma, FOXP3$^+$ Treg infiltrates correlated with shorter OS whereas they were associated with improved survival in patients with colorectal, head and neck, and esophageal cancers (124). In recent years, several studies have described the heterogeneity in FOXP3-expressing cell populations (125). In 2016, Saito et al. showed that human CRCs could be distinguished by the extent of infiltration of two distinct FOXP3$^+$CD4$^+$ T cell populations (126). Type A CRCs had low frequencies (<9.8%) while Type B had comparatively higher frequencies (>9.8%) of infiltrating non-suppressive FOXP3^{lo}CD45$^-$ T cells. Infiltration by these non-suppressive T cells was correlated with the presence of intestinal bacteria, in particular *Fusobacterium nucleatum* within the tumor (126). Furthermore, Type B CRCs were marked by high mRNA expression of *IL12A* and *TGFB1* compared with Type A and tumors with high expression of these mRNAs exhibited significantly longer disease-free survival versus low expressing tumors. Thus, FOXP3$^+$ T cell infiltration must be considered in combination with other immune signatures while determining the immune status of a tumor. In addition to T cells, the roles of B cells in the TME are being currently explored as they have both APC and effector lymphocyte functions (127). Studies in melanoma have demonstrated that CD20$^+$ infiltrating B cells are found in most tumors and higher levels of these infiltrates correlated with improved patient survival (127). Furthermore, B cells are known to produce IgG antibodies that can recognize tumor cells and within a murine model of organ transplantation have been observed to promote chronic allograft rejection through antigen presentation rather than their antibody secreting functions (127, 128). Finally, recent studies have also focused on the roles of putative regulatory B cells in the context of transplantation and autoimmunity, as these cells can produce potent immunosuppressive mediators such as IL-10 and TGFβ (129). The multiple immunoregulatory mechanisms that effect TIL are the targets of a majority of current immunotherapies. However, as the aforementioned observations indicate, there are several functionally redundant pathways that allow for immunological escape of tumors in immunocompetent individuals. Thus, to be successful, the field of immunotherapy must move toward combinatorial and multipronged approaches for tumor treatment. This involves investigation of the mechanisms of innate immune cells such as NK cells, TAM, and TIDC within the TME.

Tumor-Infiltrating Dendritic Cells

Despite their discovery over 40 years ago, the exact mechanisms underlying DC dysfunction in cancer remain poorly understood (107). In both mice and humans, DC are classified into two major subsets comprised of conventional or cDC, and plasmacytoid DC (pDC) (130). In non-steady state conditions such as cancer or autoimmune disease, inflammatory DC derived from monocytes have also been described in humans and in mice (130, 131). Despite the fact that nearly all DC subsets express the surface marker CD11c, there are unique transcription factors and surface proteins that characterize the major DC subsets in human and mice. These markers have been extensively reviewed in the literature, but further study is needed to accurately profile each subset (130, 132, 133). DC canonically present extracellular antigens on MHC class II while intracellular or self-antigens are presented on MHC class I (134). However, murine and human DC also possess the capacity to cross-present antigens of extracellular origin on MHC class I to activate CD8$^+$ CTL (135, 136). In humans, the primary cross-presenting DC subset is characterized by CD141 (BDCA-3) while in mice this subset is marked by surface expression of CD8α or CD103 (137). The mechanistic roles played by various DC subsets in both tumor progression and the response to treatment are a key area of research for cancer immunotherapy with little consensus as to their frequencies and functions (102, 107). In 2008, it was reported that knocking out *Batf3* in mice eliminated CD8α^+ DC, and consequently it was demonstrated that these mice were incapable of cross-presenting antigen or rejecting highly immunogenic fibrosarcomas (138). Although pDC are purportedly not efficient at cross-presentation, studies have shown their capacity to mediate direct tumor killing and to activate NK cells via the production of type I IFN (139). Despite the key roles played by TIDC in promoting antitumor responses, generally TIDC are skewed in both phenotype and function toward an immunosuppressive role in the microenvironment (107). These alterations in TIDC have been mechanistically studied in murine models (107, 140). The TME has been reported to induce a "paralyzed" state in TIDC resembling an immature phenotype with reduced expression of costimulatory CD80 and CD86 molecules and a diminished capacity to present antigens (107). This induction is a result of various immunosuppressive factors such as VEGF, TGFβ, IDO produced by tumor cells as well as by other cells in the TME (72, 107). Furthermore, DC paralysis in mouse models has been observed to be associated with upregulation of immune checkpoint receptors such as PD-1 and T cell immunoglobulin and mucin-domain containing-3 (TIM-3), which was reported to interact with the alarmin protein high mobility group box 1 (HMGB1) resulting in reduced DC sensing of tumor-derived nucleic acids (107). TIDC with immature and paralyzed phenotypes themselves suppress immune cells in the TME through various mechanisms such as but not limited to, expression of inhibitory molecules (PD-L1), production of regulatory cytokines such as IDO and induction of Tregs (107, 141).

As previously noted, there has been significant research on TIL in melanoma. On the other hand, the mechanistic roles of TIDC in melanoma are not well studied. Melanoma is of particular interest due to the fact that skin contains multiple DC subsets.

The five major DC subsets found in human skin are Langerhans cells, CD14$^+$ DC, CD1c$^+$ DC, CD1a$^+$ DC, and CD141$^+$ DC (133). The correlations between various TIDC subsets and disease outcome, their association with other cells and specific functions have not yet been fully elucidated (102). However, recently it was demonstrated that intratumoral CD103$^+$ DC in mice were crucial for trafficking of melanoma tumor antigen to LN and were dependent on surface expression of CCR7 (142). Enhanced CCR7 mRNA expression in human melanoma samples was also correlated to increased T cell infiltrates and improved patient outcomes (142). In general, it is observed that there are higher frequencies of TIDC in the peritumoral region than within the tumor (102). These peritumoral DC include arguably the most mature population of DC-LAMP$^+$CD83$^+$fascin$^+$ cells (102). In fact, DC-LAMP expression is associated with positive prognosis in not only melanoma but also lung, breast, and metastatic CRC (120). On the other hand, CD123$^+$ pDC that do in principle possess the capacity to promote antitumor responses are found to be associated with early relapse and poor prognosis in human melanoma (102, 143). It was shown in both *ex vivo* patient samples and in that a humanized melanoma mouse model that pDC in melanoma are directed toward a T$_H$2 promoting phenotype by induction of the molecules OX-40L (TNFSF4) and ICOSL (inducible T cell costimulator ligand), which then drive tumor progression (143). To comprehensively characterize TIDC in melanoma, it is crucial to obtain genomic data to appropriately distinguish and profile TIDC subsets. Pyfferoen et al. performed transcriptomic profiling of DC in a murine model of lung carcinoma and demonstrated that TIDC had significantly increased expression of PD-L1, acquisition of TAM surface markers and a pro-metastatic microRNA signature (144). To date, similar studies have not been performed in human melanoma. There have been several studies in murine models that have demonstrated the therapeutic reprogramming of TIDC (107). Thus, manipulation of TIDC represents a hitherto unexplored target for future melanoma immunotherapies. Many of the same agents that have been shown to induce DC activation and maturation *in vitro* have been tested for direct targeting of DC *in vivo* (133, 145). For instance, direct administration of BCG has been utilized for the treatment of bladder cancer for over 30 years although its precise mechanisms of action *in vivo* are still under study (146). Direct modulation of DC *in vivo* using DC maturation agents and mAbs is a highly desirable goal in tumor immunotherapy. This is due to the excessive costs, safety considerations, and practical limitations of using cellular products (147). As such, the identification of both targetable DC receptors and maturation stimuli continues to be an active area of research interest. In particular, targeting antigen-coupled antibodies to DC C-type lectin receptors (CLRs) such as DEC205 (CD205), Clec9A, and DC-SIGN in murine and *in vitro* studies resulted in effective CD4$^+$ and CD8$^+$ T cell responses (145, 148). Additional receptors such as XCR1 (expressed entirely on CD141$^+$ DC) are also being studied for their effects on DC function (133). Clinical trials for multiple cancer types are presently underway to investigate the efficacy of anti-DEC205 conjugated to the cancer–testis antigen NY-ESO-1, which is also used for melanoma immunotherapy (133, 149). Recently, a series of seminal papers have shown the importance of the cytosolic DNA sensor cyclic GMP-AMP (cGAMP) synthase (cGAS) in promoting antitumor immunity (150–152). DNA introduced to the cytosol as a result of viral infections or cellular damage is a potent immune activator that leads to the production of type I IFN (153). Upon detection of DNA by cGAS, it catalyzes the production of cGAMP that binds to the adaptor protein stimulator of interferon genes (STING) ultimately resulting in the production of type I IFN (153). In 2014, Woo et al. demonstrated in a mouse model that tumor-derived DNA was responsible for inducing IFNβ production and the consequent activation of APC and CD8[+] T cells versus melanoma *in vivo* (150). Alternately, mice deficient in STING failed to reject these tumors highlighting the crucial role played by this pathway in the immune response to cancer (150, 151). In a more recent paper, Wang et al. showed the role of cGAMP in mediating the effects of ICB (152). It was reported that in mice lacking either cGAS or STING, PD-L1 blockade did not result in significant shrinkage of tumor volume or increase in survival compared with WT mice. Moreover, intramuscular injection of cGAMP in combination with PD-L1 significantly enhanced survival, compared with PD-L1 or cGAMP alone (152). Finally, it was also shown that cGAMP treatment of BMDC enhanced expression of DC activation markers and increased DC antigen cross-presentation. Another molecule that has recently gained interest for its effects on DC is IL-32. In 2012, Schenk et al., identified an IL-32-dependent mechanism for DC differentiation in response to nucleotide-binding oligomerization domain containing protein (NOD2) activation through its ligand muramyl dipeptide (154). DC obtained from IL-32 differentiation were found to express higher levels of MHC class I and CD86, as well as, present antigen to CD8[+] T cells more effectively than GM-CSF differentiated DC (154). These studies highlight the multiple pathways that may be targeted to generate effective DC *in vivo*, which is essential for antitumor immunity.

NK Cells

Natural killer cells were characterized over 40 years and are the first population of ILC to be described and studied (155, 156). NK cell defects lead to enhanced susceptibility to viruses and many forms of cancer in humans and in mouse models (156). NK cell functions are modulated by a number of surface receptors that provide either NK activating or inhibitory signals (156, 157). NK cells are broadly defined as CD3[−]CD56[+] in humans and CD3[−]NK1.1[+] in mice while both murine and human NK cells express the surface receptor NKp46 (CD335) (156). In humans, NK cells are further divided into CD16[+]CD56[dim] which predominate in blood, and CD16[−]CD56[bright] populations (156). Canonically, NK cells can recognize tumor cells that have downregulated MHC class I molecules or upregulated induced stress molecules (155, 156). NK cells can also bind to antibodies bound to tumor antigens and mediate antibody-dependent cellular cytotoxicity (156). As with CD8[+] CTL, NK cells mediate their cytotoxic functions through perforin and granzymes, as well as, by expressing death mediating ligands such as FasL (CD95L) and TRAIL (TNF-related apoptosis inducing ligand) (156). Activated NK cells also produce IFNγ, among other cytokines, which leads to recruitment of other immune cell populations (156).

The roles of NK cells in the TME are currently not fully described (155, 157). Several studies have indicated that NK cell infiltration is generally a positive prognostic factor in various types of cancer (155). In the context of melanoma, the roles of NK cells are an important venue of research. Analysis of several melanoma cell lines indicated that a high percentage of melanoma cells possess ligands for a NK activating receptors such as NKG2D and DNAM1, while ligands have also been identified for NK-bound NCR (natural cytotoxicity receptors) such as NKp30 (157). Melanoma cells are also known to have decreased MHC class I expression as a mechanism to escape CD8[+] T cells, thus making them targets for NK cells (157). Despite these observations, melanoma immunoediting leads to tumor escape from NK cells via multiple mechanisms (157). Melanoma immunoediting by NK cells increases expression of MHC I, or downregulates NK ligands supported by the decreased expression of MICA reported in metastatic versus primary melanoma (157). IDO and prostaglandin E2 (PGE2) produced by melanoma cells act directly to inhibit NK cells while increased expression of ligands to regulatory receptors such as TIGIT modulate NK cell activity (157). In light of these observations, it will be important to identify NK populations that have persistent antitumor activity and characterize their phenotypes to better understand the mechanism involved in effective NK immunity. Recently, it was reported that tumor-bearing/infiltrated LN in melanoma patients contained twice as many NK cells as ipsilateral tumor-free LN (158). These tumor-infiltrated LN also contained a population of highly cytotoxic CD56[dim]KIR[+]CCR7[+] NK cells that may have prognostic potential for melanoma (158). Conversely, melanoma, breast, and colon cancers were found to be infiltrated by CD56[bright] NK subsets, which are similar to decidual NK cells during pregnancy thus implying a potentially regulatory role for this subset (159). NK cells remain an important target for immunotherapy. Along with T cells, NK cells were used early on for adoptive cell transfer therapy of melanoma in the 1980s and both autologous and allogeneic NK cell adoptive transfers are being studied in clinical trials (156, 157). Currently, two antibodies for the blockade of NK checkpoints are under clinical development, namely, lirilumab (anti-KIR-studied in combination with ipilimumab) and IPH2201 (anti-NKG2A) for various types of cancers including melanoma (157). However, further study of NK cells in the melanoma TME is required to understand the several mechanisms of immune escape from NK cells and CD8[+] CTL and thus devise, rational combinatorial immunotherapies.

MELANOMA IMMUNOTHERAPY

In 2013, the journal *Science* hailed cancer immunotherapy as the breakthrough of the year (56). This was in recognition of the promising clinical responses that can be achieved by directing the immune system to fight cancer. Despite highly encouraging advances, current immunotherapies only result in clinical benefit for a subset of patients (160, 161). Thus, there is a significant scientific effort to understand the tumor cell-intrinsic and extrinsic mechanisms of resistance to immunotherapy (162). The three major mechanisms of resistance to immunotherapies have been conceptualized as follows. *Primary* resistance denotes a clinical setting where the initial immunotherapy is unsuccessful. This can be due to *adaptive* resistance which defines a mechanism whereby there are initial antitumor immune responses but are inhibited by adaptation and immune escape of the tumor (162). Clinically, adaptive resistance may be seen as primary resistance, mixed responses or *acquired* resistance. Acquired resistance describes a clinical scenario where the tumor initially responded to immunotherapy but has eventually progressed and acquired resistance to the therapy (162). To overcome resistance to various forms of immunotherapy, it will be important to understand the mechanisms that allow tumor cells to escape immune attack. The clinical experience with melanoma immunotherapies has shown significant promise and there is increasing evidence that a multipronged approach may be required to ensure durable responses in a majority of patients. This section describes the major immunotherapies that have already been developed or are under clinical development for the treatment of metastatic melanoma (summarized in **Table 1**). Advances in immunotherapy for other types of cancers, as well as, the use of mAbs to specifically target tumors have been previously reviewed in detail (163–166).

Early Advances in Melanoma Immunotherapy

As previously noted, the mechanistic basis for Coley's observations remained unknown for some time and during this time, surgery, radiation treatment, and cytotoxic chemotherapy became the primary means of cancer treatment. However, in the context of melanoma, two major forms of immunotherapy witnessed encouraging breakthroughs starting in the 1980s and led to renewed interest in the entire field. These breakthroughs occurred in systemic cytokine therapy with IL-2 and adoptive cell transfer using TIL (183). In 1985, Rosenberg et al., demonstrated in C57BL/6 mice that intraperitoneal injections of recombinant IL-2 were capable of significantly attenuating pulmonary metastases from tumors generated by the MCA-105 and -106 syngeneic sarcoma and B16 syngeneic melanoma lines (184). Retrospective analyses of metastatic melanoma patients who had been treated with IL-2 demonstrated an ORR of 16% and represented a significant advance in the treatment (185). IL-2 received FDA approval in 1998 for metastatic melanoma. However, as systemic treatment of IL-2 resulted in various toxicities, several groups have shifted to intralesional administration of IL-2, which resulted in CR rates of between 41 and 76% in various trials (48). In parallel to the successes achieved with IL-2, Rosenberg and colleagues reported the first successful use of adoptive T cell transfer for the treatment of solid cancers (186). Patients were treated with IL-2 and autologous TIL expanded from surgically resected melanomas. Objective responses were observed in 60% (9/15) of treated patients (186). Subsequently, in 2002, this approach was combined with lymphodepletion prior T cell transfer and demonstrated enhanced responses in patients (50). Currently, adoptive cell therapy (ACT) using TIL remains one of the most effective therapies for metastatic melanoma (183).

Immune Checkpoint Blockade

Drugs that mediate ICB by targeting the inhibitory receptors CTLA-4 and PD-1 (**Figure 2** *inset panel*) have been shown to induce durable responses in subsets of patients with various types of cancer including melanoma, NSCLC, and renal cell cancer

TABLE 1 | Key immunotherapeutics and their primary mechanisms of action.

Treatment	Clinically tested agents	Mechanism(s) of action	Reference
Immune activating mAbs			
αCTLA-4	Ipilimumab (Yervoy®)	– Blockade of T cell checkpoint receptor – Depletion of intratumoral Treg	(160, 167)
αPD-1	Nivolumab (Opdivo®), pembrolizumab (Keytruda®)	– Blockade of T cell checkpoint receptor	(167, 168)
αPD-L1	Atezolizumab, durvalumab, avelumab	– Blockade of inhibitory checkpoint ligand expressed on immune cells and tumor cells	(167, 169)
αCD137 (4-1BB)	Urelumab	– Agonist of T cell costimulatory receptor	(170)
αKIR	Lirilumab	– Blockade of NK cell inhibitory receptor	(157, 171)
αLAG-3	BMS986016	– Blockade of T cell surface inhibitory molecule	(167)
Adoptive T cell therapy			
TIL	*Ex vivo* expanded TIL	– Infusion of pool of antitumor T cells	(50, 172)
Engineered T cells	Transgenic TCR or CAR bearing T lymphocytes	– Infusion of engineered T cells specific for tumor antigens	(50, 173)
Vaccines			
Cell-based vaccines	Tumor cells or activated DC/APC	– Induction of tumor-specific adaptive immunity	(87, 174, 175)
Peptide vaccines	Various tumor antigen peptides/lysates + adjuvant	– Induction of tumor-specific adaptive immunity	(165, 176)
Oncolytic viral vaccines	Talimogene laherparepvec (T-VEC/Imlygic™)	– Viral induction of tumor cell lysis and adjuvant mediated host immune activation	(177, 178)
Cytokines			
Interleukin-2	Aldesleukin (Proleukin®)	– Activates and expands T cells	(179, 180)
Interferon alpha	Interferon alfa 2b (Intron® A, Sylatron™)	– Activates multiple facets of immunity and has direct effects on tumor cells	(181, 182)

An overview of current immunotherapy approaches and their proposed mechanisms of action as discussed in this review.
Trade names are provided for drugs that have received clinical approval in melanoma. References provided for further description of each approach.
KIR, killer-cell immunoglobulin-like receptor; DC, dendritic cells; APC, antigen-presenting cell; TCR, T cell receptor; CAR, chimeric antigen receptor;
TIL, tumor-infiltrating lymphocyte; NK, natural killer; Treg, regulatory T cells.

(RCC) (187–190). Furthermore, antibodies targeted to the PD-1 ligand, PD-L1, are undergoing clinical trials and have resulted in objective responses for multiple cancer types (51, 191). To date, the FDA has approved four mAbs for ICB therapy: (1) ipilimumab (αCTLA-4); (2) nivolumab (αPD-1); (3) pembrolizumab (αPD-1); and (4) atezolizumab (αPD-L1) (192). They have been approved for various advanced and metastatic cancers ranging from unresectable or metastatic melanoma to urothelial carcinoma (atezolizumab) (168, 192). Currently, only ipilimumab, nivolumab, and pembrolizumab have received FDA approval for melanoma (167). Due to the fact that checkpoint receptors play important roles in regulating autoimmunity, the major toxicities associated with the use of ICB drugs include a range of autoimmune symptoms labeled immune-related adverse events (IRAEs) (193). The incidence of IRAEs is quite high, ranging from 70% in patients treated with αPD-1/αPD-L1 antibodies to as high as 90% in patients treated with αCTLA-4 and require careful management in the clinic with immunosuppressive medications (193). As ICB results in objective responses for only a subset of patients, there is a crucial need to identify biomarkers that can potentially predict the efficacy of a particular ICB treatment or designate a particular subset of patients who may benefit from ICB therapy (194).

CTLA-4

Cytotoxic T lymphocyte antigen-4 (also termed cytotoxic T-lymphocyte-associated protein 4), is a crucial regulator of T cell activation and ipilimumab, a human IgG1 mAb targeted to this molecule was the first ICB drug to show clinical efficacy in advanced melanoma and a number of other cancer types (48, 195). CTLA-4 plays a key role in T cell immunity and its molecular biology has been recently reviewed elsewhere (167, 196). However, to understand the clinical role of CTLA-4 blockade, a brief summary of its mechanism of action is warranted. Naive T cells are modulated by APC through the interaction of multiple surface receptors in a region referred to as the "immunological synapse" (197). Canonically, naive T cells require 3 signals for complete activation (**Figure 2** *inset panel*) (198). The engagement of the TCR by peptide antigen presented in the context of MHC, provides the first signal of T cell activation (signal 1) (198, 199). T cells require further signaling from the binding of costimulatory molecules on T cells such as CD28, to its respective ligands CD80/86 on APC (signal 2). Finally, the complete activation requires cytokines (IL-2) binding to their cognate receptors on T cells (Signal 3) (199). As an evolutionary checkpoint to autoimmunity, activated T cells induce surface CTLA-4 expression, which binds with greater affinity to CD80/86 and mediates T cell inhibition and cell cycle arrest (195, 200). CTLA-4 is also expressed constitutively on Treg (167). The crucial role of CTLA-4 in maintaining tolerance is demonstrated by the severe multiorgan autoimmune pathologies and early mortality (3–4 weeks) observed in CTLA-4$^{-/-}$ mice (201). Humans with heterozygous germline mutations in CTLA-4 also exhibit autoantibodies, increased intra-organ lymphocyte infiltration and other symptoms of immune dysregulation (167).

In 2010, Hodi et al. demonstrated the clinical efficacy of ipilimumab in patients with stage III and IV unresectable and metastatic melanoma whose tumors were refractory to prior treatments (187). The treatment subjects received ipilimumab alone, ipilimumab plus the peptide gp100 or gp100 alone. Patients receiving ipilimumab alone or ipilimumab plus gp100 had significantly increased median OS compared with those receiving gp100 alone (roughly 10 versus 6 months) (187). Currently, ipilimumab has only received FDA approval for melanoma. However, a number of studies have shown modest responses to ipilimumab in other tumor types such as metastatic RCC and NSCLC, and it continues to be studied in clinical trials as combination therapy with PD-1/PD-L1 (discussed below) (160, 167). As mentioned previously, a number of immunological toxicities (IRAEs) are commonly observed to occur in patients treated with ipilimumab primarily in the skin, GI tract, and the endocrine system and in some rare cases result in deaths (193). The frequency of severe toxicities (grade 3 or 4) in the preliminary phase III trials of ipilimumab was demonstrated to be 20%, but this value was not significantly higher than the toxicities associated with many chemotherapy or targeted therapy drugs (163, 195). Most IRAEs can be resolved within 6–12 weeks of steroid therapy but for steroid-resistant adverse events, patients can also be treated with immunosuppressive antimetabolite drugs such as azathioprine and mycophenolate mofetil (193). Novel CTLA-4 blockade agents including modified versions of ipilimumab are also currently under study for a number of advanced solid tumors with the aim of improving safety profiles and tumor-specific delivery (202).

PD-1/PD-1 Ligand (PD-L1)

The most clinically successful agents for ICB to date target the inhibitory PD-1/PD-L1 axis (169, 195). The transmembrane receptor PD-1 (CD279) plays a crucial role in regulating antigen-specific T cell responses (169, 203). PD-1 is not only expressed on activated effector T cells but also on NK cells, B cells, macrophages, and Tregs (167, 203). Similar to the activating co-receptor CD28, PD-1 is acted upon by two distinct ligands PD-L1 (B7-H1, CD274) and PD-L2 (B7-DC, CD273) (203). Whereas PD-L2 expression has hitherto been observed only on professional APC (including B cells), PD-L1 is expressed on various tissue types such as epithelial tissue, vascular endothelium, stromal cells as well as tumor cells and virus-infected cells (167, 203). The induction of PD-L1 expression is generally in response to pro-inflammatory cytokines such as interferons, TNF-α, and VEGF (167, 169). PD-1 does not, as its name implies, directly induce cell death. The binding of PD-1 to its ligands instead serves to attenuate T cell activation by recruiting the tyrosine phosphatase SHP-2, which interferes with signaling downstream of the TCR and leading to decreased T cell growth and reduced cytokine production (203). However, PD-1 signaling can also reduce the expression of antiapoptotic genes while upregulating proapoptotic gene expression thus impairing T cell survival (167).

PD-1-deficient mice do not display as severe a phenotype as CTLA-4$^{-/-}$ mice, developing glomerulonephritis and arthritis in a C57BL/6 background and autoantibody induced dilated cardiomyopathy in BALB/c mice as they age (204, 205). This is arguably due to the more direct inhibitory and Treg-related functions of CTLA-4, whereas PD-1 serves to limit T cell activation indirectly and prevent peripheral autoimmunity (169). As noted previously, in certain conditions of persistent antigen exposure such as in chronic viral infections or in cancer, T cells are observed to develop a dysfunctional or "exhausted" phenotype (72, 167). Such T cells are also marked by elevated expression of PD-1 and other inhibitory receptors such as TIM-3 and LAG3 (72). Furthermore, PD-L1 and/or PD-L2 are both observed to be expressed on a number of tumor-infiltrating APC and tumor cells themselves, not only as a result of cytokines but also due to alternative factors such as gain of chromosomes carrying PD-L1 and PD-L2 or the signaling of the epidermal growth factor pathway (167). Recent studies have shown that APC and tumor cells bearing PD-L1 play additive non-redundant roles in the suppression of antitumor immunity (206). Thus, blockade of the PD-1/PD-L1 axis remains a critical area of interest in tumor immunotherapy with studies on its efficacy in nearly 20 types of solid tumors and hematological cancers (169).

In the context of melanoma, nivolumab, and pembrolizumab, both of which target PD-1 have been shown to have significant clinical efficacies (160, 169, 195). In 2012, results from a phase I study comparing various doses of nivolumab in NSCLC, prostate cancer, CRC, renal cell carcinoma, and melanoma patients were reported (188). The highest activity was demonstrated in melanoma patients where the cumulative response rate (for all doses) was 28% compared with 27% for renal carcinoma and 18% for NSCLC (188). In the same year, an αPD-L1 antibody (BMS-963559) was tested in advanced cancers ranging from melanoma to RCC and was shown to have comparatively low response rates (6–17%) (191). A number of recently concluded trials have also demonstrated the potency of pembrolizumab. The large multicenter phase II trial KEYNOTE-002 examined the efficacy and safety of pembrolizumab in patients who had progressed on ipilimumab therapy, and in patients with BRAF mutations, those who had received either BRAF or MEK inhibitor treatment (207). Patients received either two separate doses of pembrolizumab (2 or 10 mg/kg) or chemotherapy of the investigators choice (carboplatin, dacarbazine, paclitaxel, and temozolomide). The results were highly encouraging as the 6-month PFS was shown to be 38% (10 mg/kg) and 34% (2 mg/kg) in the pembrolizumab group compared with only 16% in the chemotherapy group (207). Similar efficacy over investigator choice chemotherapy (32 versus 11%) has also been reported from an open-label phase III trial of nivolumab in patients who had progressed on ipilimumab (195). Furthermore, pembrolizumab was shown to have significantly higher activity than ipilimumab in patients with advanced melanoma. Robert et al. compared two dosing schedules (every 2 or 3 weeks) of pembrolizumab to ipilimumab and reported 6-month PFS in the range of 46–47% (response rates of roughly 33%) for the pembrolizumab group versus 26.5% (RR of 11.9%) for the ipilimumab-treated patients (208). Finally, in a phase III trial of nivolumab in previously untreated advanced melanoma patients (without BRAF mutations), ICB therapy was demonstrated to have significantly higher efficacy compared with dacarbazine with a 1 year survival rate of 72.9% in the nivolumab treated group versus 42% in the dacarbazine group (189). The successes of αPD-1 in melanoma treatment have also been

observed (albeit at lower rates) in a range of other cancer types (167, 169). Furthermore, the rate of grade 3 or 4 treatment related adverse events is lower in patients receiving PD-1 blockade therapy versus ipilimumab which is similar to the decreased severity of autoimmune pathologies observed in PD-1 versus CTLA-4 knockout mice (169, 193). In contrast to PD-1 blockade antibodies, the αPD-L1 agent atezolizumab (MPDL3280A) has thus far received FDA approval only for urothelial bladder cancer and lung cancer (169, 209). Recently, studies have further complicated the role of PD-L1 by demonstrating that it binds to CD80 on T cells and provides another inhibitory signal (210). Thus, further studies are warranted to determine the role of PD-L1 in T cell inhibition in tumors and investigate which tumor types may benefit most from PD-L1 versus PD-1 blockade. A large number of clinical trials are currently underway targeting PD-1/PD-L1 as well as novel combination approaches (169). As previously mentioned, further study will be required to determine biomarkers of response to ICB and further mechanistic knowledge will be necessary to design effective combinatorial immunotherapies. Four clinical biomarker profiles for ICB treatment have already been proposed based on the presence of PD-L1 and TIL (211). The tumor are characterized as type I (PD-L1$^+$TIL$^+$), type II (PD-L1$^-$TIL$^-$), type III (PD-L1$^+$TIL$^-$), and type IV (PD-L1$^-$TIL$^+$) (211). In melanoma, where the data are most complete, the majority of patients are either type I (~38%) or type II (~41%). Type I patients are deemed to be the best responders to PD-1 blockade whereas type II tumors are estimated to have very poor prognosis due to their lack of immune cell infiltrates (211). Currently, the mechanisms that regulate the immune composition of a tumor are not well understood and there is a significant interest in treatments that can convert T cell non-inflamed (non-infiltrated) tumors to T cell inflamed (infiltrated) tumors (212).

Combinatorial Checkpoint Blockade

Despite the tremendous successes of ICB, to date, only a subset of patients achieve durable clinical responses (160, 167). However, the potency of immune checkpoint therapies has ushered in a new era of cancer treatment by offering the possibility of combining these drugs with conventional cancer treatments such as radiation, chemotherapy, and targeted molecular therapy (e.g., BRAF/MEK inhibitors). The prospects for such combination treatments in melanoma and other cancer types, as well as the clinical findings to date using such approaches have been expertly reviewed this year (213–215). The primary focus of this section will be to discuss the approaches involving combination checkpoint blockade therapies for melanoma that have demonstrated efficacy thus far. Nevertheless, it is pertinent to note that currently there are no clinical data to distinguish between ICB or BRAFi/MEKi targeted therapy as first line treatment for melanoma and a clinical trial (NCT02224781) is being conducted to provide direct comparisons between clinical outcomes in patients receiving checkpoint blockade drugs following targeted therapies and vice versa (215).

The success of combined ipilimumab and nivolumab has also been recently reported in a number of clinical trials. In 2015, Postow et al. reported the results of a study where previously untreated patients with metastatic melanoma received either ipilimumab in combination with nivolumab or with placebo preceding a subsequent treatment with nivolumab or placebo (216). The ORR was 61% in the combination treatment group versus 11% in the ipilimumab plus placebo group. Moreover, nearly 22% of patients treated with combination therapy achieved CR compared with none of the patients given ipilimumab and placebo (216). In the same year, results were published from a phase III trial in 945 patients with unresectable stage III or IV melanoma treated with nivolumab alone, nivolumab plus ipilimumab, or ipilimumab alone. The median PFS was 11.5 months for the combination group, 6.9 months for the nivolumab group, and 2.9 months for the ipilimumab group (217). However, serious (grade 3 or 5) treatment related adverse events in the combination treatment group were significantly higher reaching 55% compared with 27% for the ipilimumab group (217). These studies also indicate the superiority of combinatorial checkpoint blockade over monotherapy leading to the approval of ipilimumab and nivolumab dual therapy for melanoma in the USA, while its efficacy in other tumor types continues to be investigated (218). The successful use of combined checkpoint blockade has also sparked clinical interest in additional immune checkpoints some of which are undergoing preclinical or clinical investigation (167, 169, 218). A target of particular interest is the CD4 homolog lymphocyte activation gene-3 (LAG-3), which is expressed on Treg, effector $CD4^+$ and $CD8^+$ T cells, NK cells, B cells, and pDC and which also binds to MHC class II (167, 219). LAG-3 is an important negative regulator of $CD4^+$ and $CD8^+$ T cells and is required for Treg activity (219). The αLAG-3 antibody BMS986016 is currently being examined in a clinical trial (NCT01968109) for several advanced tumors both as a monotherapy and in combination with nivolumab (167). Another immune checkpoint that has exciting potential for tumor immunotherapy is TIGIT (T cell immunoreceptor with immunoglobulin and ITIM domain) (167). TIGIT is expressed by activated T cells, NK cells and is also expressed on highly functional subsets of Treg (219, 220). TIGIT has two ligands, namely, CD155 (poliovirus receptor, PVR) and CD112 (PVRL2) that are expressed on APC as well as on tumor cells (167). Likewise, TIGIT is reportedly expressed on TIL (219). The immunoregulatory functions of TIGIT are only recently beginning to be described (221). TIGIT can bind to CD155 on DC resulting in increased IL-10 and decreased IL-12 secretion (167). Ligation of TIGIT on Treg results in the expression of fibrinogen-like protein 2 (Fgl2), a Treg effector molecule that has broad immunosuppressive effects such as mediating Th1 and Th17 phenotype suppression in favor of Th2 (167, 222). In human melanoma, tumor-specific $CD8^+$ T cells in peripheral circulation and $CD8^+$ TIL were found to express both TIGIT and PD-1 and furthermore, TIGIT was upregulated in response to PD-1 blockade (223). Thus, the described functions of TIGIT further complicate our understanding of the immune response to αPD-1 treatment and provides further proof of the need of combinatorial approaches to overcome current barriers to ICB treatment. The positive results associated with ICB treatment have also renewed interest in a parallel treatment approach involving the development of agonistic antibodies for T cell costimulatory molecules such as CD137 (4-1BB), GITR (glucocorticoid-induced TNFR family related gene), and OX40

(CD134) many of which are currently undergoing clinical trials in combination with nivolumab (167, 169, 218). In 2016, early results were showcased for the antibody urelumab (αCD137) in combination with nivolumab (202). In melanoma, the ORR was observed to be 50% in patients who had not previously received checkpoint blockade therapy and was found to be independent of tumor PD-L1 status (202). Thus immune agonistic antibodies have revealed a plethora of novel possibilities for cancer treatment. Future studies will involve analyses of various combinations aimed at developing immunotherapies tailored to the specific tumor immune microenvironment (224).

Adoptive Cell Therapy

Adoptive cell therapy involves the use of *ex vivo* manipulated cells transferred directly to patients to mediate antitumor immunity (50, 172). Thus far, the majority of clinical research in ACT has been conducted using autologous tumor-specific T cells (TIL) harvested and cultured from resected melanoma tissue (161, 173). Other cell types such as NK cells have also been investigated since the 1980s for their use in adoptive transfer therapy but have yet to be as widely studied as T cells (156). Thus, the primary focus of this section will be on studies with T cell ACT. The benefits of this approach are that it allows for the *ex vivo* expansion of tumor-specific cells that are not modulated by the immunosuppressive TME and can be administered in sufficient numbers to induce tumor regressions (50). As mentioned previously, this field was pioneered by Rosenberg and colleagues using autologous TIL from patients with metastatic melanoma and resulted in durable antitumor responses (186). Since that time, developments in molecular biology allowed for the elucidation of various tumor antigens and the development of genetically engineered T cell products with tumor-specific TCR or chimeric antigen receptors (CARs) (50, 225). To date, successful ACT through TIL transfer has been largely limited to melanoma although it is currently being studied in metastatic HPV-associated cancer and has been demonstrated to induce potent prophylactic clinical responses in HSCT recipients against Epstein–Barr virus-associated lymphoproliferative disorders (225). Lymphodepletion before TIL therapy has been shown to significantly augment clinical response, and although its precise mechanisms of action are not well understood, it is posited to complement TIL transfer by eliminating suppressive Treg and myeloid cells (50). In patients treated with autologous TIL therapy post lymphodepletion, the group of Rosenberg and colleagues at the NCI (Bethesda, MD, USA) has reported OR rates of 55% (226). These results are similar to those observed in patients from other centers that perform ACT using TIL such as MD Anderson (Houston, TX, USA) with an ORR of 48% in their patient cohort and Ella Cancer Institute (Raman Gat, Israel) with an ORR of 40% (50, 227). Overall, TIL therapy is not reported to be associated with severe adverse events, and the major toxic side effects are associated with the lymphoablative conditioning regimens (226). The primary hematological pathologies observed are anemia and thrombocytopenia necessitating transfusion in these patients, while patients in cohorts that receive TIL and IL-2 may report to develop grade 3 and 4 non-hematological toxicities (228). Currently, the predominant clinical form of ACT for melanoma is TIL therapy (50, 173). Nevertheless, there is also significant clinical interest in the use of highly specific T cells expressing TCRs specific to tumor antigens. These T cells can be generated through *in vitro* selection and expansion of specific antitumor clones (173). However, engineered T cells bearing conventional antitumor alpha beta TCRs or CARs have generated significant interest in the field of adoptive cell therapies (229). CARs are artificial receptors that were developed to circumvent the requirement of MHC–TCR interactions as many tumor cells downregulate MHC expression to escape the immune system (173). CARs consist of an extracellular ligand-binding domain constructed with immunoglobulin heavy and light chain variable regions fused through a transmembrane domain to intracellular CD3 zeta signaling chains in addition to CD28 or CD137 costimulatory domains for induction of complete T cell activation (50, 229). Currently, CAR T cells have demonstrated efficacy only in B cell malignancies using anti-CD19 CARs, to achieve response rates of up to 90% (173). However, a number of studies are currently underway investigating the use of CAR T cells in solid tumors (173). On the other hand, studies using transgenic tumor-specific TCRs have been tested in melanoma with the first proof-of-concept study being performed in 2006 using T cells transduced with a TCR against the melanoma differentiation antigen MART-1 (230). This early study showed evidence of clinical activity in only 2 out of 17 patients but a more recent report by Chodon et al. (231) demonstrated that MART-1 specific T cells in combination with MART-1 pulsed DC vaccine were able to induce tumor regression in 9 out of 13 studied patients (231). Thus, combining ACT with other immunotherapies may unveil potentially novel synergistic treatments that can overcome the current barriers to ACT. A number of clinical trials using ACT in conjunction with checkpoint blockade agents (nivolumab-NCT02652455) or targeted therapy (vemurafenib-NCT01659151) are being tested in patients with melanoma (173). A number of salient factors warrant consideration when discussing the merits of ACT immunotherapies for cancer. First, it is pertinent to mention that ACT requires *ex vivo* manipulation of cells, which is both expensive and labor intensive (173). Therefore ACT currently remains limited to a few specialized centers around the world (50). Furthermore, engineered T cells have the potential to induce stronger toxicities versus conventional TIL due to their clonal specificity toward a single antigen. This is a particular concern with TCRs targeted to antigens that are shared by tumor and normal tissue resulting in an immune activation versus the target but not necessarily against the tumor (on-target, off-tumor toxicity) (173). This effect has been observed in a number of trials. In a study treating patients with T cells bearing transgenic TCRs specific to MART-1 and gp100, several patients developed toxicities in the skin, ears, and eyes due to the presence of melanocytes in these organs (232). This effect has also been seen in other tumor types such as metastatic renal cancer where in a recent report, 4 out of 12 patients treated with CAR T cells specific to carbonic anhydrase IX (CAIX), developed liver toxicity due to the presence of this antigen in the bile duct (233). Thus, strategies will need to be developed to overcome such off-target effects of engineered lymphocytes and in the case of the aforementioned CAIX trial,

hepatic T cell mediated toxicity was significantly lowered by treatment with blocking anti-CAIX antibodies (233). Although early studies showed that MART-1 and gp100 are among the major tumor antigens recognized by anti-melanoma TIL, recent advances in whole-exome sequencing offer the potential to reveal novel antigens (i.e. neoantigens) resulting from mutations that may be highly immunogenic but also safe due to their absence from the rest of the body (50). Another concerning immune-related toxicity observed in CAR and conventional T cell therapy is cytokine release syndrome, which presents as a systemic multisymptomatic inflammation causing fever, hypotension, and tachycardia (173). In terms of efficacy, a key concern using CAR T cells is that while they have shown remarkable results for hematological cancers, solid tumors are more difficult to treat and have a highly suppressive TME (173, 229). Nevertheless, advances in lymphocyte engineering have allowed for the conceptualization of a number of novel types of CAR T cells which can be switched on conditionally, or lack checkpoint molecules to prevent suppression. These novel CARs may have high utility for solid cancers and have been reviewed expertly elsewhere (229). Similarly, a novel type of molecule that has recently gained attention is a bispecific antibody construct that can bind to CD3 thus activating T cells as well as, a tumor antigen and is termed a bispecific T cell engager (BiTE®) (234). The anti-CD19 BiTE® blinatumomab was approved by the FDA after showing activity in acute lymphoblastic leukemia but to date, none of the tested BiTE® constructs tested in solid tumors have exhibited noteworthy antitumor responses (234). Novel developments in the field of genomic sequencing as well as T cell engineering have allowed for the conceptualization of highly personalized ACT treatment for cancer. Nevertheless, as discussed previously, without breakthroughs in *ex vivo* cell handling and automation, this therapy will remain highly costly and be limited to a few centers of excellence around the world.

Cancer Vaccines

Vaccination for infectious disease represents a landmark of human medical achievement. Cancer vaccines seek to activate the immune system, in particular the T cells, to attack the tumor with the presentation of the tumor antigen in combination with an adjuvant (176). The vaccines may be univalent incorporating a single target antigen or polyvalent, consisting of allogeneic whole cells, or autologous tumor lysates (48). To date, none of the vaccine combinations tested in established tumors have shown the same efficacy as checkpoint blockade or ACT (165, 176). A number of studies have shown modest increases in clinical activity such as the study by Schwartzentruber et al. in 2011 that showed that patients with advanced melanoma treated with IL-2 and a gp100 peptide vaccine fared better than patients treated with IL-2 alone (median OS 18 versus 11 months, respectively) (48, 235). Nevertheless, cancer vaccination for solid tumors becomes particularly challenging due to the immunosuppressive TME and a constantly evolving tumor geared toward immune escape (165). In the past 30 years, as research unveiled the crucial role of DC in antigen processing and T cell activation, DC-targeted vaccines also became a major focus of cancer vaccination research (161). DC are considered to be ideal tools for inducing effective anticancer immunity due to their central role in antigen presentation and their ability to produce crucial effector cytokines (174, 236). The use of DC as anticancer vaccines has been comprehensively reviewed elsewhere (133, 145, 174, 237). Generally, this approach involves the generation of DC from isolated patient PBMC, which are then loaded with antigen and reinfused into the patient (161). Clinically a widely accepted DC maturation protocol involves the use of a cocktail containing TNFα, IL-1β, IL-6, and PGE2, resulting in the upregulation of MHC class I and II and costimulatory molecules (133). Other approaches in the clinic have used mixtures of prophylactic vaccines (which contain TLR agonists) containing Bacillus Calmette–Guerin (BCG)-SSI, Influvac, and Typhim (133, 238). DC maturation can also be induced by targeting the costimulatory receptor CD40 with CD40L (which is expressed by a range of immune cells but its most functionally important expression is on activated T cells *in vivo*) or anti-CD40 mAbs, resulting in the upregulation of costimulatory molecules and production of IL-12 (133, 237, 239). Currently, there is no gold standard in terms of maturation cocktails for DC and novel combinations continue to be tested both preclinically and in clinical trials (174). GVAX® (Cell Genesys, San Francisco, CA, USA) are a cell product composed of irradiated autologous or allogeneic, tumor cells engineered to produce GM-CSF (240). GVAX® vaccines were shown to elicit antitumor immune responses in a number of early clinical studies (241). However, a phase III trial using allogeneic GVAX® in prostate cancer observed that this approach was not superior to current treatments (241). In melanoma, the GVAX® approach has not shown significant clinical activity including a recent study by Lipson et al. that demonstrated that although melanoma GVAX® was safely tolerated, it did not result in markedly increased anti-melanoma responses in peripheral blood T cells (175, 241). These early and currently ongoing studies demonstrate the difficulty of using cell-based approaches for cancer vaccination. Currently, Sipuleucel-T (Provenge®) is the only cell-based vaccine to be approved by the FDA for its observed clinically significant but modest increases in the OS of patients with prostate cancer (174). No such vaccine has yet received FDA approval for melanoma (161). In 2013, Carreno et al. reported the use of an autologous CD40L/IFNγ-matured DC vaccine pulsed with gp100-derived peptides and capable of producing IL-12 (242). In six out seven patients, this treatment successfully induced immune responses with three out of the six responding patients exhibiting tumor remissions (242). Despite these encouraging results, a number of concerns with cancer vaccination still exist, in particular with the choice of target antigen as tumors continue to continuously evade the immune response while novel mutated epitopes may not be sufficient for inducing potent antitumor T cell responses (161). Thus, there has been a significant clinical interest in the use of oncolytic viral vaccines for directly inducing cell death in tumors (48, 161). This approach attempts to harness the specificity of some oncolytic viruses for tumor cells as well as the induction of tumor cytolysis as an immune activating stimulus against non-infected tumor cells (177, 161). The first viral product to receive FDA approval is talimogene laherparepvec (T-VEC) which is

a construct derived from herpes simplex virus 1 with deleted ICP34.5 and ICP47 genes and coding for human GM-CSF (177). In 2015, T-VEC was the first virotherapy that showed durable antitumor responses in patients with melanoma (178). Over 400 patients were treated with intralesional T-VEC or subcutaneous GM-CSF, and median OS was demonstrably higher in the T-VEC group versus the GM-CSF group (23 versus 19 months, respectively) (178). Moreover, the durable response rates and overall response rates were also higher in the T-VEC group than in the GM-CSF group with very limited toxicities associated with T-VEC treatment (178). As a result of these findings, the field of cancer vaccine research has been energized, and currently trials are underway to examine potential combination approaches using ICB in combination with oncolytic vaccine regimens to induce a long-lasting antitumor immune response (39, 161). The major limitation of the T-VEC approach is that it was found to be more effective in patients with less advanced (stage III and locally metastatic) melanoma than in patients with visceral metastatic disease (178, 161). Thus, in patients with established and advanced tumors, cancer vaccination approaches at best provide part of the solution for complete cure. With the complex immunoregulatory pathways that are established in advanced tumors, it may be difficult to achieve continued DC stimulation and activation through vaccines. Thus, a number of studies have begun to investigate the targeting of DC *in vivo* as crucial for the success for future immunotherapies (133). The success of T cell checkpoint therapy has already demonstrated the utility of treatments that mediate *in vivo* activation of antitumor immunity. Although a number of other cell types such as NK cells and MDSC have recently gained interest as targetable populations, DC remain a primary cell of interest for *in vivo* targeted immunotherapy due to their crucial roles as APC and in cytokine production (237, 243, 244).

Nanoparticles as Multifunctional Immunotherapeutics

The past two decades have witnessed significant advances in our understanding of tumor immunology and the development of immunotherapeutic drugs (56, 163). In parallel, improvements in the field of nanomedicine provides us with a number of opportunities that can be used in combination with modern immunotherapies to enhance their antitumor efficacy (245–248). The primary advantage to NP is the supreme versatility in their design as their size, shape, constituent biomaterials, and surface modifications can be tailored for specific uses in tumor immunotherapy (**Figure 3**) (245, 247). Liposomes are self-assembling nanosized vesicles comprised of phospholipids and cholesterol arranged in one or more lipid bilayers enclosing an aqueous core (246, 249). Liposome-encapsulated drugs have been demonstrated to have reduced systemic toxicity profiles owing to improved pharmacokinetics and biodistribution (247, 249). Liposomal doxorubicin (Doxil) first received FDA approval in 1995, and even though it did not enhance OS, it is associated with improved toxicity profiles (247). This is of particular use for immunotherapy as many powerful adjuvants such as IL-2 and IFN-α have serious toxic side effects (161). In 2012, Park et al.

NANOPARTICLES AS MULTIFUNCTIONAL IMMUNOTHERAPEUTICS IN CANCER TREATMENT

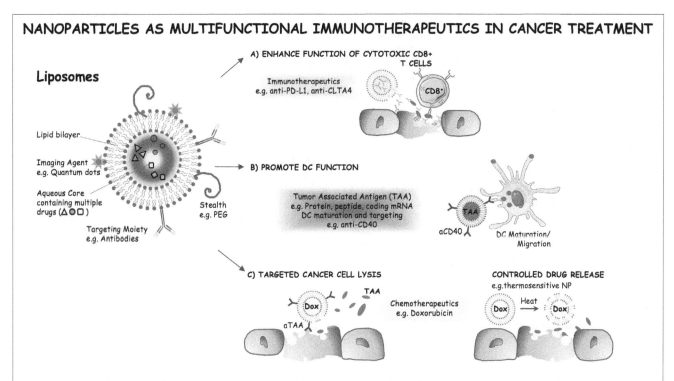

FIGURE 3 | Multifunctional nanoparticles (NP) in cancer treatment. NP can be tailored to specific applications in tumor immunotherapy using versatile designs of various sizes, constituent biomaterials, and surface modifications. The surface of NP can be functionalized with specific polymers and antibodies to increase their targeting to certain types of cells. Liposomes are self-assembling nanosized vesicles comprised of phospholipids and cholesterol arranged in one or more lipid bilayers enclosing an aqueous core. NP such as liposomes can be used as platforms for the simultaneous delivery of multiple agents, such as **(A)** immunotherapeutics, e.g., anti-PD-L1 and anti-cytotoxic T lymphocyte antigen-4 (CTLA-4), to enhance the function of tumor-specific effector T cells; **(B)** tumor-associated antigens (TAA) and adjuvant targeted to dendritic cells (DC) to promote their function; **(C)** chemotherapeutics and targeted release thereof, for instance, using thermosensitive NP, to promote cancer cell death.

demonstrated the utility of a biodegradable liposome and solid polymer hybrid gel as a dual delivery platform for IL-2 as well as an inhibitor of the immunoregulatory cytokine TGF-β (250). Treatment with this platform showed no significant toxicity in treated animals and more importantly delayed tumor growth was mediated via increased intratumoral NK and CD8⁺ T cell infiltration (250). Thus, NP can not only deliver drugs but also serve as platforms for simultaneous delivery of multiple agents. In the context of immunotherapy, NP can deliver tumor antigens, nucleic acids, and adjuvants (246, 248). There has also been research in the field of artificial APC NP platforms that present antigen loaded MHC I in combination with antibodies to the T cell costimulatory molecule CD28 (246). Finally, the surfaces of NP can be functionalized with specific polymers and antibodies to increase their targeting to certain types of cells (245). Even without direct targeting, systemically treated NP can accumulate at tumor sites due to "leaky" tumor vasculature (247). Earlier this year, Koshy et al. reported the antitumor potency of liposome-encapsulated cGAMP (251). The authors showed that cationic liposome loaded with cGAMP resulted in passive lung-specific delivery in metastatic B16F10 melanoma lung tumors leading to pronounced antitumor activity and the formation of immune memory (251). Currently, a number of unique immunotherapeutic NP are being investigated in Phase I–III clinical trials (247). However, to date no directly DC-targeted NP formulation has

reached clinical trials. As DC play central roles in priming antitumor immunity as well as directly influencing the immune infiltration of T cells into cancer (212), NP targeted to DC warrant inclusion in future combinatorial immunotherapies (252). In 2016, Kranz et al. developed a strategy to deliver RNA-NP to DC in a pilot study with three melanoma patients (105). The RNA encoded for the melanoma antigens NY-ESO-1, MAGE-A3, tyrosinase, and TPTE (transmembrane phosphatase with tensin homology) and resulted in IFNα and antigen-specific T cell responses in all three patients (105). This approach was administered systemically and was not found to be associated with any adverse effects. This study thus opens a new field of DC-targeted, highly potent immunotherapies for cancer. NP are biodegradable, relatively cost-effective (compared with *ex vivo* manipulated cells) (133) and highly multifunctional platforms for enhancing modern immunotherapies or developing independent DC-targeted treatments (247).

SUMMARY

Currently, the field of immunotherapy is one of the most promising avenues of research in the quest to develop long-term broadly acting treatments for cancer (55, 161, 253). The possibilities for synergistic combinations with radiation, chemotherapy, and small molecule targeted treatments have also unveiled countless possibilities for tailoring individualized therapies in the drive towards "precision medicine" (213, 214, 254). However, evolutionary checkpoints against autoimmunity and the fact that cancer arises from self-tissue presents a particularly challenging landscape for developing multitargeted immunotherapies that are cost-effective, safe, and efficacious. Conceptually, there are four general facets of tumor immunity that must be achieved for successful immunotherapy (253). These are the removal of immunosuppressive cues, the induction of immunogenic cell death in tumors, improved activity of APC and increased T cell effector functions (253). In addition to a comprehensive overview of the immune contexture of a tumor, other host specific factors such as genetics and individual microbiota must be further dissected to determine their interplay with immunotherapeutic agents (255). In recent years, advances in high-throughput techniques such as next-generation sequencing and mass cytometry (CyTOF) have enabled highly detailed phenotyping of cancer (256, 257). However, there is still an unmet need for bioinformatics platforms and deep-learning algorithms that can assist biologists with mining and analyzing such massive datasets (258). Finally, due to the need to finely target various facets of tumor immunology in immunotherapy, NP technology may become indispensable as the delivery vectors and the platforms upon which these multifunctional therapeutics are designed (248).

AUTHOR CONTRIBUTIONS

MS conceptualized the manuscript and oversaw all aspects of its completing including writing, figure design, and literature review. HS and TG contributed equally to this manuscript by performing literature review and writing of the manuscript. RH provided medical expertise in the subject matter during writing of the manuscript and contributed clinical images.

REFERENCES

1. Miller AJ, Mihm MC. Melanoma. *N Engl J Med* (2006) 355(1):51–65. doi:10.1056/NEJMra052166
2. Bandarchi B, Jabbari CA, Vedadi A, Navab R. Molecular biology of normal melanocytes and melanoma cells. *J Clin Pathol* (2013) 66(8):644–8. doi:10.1136/jclinpath-2013-201471
3. Madan V, Lear JT, Szeimies R-M. Non-melanoma skin cancer. *Lancet* (2010) 375(9715):673–85. doi:10.1016/S0140-6736(09)61196-X
4. Shain AH, Bastian BC. From melanocytes to melanomas. *Nat Rev Cancer* (2016) 16(6):345–58. doi:10.1038/nrc.2016.37
5. Tsao H, Chin L, Garraway LA, Fisher DE. Melanoma: from mutations to medicine. *Genes Dev* (2012) 26(11):1131–55. doi:10.1101/gad.191999.112
6. Bertolotto C. Melanoma: from melanocyte to genetic alterations and clinical options. *Scientifica (Cairo)* (2013) 2013:635203. doi:10.1155/2013/635203
7. Mort RL, Jackson IJ, Patton EE. The melanocyte lineage in development and disease. *Development* (2015) 142(4):620–32. doi:10.1242/dev.106567
8. Slominski A, Tobin DJ, Shibahara S, Wortsman J. Melanin pigmentation in mammalian skin and its hormonal regulation. *Physiol Rev* (2004) 84(4):1155–228. doi:10.1152/physrev.00044.2003
9. Ali Z, Yousaf N, Larkin J. Melanoma epidemiology, biology and prognosis. *EJC Suppl* (2013) 11(2):81–91. doi:10.1016/j.ejcsup.2013.07.012
10. Siegel RL, Miller KD, Jemal A. Cancer statistics, 2017. *CA Cancer J Clin* (2017) 67(1):7–30. doi:10.3322/caac.21387
11. Erdmann F, Lortet-Tieulent J, Schuz J, Zeeb H, Greinert R, Breitbart EW, et al. International trends in the incidence of malignant melanoma 1953-2008 – are recent generations at higher or lower risk? *Int J Cancer* (2013) 132(2):385–400. doi:10.1002/ijc.27616
12. Karimkhani C, Green AC, Nijsten T, Weinstock MA, Dellavalle RP, Naghavi M, et al. The global burden of melanoma: results from Global Burden of Disease study 2015. *Br J Dermatol* (2017) 177(1):134–40. doi:10.1111/bjd.15510
13. Global Burden of Disease Cancer Collaboration, Fitzmaurice C, Allen C, Barber RM, Barregard L, Bhutta ZA, et al. Global, regional, and national cancer incidence, mortality, years of life lost, years lived with disability, and disability-adjusted life-years for 32 cancer groups, 1990 to 2015: a systematic analysis for the global burden of disease study. *JAMA Oncol* (2016) 3(4):524–48. doi:10.1001/jamaoncol.2016.5688
14. Smoller BR. Histologic criteria for diagnosing primary cutaneous malignant melanoma. *Mod Pathol* (2006) 19(S2):S34–40. doi:10.1038/modpathol.3800508
15. Bastian BC. The molecular pathology of melanoma: an integrated taxonomy of melanocytic neoplasia. *Annu Rev Pathol* (2014) 9:239–71. doi:10.1146/annurev-pathol-012513-104658
16. Viros A, Fridlyand J, Bauer J, Lasithiotakis K, Garbe C, Pinkel D, et al. Improving melanoma classification by integrating genetic and morphologic features. *PLoS Med* (2008) 5(6):e120. doi:10.1371/journal.pmed.0050120
17. Hussein MR. Melanocytic dysplastic naevi occupy the middle ground between benign melanocytic naevi and cutaneous malignant melanomas: emerging clues. *J Clin Pathol* (2005) 58(5):453–6. doi:10.1136/jcp.2004.019422
18. Eggermont AMM, Spatz A, Robert C. Cutaneous melanoma. *Lancet* (2014) 383(9919):816–27. doi:10.1016/S0140-6736(13)60802-8
19. Balch CM, Gershenwald JE, Soong S, Thompson JF, Atkins MB, Byrd DR, et al. Final version of 2009 AJCC melanoma staging and classification. *J Clin Oncol* (2009) 27(36):6199–206. doi:10.1200/JCO.2009.23.4799
20. Bichakjian CK, Halpern AC, Johnson TM, Foote Hood A, Grichnik JM, Swetter SM, et al. Guidelines of care for the management of primary cutaneous melanoma. American Academy of Dermatology. *J Am Acad Dermatol* (2011) 65(5):1032–47. doi:10.1016/j.jaad.2011.04.031
21. Clark WHJ, From L, Bernardino EA, Mihm MC. The histogenesis and biologic behavior of primary human malignant melanomas of the skin. *Cancer Res* (1969) 29(3):705–27.
22. Scolyer RA, Long GV, Thompson JF. Evolving concepts in melanoma classification and their relevance to multidisciplinary melanoma patient care. *Mol Oncol* (2011) 5(2):124–36. doi:10.1016/j.molonc.2011.03.002
23. Bandarchi B, Ma L, Navab R, Seth A, Rasty G. From melanocyte to metastatic malignant melanoma. *Dermatol Res Pract* (2010) 2010:583748. doi:10.1155/2010/583748
24. McCourt C, Dolan O, Gormley G. Malignant melanoma: a pictorial review. *Ulster Med J* (2014) 83(2):103–10.
25. Reddy BY, Miller DM, Tsao H. Somatic driver mutations in melanoma. *Cancer* (2017) 123(S11):2104–17. doi:10.1002/cncr.30593
26. Rastrelli M, Tropea S, Rossi CR, Alaibac M. Melanoma: epidemiology, risk factors, pathogenesis, diagnosis and classification. *In Vivo* (2014) 28(6):1005–11.
27. Le Clair MZ, Cockburn MG. Tanning bed use and melanoma: establishing risk and improving prevention interventions. *Prev Med Reports* (2016) 14(3):139–44. doi:10.1016/j.pmedr.2015.11.016
28. Liu Y, Sheikh MS. Melanoma: molecular pathogenesis and therapeutic management. *Mol Cell Pharmacol* (2014) 6(3):228.
29. Stratton MR, Campbell PJ, Futreal PA. The cancer genome. *Nature* (2009) 458(7239):719–24. doi:10.1038/nature07943

30. Cancer Genome Atlas Network. Genomic classification of cutaneous melanoma. *Cell* (2015) 161(7):1681–96. doi:10.1016/j.cell.2015.05.044

31. Hawryluk EB, Tsao H. Melanoma: clinical features and genomic insights. *Cold Spring Harb Perspect Med* (2014) 4(9):a015388. doi:10.1101/cshperspect.a015388

32. Fiskus W, Mitsiades N. B-Raf inhibition in the clinic: present and future. *Annu Rev Med* (2016) 67:29–43. doi:10.1146/annurev-med-090514-030732

33. Samatar AA, Poulikakos PI. Targeting RAS-ERK signalling in cancer: promises and challenges. *Nat Rev Drug Discov* (2014) 13(12):928–42. doi:10.1038/nrd4281

34. Heider D, Hauke S, Pyka M, Kessler D. Insights into the classification of small GTPases. *Adv Appl Bioinform Chem* (2010) 21(3):15–24.

35. Leicht DT, Balan V, Kaplun A, Singh-Gupta V, Kaplun L, Dobson M, et al. Raf kinases: function, regulation and role in human cancer. *Biochim Biophys Acta* (2007) 1773(8):1196–212. doi:10.1016/j.bbamcr.2007.05.001

36. Haluska F, Pemberton T, Ibrahim N, Kalinsky K. The RTK/RAS/BRAF/PI3K pathways in melanoma: biology, small molecule inhibitors, and potential applications. *Semin Oncol* (2007) 34(6):546–54. doi:10.1053/j.seminoncol.2007.09.011

37. McCain J. The MAPK (ERK) pathway: investigational combinations for the treatment of BRAF-mutated metastatic melanoma. *PT* (2013) 38(2):96–108.

38. Mehnert JM, Kluger HM. Driver mutations in melanoma: lessons learned from bench-to-bedside studies. *Curr Oncol Rep* (2012) 14(5):449–57. doi:10.1007/s11912-012-0249-5

39. DB J, JA S. Therapeutic advances and treatment options in metastatic melanoma. *JAMA Oncol* (2015) 1(3):380–6. doi:10.1001/jamaoncol.2015.0565

40. Kiuru M, Busam KJ. The NF1 gene in tumor syndromes and melanoma. *Lab Invest* (2017) 97:146–57. doi:10.1038/labinvest.2016.142

41. Larribère L, Utikal J. Multiple roles of NF1 in the melanocyte lineage. *Pigment Cell Melanoma Res* (2016) 29(4):417–25. doi:10.1111/pcmr.12488

42. Haq R, Fisher DE. Biology and clinical relevance of the micropthalmia family of transcription factors in human cancer. *J Clin Oncol* (2011) 29(25):3474–82. doi:10.1200/JCO.2010.32.6223

43. Hartman ML, Czyz M. MITF in melanoma: mechanisms behind its expression and activity. *Cell Mol Life Sci* (2015) 72(7):1249–60. doi:10.1007/s00018-014-1791-0

44. Wellbrock C, Arozarena I. Microphthalmia-associated transcription factor in melanoma development and MAP-kinase pathway targeted therapy. *Pigment Cell Melanoma Res* (2015) 28(4):390–406. doi:10.1111/pcmr.12370

45. Aguissa-Toure A-H, Li G. Genetic alterations of PTEN in human melanoma. *Cell Mol Life Sci* (2012) 69(9):1475–91. doi:10.1007/s00018-011-0878-0

46. Benafif S, Hall M. An update on PARP inhibitors for the treatment of cancer. *Onco Targets Ther* (2015) 26(8):519–28. doi:10.2147/OTT.S30793

47. Bhatia S, Tykodi SS, Thompson JA. Treatment of metastatic melanoma: an overview. *Oncology (Williston Park)* (2009) 23(6):488–96.

48. Maverakis E, Cornelius LA, Bowen GM, Phan T, Patel FB, Fitzmaurice S, et al. Metastatic melanoma – a review of current and future treatment options. *Acta Derm Venereol* (2015) 95(5):516–24. doi:10.2340/00015555-2035

49. Wong DJL, Ribas A. Targeted therapy for melanoma BT. In: Kaufman HL, Mehnert JM, editors. *Melanoma*. Cham: Springer International Publishing (2016). p. 251–62.

50. Rosenberg SA, Restifo NP. Adoptive cell transfer as personalized immunotherapy for human cancer. *Science* (2015) 348(6230):62–8. doi:10.1126/science.aaa4967

51. Herbst RS, Soria J-C, Kowanetz M, Fine GD, Hamid O, Gordon MS, et al. Predictive correlates of response to the anti-PD-L1 antibody MPDL3280A in cancer patients. *Nature* (2014) 515(7528):563–7. doi:10.1038/nature14011

52. Swaika A, Hammond WA, Joseph RW. Current state of anti-PD-L1 and anti-PD-1 agents in cancer therapy. *Mol Immunol* (2015) 67(2, Pt A):4–17. doi:10.1016/j.molimm.2015.02.009

53. Eisenhauer EA, Therasse P, Bogaerts J, Schwartz LH, Sargent D, Ford R, et al. New response evaluation criteria in solid tumours: revised RECIST guideline (version 1.1). *Eur J Cancer* (2009) 45(2):228–47. doi:10.1016/j.ejca.2008.10.026

54. Villaruz LC, Socinski MA. The clinical viewpoint: definitions, limitations of RECIST, practical considerations of measurement. *Clin Cancer Res* (2013) 19(10):2629–36. doi:10.1158/1078-0432.CCR-12-2935

55. Khalil DN, Smith EL, Brentjens RJ, Wolchok JD. The future of cancer treatment: immunomodulation, CARs and combination immunotherapy. *Nat Rev Clin Oncol* (2016) 13(5):273–90. doi:10.1038/nrclinonc.2016.25

56. Couzin-Frankel J. Cancer Immunotherapy. *Science* (2013) 342(6165):1432–3. doi:10.1126/science.342.6165.1432

57. Parish CR. Cancer immunotherapy: the past, the present and the future. *Immunol Cell Biol* (2003) 81:106–13. doi:10.1046/j.0818-9641.2003.01151.x

58. Coley WB. The treatment of inoperable sarcoma by bacterial toxins (the mixed toxins of the *Streptococcus* erysipelas and the *Bacillus prodigiosus*). *Proc R Soc Med* (1910) 3(Surg Sect):1–48.

59. Dunn GP, Bruce AT, Ikeda H, Old LJ, Schreiber RD. Cancer immunoediting: from immunosurveillance to tumor escape. *Nat Immunol* (2002) 3(11):991–8. doi:10.1038/ni1102-991

60. Burnet FM. The concept of immunological surveillance. *Prog Exp Tumor Res* (1970) 13:1–27. doi:10.1159/000386035

61. Dunn GP, Old LJ, Schreiber RD. The immunobiology of cancer immunosurveillance and immunoediting. *Immunity* (2004) 21(2):137–48. doi:10.1016/j.immuni.2004.07.017

62. Schreiber RD, Old LJ, Smyth MJ. Cancer immunoediting: integrating immunity's roles in cancer suppression and promotion. *Science* (2011) 331(6024):1565–70. doi:10.1126/science.1203486

63. Mittal D, Gubin MM, Schreiber RD, Smyth MJ. New insights into cancer immunoediting and its three component phases—elimination, equilibrium and escape. *Curr Opin Immunol* (2014) 27:16–25. doi:10.1016/j.coi.2014.01.004

64. Teng MWL, Galon J, Fridman W-H, Smyth MJ. From mice to humans: developments in cancer immunoediting. *J Clin Invest* (2015) 125(9):3338–46. doi:10.1172/JCI80004

65. Vesely MD, Kershaw MH, Schreiber RD, Smyth MJ. Natural innate and adaptive immunity to cancer. *Annu Rev Immunol* (2011) 29:235–71. doi:10.1146/annurev-immunol-031210-101324

66. Koebel CM, Vermi W, Swann JB, Zerafa N, Rodig SJ, Old LJ, et al. Adaptive immunity maintains occult cancer in an equilibrium state. *Nature* (2007) 450(7171):903–7. doi:10.1038/nature06309

67. Merlo A, Dalla Santa S, Dolcetti R, Zanovello P, Rosato A. Reverse immunoediting: when immunity is edited by antigen. *Immunol Lett* (2016) 175:16–20. doi:10.1016/j.imlet.2016.04.015

68. Chen DS, Mellman I. Oncology meets immunology: the cancer-immunity cycle. *Immunity* (2013) 39:1–10. doi:10.1016/j.immuni.2013.07.012

69. Palucka AK, Coussens LM. The basis of oncoimmunology. *Cell* (2017) 164(6):1233–47. doi:10.1016/j.cell.2016.01.049

70. Harris TJ, Drake CG. Primer on tumor immunology and cancer immunotherapy. *J Immunother Cancer* (2013) 1(1):12. doi:10.1186/2051-1426-1-12

71. Woo S-R, Corrales L, Gajewski TF. Innate immune recognition of cancer. *Annu Rev Immunol* (2015) 33:445–74. doi:10.1146/annurev-immunol-032414-112043

72. Speiser DE, Ho P-C, Verdeil G. Regulatory circuits of T cell function in cancer. *Nat Rev Immunol* (2016) 16(10):599–611. doi:10.1038/nri.2016.80

73. Mattner J, Wirtz S. Friend or foe? The ambiguous role of innate lymphoid cells in cancer development. *Trends Immunol* (2017) 38(1):29–38. doi:10.1016/j.it.2016.10.004

74. Kumar V, Patel S, Tcyganov E, Gabrilovich DI. The nature of myeloid-derived suppressor cells in the tumor microenvironment. *Trends Immunol* (2017) 37(3):208–20. doi:10.1016/j.it.2016.01.004

75. Mantovani A, Marchesi F, Malesci A, Laghi L, Allavena P. Tumour-associated macrophages as treatment targets in oncology. *Nat Rev Clin Oncol* (2017) 14(7):399–416. doi:10.1038/nrclinonc.2016.217

76. Wang H, Yang L, Wang D, Zhang Q, Zhang L. Pro-tumor activities of macrophages in the progression of melanoma. *Hum Vaccin Immunother* (2017) 25:1–7. doi:10.1080/21645515.2017.1312043

77. Robertson FC, Berzofsky JA, Terabe M. NKT cell networks in the regulation of tumor immunity. *Front Immunol* (2014) 5:543. doi:10.3389/fimmu.2014.00543

78. Klein L, Kyewski B, Allen PM, Hogquist KA. Positive and negative selection of the T cell repertoire: what thymocytes see (and don't see). *Nat Rev Immunol* (2014) 14(6):377–91. doi:10.1038/nri3667

79. Coulie PG, Van den Eynde BJ, van der Bruggen P, Boon T. Tumour antigens recognized by T lymphocytes: at the core of cancer immunotherapy. *Nat Rev Cancer* (2014) 14(2):135–46. doi:10.1038/nrc3670

80. De Plaen E, Lurquin C, Van Pel A, Mariame B, Szikora JP, Wolfel T, et al. Immunogenic (tum-) variants of mouse tumor P815: cloning of the gene of tum- antigen P91A and identification of the tum- mutation. *Proc Natl Acad Sci U S A* (1988) 85(7):2274–8. doi:10.1073/pnas.85.7.2274

81. van der Bruggen P, Traversari C, Chomez P, Lurquin C, De Plaen E, Van den Eynde B, et al. A gene encoding an antigen recognized by cytolytic T lymphocytes on a human melanoma. *Science* (1991) 254(5038):1643–7. doi:10.1126/science.1840703

82. Vigneron N. Human tumor antigens and cancer immunotherapy. *Biomed Res Int* (2015) 2015:948501. doi:10.1155/2015/948501

83. Yarchoan M, Johnson BA III, Lutz ER, Laheru DA, Jaffee EM. Targeting neoantigens to augment antitumour immunity. *Nat Rev Cancer* (2017) 17(4):209–22. doi:10.1038/nrc.2016.154

84. Desrichard A, Snyder A, Chan TA. Cancer neoantigens and applications for immunotherapy. *Clin Cancer Res* (2016) 22(4):807–12. doi:10.1158/1078-0432.CCR-14-3175

85. Yan M, Schwaederle M, Arguello D, Millis SZ, Gatalica Z, Kurzrock R. HER2 expression status in diverse cancers: review of results from 37,992 patients. *Cancer Metastasis Rev* (2015) 25(34):157–64. doi:10.1007/s10555-015-9552-6

86. Pitcovski J, Shahar E, Aizenshtein E, Gorodetsky R. Melanoma antigens and related immunological markers. *Crit Rev Oncol/Hematol* (2017) 15(115):36–49. doi:10.1016/j.critrevonc.2017.05.001

87. Wong KK, Li WA, Mooney DJ, Dranoff G. Advances in therapeutic cancer vaccines. *Adv Immunol* (2016) 130:191–249. doi:10.1016/bs.ai.2015.12.001

88. Hinrichs CS, Restifo NP. Reassessing target antigens for adoptive T-cell therapy. *Nat Biotechnol* (2013) 31(11):999–1008. doi:10.1038/nbt.2725

89. Hadrup S, Donia M, thor Straten P. Effector CD4 and CD8 T cells and their role in the tumor microenvironment. *Cancer Microenviron* (2013) 6(2):123–33. doi:10.1007/s12307-012-0127-6

90. Weon JL, Potts PR. The MAGE protein family and cancer. *Curr Opin Cell Biol* (2015) 37:1–8. doi:10.1016/j.ceb.2015.08.002

91. Sang M, Wang L, Ding C, Zhou X, Wang B, Wang L, et al. Melanoma-associated antigen genes – an update. *Cancer Lett* (2011) 302(2):85–90. doi:10.1016/j.canlet.2010.10.021

92. Saiag P, Gutzmer R, Ascierto PA, Maio M, Grob J-J, Murawa P, et al. Prospective assessment of a gene signature potentially predictive of clinical benefit in metastatic melanoma patients following MAGE-A3 immuno-therapeutic (PREDICT). *Ann Oncol* (2016) 27(10):1947–53. doi:10.1093/annonc/mdw291

93. Nicholaou T, Ebert L, Davis ID, Robson N, Klein O, Maraskovsky E, et al. Directions in the immune targeting of cancer: lessons learned from the cancer-testis Ag NY-ESO-1. *Immunol Cell Biol* (2006) 84(3):303–17. doi:10.1111/j.1440-1711.2006.01446.x

94. Aung PP, Liu Y-C, Ballester LY, Robbins PF, Rosenberg SA, Lee C-CR. Expression of NY-ESO-1 in primary and metastatic melanoma. *Hum Pathol* (2014) 45(2):259–67. doi:10.1016/j.humpath.2013.05.029

95. Adams S, O'Neill DW, Nonaka D, Hardin E, Chiriboga L, Siu K, et al. Immunization of malignant melanoma patients with full-length NY-ESO-1 protein using toll-like receptor 7 agonist imiquimod as vaccine adjuvant. *J Immunol* (2008) 181(1):776–84. doi:10.4049/jimmunol.181.1.776

96. Robbins PF, Kassim SH, Tran TLN, Crystal JS, Morgan RA, Feldman SA, et al. A pilot trial using lymphocytes genetically engineered with an NY-ESO-1-reactive T-cell receptor: long-term follow-up and correlates with response. *Clin Cancer Res* (2015) 21(5):1019–27. doi:10.1158/1078-0432.CCR-14-2708

97. Ramirez-Montagut T, Turk MJ, Wolchok JD, Guevara-Patino JA, Houghton AN. Immunity to melanoma: unraveling the relation of tumor immunity and autoimmunity. *Oncogene* (2003) 22(20):3180–7. doi:10.1038/sj.onc.1206462

98. Ghanem G, Fabrice J. Tyrosinase related protein 1 (TYRP1/gp75) in human cutaneous melanoma. *Mol Oncol* (2011) 5(2):150–5. doi:10.1016/j.molonc.2011.01.006

99. Weinstein D, Leininger J, Hamby C, Safai B. Diagnostic and prognostic biomarkers in melanoma. *J Clin Aesthet Dermatol* (2014) 7(6):13–24.

100. Wagner SN, Wagner C, Schultewolter T, Goos M. Analysis of Pmel17/gp100 expression in primary human tissue specimens: implications for melanoma immuno- and gene-therapy. *Cancer Immunol Immunother* (1997) 44(4):239–47. doi:10.1007/s002620050379

101. Kuzu OF, Nguyen FD, Noory MA, Sharma A. Current state of animal (mouse) modeling in melanoma research. *Cancer Growth Metastasis* (2015) 8 (Suppl 1):81–94. doi:10.4137/CGM.S21214

102. Klarquist JS, Janssen EM. Melanoma-infiltrating dendritic cells: limitations and opportunities of mouse models. *Oncoimmunology* (2012) 1(9):1584–93. doi:10.4161/onci.22660

103. Tarhini AA, Leng S, Moschos SJ, Yin Y, Sander C, Lin Y, et al. Safety and immunogenicity of vaccination with MART-1 (26-35, 27L), gp100 (209-217, 210M), and tyrosinase (368-376, 370D) in-adjuvant with PF-3512676 and GM-CSF in metastatic melanoma. *J Immunother* (2012) 35(4):359–66. doi:10.1097/CJI.0b013e31825481fe

104. Butterfield LH, Zhao F, Lee S, Tarhini AA, Margolin KA, White RL, et al. Immune correlates of GM-CSF and melanoma peptide vaccination in a randomized trial for the adjuvant therapy of resected high-risk melanoma (E4697). *Clin Cancer Res* (2017) 23(17):5034–43. doi:10.1158/1078-0432.CCR-16-3016

105. Kranz LM, Diken M, Haas H, Kreiter S, Loquai C, Reuter KC, et al. Systemic RNA delivery to dendritic cells exploits antiviral defence for cancer immunotherapy. *Nature* (2016) 534(7607):396–401. doi:10.1038/nature18300

106. Hanahan D, Weinberg RA. Hallmarks of cancer: the next generation. *Cell* (2011) 144:646–74. doi:10.1016/j.cell.2011.02.013

107. Tran Janco JM, Lamichhane P, Karyampudi L, Knutson KL. Tumor-infiltrating dendritic cells in cancer pathogenesis. *J Immunol* (2015) 194(7): 2985–91. doi:10.4049/jimmunol.1403134

108. Speiser DE, Utzschneider DT, Oberle SG, Munz C, Romero P, Zehn D. T cell differentiation in chronic infection and cancer: functional adaptation or exhaustion? *Nat Rev Immunol* (2014) 14(11):768–74. doi:10.1038/nri3740

109. Jiang Y, Li Y, Zhu B. T-cell exhaustion in the tumor microenvironment. *Cell Death Dis* (2015) 18(6):e1792. doi:10.1038/cddis.2015.162

110. Uppaluri R, Dunn GP, Lewis JS. Focus on TILs: prognostic significance of tumor infiltrating lymphocytes in head and neck cancers. *Cancer Immun* (2008) 8:16.

111. Fridman WH, Pagès F, Sautès-Fridman C, Galon J. The immune contexture in human tumours: impact on clinical outcome. *Nat Rev Cancer* (2012) 12(4):298–306. doi:10.1038/nrc3245

112. Takenaka M, Seki N, Toh U, Hattori S, Kawahara A, Yamaguchi T, et al. FOXP3 expression in tumor cells and tumor-infiltrating lymphocytes is associated with breast cancer prognosis. *Mol Clin Oncol* (2013) 1(4):625–32. doi:10.3892/mco.2013.107

113. Huang Y, Liao H, Zhang Y, Yuan R, Wang F, Gao Y, et al. Prognostic value of tumor-infiltrating FoxP3+ T cells in gastrointestinal cancers: a meta analysis. *PLoS One* (2014) 9(5):e94376. doi:10.1371/journal.pone.0094376

114. Lee N, Zakka LR, Mihm MC, Schatton T. Tumour-infiltrating lymphocytes in melanoma prognosis and cancer immunotherapy. *Pathology* (2016) 48(2):177–87. doi:10.1016/j.pathol.2015.12.006

115. Mihm MC, Mulé JJ. Reflections on the histopathology of tumor-infiltrating lymphocytes in melanoma and the host immune response. *Cancer Immunol Res* (2015) 3(8):827–35. doi:10.1158/2326-6066.CIR-15-0143

116. Weiss SA, Han SW, Lui K, Tchack J, Shapiro R, Berman R, et al. Immunologic heterogeneity of tumor-infiltrating lymphocyte composition in primary melanoma. *Hum Pathol* (2016) 57:116–25. doi:10.1016/j.humpath.2016.07.008

117. Galon J, Pagès F, Marincola FM, Angell HK, Thurin M, Lugli A, et al. Cancer classification using the immunoscore: a worldwide task force. *J Transl Med* (2012) 10:205. doi:10.1186/1479-5876-10-205

118. Capone M, Madonna G, Sebastiao N, Bird J, Ayala F, Caracò C, et al. Immunoscore: a new possible approach for melanoma classification. *J Immunother Cancer* (2014) 2(Suppl 3):193–193. doi:10.1186/2051-1426-2-S3-P193

119. Jones GW, Hill DG, Jones SA. Understanding immune cells in tertiary lymphoid organ development: it is all starting to come together. *Front Immunol* (2016) 7:401. doi:10.3389/fimmu.2016.00401

120. Sautès-Fridman C, Lawand M, Giraldo NA, Kaplon H, Germain C, Fridman WH, et al. Tertiary lymphoid structures in cancers: prognostic value, regulation, and manipulation for therapeutic intervention. *Front Immunol* (2016) 7:407. doi:10.3389/fimmu.2016.00407

121. Messina JL, Fenstermacher DA, Eschrich S, Qu X, Berglund AE, Lloyd MC, et al. 12-chemokine gene signature identifies lymph node-like structures in melanoma: potential for patient selection for immunotherapy? *Sci Rep* (2012) 2:765. doi:10.1038/srep00765

122. Melero I, Rouzaut A, Motz G, Coukos G. T-cell and NK-cell infiltration into solid tumors: a key limiting factor for efficacious cancer immunotherapy. *Cancer Discov* (2014) 4(5):522–6. doi:10.1158/2159-8290.CD-13-0985

123. Spranger S, Luke JJ, Bao R, Zha Y, Hernandez KM, Li Y, et al. Density of immunogenic antigens does not explain the presence or absence of the T-cell–inflamed tumor microenvironment in melanoma. *Proc Natl Acad Sci U S A* (2016) 113(48):E7759–68. doi:10.1073/pnas.1609376113

124. Shang B, Liu Y, Jiang S, Liu Y. Prognostic value of tumor-infiltrating FoxP3+ regulatory T cells in cancers: a systematic review and meta-analysis. *Sci Rep* (2015) 5:15179. doi:10.1038/srep15179

125. Ward-Hartstonge KA, Kemp RA. Regulatory T-cell heterogeneity and the cancer immune response. *Clin Transl Immunol* (2017) 6(9):e154. doi:10.1038/cti.2017.43

126. Saito T, Nishikawa H, Wada H, Nagano Y, Sugiyama D, Atarashi K, et al. Two FOXP3+CD4+ T cell subpopulations distinctly control the prognosis of colorectal cancers. *Nat Med* (2016) 22(6):679–84. doi:10.1038/nm.4086

127. Chiaruttini G, Mele S, Opzoomer J, Crescioli S, Ilieva KM, Lacy KE, et al. B cells and the humoral response in melanoma: the overlooked players of the tumor microenvironment. *Oncoimmunology* (2017) 6(4):e1294296. doi:10.1080/2162402X.2017.1294296

128. Zeng Q, Ng Y-H, Singh T, Jiang K, Sheriff KA, Ippolito R, et al. B cells mediate chronic allograft rejection independently of antibody production. *J Clin Invest* (2014) 124(3):1052–6. doi:10.1172/JCI70084

129. Mauri C, Menon M. The expanding family of regulatory B cells. *Int Immunol* (2015) 27(10):479–86. doi:10.1093/intimm/dxv038

130. Veglia F, Gabrilovich DI. Dendritic cells in cancer: the role revisited. *Curr Opin Immunol* (2017) 45:43–51. doi:10.1016/j.coi.2017.01.002

131. Segura E, Amigorena S. Inflammatory dendritic cells in mice and humans. *Trends Immunol* (2013) 34:440–5. doi:10.1016/j.it.2013.06.001

132. Radford KJ, Tullett KM, Lahoud MH. Dendritic cells and cancer immunotherapy. *Curr Opin Immunol* (2014) 27:26–32. doi:10.1016/j.coi.2014.01.005

133. Sabado RL, Balan S, Bhardwaj N. Dendritic cell-based immunotherapy. *Cell Res* (2017) 27:74–95. doi:10.1038/cr.2016.157

134. Vyas JM, Van der Veen AG, Ploegh HL. The known unknowns of antigen processing and presentation. *Nat Rev Immunol* (2008) 8(8):607–18. doi:10.1038/nri2368

135. Joffre OP, Segura E, Savina A, Amigorena S. Cross-presentation by dendritic cells. *Nat Rev Immunol* (2012) 12(8):557–69. doi:10.1038/nri3254

136. Segura E, Amigorena S. Cross-presentation in mouse and human dendritic cells. *Adv Immunol* (2015) 127:1–31. doi:10.1016/bs.ai.2015.03.002

137. Gardner A, Ruffell B. Dendritic cells and cancer immunity. *Trends Immunol* (2016) 37:855–65. doi:10.1016/j.it.2016.09.006

138. Hildner K, Edelson BT, Purtha WE, Diamond M, Matsushita H, Kohyama M, et al. Batf3 deficiency reveals a critical role for CD8alpha+ dendritic cells in cytotoxic T cell immunity. *Science* (2008) 322(5904):1097–100. doi:10.1126/science.1164206

139. Lombardi VC, Khaiboullina SF, Rizvanov AA. Plasmacytoid dendritic cells, a role in neoplastic prevention and progression. *Eur J Clin Invest* (2015) 45:1–8. doi:10.1111/eci.12363

140. Ma Y, Shurin GV, Peiyuan Z, Shurin MR. Dendritic cells in the cancer microenvironment. *J Cancer* (2013) 4:36–44. doi:10.7150/jca.5046

141. Chevalier N, Mueller M, Mougiakakos D, Ihorst G, Marks R, Schmitt-Graeff A, et al. Analysis of dendritic cell subpopulations in follicular lymphoma with respect to the tumor immune microenvironment. *Leuk Lymphoma* (2016) 57(9):2150–60. doi:10.3109/10428194.2015.1135432

142. Roberts EW, Broz ML, Binnewies M, Headley MB, Nelson AE, Wolf DM, et al. Critical role for CD103(+)/CD141(+) dendritic cells bearing CCR7 for tumor antigen trafficking and priming of T cell immunity in melanoma. *Cancer Cell* (2016) 30(2):324–36. doi:10.1016/j.ccell.2016.06.003

143. Aspord C, Leccia M-T, Charles J, Plumas J. Melanoma hijacks plasmacytoid dendritic cells to promote its own progression. *Oncoimmunology* (2014) 1(3):e27402. doi:10.4161/onci.27402

144. Pyfferoen L, Brabants E, Everaert C, De Cabooter N, Heyns K, Deswarte K, et al. The transcriptome of lung tumor-infiltrating dendritic cells reveals a tumor-supporting phenotype and a microRNA signature with negative impact on clinical outcome. *Oncoimmunology* (2017) 6(1):e1253655. doi:10.1080/2162402X.2016.1253655

145. Palucka K, Banchereau J. Dendritic-cell-based therapeutic cancer vaccines. *Immunity* (2013) 39:38–48. doi:10.1016/j.immuni.2013.07.004

146. Redelman-Sidi G, Glickman MS, Bochner BH. The mechanism of action of BCG therapy for bladder cancer – a current perspective. *Nat Rev Urol* (2014) 11(3):153–62. doi:10.1038/nrurol.2014.15

147. Tacken PJ, Figdor CG. Targeted antigen delivery and activation of dendritic cells in vivo: steps towards cost effective vaccines. *Semin Immunol* (2011) 23:12–20. doi:10.1016/j.smim.2011.01.001

148. Lehmann CHK, Heger L, Heidkamp GF, Baranska A, Lühr JJ, Hoffmann A, et al. Direct delivery of antigens to dendritic cells via antibodies specific for endocytic receptors as a promising strategy for future therapies. *Vaccines (Basel)* (2016) 4(2):8. doi:10.3390/vaccines4020008

149. Apostolopoulos V, Pietersz GA, Tsibanis A, Tsikkinis A, Stojanovska L, McKenzie IFC, et al. Dendritic cell immunotherapy: clinical outcomes. *Clin Trans Immunol* (2014) 18(3):e21. doi:10.1038/cti.2014.14

150. Woo S-R, Fuertes MB, Corrales L, Spranger S, Furdyna MJ, Leung MYK, et al. STING-dependent cytosolic DNA sensing mediates innate immune recognition of immunogenic tumors. *Immunity* (2014) 41(5):830–42. doi:10.1016/j.immuni.2014.10.017

151. Demaria O, De Gassart A, Coso S, Gestermann N, Di Domizio J, Flatz L, et al. STING activation of tumor endothelial cells initiates spontaneous and therapeutic antitumor immunity. *Proc Natl Acad Sci* (2015) 112(50):15408–13. doi:10.1073/pnas.1512832112

152. Wang H, Hu S, Chen X, Shi H, Chen C, Sun L, et al. cGAS is essential for the antitumor effect of immune checkpoint blockade. *Proc Natl Acad Sci U S A* (2017) 114(7):1637–42. doi:10.1073/pnas.1621363114

153. Cai X, Chiu Y-H, Chen ZJ. The cGAS-cGAMP-STING pathway of cytosolic DNA sensing and signaling. *Mol Cell* (2014) 54(2):289–96. doi:10.1016/j.molcel.2014.03.040

154. Schenk M, Krutzik SR, Sieling PA, Lee DJ, Teles RMB, Ochoa MT, et al. NOD2 triggers an interleukin-32-dependent human dendritic cell program in leprosy. *Nat Med* (2012) 18(4):555–63. doi:10.1038/nm.2650

155. Larsen SK, Gao Y, Basse PH. NK cells in the tumor microenvironment. *Crit Rev Oncog* (2014) 19(0):91–105. doi:10.1615/CritRevOncog.2014011142

156. Morvan MG, Lanier LL. NK cells and cancer: you can teach innate cells new tricks. *Nat Rev Cancer* (2016) 16(1):7–19. doi:10.1038/nrc.2015.5

157. Tarazona R, Duran E, Solana R. Natural killer cell recognition of melanoma: new clues for a more effective immunotherapy. *Front Immunol* (2015) 7(6):649. doi:10.3389/fimmu.2015.00649

158. Ali TH, Pisanti S, Ciaglia E, Mortarini R, Anichini A, Garofalo C, et al. Enrichment of CD56dimKIR+CD57+ highly cytotoxic NK cells in tumour-infiltrated lymph nodes of melanoma patients. *Nat Com* (2014) 5:5639. doi:10.1038/ncomms6639

159. Levi I, Amsalem H, Nissan A, Darash-Yahana M, Peretz T, Mandelboim O, et al. Characterization of tumor infiltrating natural killer cell subset. *Oncotarget* (2015) 6(15):13835–43. doi:10.18632/oncotarget.3453

160. Topalian SL, Drake CG, Pardoll DM. Immune checkpoint blockade: a common denominator approach to cancer therapy. *Cancer Cell* (2015) 27(4):450–61. doi:10.1016/j.ccell.2015.03.001

161. Farkona S, Diamandis EP, Blasutig IM. Cancer immunotherapy: the beginning of the end of cancer? *BMC Med* (2016) 14(1):73. doi:10.1186/s12916-016-0623-5

162. Sharma P, Hu-Lieskovan S, Wargo JA, Ribas A. Primary, adaptive, and acquired resistance to cancer immunotherapy. *Cell* (2017) 168(4):707–23. doi:10.1016/j.cell.2017.01.017

163. Drake CG, Lipson EJ, Brahmer JR. Breathing new life into immunotherapy: review of melanoma, lung and kidney cancer. *Nat Rev Clin Oncol* (2014) 11(1):24–37. doi:10.1038/nrclinonc.2013.208

164. Schweizer MT, Drake CG. Immunotherapy for prostate cancer: recent developments and future challenges. *Cancer Metastasis Rev* (2014) 33:641–55. doi:10.1007/s10555-013-9479-8

165. van der Burg SH, Arens R, Ossendorp F, van Hall T, Melief CJM. Vaccines for established cancer: overcoming the challenges posed by immune evasion. *Nat Rev Cancer* (2016) 16(4):219–33. doi:10.1038/nrc.2016.16

166. Scott AM, Wolchok JD, Old LJ. Antibody therapy of cancer. *Nat Rev Cancer* (2012) 12(4):278–87. doi:10.1038/nrc3236

167. Baumeister SH, Freeman GJ, Dranoff G, Sharpe AH. Coinhibitory pathways in immunotherapy for cancer. *Annu Rev Immunol* (2016) 34(1):539–73. doi:10.1146/annurev-immunol-032414-112049

168. Zou W, Wolchok JD, Chen L. PD-L1 (B7-H1) and PD-1 pathway blockade for cancer therapy: mechanisms, response biomarkers, and combinations. *Sci Transl Med* (2016) 8(328):328rv4. doi:10.1126/scitranslmed.aad7118

169. Iwai Y, Hamanishi J, Chamoto K, Honjo T. Cancer immunotherapies targeting the PD-1 signaling pathway. *J Biomed Sci* (2017) 24(1):26. doi:10.1186/s12929-017-0329-9

170. Chester C, Ambulkar S, Kohrt HE. 4-1BB agonism: adding the accelerator to cancer immunotherapy. *Cancer Immunol Immunother* (2016) 65:1243–8. doi:10.1007/s00262-016-1829-2

171. Adusumilli PS, Cha E, Cornfeld M, Davis T, Diab A, Dubensky TW, et al. New cancer immunotherapy agents in development: a report from an associated program of the 31stAnnual Meeting of the Society for Immunotherapy of Cancer, 2016. *J Immunother Cancer* (2017) 5(1):50. doi:10.1186/s40425-017-0253-2

172. Yang JC, Rosenberg SA. Adoptive T-cell therapy for cancer. *Adv Immunol* (2016) 130:279–94. doi:10.1016/bs.ai.2015.12.006

173. Baruch EN, Berg AL, Besser MJ, Schachter J, Markel G. Adoptive T cell therapy: an overview of obstacles and opportunities. *Cancer* (2017) 123(S11):2154–62. doi:10.1002/cncr.30491

174. Constantino J, Gomes C, Falcão A, Cruz MT, Neves BM. Antitumor dendritic cell–based vaccines: lessons from 20 years of clinical trials and future perspectives. *Transl Res* (2016) 168:74–95. doi:10.1016/j.trsl.2015.07.008

175. Lipson EJ, Sharfman WH, Chen S, McMiller TL, Pritchard TS, Salas JT, et al. Safety and immunologic correlates of Melanoma GVAX, a GM-CSF secreting allogeneic melanoma cell vaccine administered in the adjuvant setting. *J Transl Med* (2015) 13:214. doi:10.1186/s12967-015-0572-3

176. Melief CJM, van Hall T, Arens R, Ossendorp F, van der Burg SH. Therapeutic cancer vaccines. *J Clin Invest* (2015) 125(9):3401–12. doi:10.1172/JCI80009

177. Rehman H, Silk AW, Kane MP, Kaufman HL. Into the clinic: talimogene laherparepvec (T-VEC), a first-in-class intratumoral oncolytic viral therapy. *J Immunother Cancer* (2016) 4(1):53. doi:10.1186/s40425-016-0158-5

178. Andtbacka RHI, Kaufman HL, Collichio F, Amatruda T, Senzer N, Chesney J, et al. Talimogene laherparepvec improves durable response rate in patients with advanced melanoma. *J Clin Oncol* (2015) 33(25):2780–8. doi:10.1200/JCO.2014.58.3377

179. Amaria RN, Reuben A, Cooper ZA, Wargo JA. Update on use of aldesleukin for treatment of high-risk metastatic melanoma. *Immunotargets Ther* (2015) 7(4):79–89. doi:10.2147/ITT.S61590

180. Boyman O, Sprent J. The role of interleukin-2 during homeostasis and activation of the immune system. *Nat Rev Immunol* (2012) 12(3):180–90. doi:10.1038/nri3156

181. Parker BS, Rautela J, Hertzog PJ. Antitumour actions of interferons: implications for cancer therapy. *Nat Rev Cancer* (2016) 16(3):131–44. doi:10.1038/nrc.2016.14

182. Pestka S, Krause CD, Walter MR. Interferons, interferon-like cytokines, and their receptors. *Immunol Rev* (2004) 202:8–32. doi:10.1111/j.0105-2896.2004.00204.x

183. Rosenberg SA. Decade in review[mdash]cancer immunotherapy: entering the mainstream of cancer treatment. *Nat Rev Clin Oncol* (2014) 11(11): 630–2. doi:10.1038/nrclinonc.2014.174

184. Rosenberg SA, Mule JJ, Spiess PJ, Reichert CM, Schwarz SL. Regression of established pulmonary metastases and subcutaneous tumor mediated by the systemic administration of high-dose recombinant interleukin 2. *J Exp Med* (1985) 161(5):1169–88. doi:10.1084/jem.161.5.1169

185. Atkins MB, Lotze MT, Dutcher JP, Fisher RI, Weiss G, Margolin K, et al. High-dose recombinant interleukin 2 therapy for patients with metastatic melanoma: analysis of 270 patients treated between 1985 and 1993. *J Clin Oncol* (1999) 17(7):2105–16. doi:10.1200/JCO.1999.17.7.2105

186. Rosenberg SA, Packard BS, Aebersold PM, Solomon D, Topalian SL, Toy ST, et al. Use of tumor-infiltrating lymphocytes and interleukin-2 in the immunotherapy of patients with metastatic melanoma. *N Engl J Med* (1988) 319(25):1676–80. doi:10.1056/NEJM198812223192527

187. Hodi FS, O'Day SJ, McDermott DF, Weber RW, Sosman JA, Haanen JB, et al. Improved survival with ipilimumab in patients with metastatic melanoma. *N Engl J Med* (2010) 363(8):711–23. doi:10.1056/NEJMoa1003466

188. Topalian SL, Hodi FS, Brahmer JR, Gettinger SN, Smith DC, McDermott DF, et al. Safety, activity, and immune correlates of anti-PD-1 antibody in cancer. *N Engl J Med* (2012) 366(26):2443–54. doi:10.1056/NEJMoa1200690

189. Robert C, Long GV, Brady B, Dutriaux C, Maio M, Mortier L, et al. Nivolumab in previously untreated melanoma without BRAF mutation. *N Engl J Med* (2015) 372(4):320–30. doi:10.1056/NEJMoa1412082

190. Omid H, Caroline R, Adil D, Stephen HF, Wen-Jen H, Richard K, et al. Safety and tumor responses with lambrolizumab (anti–PD-1) in melanoma. *N Engl J Med* (2013) 369:134–44. doi:10.1056/NEJMoa1305133

191. Brahmer JR, Tykodi SS, Chow LQM, Hwu W-J, Topalian SL, Hwu P, et al. Safety and activity of anti-PD-L1 antibody in patients with advanced cancer. *N Engl J Med* (2012) 366(26):2455–65. doi:10.1056/NEJMoa1200694

192. Pitt JM, Vétizou M, Daillère R, Roberti MP, Yamazaki T, Routy B, et al. Resistance mechanisms to immune-checkpoint blockade in cancer: tumor-intrinsic and -extrinsic factors. *Immunity* (2016) 44(6):1255–69. doi:10.1016/j.immuni.2016.06.001

193. Michot JM, Bigenwald C, Champiat S, Collins M, Carbonnel F, Postel-Vinay S, et al. Immune-related adverse events with immune checkpoint blockade: a comprehensive review. *Eur J Cancer* (2016) 54:139–48. doi:10.1016/j.ejca.2015.11.016

194. Topalian SL, Taube JM, Anders RA, Pardoll DM. Mechanism-driven biomarkers to guide immune checkpoint blockade in cancer therapy. *Nat Rev Cancer* (2016) 16(5):275–87. doi:10.1038/nrc.2016.36%5Cn

195. Postow MA, Callahan MK, Wolchok JD. Immune checkpoint blockade in cancer therapy. *J Clin Oncol* (2015) 33(17):1974–82. doi:10.1200/JCO.2014.59.4358

196. Gardner D, Jeffery LE, Sansom DM. Understanding the CD28/CTLA-4 (CD152) pathway and its implications for costimulatory blockade. *Am J Transplant* (2014) 14(9):1985–91. doi:10.1111/ajt.12834

197. Dustin ML, Choudhuri K. Signaling and polarized communication across the T cell immunological synapse. *Annu Rev Cell Dev Biol* (2016) 32(1): 303–25. doi:10.1146/annurev-cellbio-100814-125330

198. Malek TR, Bayer AL. Tolerance, not immunity, crucially depends on IL-2. *Nat Rev Immunol* (2004) 4(9):665–74. doi:10.1038/nri1435

199. Gutcher I, Becher B. APC-derived cytokines and T cell polarization in autoimmune inflammation. *J Clin Invest* (2007) 117(5):1119–27. doi:10.1172/JCI31720

200. Postow MA, Callahan MK, Wolchok JD. The antitumor immunity of ipilimumab: (T-cell) memories to last a lifetime? *Clin Cancer Res* (2012) 18(7):1821–3. doi:10.1158/1078-0432.CCR-12-0409

201. Tivol EA, Borriello F, Schweitzer AN, Lynch WP, Bluestone JA, Sharpe AH. Loss of CTLA-4 leads to massive lymphoproliferation and fatal multiorgan tissue destruction, revealing a critical negative regulatory role of CTLA-4. *Immunity* (1995) 3(5):541–7. doi:10.1016/1074-7613(95)90125-6

202. Gulley JL, Repasky EA, Wood LS, Butterfield LH. Highlights of the 31st annual meeting of the society for immunotherapy of cancer (SITC), 2016. *J Immunother Cancer* (2017) 5(1):55. doi:10.1186/s40425-017-0262-1

203. Okazaki T, Chikuma S, Iwai Y, Fagarasan S, Honjo T. A rheostat for immune responses: the unique properties of PD-1 and their advantages for clinical application. *Nat Immunol* (2013) 14(12):1212–8. doi:10.1038/ni.2762

204. Nishimura H, Nose M, Hiai H, Minato N, Honjo T. Development of lupus-like autoimmune diseases by disruption of the PD-1 gene encoding an ITIM motif-carrying immunoreceptor. *Immunity* (1999) 11:141–51. doi:10.1016/S1074-7613(00)80089-8

205. Nishimura H, Okazaki T, Tanaka Y, Nakatani K, Hara M, Matsumori A, et al. Autoimmune dilated cardiomyopathy in PD-1 receptor-deficient mice. *Science* (2001) 291:319–22. doi:10.1126/science.291.5502.319

206. Lau J, Cheung J, Navarro A, Lianoglou S, Haley B, Totpal K, et al. Tumour and host cell PD-L1 is required to mediate suppression of anti-tumour immunity in mice. *Nat Commun* (2017) 21(8):14572. doi:10.1038/ncomms14572

207. Ribas A, Puzanov I, Dummer R, Schadendorf D, Hamid O, Robert C, et al. Pembrolizumab versus investigator-choice chemotherapy for ipilimumab-refractory melanoma (KEYNOTE-002): a randomised, controlled, phase 2 trial. *Lancet Oncol* (2015) 16(8):908–18. doi:10.1016/S1470-2045(15)00083-2

208. Robert C, Schachter J, Long GV, Arance A, Grob JJ, Mortier L, et al. Pembrolizumab versus ipilimumab in advanced melanoma. *N Engl J Med* (2015) 372(26):2521–32. doi:10.1056/NEJMoa1503093

209. Powles T, Eder JP, Fine GD, Braiteh FS, Loriot Y, Cruz C. MPDL3280A (anti-PD-L1) treatment leads to clinical activity in metastatic bladder cancer. *Nature* (2014) 515(7528):558–62. doi:10.1038/nature13904

210. Park JJ, Omiya R, Matsumura Y, Sakoda Y, Kuramasu A, Augustine MM, et al. B7-H1/CD80 interaction is required for the induction and maintenance of peripheral T-cell tolerance. *Blood* (2010) 116(8):1291–8. doi:10.1182/blood-2010-01-265975

211. Teng MWL, Ngiow SF, Ribas A, Smyth MJ. Classifying cancers based on T cell infiltration and PD-L1. *Cancer Res* (2015) 75(11):2139–45. doi:10.1158/0008-5472.CAN-15-0255

212. Spranger S. Mechanisms of tumor escape in the context of the T-cell-inflamed and the non-T-cell-inflamed tumor microenvironment. *Int Immunol* (2016) 28(8):383–91. doi:10.1093/intimm/dxw014

213. Sindoni A, Minutoli F, Ascenti G, Pergolizzi S. Combination of immune checkpoint inhibitors and radiotherapy: review of the literature. *Crit Rev Oncol Hematol* (2017) 113:63–70. doi:10.1016/j.critrevonc.2017.03.003

214. Gotwals P, Cameron S, Cipolletta D, Cremasco V, Crystal A, Hewes B, et al. Prospects for combining targeted and conventional cancer therapy with immunotherapy. *Nat Rev Cancer* (2017) 17(5):286–301. doi:10.1038/nrc.2017.17

215. Luke JJ, Flaherty KT, Ribas A, Long GV. Targeted agents and immunotherapies: optimizing outcomes in melanoma. *Nat Rev Clin Oncol* (2017) 14(8):463–82. doi:10.1038/nrclinonc.2017.43

216. Postow MA, Chesney J, Pavlick AC, Robert C, Grossmann K, McDermott D, et al. Nivolumab and ipilimumab versus ipilimumab in untreated melanoma. *N Engl J Med* (2015) 372(21):2006–17. doi:10.1056/NEJMoa1414428

217. Larkin J, Chiarion-Sileni V, Gonzalez R, Grob JJ, Cowey CL, Lao CD, et al. Combined nivolumab and ipilimumab or monotherapy in untreated melanoma. *N Engl J Med* (2015) 337(1):23–34. doi:10.1056/NEJMoa1504030

218. Swart M, Verbrugge I, Beltman JB. Combination approaches with immune-checkpoint blockade in cancer therapy. *Front Oncol* (2016) 6:233. doi:10.3389/fonc.2016.00233

219. Tsai H-F, Hsu P-N. Cancer immunotherapy by targeting immune checkpoints: mechanism of T cell dysfunction in cancer immunity and new therapeutic targets. *J Biomed Sci* (2017) 24(1):35. doi:10.1186/s12929-017-0341-0

220. Joller N, Lozano E, Burkett PR, Patel B, Xiao S, Zhu C, et al. Treg cells expressing the coinhibitory molecule TIGIT selectively inhibit proinflammatory Th1 and Th17 cell responses. *Immunity* (2014) 40(4):569–81. doi:10.1016/j.immuni.2014.02.012

221. Manieri NA, Chiang EY, Grogan JL. TIGIT: a key inhibitor of the cancer immunity cycle. *Trends Immunol* (2016) 38(1):20–8. doi:10.1016/j.it.2016.10.002

222. Chruscinski A, Sadozai H, Rojas-Luengas V, Bartczak A, Khattar R, Selzner N, et al. Role of regulatory T cells (Treg) and the Treg effector molecule fibrinogen-like protein 2 in alloimmunity and autoimmunity. *Rambam Maimonides Med J* (2015) 6(3):e0024. doi:10.5041/RMMJ.10209

223. Chauvin J-M, Pagliano O, Fourcade J, Sun Z, Wang H, Sander C, et al. TIGIT and PD-1 impair tumor antigen-specific CD8⁺ T cells in melanoma patients. *J Clin Invest* (2015) 125(5):2046–58. doi:10.1172/JCI80445

224. Becht E, Giraldo NA, Dieu-Nosjean M-C, Sautès-Fridman C, Fridman WH. Cancer immune contexture and immunotherapy. *Curr Opin Immunol* (2016) 39:7–13. doi:10.1016/j.coi.2015.11.009

225. Hinrichs CS, Rosenberg SA. Exploiting the curative potential of adoptive T-cell therapy for cancer. *Immunol Rev* (2014) 257(1):56–71. doi:10.1111/imr.12132

226. Rosenberg SA, Yang JC, Sherry RM, Kammula US, Hughes MS, Phan GQ, et al. Durable complete responses in heavily pretreated patients with metastatic melanoma using T-cell transfer immunotherapy. *Clin Cancer Res* (2011) 17(13):4550–7. doi:10.1158/1078-0432.CCR-11-0116

227. Radvanyi LG, Bernatchez C, Zhang M, Fox PS, Miller P, Chacon J, et al. Specific lymphocyte subsets predict response to adoptive cell therapy using expanded autologous tumor-infiltrating lymphocytes in metastatic melanoma patients. *Clin Cancer Res* (2012) 15(1824):6758–70. doi:10.1158/1078-0432.CCR-12-1177

228. Pilon-Thomas S, Kuhn L, Ellwanger S, Janssen W, Royster E, Marzban S, et al. Brief communication: efficacy of adoptive cell transfer of tumor infiltrating lymphocytes after lymphopenia induction for metastatic melanoma. *J Immunother* (2012) 35(8):615–20. doi:10.1097/CJI.0b013e31826e8f5f

229. Fesnak AD, June CH, Levine BL. Engineered T cells: the promise and challenges of cancer immunotherapy. *Nat Rev Cancer* (2016) 16(9):566–81. doi:10.1038/nrc.2016.97

230. Morgan RA, Dudley ME, Wunderlich JR, Hughes MS, Yang JC, Sherry RM, et al. Cancer regression in patients after transfer of genetically

231. engineered lymphocytes. *Science* (2006) 314(5796):126–9. doi:10.1126/science.1129003

231. Chodon T, Comin-Anduix B, Chmielowski B, Koya RC, Wu Z, Auerbach M, et al. Adoptive transfer of MART-1 T-cell receptor transgenic lymphocytes and dendritic cell vaccination in patients with metastatic melanoma. *Clin Cancer Res* (2014) 20(9):2457–65. doi:10.1158/1078-0432.CCR-13-3017

232. Johnson LA, Morgan RA, Dudley ME, Cassard L, Yang JC, Hughes MS, et al. Gene therapy with human and mouse T-cell receptors mediates cancer regression and targets normal tissues expressing cognate antigen. *Blood* (2009) 114(3):535–46. doi:10.1182/blood-2009-03-211714

233. Lamers CH, Sleijfer S, van Steenbergen S, van Elzakker P, van Krimpen B, Groot C, et al. Treatment of metastatic renal cell carcinoma with CAIX CAR-engineered T cells: clinical evaluation and management of on-target toxicity. *Mol Ther* (2013) 21(4):904–12. doi:10.1038/mt.2013.17

234. Klinger M, Benjamin J, Kischel R, Stienen S, Zugmaier G. Harnessing T cells to fight cancer with BiTE® antibody constructs – past developments and future directions. *Immunol Rev* (2016) 270(1):193–208. doi:10.1111/imr.12393

235. Schwartzentruber DJ, Lawson DH, Richards JM, Conry RM, Miller DM, Treisman J, et al. gp100 peptide vaccine and interleukin-2 in patients with advanced melanoma. *N Engl J Med* (2011) 364(22):2119–27. doi:10.1056/NEJMoa1012863

236. Merad M, Sathe P, Helft J, Miller J, Mortha A. The dendritic cell lineage: ontogeny and function of dendritic cells and their subsets in the steady state and the inflamed setting. *Annu Rev Immunol* (2013) 31:563–604. doi:10.1146/annurev-immunol-020711-074950

237. Bol KF, Schreibelt G, Gerritsen WR, De Vries IJM, Figdor CG. Dendritic cell-based immunotherapy: state of the art and beyond. *Clin Cancer Res* (2016) 22(8):1897–906. doi:10.1158/1078-0432.CCR-15-1399

238. Schreibelt G, Benitez-Ribas D, Schuurhuis D, Lambeck AJA, Van Hout-Kuijer M, Schaft N, et al. Commonly used prophylactic vaccines as an alternative for synthetically produced TLR ligands to mature monocyte-derived dendritic cells. *Blood* (2010) 116(4):564–74. doi:10.1182/blood-2009-11-251884

239. Bol KF, Aarntzen EHJG, Pots JM, Olde Nordkamp MAM, van de Rakt MWMM, Scharenborg NM, et al. Prophylactic vaccines are potent activators of monocyte-derived dendritic cells and drive effective anti-tumor responses in melanoma patients at the cost of toxicity. *Cancer Immunol Immunother* (2016) 65(3):327–39. doi:10.1007/s00262-016-1796-7

240. Simons JW, Sacks N. Granulocyte-macrophage colony-stimulating factor-transduced allogeneic cancer cellular immunotherapy: the GVAX vaccine for prostate cancer. *Urol Oncol* (2006) 24:419–24. doi:10.1016/j.urolonc.2005.08.021

241. Jinushi M, Tahara H. Cytokine gene-mediated immunotherapy: current status and future perspectives. *Cancer Sci* (2009) 100:1389–96. doi:10.1111/j.1349-7006.2009.01202.x

242. Carreno BM, Becker-Hapak M, Huang A, Chan M, Alyasiry A, Lie WR, et al. IL-12p70-producing patient DC vaccine elicits Tc1-polarized immunity. *J Clin Invest* (2013) 123(8):3383–94. doi:10.1172/JCI68395

243. Diaz-Montero CM, Salem ML, Nishimura MI, Garrett-Mayer E, Cole DJ, Montero AJ. Increased circulating myeloid-derived suppressor cells correlate with clinical cancer stage, metastatic tumor burden, and doxorubicin-cyclophosphamide chemotherapy. *Cancer Immunol Immunother* (2009) 58:49–59. doi:10.1007/s00262-008-0523-4

244. Guillerey C, Huntington ND, Smyth MJ. Targeting natural killer cells in cancer immunotherapy. *Nat Immunol* (2016) 17(9):1025–36. doi:10.1038/ni.3518

245. Toy R, Roy K. Engineering nanoparticles to overcome barriers to immunotherapy. *Bioeng Transl Med* (2016) 1(1):47–62. doi:10.1002/btm2.10005

246. Fontana F, Liu D, Hirvonen J, Santos HA. Delivery of therapeutics with nanoparticles: what's new in cancer immunotherapy? *Wiley Interdiscip Rev Nanomed Nanobiotechnol* (2017) 9(1):e1421. doi:10.1002/wnan.1421

247. Shi J, Kantoff PW, Wooster R, Farokhzad OC. Cancer nanomedicine: progress, challenges and opportunities. *Nat Rev Cancer* (2017) 17(1):20–37. doi:10.1038/nrc.2016.108

248. Shao K, Singha S, Clemente-Casares X, Tsai S, Yang Y, Santamaria P. Nanoparticle-based immunotherapy for cancer. *ACS Nano* (2015) 9(1):16–30. doi:10.1021/nn5062029

249. Conniot J, Silva JM, Fernandes JG, Silva LC, Gaspar R, Brocchini S, et al. Cancer immunotherapy: nanodelivery approaches for immune cell

targeting and tracking. *Front Chem* (2014) 2(November):105. doi:10.3389/fchem.2014.00105

250. Park J, Wrzesinski SH, Stern E, Look M, Criscione J, Ragheb R, et al. Combination delivery of TGF-β inhibitor and IL-2 by nanoscale liposomal polymeric gels enhances tumour immunotherapy. *Nat Mater* (2012) 11(10):895–905. doi:10.1038/nmat3355

251. Koshy ST, Cheung AS, Gu L, Graveline AR, Mooney DJ. Liposomal delivery enhances immune activation by STING agonists for cancer immunotherapy. *Adv Biosyst* (2017) 1(1–2):1600013. doi:10.1002/adbi.201600013

252. Shi G-N, Zhang C-N, Xu R, Niu J-F, Song H-J, Zhang X-Y, et al. Enhanced antitumor immunity by targeting dendritic cells with tumor cell lysate-loaded chitosan nanoparticles vaccine. *Biomaterials* (2017) 113:191–202. doi:10.1016/j.biomaterials.2016.10.047

253. Smyth MJ, Ngiow SF, Ribas A, Teng MWL. Combination cancer immunotherapies tailored to the tumour microenvironment. *Nat Rev Clin Oncol* (2016) 13(3):143–58. doi:10.1038/nrclinonc.2015.209

254. Bahcall O. Precision medicine. *Nature* (2015) 526(7573):335–335. doi:10.1038/526335a

255. Chen DS, Mellman I. Elements of cancer immunity and the cancer-immune set point. *Nature* (2017) 541(7637):321–30. doi:10.1038/nature21349

256. Mardis ER. Next-generation sequencing platforms. *Annu Rev Anal Chem* (2013) 6:287–303. doi:10.1146/annurev-anchem-062012-092628

257. Dempsey LA. CyTOF analysis of anti-tumor responses. *Nat Immunol* (2017) 18(3):254–254. doi:10.1038/ni.3701

258. Min S, Lee B, Yoon S. Deep learning in bioinformatics. *Brief Bioinform* (2016) 18(5):851–69. doi:10.1093/bib/bbw068

5

Continued Chemotherapy After Concurrent Chemoradiotherapy Improves Treatment Outcomes for Unresectable Cutaneous Squamous Cell Carcinoma: An Analysis of 13 Cases

Azusa Hiura[1]*, Koji Yoshino[1], Takuya Maeda[1], Kojiro Nagai[1], Satoe Oaku[1], Chisato Yamashita[1], Megumi Kato[1], Jiro Uehara[1] and Yasuhiro Fujisawa[2]

[1] Department of Dermatologic Oncology, Tokyo Metropolitan Cancer and Infectious Diseases Center Komagome Hospital, Tokyo, Japan, [2] Department of Dermatology, University of Tsukuba, Tsukuba, Japan

*Correspondence:
Azusa Hiura
azukiazusazzzzz@yahoo.co.jp

Background: There is no standard systemic therapy for unresectable cutaneous squamous cell carcinoma (ucSCC), although various chemotherapy regimens have been reported. In our department, concurrent chemoradiotherapy (CCRT) for ucSCC resulted in a 1-year survival rate similar to that of resectable cutaneous squamous cell carcinoma (cSCC). Treatment involves continued chemotherapy after CCRT. Here, we report the importance of continued chemotherapy after CCRT, based on treatment outcomes.

Patients and Methods: We retrospectively evaluated 13 patients with ucSCC, assessing the overall survival, overall response rate (ORR), and disease control rate (DCR).

Results: CCRT with continued chemotherapy resulted in an ORR of 84.6%, DCR of 92.3%, and 1-year survival rate of 75%. Of the 13 patients treated with CCRT with continued chemotherapy, 6 had no metastasis. The remaining 7 patients developed metastasis to other organs or lymph nodes beyond the regional lymph nodes, although most sites of metastasis were outside the irradiation area.

Conclusion: We conclude that CCRT with continued chemotherapy was effective in treating the irradiation site (primary lesion and regional lymph nodes) and any organ metastasis, although, it is unclear for how long the treatment remains effective.

Keywords: concurrent chemoradiotherapy (CCRT), low-dose cisplatin and 5-fluorouracil, overall response rate, OS, disease control rates, 1-year survival rate, continued chemotherapy, unresectable cutaneous squamous cell carcinoma (ucSCC)

INTRODUCTION

Cutaneous squamous cell carcinoma (cSCC) is the second most common type of non-melanoma skin cancer (1). We consider surgery as an option for treating cSCC during the early stages, but exclude surgical excision as a treatment option for unresectable cSCC (ucSCC) in advanced stages. We define ucSCC as an unresectable case of either the primary site and/or regional lymph nodes (2–6). Currently, there is no standard treatment for ucSCC, although various chemotherapy regimens have been reported.

In our department, concurrent chemoradiotherapy (CCRT) is performed for ucSCC. Chemotherapy and radiotherapy (RT) begin after surgical excision. If either the primary site or regional lymph nodes are unresectable, RT is performed.

We mainly administer chemotherapy regimens of low-dose cisplatin and 5-fluorouracil (low-dose FP) or carboplatin and 5-fluorouracil (FP') (7). In addition, in our department, we continue chemotherapy if the tumor clearly remains at the primary site and/or regional lymph nodes after CCRT.

The treatment outcomes and 1-year survival rates of CCRT for stage IV cSCC in our department are not significantly different from the outcomes for surgical excision cases and unresectable cases with CCRT with continued chemotherapy (8). Here, we report the importance of continued chemotherapy after CCRT.

METHODS

Staging of cSCC was performed using the TNM classification (8th UICC) (9). The first-line treatment for cSCC was determined on the basis of whether the primary site and regional lymph nodes were resectable. If the primary site and regional lymph nodes were resectable, surgical excision was performed. If the primary site and/or regional lymph nodes were not resectable, CCRT was performed. If surgical excision of the regional lymph nodes was difficult, we surgically excised the primary site, and treated the regional lymph nodes with CCRT. If surgical excision of the primary site was difficult, we surgically excised the regional lymph nodes and treated the primary site by CCRT. Patients who had a performance status score ≥3 were not selected for CCRT, and instead underwent RT monotherapy and palliative treatment (**Figure 1**). No patients underwent chemotherapy monotherapy as a first-line therapy in our department.

The study included 13 patients who were diagnosed with ucSCC and who underwent CCRT with continued chemotherapy. RT irradiation was performed at the primary site

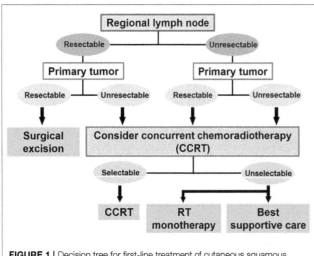

FIGURE 1 | Decision tree for first-line treatment of cutaneous squamous cell carcinoma.

and/or regional lymph nodes. The radiation dose was ≥50 Gy. In addition, for chemotherapy during CCRT, we used low-dose FP [(days 1–5) 15 mg/m2 cisplatin plus 800 mg/m2 5-fluorouracil; every 4 weeks] or FP' [(day 1) carboplatin area under the blood concentration-time curve (AUC): 5 (days 1–5) 600 mg/m2 5-fluorouracil; every 4 weeks]. We administered FP' in renal dysfunction cases.

Clinical data included age, sex, primary tumor site, metastasis site, N phase, M phase, histopathological differentiation type, irradiation dose, treatment effect [overall response rate (ORR), disease control rate (DCR)], progression-free survival (PFS), and overall survival (OS). The treatment effect was determined by using computed tomography (CT) every 1 to 3 months based on RECIST (version 1.1) (10) for solid tumors. The PFS and OS were analyzed retrospectively using the Kaplan-Meier method. All statistical analyses were conducted using Microsoft Excel 2016. This study was approved by the Ethics Committee of the Tokyo Metropolitan Cancer and Infectious Disease Center, Komagome Hospital, in accordance with the Declaration of Helsinki. We obtained informed consent from each patient before the treatment.

RESULTS

The patients' age ranged from 44 to 87 years (mean age, 72.1 years); the study included 8 men and 5 women. Primary lesions were present in the head and neck in 2 cases, in the lower limbs in 6 cases, and in the perineal region in 5 cases. The clinical stage was 4, and PS was 2 or less for all patients (**Figure 2**). Analysis for the 13 cases was performed retrospectively using the Kaplan-Meier method. **Figure 3** shows the survival curves in the 13 cases according to treatment with CCRT with continued chemotherapy as the first-line therapy for ucSCC. The patients treated with CCRT with continued chemotherapy showed an ORR of 84.6%, DCR of 92.3%, 1-year survival rate of 75 %, 2-year survival rate of 58.3 %, and a median survival time of 768 days.

Of the 13 patients treated with CCRT with continued chemotherapy, 5 patients had lymph node metastases beyond the regional lymph nodes without other organ metastasis before CCRT, and 8 patients had metastases only in the regional lymph nodes before CCRT. Three of 5 patients with lymph node metastases beyond the regional lymph nodes, had no progressive disease during continued chemotherapy, after CCRT. Three of 8 patients with metastases within the regional lymph nodes, had no progressive disease during continued chemotherapy, after CCRT. In 6 patients, who had no progressive disease, there was no difference in histopathological differentiation. Seven patients had lymph node metastasis beyond the regional lymph nodes or other organ metastases during continued chemotherapy (after CCRT), but most sites of metastasis were outside the irradiation area. Seven patients with metastasis during continued chemotherapy showed a 1-year PFS of 64.3 %, and median PFS of 262 days.

In our hospital, 3 patients requested to stop chemotherapy after CCRT, and 1 patient stopped chemotherapy during CCRT due to side effects of chemotherapy. Three patients who were administered low-dose FP stopped chemotherapy after 2, 6, and

No.	PS	Primary site	T	N	M	histopathological differentiation	RT (Gy)	Chemotherapy	Adverse event (>Grade3)	Vital status
1	44M	1	Lower limb	X	2	1	Moderately	50	Low-dose FP	G3 : Neutrophil count decreased	Dead on disease
2	74F	1	Lower limb	2	3	0	Well	50	TS-1		Dead on disease
3	78F	1	Perineal	3	2	0	Poorly	50.4	Low-dose FP		Alive with disease
4	75M	1	Lower limb	3	2	1	Poorly	60	Low-dose FP		Alive with disease
5	67M	1	Perineal	X	2	0	Poorly	59.4	Low-dose FP	G3 : Neutrophil count decreased	Dead on disease
6	74F	1	Perineal	2	2	1	Poorly	59.4	Low-dose FP	G3 : Neutrophil count decreased G3 : Anemia	Alive with disease
7	59M	1	Perineal	X	3	1	Poorly	60	Low-dose FP	G3 : Neutrophil count decreased G3 : Anemia	Dead on disease
8	78F	1	Perineal	3	2	0	Well	66	Low-dose FP	G3 : Neutrophil count decreased	Alive with disease
9	71M	1	Face	3	2	0	Well	60	Low-dose FP	G3 : Neutrophil count decreased	Alive with disease
10	77M	1	Lower limb	X	3	0	Well	60	Low-dose FP	G3 : Neutrophil count decreased	Alive with disease
11	87M	1	Face	3	2	0	Moderately	60	FP'		Dead on other disease
12	76M	1	Lower limb	X	2	1	Well	50	Low-dose FP		Dead on other disease
13	77F	2	Lower limb	3	2	0	Well	60	FP'		Alive with disease

FIGURE 2 | Patients characteristics.

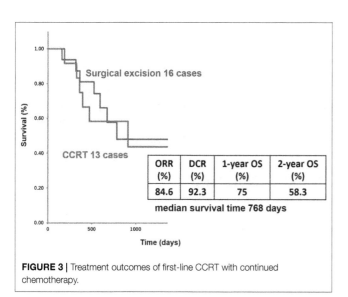

ORR (%)	DCR (%)	1-year OS (%)	2-year OS (%)
84.6	92.3	75	58.3

median survival time 768 days

FIGURE 3 | Treatment outcomes of first-line CCRT with continued chemotherapy.

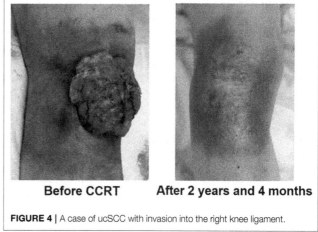

Before CCRT   After 2 years and 4 months

FIGURE 4 | A case of ucSCC with invasion into the right knee ligament.

8 times, but 6, 10, and 13 months later (respectively), they had recurrence within the irradiation area or other organ metastasis. One patient who stopped due to side effects from chemotherapy had organ metastasis during CCRT.

In our study, among the 13 patients treated with CCRT with continued chemotherapy, 10 patients received low-dose FP therapy, 2 patients received FP' therapy, and 1 patient received other chemotherapy regimens. The results showed low-dose FP and FP' therapy as effective with an ORR of 91.7%, DCR of 91.7%, 1-year survival rate of 72.7%, 2-year survival rate of 63.6%, and median survival time of 804 days. **Figure 4** shows an ucSCC with invasion into the right knee ligament and several regional lymph node metastases. It was successfully treated with CCRT with continued chemotherapy. Surgery in this case would have required the patient to undergo an amputation above the knee. Currently, 2 years and 4 months since treatment, the primary lesion has not been observed. The only remnant of the lesion at that location is a scar, moreover, his leg remains and allows the patient to walk normally. Thus, CCRT with continued chemotherapy is a suitable treatment option for ucSCC, as it can improve the quality of life regarding appearance and function.

CONCLUSION

Surgical excision is the first choice for the treatment of resectable cSCC, but there is no established treatment for unresectable cases. However, the results of our study show that CCRT with continued chemotherapy was an effective treatment method for unresectable cases. While there are several effective chemotherapy regimens for cSCC, our department mainly uses low-dose FP therapy.

The administration of neoadjuvant chemotherapy with FP therapy significantly improves the overall survival of patients with resectable stage II/III esophageal cancer (11). Moreover, FP therapy is an effective treatment for squamous cell carcinoma.

The age at the onset of cSCC is high, and the mean age of patients in our department was 72.1 years. Cisplatin can cause kidney dysfunction owing to age-related decline in kidney function. Therefore, we believe it is better to use low-dose FP therapy, which enhances the action of 5-fluorouracil as a biochemical modulator with low doses of cisplatin. For patients with renal dysfunction, carboplatin should be used instead of cisplatin.

For most cases of ucSCC after CCRT, the tumor clearly remained at the primary site and/or regional lymph nodes. One patient who stopped chemotherapy during CCRT had an organ metastasis immediately. Three patients who stopped continued chemotherapy after CCRT had recurrence within the irradiation area or other organ metastasis.

Although cutaneous angiosarcoma is a type of skin cancer, patients who received CRT for maintenance chemotherapy showed a significant improvement in OS over patients who received CRT alone (12). From these results, we considered continuing treatment after CCRT using the same chemotherapy regimen.

During continued chemotherapy, 7 of 13 patients had lymph node metastasis beyond the regional lymph nodes or other organ metastasis. Metastasis occurred in 7 patients during continued chemotherapy. This group had a 1-year PFS of 64.3%, and a median PFS of 262 days. Because of these results, we believe that it is important to continue chemotherapy after CCRT. Seven patients who had progressive disease changed to other chemotherapy regimens. Six other patients who had no recurrence within the irradiation range or other organ metastasis continued receiving low-dose FP or FP' therapy.

We recognize it is difficult to control ucSCC with CCRT alone during long-term observation. Thus, although CCRT with continued chemotherapy is effective, metastasis may be observed later. By continuing chemotherapy after CCRT,

recurrence within an irradiation area and other organ metastasis were suppressed. Therefore, the treatment outcome of CCRT with continued chemotherapy for ucSCC and that of surgical excision for resectable cSCC were similar (8). Additionally, we understood that continued chemotherapy after CCRT improved the treatment outcome of ucSCC.

In recent years, treatment with immune checkpoint inhibitors has become another option for advanced cSCC. Treatment response for SCC with metastases was 47 and 7% of the patients discontinued the treatment because of an immune-related adverse event (13). Our treatment of CCRT with continued chemotherapy is rarely discontinued due to side effects. We consider chemotherapy as a reasonable treatment option to administer to patients who are elderly. The response rate of CCRT with continued chemotherapy was 84.6%, suggesting that it is an effective treatment for ucSCC.

We evaluated the effectiveness of CCRT with continued chemotherapy for the treatment of ucSCC. We conclude CCRT with continued chemotherapy was effective for treating the irradiation site (primary lesion and regional lymph nodes) and the other organ metastasis.

At this time, due to the small number of cases in this study, the optimal duration of chemotherapy therapy is unknown for patients who receive CCRT with continued chemotherapy without progressive disease. We intend to investigate this in the future.

ETHICS STATEMENT

The studies involving human participants were reviewed and approved by the Ethics Committee of the Tokyo Metropolitan Cancer and Infectious Disease Center Komagome Hospital. The patients/participants provided their written informed consent to participate in this study.

AUTHOR CONTRIBUTIONS

AH held primary responsibility for communication with the journal and editorial office during the submission process, throughout peer review and during publication. AH was also responsible for ensuring that the submission adheres to all journal requirements including, but not exclusive to, details of authorship, study ethics and ethics approval, clinical trial registration documents and conflict of interest declaration. AH should also be available post-publication to respond to any queries or critiques. All authors contributed conception and design of the study. All authors contributed to manuscript revision, read and approved the submitted version.

REFERENCES

1. Alam M, Ratner D. Cutaneous squamous-cell carcinoma. *N Engl J Med.* (2001) 344:975–83. doi: 10.1056/NEJM200103293441306

2. Eigentler TK, Leiter U, Häfner HM, Garbe C, Röcken M, Breuninger H. Survival of patients with cutaneous squamous cell carcinoma: results of a prospective cohort study. *J Invest Dermatol.* (2017) 137:2309–15. doi: 10.1016/j.jid.2017.06.025

3. Schmults CD, Karia PS, Carter JB, Han J, Qureshi AA. Factors predictive of recurrence and death from cutaneous squamous cell carcinoma: a 10-year, single-institution cohort study. *JAMA Dermatol.* (2013) 149:541–7. doi: 10.1001/jamadermatol.2013.2139

4. Brantsch KD, Meisner C, Schönfisch B, Trilling B, Wehner-Caroli J, Röcken M, et al. Analysis of risk factors determining prognosis of cutaneous squamous-cell carcinoma: a prospective study. *Lancet Oncol.* (2008) 9:713–20. doi: 10.1016/S1470-2045(08)70178-5

5. Hillen U, Leiter U, Haase S, Kaufmann R, Becker J, Gutzmer R, et al. Advanced cutaneous squamous cell carcinoma: a retrospective analysis of patient profiles and treatment patterns-Results of a non-interventional study of the DeCOG. *Eur J Cancer.* (2018) 96:34–43. doi: 10.1016/j.ejca.2018.01.075

6. Stratigos A, Garbe C, Lebbe C, Malvehy J, del Marmol V, Pehamberger H, et al. Diagnosis and treatment of invasive squamous cell carcinoma of the skin: European consensus-based interdisciplinary guideline. *Eur J Cancer.* (2015) 51:1989–2007. doi: 10.1016/j.ejca.2015.06.110

7. Fujisawa Y, Umebayashi Y, Ichikawa E, Kawachi Y, Otsuka F. Chemoradiation using low-dose cisplatin and 5-fluorouracil in locally advanced squamous cell carcinoma of the skin: a report of two cases. *J Am Acad Dermatol.* (2006) 55:S81–5. doi: 10.1016/j.jaad.2005.12.035

8. Hiura A, Yoshino K, Maeda T, Nagai K, Oaku S, Kato M, et al. Chemoradiotherapy could improve overall survival of patients with stage IV cutaneous squamous cell carcinoma: analysis of 34 cases. *Br J Dermatol.* (2019) 180:1557–8. doi: 10.1111/bjd.17792

9. Brierley, JD, Gospodarowicz, MK, Wittekind, C. *TNM Classification of Malignant Tumours.* 8th ed. John Wiley & Sons, Ltd. (2017).

10. Eisenhauer E, Therasse P, Bogaerts J, Schwartz LH, Sargent D, Ford R, et al. New response evaluation criteria in solid tumours: revised RECIST guideline (version 1.1). *Eur J Cancer.* (2009) 45:228–47. doi: 10.1016/j.ejca.2008.10.026.

11. Ando N, Kato H, Igaki H, Shinoda M, Ozawa S, Shimizu H, et al. A randomized trial comparing postoperative adjuvant chemotherapy with cisplatin and 5-fluorouracil versus preoperative chemotherapy for localized advanced squamous cell carcinoma of the thoracic esophagus (JCOG9907). *Ann Surg Oncol.* (2012) 19:68–74. doi: 10.1245/s10434-011-2049-9

12. Fujisawa Y, Yoshino K, Kadono T, Miyagawa T, Nakamura Y, Fujimoto M. Chemoradiotherapy with taxane is superior to conventional surgery and radiotherapy in the management of cutaneous angiosarcoma: a multicentre, retrospective study. *Br J Dermatol.* (2014) 171:1493–500. doi: 10.1111/bjd.13110

13. Migden MR, Rischin D, Schmults CD, Guminski A, Hauschild A, Lewis KD, et al. PD-1 Blockade with Cemiplimab in Advanced Cutaneous Squamous-Cell Carcinoma. *N Engl J Med.* (2018) 379:341–51. doi: 10.1056/NEJMoa1805131

6

Tumor-Associated Macrophages: Therapeutic Targets for Skin Cancer

Taku Fujimura[1]*, Yumi Kambayashi[1], Yasuhiro Fujisawa[2], Takanori Hidaka[1] and Setsuya Aiba[1]

[1] *Department of Dermatology, Tohoku University Graduate School of Medicine, Sendai, Japan,* [2] *Department of Dermatology, University of Tsukuba, Tsukuba, Japan*

*Correspondence:
Taku Fujimura
tfujimura1@mac.com

Tumor-associated macrophages (TAMs) and regulatory T cells (Tregs) are significant components of the microenvironment of solid tumors in the majority of cancers. TAMs sequentially develop from monocytes into functional macrophages. In each differentiation stage, TAMs obtain various immunosuppressive functions to maintain the tumor microenvironment (e.g., expression of immune checkpoint molecules, production of Treg-related chemokines and cytokines, production of arginase I). Although the main population of TAMs is immunosuppressive M2 macrophages, TAMs can be modulated into M1-type macrophages in each differential stage, leading to the suppression of tumor growth. Because the administration of certain drugs or stromal factors can stimulate TAMs to produce specific chemokines, leading to the recruitment of various tumor-infiltrating lymphocytes, TAMs can serve as targets for cancer immunotherapy. In this review, we discuss the differentiation, activation, and immunosuppressive function of TAMs, as well as their benefits in cancer immunotherapy.

Keywords: tumor-associated macrophages, immunosuppression, M2 polarization, chemokines, angiogenetic factors, regulatory T cells

INTRODUCTION

Tumor-associated macrophages (TAMs) and regulatory T cells (Tregs) are significant components of the tumor microenvironment (1, 2). TAMs express immune checkpoint modulators [e.g., B7 family, B7-homolog family including programmed death ligand 1 (PD-L1)] (3) that directly suppress activated T cells. In addition, TAMs produce various chemokines that attract other immunosuppressive cells such as Tregs, myeloid-derived suppressor cells (MDSCs), and type 2 helper (Th2) T cells, which maintain the immunosuppressive factors of the tumor microenvironment (1, 2, 4). Moreover, TAMs also produce matrix metalloproteinases (MMPs), which play critical roles in tissue remodeling associated with various physiological processes such as morphogenesis, angiogenesis, tissue repair, local invasion, and metastasis (1, 5, 6). TAMs have been detected in various skin cancers such as melanoma, squamous cell carcinoma (SCC), extramammary Paget's disease (EMPD), Merkel cell carcinoma, basal cell carcinoma, and mycosis fungoides (MFs) (1, 2, 7–15) (**Table 1**). Because the stromal factor on each cancer stem cell is an important factor for TAM stimulation, leading to the induction of specific TAM phenotypes, investigating the immunomodulatory stromal cells in the tumor microenvironment is important for establishing the appropriate immunotherapy for each type of cancer (1, 8, 9, 16, 17). In addition, it may be possible to repolarize TAMs into anti-tumor macrophages, such as M1-phenotype macrophages, to suppress tumor progression by modifying the profiles of tumor-infiltrating lymphocytes (TILs) (7, 18, 19). Thus, TAMs could be a target for immunotherapy in skin cancers (1, 2). In this review, we discuss the differentiation, activation, and

TABLE 1 | Tumor-associated macrophages in skin cancer: mouse and human models.

Cancer species	Mouse (reference)	Human (reference)	Depletion	Reprogrammed	Biomarkers
Malignant melanoma	(3, 7, 13, 19, 20, 22, 39, 51, 62, 63, 64, 65)	(7, 35, 59, 60)	(13, 65)	(5, 19, 20, 22, 35, 39)	(3, 59, 60, 61)
Cutaneous squamous cell carcinoma	(23, 24, 32)	(11, 12, 34)	(23)	(24, 32)	(11, 12)
Merkel cell carcinoma	–	(14, 36)			(14, 36)
Extramammary Paget's disease	–	(8, 17)		(17)	(8)
Basal cell carcinoma	(26)	(15)	(26)		(15)
Dermatofibrosarcoma protuberans	–	(5)			(5)
Cutaneous T cell lymphoma	(25)	(9, 18, 28, 29, 30, 31, 57)	(25)	(18, 57)	(9, 28, 29, 30)

immunosuppressive function of TAMs, as well as their benefit in cancer immunotherapy.

DIFFERENTIATION AND ACTIVATION OF TAMs IN TUMORS

Tumor-associated macrophages are characterized by their heterogeneity and plasticity, as they can be functionally reprogrammed to polarized phenotypes by exposure to cancer-related factors, stromal factors, infections, or even drug interventions (1, 2, 7, 9, 11, 17, 19). Because TAMs sequentially differentiate from monocytes into functional macrophages through multiple steps, they have heterogeneity and plasticity in cancer (**Figure 1**). Monocytes recruited from the circulation differentiate into tissue macrophages by macrophage colony-stimulating factor (M-CSF), and are primed with several cytokines such as interferon gamma (IFN-γ), interleukin 4 (IL-4), and IL-13 (2). Thereafter, macrophages change their functional phenotype in response to environmental factors or even tumor-derived protein stimulation (2, 8, 17). In skin cancer, for example, targeting the M-CSF receptor with anti-CSF short interfering RNA (siCD115) in TAMs led to modulation of the TIL profile, resulting in growth suppression of B16 melanoma *in vivo* (20). In the second phase of priming, type I IFN (IFN-α, IFN-β) and type II IFN (IFN-γ) modulate the production of chemokines from TAMs, suggesting that these cytokines repolarize TAMs in several skin cancers (7, 18). Cancer stromal factors such as soluble receptor activator of nuclear factor kappa-B ligand (RANKL) derived from cancer cells could be a third mode of stimulation that activates mature M2 macrophages to produce a series of chemokines that recruit immunosuppressive cells such as Tregs and Th2, leading to maintenance of the tumor microenvironment (8, 10, 17). These reports suggest that each of these three differentiation steps could serve as a target for immunotherapies.

ROLES OF TAMs IN MAINTAINING THE IMMUNOSUPPRESSIVE MICROENVIRONMENT

Chemokines from TAMs Determine the Immunological Microenvironment in Tumors

Chemokines play crucial roles in determining the profiles of TILs in the tumor microenvironment, and the profiles of chemokines

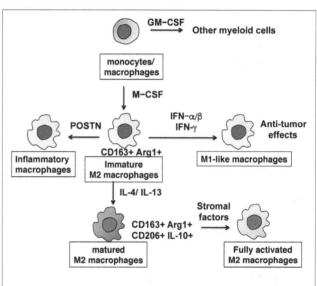

FIGURE 1 | Differentiation of M2-polarized tumor-associated macrophages. The multiple steps of the development of monocytes into fully functional macrophages.

from TAMs are determined by stromal factors of each skin cancer (1). For example, immune cells in the tumor microenvironment determine the aggressiveness of melanoma (21). In metastatic melanoma, periostin (POSTN) is expressed in the region surrounding melanoma cell nests in metastatic melanoma lesions that develop at the wound site (16). In addition, TAMs are prominent in the tumor stroma in melanoma (7, 19, 22), and POSTN stimulates CD163+ macrophages to produce several specific cytokines including Treg-related chemokines [chemokine ligand 17 (CCL17), CCL22] (9). Because CCL17 and CCL22 from TAMs attracts Tregs to the tumor site in melanoma (7, 21, 22), repolarization of TAMs by immunomodulatory reagents such as IFN-β and imiquimod are useful for suppressing tumor growth in melanoma (7, 22). The downregulation of CCL22 production was also observed in B16F10 melanoma mouse treated with classical cytotoxic anti-melanoma drugs such as dacarbazine, nimustine hydrochloride, and vincristine, all of which have been used in the adjuvant setting for advanced melanoma for the last 30 years (19). Other reports have suggested that a series of chemokines (CCL17, CXCL10, CCL4, and IL-8) in cerebrospinal fluid may be useful for predicting brain metastasis in melanoma patients (21). Together, these reports suggest the significance of chemokines from TAMs that can be induced by POSTN in the tumor stroma to induce melanoma-specific TILs in patients with melanoma.

Tumor-associated macrophages in non-melanoma skin cancer also secrete an array of chemokines in lesional skin to regulate the tumor microenvironment (1). In EMPD, for example, soluble RANKL released by Paget cells increases the production of CCL5, CCL17, and CXCL10 from RANK⁺ M2 polarized TAMs (8, 10, 17), suggesting that Paget cells can determine the immunological microenvironment by the stimulation of TAMs. The results of this study led to the hypothesis that denosumab, a full human monoclonal antibody for RANKL, has therapeutic effects in invasive EMPD. In cutaneous squamous cell carcinoma (cSCC), according to its heterogeneity of differentiation of cancer cells, TAMs in cSCC heterogeneously polarized from M1 to M2 (11). Indeed, Petterson et al. (11) reported that CD163⁺ TAMs not only express CCL18 (11), an M2 chemokine involved in remodeling of the tumor microenvironment but are also colocalized with phosphorylated signal transducer and activator of transcription 1 (11), suggesting the heterogeneous activation states of TAMs. Although the exact stimulator of cSCC is unknown, the depletion of TAMs such as antibody-mediated depletion (e.g., anti-CSF1R Ab) or bisphosphonate could be a useful therapy for unresectable cSCC (23–26).

Not only solid tumors but also hematopoietic malignancies in the skin contain CD163⁺ TAMs (25, 27–29), which produce chemokines that direct to specific anatomic sites to form metastases (25). Indeed recently, Wu et al. (9) used a human xenograft CTCL cell model to demonstrate that chemokines from TAMs play crucial roles in tumor formation in MF lesions. In another report, it was shown that the cancer stroma of MF containing POSTN and IL-4 might stimulate TAMs to produce chemokines that correlate with tumor formation in MF (25), and that chemokines from TAMs can be modified by immunomodulatory agents such as IFN-α and IFN-γ, leading to their therapeutic effects (18). Furthermore, CCL18 produced by TAMs in MF at the invasive margin of the tumor promote the recruitment of CTCL cells, leading to cancer progression (30). These reports suggest the significance of chemokines from TAMs for the development of CTCL.

Direct Suppressive Function of TAMs

Immunomodulatory costimulatory molecules, such as B7 homologs, play representative roles in the direct cell-mediated suppressive mechanism of TAMs. Recently, several reports have suggested that the expression of PD-L1 (also known as B7H1) in TAMs is necessary for antigen-specific tolerance induction (1, 3, 31) in tumor-bearing hosts. For example, the expression of PD-L1 on TAMs is augmented by autocrine IL-10 from M2-polarized TAMs stimulated by specific antigens (31). Another report showed that the decrease of IL-10 in MDSCs led to the downregulation of PD-L1 expression in MDSC in a mouse melanoma model (3). Linde et al. (32) reported that IL-10-polarized TAMs into M2 phenotypes in the presence of IL-4 and vascular endothelial growth factor A (VEGF-A) in cSCC. These reports suggest that IL-10 upregulates PD-L1 expression on TAMs, inducing immunosuppression in the tumor microenvironment in the skin. Arginase 1 is one of the key factors

for the suppressive function of TAMs. Its expression is widely detected in immature and functional M2 macrophages (1, 8, 17), leading to suppression of T cell activity by L-arginine catabolism (33). Indeed, CD163⁺ TAMs expresses arginase 1 in several skin cancers such as EMPD and SCC (8, 34). More recently, Pico de Coaña et al. (35) reported the additional immunomodulatory effects of ipilimumab on granulocytic MDSCs, which are circulating macrophages in tumor-bearing hosts, suggesting the crosstalk between Tregs and granulocytic MDSCs through the CTLA4/B7 homolog pathway and the significance of the direct suppressive function of TAMs (35).

Angiogenetic Factors from TAMs

Tumor-associated macrophages produce angiogenetic factors such as VEGF, platelet-derived growth factor, and transforming growth factor β, or by expressing MMPs to induce neovascularization (10, 28, 32, 36–38). Linde et al. (32) reported that VEGF-A augments the recruitment of TAMs at a tumor site by promoting neovascularization in a mouse skin tumor model (32). In a human skin cancer model, Werchau et al. (36) reported that VEGF-C expressed by TAMs contributes to lymphangiogenesis and the progression of Merkel cell carcinoma (36). In angiosarcoma, TAMs express MMP9, which might be a target for amino bisphosphonate (37). Another report suggested that inhibition of the VEGF/VEGF receptor pathway inhibits M2 polarization in TAMs, leading to reduced vascular density and tumor growth in MCA205 mouse sarcoma (38). In addition, more recently, Yamada et al. (39) reported that the expression of MGF-E8 on mesenchymal stromal cells plays crucial roles in inducing M2 macrophage polarization, leading to suppression of tumor growth by the reduction of VEGF expression in TAMs in B16F10 melanoma. These reports indicate the significance of VEGF produced by M2 macrophages in tumor progression, and show that both VEGF and MMPs are key markers for M2 macrophages in skin cancers (11, 40, 41). For example, in a melanoma model, osteopontin signaling promoted macrophage recruitment by the secretion of prostaglandin E2 and MMP-9 from TAMs, leading to angiogenesis and tumor progression (41). These reports suggest that MMPs play crucial roles in tumor progression. MMPs can also be produced by TAMs upon stimulation of stromal proteins in skin cancer (9, 10). For example, the stimulation of POSTN augments the production of MMP1 and MMP12 from monocyte-derived immature M2 macrophages (9). Because POSTN is abundant in the tumor stroma of MF and dermatofibrosarcoma protuberans (DFSP) (5, 9), and because substantial numbers of CD163⁺ TAMs have been detected in the POSTN-rich area in the lesional skin of skin tumors (5, 9), the production of MMP1 and MMP12 is prominent in the lesional skin of MF and DFSP. Notably, as reported by Livtinov et al. (42), among the MMPs, only MMP12 is a risk factor for CTCL progression, as determined by transcriptional profiling (42). RANKL is expressed in skin cancers of apocrine origin such as EMPD and apocrine carcinoma (8, 37), and is released in its soluble form. Because monocyte-derived M2 macrophages produce MMP1 and MMP25 by RANKL stimulation, TAMs in skin cancer of apocrine origin produce MMP1 and MMP25 at the tumor site (37). These reports suggest that TAMs stimulated by tumor stromal factors play roles in the carcinogenesis of these skin cancers, and might be targets for molecular-targeted therapy in the future.

CLINICAL BENEFITS OF TAMs

The Effects of Anticancer Drug for TAMs

Because TAMs comprise the immunosuppressive microenvironment at the tumor site, they may be optimal therapeutic targets in cancer (1, 2, 4, 43–46). For example, Rogers et al. (44) reported the immunomodulatory effects of bisphosphonate on TAMs in patients with breast and prostate cancers upon the repolarization of TAMs into tumoricidal macrophages (44). More recently, several reports have also focused on the immunomodulatory effects of chemotherapeutic reagents on TAMs (19, 47, 48). For example, a non-cytotoxic dose of paclitaxel decreased MDSCs and even blocked the immunosuppressive potential of MDSCs in a mouse melanoma model (47). More recently, Fujimura et al. (19) reported the immunomodulatory effects of cytotoxic anti-melanoma drugs, dacarbazine, nimustine hydrochloride, and vincristine, on TAMs both *in vitro* and *in vivo* by inhibition of STAT3 signals (19). The authors concluded that their immunomodulatory effects could explain their antitumor effects in postoperative melanoma patients. Peplomycin administered through a superficial temporal artery using an intravascular indwelling catheter, which can cause dose-independent interstitial pneumonia (49), decreased the number of TAMs and Tregs in cSCC on the lips, leading to an increase in the number of immunoreactive cells at the tumor sites (50), and possible autoimmune-like interstitial pneumonia (49, 50). More recently, not only cytotoxic chemotherapeutic drugs but also low molecular weight compounds were reported to co-localize with TAMs at tumor sites. Indeed, Hu-Lieskovan et al. (13) reported that single-agent dabrafenib increased TAMs and Tregs in melanoma, which decreased with the addition of trametinib, leading to the synergistic effects of immune checkpoints inhibitors with dabrafenib and trametinib combination therapy. In another report, the anti-macrophage receptor with collagenous structure was reported to polarize TAMs into proinflammatory phenotypes to induce anti-melanoma immune response in B16 melanomas (51). In addition, Gordon et al. (52) reported that inhibition of PD-1/PD-L1 *in vivo* increased macrophage phagocytosis, reduced tumor growth, and prolonged the survival of macrophages. In another report, increasing expression levels of PD-L1 in TAMs, 2 months after the administration of anti-PD-1 Abs in patients with advanced melanoma, was correlated with the response to immunotherapy (53), suggesting that PD-L1 expression in TAMs could be a biomarker that predicts the effectiveness of anti-PD-1 Ab therapy. Because the anti-PD-1 Abs nivolumab and pembrolizumab are widely used to treat advanced cancer, including melanoma (53), one target of anti-PD-1 Abs in patients with advanced melanoma could be an immunomodulatory effect on TAM, which, in turn, might be correlated with both their effectiveness and the development of adverse events. TAMs produce not only chemokines that directly recruit immunosuppressive cells to the tumor microenvironment but also produce cytokines that stimulate other stromal cells such as fibroblasts to produce chemokines (54, 55). Indeed, Young et al. (54) reported that IL-1β from TAMs stimulate fibroblasts to produce CXCR2 ligand,

which plays crucial roles in recruiting granulocytic MDSCs to tumor sites (55, 56). The authors concluded that CXCR2 agonists in combination with anti-CD115 Abs could suppress B16F10 melanoma *in vivo* by inhibiting the recruitment of granulocytic MDSCs and depletion of immature TAMs (56). Interestingly, the antihuman CD115 Ab, emactuzumab, decreased the number of CD163+ CD206+ M2 macrophages in patients with melanoma by depleting immature TAMs before the IL-4 stimulation phase (57). Together, these reports suggest that anti-CXCR2 agonists in combination with emactuzumab might induce the antimelanoma immune response by reducing the number of M2 polarized TAMs. These reports suggest the significance of assessing the effects of chemotherapeutic drugs on TAMs (13, 19, 47, 49, 50).

TAMs as a Biomarker for Disease Activity and Adverse Events

As described above, because TAMs produce tumor-specific chemokines by the stimulation of stromal factors, chemokines might serve as biomarkers that reflect disease activity. For example, TAMs produced CCL18 in the lesional skin of CTCL (26), which reflect disease severity and prognosis (58). Immunomodulatory reagents such as IFNs and imiquimod reduce CCL22 from TAMs, leading to the therapeutic effects of them in mouse B16F10 melanoma models (7, 22). CCL5, which induces Th2 cells from naive T cells (59), reflects the cancer stage and disease progression in gastric cancers (60). Another TAM-associated factor, sCD163, could be a useful biomarker for cancer treatment, as it is an activation marker for CD163+ tissue macrophages that is present in the serum as a result of proteolytic shedding (61). Serum sCD163 levels increase in autoimmune diseases such as atherosclerosis, rheumatoid arthritis, moyamoya disease, pemphigus vulgaris, and bullous pemphigoid (62–64), and reflect disease activity (61). Therefore, as we previously reported, sCD163 is a possible marker for predicting immune-related adverse events caused by immune checkpoints inhibitors (64, 65). These reports suggested that the production derived from TAMs could be a biomarker for cancer treatment in the future.

CONCLUDING REMARKS

Although several studies have suggested that high numbers of TAMs in tumor-bearing individuals are associated with a poor prognosis, making them useful as prognostic markers in cancer, further studies are needed to quantify their impact in different cancers.

AUTHOR CONTRIBUTIONS

FT designed the study. FT, KY, and HT wrote the article. FT, FY, and AS supervised the study.

REFERENCES

1. Fujimura T, Kakizaki A, Furudate S, Kambayashi Y, Aiba S. Tumor-associated macrophages in skin: how to treat their heterogeneity and plasticity. *J Dermatol Sci* (2016) 83(3):167–73. doi:10.1016/j.jdermsci.2016.05.015

2. Noy R, Pollard JW. Tumor-associated macrophages: from mechanisms to therapy. *Immunity* (2014) 41:49–61. doi:10.1016/j.immuni.2014.06.010

3. Fujimura T, Ring S, Umansky V, Mahnke K, Enk AH. Regulatory T cells (Treg) stimulate B7-H1 expression in myeloid derived suppressor cells (MDSC) in *ret* melanomas. *J Invest Dermatol* (2012) 132(4):1239–46. doi:10.1038/jid.2011.416

4. Fujimura T, Mahnke K, Enk AH. Myeloid derived suppressor cells and their role in tolerance induction in cancer. *J Dermatol Sci* (2010) 59(1):1–6. doi:10.1016/j.jdermsci.2010.05.001

5. Fujimura T, Kakizaki A, Sato Y, Tanita K, Furudate S, Aiba S. The immunological roles of periostin/tumor-associated macrophage axis in development of dermatofibrosarcoma protuberans. *Anticancer Res* (2017) 37(6):2867–73. doi:10.21873/anticanres.11639

6. Baay M, Brouwer A, Pauwels P, Peeters M, Lardon F. Tumor cells and tumor-associated macrophages: secreted proteins as potential targets for therapy. *Clin Dev Immunol* (2011) 2011:565187. doi:10.1155/2011/565187

7. Kakizaki A, Fujimura T, Furudate S, Kambayashi Y, Yamauchi T, Yagita H, et al. Immunomodulatory effect of peritumoral administration of interferon-beta on melanoma through tumor-associated macrophages. *Oncoimmunology* (2015) 4(11):e1047584. doi:10.1080/2162402X.2015.1047584

8. Kambayashi Y, Fujimura T, Furudate S, Asano M, Kakizaki A, Aiba S. The possible interaction between receptor activator of nuclear factor kappa-B ligand (RANKL) expressed by extramammary Paget cells and its ligand on dermal macrophages. *J Invest Dermatol* (2015) 135(10):2547–50. doi:10.1038/jid.2015.199

9. Furudate S, Fujimura T, Kakizaki A, Kambayashi Y, Asano M, Watabe A, et al. The possible interaction between periostin expressed by cancer stroma and tumor-associated macrophages in developing mycosis fungoides. *Exp Dermatol* (2016) 25(2):107–12. doi:10.1111/exd.12873

10. Fujimura T, Kambayashi Y, Furudate S, Kakizaki A, Hidaka T, Asano M, et al. Receptor activator of nuclear factor kappa-B ligand (RANKL)/RANK signaling promotes cancer-related inflammation through M2 macrophages. *Exp Dermatol* (2016) 25(5):397–9. doi:10.1111/exd.12949

11. Pettersen JS, Fuentes-Duculan J, Suárez-Fariñas M, Pierson KC, Pitts-Kiefer A, Fan L, et al. Tumor-associated macrophages in the cutaneous SCC microenvironment are heterogeneously activated. *J Invest Dermatol* (2011) 131(6):1322–30. doi:10.103/jid.2011.9

12. Kambayashi Y, Fujimura T, Aiba S. Comparison of immunosuppressive and immunomodulatory cells in keratoacanthoma and cutaneous squamous cell carcinoma. *Acta Derm Venereol* (2013) 93(6):663–8. doi:10.2340/00015555-1597

13. Hu-Lieskovan S, Mok S, Homet Moreno B, Tsoi J, Robert L, Goedert L, et al. Improved antitumor activity of immunotherapy with BRAF and MEK inhibitors in BRAF(V600E) melanoma. *Sci Transl Med* (2015) 7(279):ra41. doi:10.1126/scitranslmed.aaa4691

14. Fujimura T, Furudate S, Kambayashi Y, Kakizaki A, Yamamoto Y, Okuhira H, et al. Phospho-STAT5B expression is a prognostic marker for Merkel cell carcinoma. *Anticancer Res* (2017) 37(5):2335–41. doi:10.21873/anticanres.11571

15. Tjiu JW, Chen JS, Shun CT, Lin SJ, Liao YH, Chu CY, et al. Tumor-associated macrophage-induced invasion and angiogenesis of human basal cell carcinoma cells by cyclooxygenase-2 induction. *J Invest Dermatol* (2009) 129(4):1016–25. doi:10.1038/jid.2008.310

16. Fukuda K, Sugihara E, Ohta S, Izuhara K, Funakoshi T, Amagai M, et al. Periostin is a key niche component for wound metastasis of melanoma. *PLoS One* (2015) 10(6):e0129704. doi:10.1371/journal.pone.0129704

17. Fujimura T, Kambayashi Y, Furudate S, Asano M, Kakizaki A, Aiba S. Receptor activator of nuclear factor kappa-B ligand (RANKL) promotes the production of CCL17 from RANK+ M2 macrophages. *J Invest Dermatol* (2015) 135(11):2884–7. doi:10.1038/jid.2015.209

18. Furudate S, Fujimura T, Kakizaki A, Hidaka T, Asano M, Aiba S. Tumor-associated M2 macrophages in mycosis fungoides acquire immunomodulatory function by interferon alpha and interferon gamma. *J Dermatol Sci* (2016) 83(3):182–9. doi:10.1016/j.jdermsci.2016.05.004

19. Fujimura T, Kakizaki A, Kambayashi Y, Sato Y, Tanita K, Lyu C, et al. Cytotoxic anti-melanoma drugs suppress the activation of M2 macrophages. *Exp Dermatol* (2018) 27(1):64–70. doi:10.1111/exd.13417

20. Qian Y, Qiao S, Dai Y, Xu G, Dai B, Lu L, et al. Molecular-targeted immuno-therapeutic strategy for melanoma via dual-targeting nanoparticles delivering small interfering RNA to tumor-associated macrophages. *ACS Nano* (2017) 11(9):9536–49. doi:10.1021/acsnano.7b05465

21. Lok E, Chung AS, Swanson KD, Wong ET. Melanoma brain metastasis globally reconfigures chemokine and cytokine profiles in patient cerebrospinal fluid. *Melanoma Res* (2014) 24(2):120–30. doi:10.1097/CMR.0000000000000045

22. Furudate S, Fujimura T, Kambayashi Y, Kakizaki A, Hidaka T, Aiba S. Immunomodulatory effect of imiquimod through CCL22 produced by tumor-associated macrophages in B16F10 melanomas. *Anticancer Res* (2017) 37(7):3461–71. doi:10.21873/anticanres.11714

23. Wang H, Liang X, Li M, Tao X, Tai S, Fan Z, et al. Chemokine (CC motif) ligand 18 upregulates Slug expression to promote stem-cell like features by activating the mammalian target of rapamycin pathway in oral squamous cell carcinoma. *Cancer Sci* (2017) 108(8):1584–93. doi:10.1111/cas.13289

24. Antsiferova M, Piwko-Czuchra A, Cangkrama M, Wietecha M, Sahin D, Birkner K, et al. Activin promotes skin carcinogenesis by attraction and reprogramming of macrophages. *EMBO Mol Med* (2017) 9(1):27–45. doi:10.15252/emmm.201606493

25. Wu X, Schulte BC, Zhou Y, Haribhai D, Mackinnon AC, Plaza JA, et al. Depletion of M2-like tumor-associated macrophages delays cutaneous T-cell lymphoma development in vivo. *J Invest Dermatol* (2014) 134(11):2814–22. doi:10.1038/jid.2014.206

26. König S, Nitzki F, Uhmann A, Dittmann K, Theiss-Suennemann J, Herrmann M, et al. Depletion of cutaneous macrophages and dendritic cells promotes growth of basal cell carcinoma in mice. *PLoS One* (2014) 9(4):e93555. doi:10.1371/journal.pone.0093555

27. Sugaya M, Miyagaki T, Ohmatsu H, Suga H, Kai H, Kamata M, et al. Association of the numbers of CD163(+) cells in lesional skin and serum levels of soluble CD163 with disease progression of cutaneous T cell lymphoma. *J Dermatol Sci* (2012) 68(1):45–51. doi:10.1016/j.jdermsci.2012.07.007

28. Kim YH, Tavallaee M, Sundram U, Salva KA, Wood GS, Li S, et al. Phase II investigator-initiated study of brentuximab vedotin in mycosis fungoides and Sézary syndrome with variable CD30 expression level: a multi-institution collaborative project. *J Clin Oncol* (2015) 33(32):3750–8. doi:10.1200/JCO.2014.60.3969

29. Kakizaki A, Fujimura T, Kambayashi Y, Furudate S, Aiba S. Comparison of CD163+ macrophages and CD206+ cells in the lesional skin of CD30+ lymphoproliferative disorders: lymphomatoid papulosis and primary cutaneous anaplastic large-cell lymphoma. *Acta Derm Venereol* (2015) 95(5):600–2. doi:10.2340/00015555-2016

30. Günther C, Zimmermann N, Berndt N, Grosser M, Stein A, Koch A, et al. Up-regulation of the chemokine CCL18 by macrophages is a potential immunomodulatory pathway in cutaneous T-cell lymphoma. *Am J Pathol* (2011) 179(3):1434–42. doi:10.1016/j.ajpath.2011.05.040

31. Getts DR, Turley DM, Smith CE, Harp CT, McCarthy D, Feeney EM, et al. Tolerance induced by apoptotic antigen-coupled leukocytes is induced by PD-L1+ and IL-10-producing splenic macrophages and maintained by T regulatory cells. *J Immunol* (2011) 7(5):2405–17. doi:10.4049/jimmunol.1004175

32. Linde N, Lederle W, Depner S, van Rooijen N, Gutschalk CM, Mueller MM. Vascular endothelial growth factor-induced skin carcinogenesis depends on recruitment and alternative activation of macrophages. *J Pathol* (2012) 227(1):17–28. doi:10.1002/path.3989

33. Rodriguez PC, Quiceno DG, Ochoa AC. L-arginine availability regulates T-lymphocyte cell-cycle progression. *Blood* (2007) 109(4):1568–73. doi:10.1182/blood-2006-06-031856

34. Cyrus N, Mai-Anh Bui C, Yao X, Kohn LL, Galan A, Rhebergen AM, et al. Density and polarization states of tumor-associated macrophages in human cutaneous squamous cell carcinomas arising in solid organ transplant recipients. *Dermatol Surg* (2016) 42(Suppl 1):S18–23. doi:10.1097/DSS.0000000000000371

35. Pico de Coaña Y, Poschke I, Gentilcore G, Mao Y, Nyström M, Hansson J, et al. Ipilimumab treatment results in an early decrease in the frequency of circulating granulocytic myeloid-derived suppressor cells as well as their Arginase1 production. *Cancer Immunol Res* (2013) 1(3):158–62. doi:10.1158/2326-6066

36. Werchau S, Toberer F, Enk A, Dammann R, Helmbold P. Merkel cell carcinoma induces lymphatic microvessel formation. *J Am Acad Dermatol* (2012) 67(2):215–25. doi:10.1016/j.jaad.2011.09.002

37. Kambayashi Y, Fujimura T, Furudate S, Hashimoto A, Haga T, Aiba S. Comparison of immunosuppressive cells and cytotoxic cells in angiosarcoma: the development of a possible supportive therapy for angiosarcoma. *Dermatology* (2013) 227(1):14–20. doi:10.1159/000351316

38. Zhu X, Yang J, Gao Y, Wu C, Yi L, Li G, et al. The dual effects of a novel peptibody on angiogenesis inhibition and M2 macrophage polarization on sarcoma. *Cancer Lett* (2017) 416:1–10. doi:10.1016/j.canlet.2017.10.043

39. Yamada K, Uchiyama A, Uehara A, Perera B, Ogino S, Yokoyama Y, et al. 6-MFG-E8 drives melanoma growth by stimulating mesenchymal stromal cell-induced angiogenesis and M2 polarization of tumor-associated macrophages. *Cancer Res* (2016) 76(14):4283–92. doi:10.1158/0008-5472.CAN-15-2812

40. Heissig B, Hattori K, Dias S, Friedrich M, Ferris B, Hackett NR, et al. Recruitment of stem and progenitor cells from the bone marrow niche requires MMP-9 mediated release of kit-ligand. *Cell* (2002) 109(5):625–37. doi:10.1016/S0092-8674(02)00754-7

41. Kale S, Raja R, Thorat D, Soundararajan G, Patil TV, Kundu GC. Osteopontin signaling upregulates cyclooxygenase-2 expression in tumor-associated macrophages leading to enhanced angiogenesis and melanoma growth via α9β1 integrin. *Oncogene* (2014) 33(42):2295–306. doi:10.1038/onc.2015.315

42. Litvinov IV, Netchiporouk E, Cordeiro B, Doré MA, Moreau L, Pehr K, et al. The use of transcriptional profiling to improve personalized diagnosis and management of cutaneous T-cell lymphoma (CTCL). *Clin Cancer Res* (2015) 21(12):2820–9. doi:10.1158/1078-0432.CCR-14-3322

43. Mantovani A, Allavena P, Sica A, Balkwill F. Cancer-related inflammation. *Nature* (2008) 454(7203):436–44. doi:10.1038/nature07205

44. Rogers TL, Holen I. Tumour macrophages as potential targets of bisphosphonates. *J Transl Med* (2011) 9:177. doi:10.1186/1479-5876-9-177

45. Melani C, Sangaletti S, Barazzetta FM, Werb Z, Colombo MP. Amino-biphosphonate-mediated MMP-9 inhibition breaks the tumor-bone marrow axis responsible for myeloid derived suppressor cell expansion and macrophage infiltration in tumor stroma. *Cancer Res* (2007) 67(23):11438–46. doi:10.1158/0008-5472.CAN-07-1882

46. Mitchem JB, Brennan DJ, Knolhoff BL, Belt BA, Zhu Y, Sanford DE, et al. Targeting tumor-infiltrating macrophages decreases tumor-initiating cells, relieves immunosuppression, and improves chemotherapeutic responses. *Cancer Res* (2013) 73(3):1128–41. doi:10.1158/0008-5472.CAN-12-2731

47. Sevko A, Michels T, Vrohlings M, Umansky L, Beckhove P, Kato M, et al. Antitumor effect of Paclitaxel is mediated by inhibition of myeloid-derived suppressor cells and chronic inflammation in the spontaneous melanoma model. *J Immunol* (2013) 190(5):2464–71. doi:10.4049/jimmunol.1202781

48. Bruchard M, Mignot G, Derangère V, Chalmin F, Chevriaux A, Végran F, et al. Chemotherapy-triggered cathepsin B release in myeloid-derived suppressor cells activates the Nlrp3 inflammasome and promotes tumor growth. *Nat Med* (2013) 19(1):57–64. doi:10.1038/nm.2999

49. Fujimura T, Takahashi K, Kambayashi Y, Furudate S, Hidaka T, Kakizaki A, et al. Retrospective study of cutaneous squamous cell carcinoma on the lip treated with peplomycin administered through a superficial temporal artery. *Anticancer Res* (2017) 37(4):1885–9. doi:10.21873/anticanres.11526

50. Fujimura T, Kambayashi Y, Furudate S, Kakizaki A, Haga T, Hashimoto A, et al. Immunomodulatory effects of peplomycin on immunosuppressive and cytotoxic cells in the lesional skin of cutaneous squamous cell carcinoma. *Dermatology* (2015) 230(3):250–5. doi:10.1159/000369166

51. Georgoudaki AM, Prokopec KE, Boura VF, Hellqvist E, Sohn S, Östling J, et al. Reprogramming tumor-associated macrophages by antibody targeting inhibits cancer progression and metastasis. *Cell Rep* (2016) 15(9):2000–11. doi:10.1016/j.celrep.2016.04.084

52. Gordon SR, Maute RL, Dulken BW, Hutter G, George BM, McCracken MN, et al. PD-1 expression by tumour-associated macrophages inhibits phagocytosis and tumour immunity. *Nature* (2017) 545(7655):495–9. doi:10.1038/nature22396

53. Vilain RE, Menzies AM, Wilmott JS, Kakavand H, Madore J, Guminski A, et al. Dynamic changes in PD-L1 expression and immune infiltrates early during

54. Young HL, Rowling EJ, Bugatti M, Giurisato E, Luheshi N, Arozarena I, et al. An adaptive signaling network in melanoma inflammatory niches confers tolerance to MAPK signaling inhibition. *J Exp Med* (2017) 214(6):1691–710. doi:10.1084/jem.20160855

55. Kumar V, Donthireddy L, Marvel D, Condamine T, Wang F, Lavilla-Alonso S, et al. Cancer-associated fibroblasts neutralize the anti-tumor effect of CSF1 receptor blockade by inducing PMN-MDSC infiltration of tumors. *Cancer Cell* (2017) 32(5):654.e–68.e. doi:10.1016/j.ccell.2017.10.005

56. Lyons YA, Pradeep S, Wu SY, Haemmerle M, Hansen JM, Wagner MJ, et al. Macrophage depletion through colony stimulating factor 1 receptor pathway blockade overcomes adaptive resistance to anti-VEGF therapy. *Oncotarget* (2017) 8(57):96496–505. doi:10.18632/oncotarget.20410

57. Pradel LP, Ooi CH, Romagnoli S, Cannarile MA, Sade H, Rüttinger D, et al. Macrophage susceptibility to emactuzumab (RG7155) treatment. *Mol Cancer Ther* (2016) 15(12):3077–86. doi:10.1158/1535-7163.MCT-16-0157

58. Miyagaki T, Sugaya M, Suga H, Ohmatsu H, Fujita H, Asano Y, et al. Increased CCL18 expression in patients with cutaneous T-cell lymphoma: association with disease severity and prognosis. *J Eur Acad Dermatol Venereol* (2013) 27(1):e60–7. doi:10.1111/j.1468-3083.2012.04495.x

59. Zhang Q, Qin J, Zhong L, Gong L, Zhang B, Zhang Y, et al. CCL5-mediated Th2 immune polarization promotes metastasis in luminal breast cancer. *Cancer Res* (2015) 75(20):4312–21. doi:10.1158/0008-5472.CAN-14-3590

60. Ding H, Zhao L, Dai S, Li L, Wang F, Shan B. CCL5 secreted by tumor associated macrophages may be a new target in treatment of gastric cancer. *Biomed Pharmacother* (2016) 77:142–9. doi:10.1016/j.biopha.2015.12.004

61. Van Gorp H, Delputte PL, Nauwynck HJ. Scavenger receptor CD163, a Jack-of-all-trades and potential target for cell-directed therapy. *Mol Immunol* (2010) 47(7–8):1650–1460. doi:10.1016/j.molimm.2010.02.008

62. Fujimura M, Fujimura T, Kakizaki A, Sato-Maeda M, Niizuma K, Tomata Y, et al. Increased serum production of soluble CD163 and CXCL5 in patients with moyamoya disease: possible involvement of autoimmunity in its pathogenesis. *Brain Res* (2017) 1679:39–44. doi:10.1016/j.brainres.2017.11.013

63. Fujimura T, Kakizaki A, Furudate S, Aiba S. A possible interaction between periostin and CD163+ skin-resident macrophages in pemphigus vulgaris and bullous pemphigoid. *Exp Dermatol* (2016) 26(12):1193–8. doi:10.1111/exd.13157

64. Fujimura T, Kambayashi Y, Furudate S, Kakizaki A, Hidaka T, Haga T, et al. Isolated ACTH deficiency possibly caused by nivolumab in a metastatic melanoma patient. *J Dermatol* (2017) 44(3):e13–4. doi:10.1111/1346-8138.13532

65. Fujimura T, Hidaka T, Kambayashi Y, Furudate S, Kakizaki A, Tono H, et al. Phase I study of nivolumab combined with IFN-β for patients with advanced melanoma. *Oncotarget* (2017) 8(41):71181–7. doi:10.18632/oncotarget.17090

treatment predict response to PD-1 blockade in melanoma. *Clin Cancer Res* (2017) 23(17):5024–33. doi:10.1158/1078-0432.CCR-16-0698

7

Aryl Hydrocarbon Receptor Modulates Carcinogenesis and Maintenance of Skin Cancers

Takanori Hidaka*, Taku Fujimura and Setsuya Aiba

Department of Dermatology, Tohoku University Graduate School of Medicine, Sendai, Japan

*Correspondence:
Takanori Hidaka
takanori-h@med.tohoku.ac.jp

The aryl hydrocarbon receptor (AHR) is a ligand-activated transcription factor that responds to a wide range of chemicals, including chemical carcinogens such as dioxins and carcinogenic polyaromatic hydrocarbons, and induces a battery of genes associated with detoxification, proliferation, and immune regulation. Recent reports suggest that AHR plays an important role in carcinogenesis and maintenance of various types of skin cancers. Indeed, AHR is a susceptibility gene for squamous cell carcinoma and a prognostic factor for melanoma and Merkel cell carcinoma. In addition, the carcinogenic effects of ultraviolet (UV) and chemical carcinogens, both of which are major environmental carcinogenetic factors of skin, are at least partly mediated by AHR, which regulates UV-induced inflammation and apoptosis, the DNA repair system, and metabolic activation of chemical carcinogens. Furthermore, AHR modulates the efficacy of key therapeutic agents in melanoma. AHR activation induces the expression of resistance genes against the inhibitors of V600E mutated B-Raf proto-oncogene, serine/threonine kinase (BRAF) in melanoma and upregulation of programmed cell death protein 1 (PD-1) in tumor-infiltrating T cells surrounding melanoma. Taken together, these findings underscore the importance of AHR in the biology of skin cancers. Development of therapeutic agents that modulate AHR activity is a promising strategy to advance chemoprevention and chemotherapy for skin cancers.

Keywords: aryl hydrocarbon (Ah) receptor, squamous cell carcinoma, melanoma, ultraviolet, air pollutant, BRAF inhibitor, PD-1

INTRODUCTION

Recently, the incident rate of skin cancer has been greatly increasing. The number of patients treated for skin cancers has increased by 44% during the past 5 years (1), and skin cancer has become the most common cancer type in Caucasians (2). Although both genetic and environmental factors contribute to the carcinogenesis of skin cancer, this rapid increase suggests the relative importance of environmental factors. The skin is the outermost interface between the body and the environment and is ineluctably exposed to environmental insults such as ultraviolet radiation (UVR) or air pollutants (3). As UVR and air pollutants can induce carcinogenesis in the skin (4), the skin contains a system that recognizes and detoxifies these carcinogenic insults, the dysregulation of which leads to the initiation of skin cancer. In addition to the increase in carcinogenesis of skin cancer, recent therapeutic aspects of skin cancer have greatly changed. In particular, the emergence of molecular targeted therapies including inhibitors for V600E mutated B-Raf proto-oncogene, serine/threonine kinase (BRAF) and checkpoint inhibitors, which attenuate suppression of the anti-tumor immune response, have drastically improved the outcome of advanced melanoma. These drugs retrogradely elucidated the critical contribution of specific proliferative signals and tumor immunity in the maintenance of melanoma. These recent changes in skin cancers imply the importance of identifying a key molecule that modulates carcinogenesis and maintains skin cancer to improve prevention of and therapy for skin cancers.

The aryl hydrocarbon receptor (AHR) is an evolutionarily conserved, ligand-activated transcription factor, which is a member of the basic helix-loop-helix/PER-ARNT-SIM family (5). Due to its broad capacity to recognize a wide range of chemicals in the environment, AHR is often described as an environmental sensor. Once activated by ligand binding, AHR translocates into the nucleus and dimerizes with ARNT (Ah receptor nuclear translocator). Then the AHR/ARNT heterodimer enhances the expression of its target genes that encode drug-metabolizing cytochrome P450s, including CYP1A1, CYP1A2, and CYP1B1 (6) (Figure 1). These target molecules of AHR facilitate the metabolic degradation of its ligands. In addition to this role in detoxification, recent works have also revealed novel roles for AHR in tumor biology. In various tumors, differential expression of AHR is indeed observed compared to normal tissue. This different expression status of AHR plays a critical role in pro- or anti-tumor activity according to the cell state (7). Regarding skin cancer, a genome-wide association study of cutaneous squamous cell carcinoma (SCC) also identified AHR as a novel susceptibility locus (8). Furthermore, among various solid tumors, the expression level of CYP1A1, CYP1A2, and CYP1B1 is associated with prognosis of melanoma (9). These findings imply that AHR also plays important roles in the biology of skin cancers. In support of this hypothesis, AHR has recently been found to be associated with UVR and air pollutant-induced carcinogenesis of skin cancer (10, 11). Furthermore, AHR may play a role in modulating the efficacy of BRAF inhibitors and checkpoint inhibitors (12, 13) (Figure 2). In the following sections, we introduce the function of AHR in the context of carcinogenesis and maintenance of skin cancer and mainly focus on environmental carcinogens and molecular targeted therapy.

ENVIRONMENTAL FACTOR-INDUCED SKIN CARCINOGENESIS VIA AHR ACTIVATION

Ultraviolet Radiation

As much as 90% of non-melanoma skin cancers are associated with exposure to UVR (14). UVR causes mutagenesis of DNA and inflammation, which may eventually lead to the formation of skin cancers. UVA radiation (400-320 nm wavelength) excites endogenous chromophores and generates reactive oxygen species, leading to modifications of oxidative bases and generation of 7,8-dihydro-8-oxoguanine at guanine bases (15). In contrast, UVB radiation (320-290 nm wavelength) activates a photochemical reaction and forms photoproducts, including cyclobutane pyrimidine dimers (CPDs) and pyrimidine 6-4 pyrimidones, at adjacent pyrimidine nucleotides (15). To keep genomic integrity, these DNA photoproducts have to be removed by DNA repair system or apoptosis, depending on the extent of DNA damage (16). However, once the incorrect repair of

these DNA modifications occurs, it may inhibit polymerases, lead to the arrest of replication or cause misreadings during transcription or replication, which results in the formation of mutations, initiation of carcinogenesis, and skin cancer (15). The importance of DNA repair enzymes is clearly evident as seen by the drastically increased risk of developing UV signature mutations and subsequent skin cancers in Xeroderma Pigmentosum patients who lack one of the DNA repair enzymes (17). In addition to mutagenesis, UVR causes the body a UV stress response, the inflammatory response at the exposed site. Increasing evidence suggests that sustained inflammation induced by UVR plays an important role in cancer initiation and progression (18).

AHR acts as a light sensor in keratinocytes following activation by UVR. UVR (in particular UVB) generates formylindolo (3,2-b)carbazole (FICZ), a tryptophan derivative, in epidermal keratinocytes (19). FICZ functions as a high-affinity ligand for AHR and induces UVR-mediated AHR activation, which is associated with UV-induced skin carcinogenesis. Pollet et al. reported that the chronic irradiation of UVB causes only a half numbers of cutaneous SCCs on AHR$^{-/-}$ mice compared to AHR$^{+/+}$ littermates, which implies a critical contribution of AHR in carcinogenesis of SCC. As a molecular mechanism, they revealed AHR activation attenuates the clearance of UVB-induced CPDs by repressing global genomic repair in a p27-dependent manner (10). In addition to the role of AHR in the attenuation of DNA repair systems, AHR works as a negative regulator of apoptosis in UVB damaged keratinocytes. Frauenstein et al. reported that chemical inhibition or knockdown of AHR sensitize keratinocytes to UVB-induced apoptosis by decreasing the expression of E2F1 and its target gene checkpoint kinase 1 (CHK1) (20). AHR also promotes the UV stress response (19). Although the concise molecular mechanism of the UV stress response remains largely unknown, the involvement of different tyrosine kinases including the epidermal growth factor receptor (EGFR) and pro-inflammatory molecules has been suggested (21). For instance, FICZ induces the internalization and subsequent activation of EGFR in an AHR-dependent manner, which is also induced by UVB radiation (19). Moreover, AHR activation in keratinocyte induces the expression of various pro-inflammatory molecules. Irradiation of UVR followed by topical application with FICZ on Ahr$^{+/+}$ mice induces cutaneous expression of a neutrophil directing chemokine (C-X-C motif) ligand 5 (Cxcl5) compared with UV alone, which cannot be observed in Ahr$^{-/-}$ mice (22). In addition, the exposure of FICZ to keratinocyte cell-line induces the activation of AHR and ROS production, which leads to the production of pro-inflammatory cytokine, IL-6 (23). Furthermore, AHR activation induced by UVB irradiation can activate the expression of cyclooxygenase-2, which is pro-inflammatory and associated with the development of skin cancer (19, 24).

These observations imply that AHR activation promotes UVR-induced skin carcinogenesis via attenuation of the DNA repair system and apoptosis and via enhancement of the UV response.

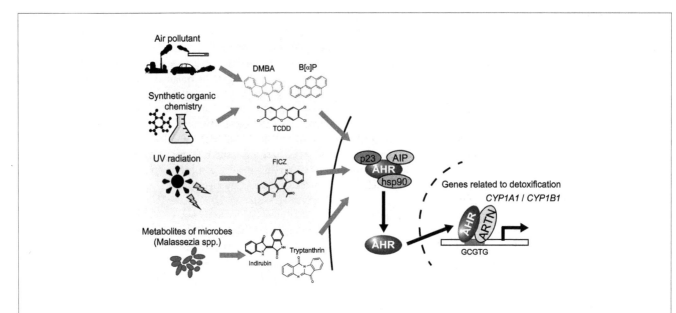

FIGURE 1 | AHR works as an environmental sensor. AHR binds to polycyclic aromatic hydrocarbons and their derivatives derived from environment. Once these ligands binded, AHR isolates from the complex in cytoplasm, translocates into nucleus and activates translation of the target genes, including CYP1A1 and CYP1B1. DMBA, 7,12-Dimethyl benz[*a*]anthracen; B[*a*]P, Benzo[*a*]pyrene; TCDD, 2,3,7,8-Tetrachloro dibenzo-*p*-dioxin; FICZ, 6-Formylindolo [3,2-*b*]carbazole.

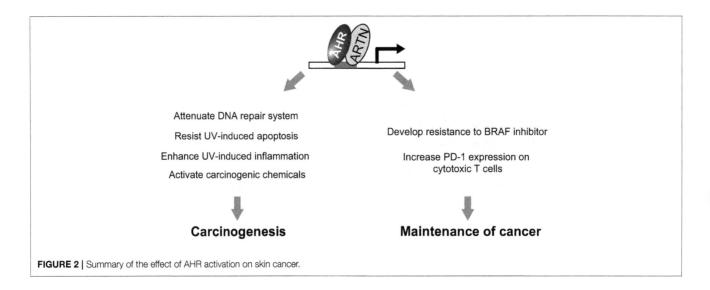

FIGURE 2 | Summary of the effect of AHR activation on skin cancer.

Carcinogenic Chemicals in Air Pollutants

Carcinogenic chemicals are another well-known type of environmental carcinogen that leads to skin cancer. Airborne particulate matter (PM) and ambient air pollution, which contain various carcinogenic chemicals, are considered group 1 human carcinogens by the International Agency for Research on Cancer (25, 26). As the skin is located at the outermost layer of the body, it is continuously exposed to air pollutants, which may increase the risk of skin cancer. Carcinogenic chemicals, including polycyclic aromatic hydrocarbons (PAHs) and dioxins, contained in PM are responsible for PM-induced carcinogenesis (27). Due to their lipophilicity, these chemicals easily penetrate through the skin (28, 29) and are retained in

the skin for a long time (30). PAHs and dioxins exert their biological effects via binding to AHR. AHR activation by these chemicals has gained a lot of attention as a mechanism that contributes to skin carcinogenesis. In fact, PAHs and dioxins cause SCC in *in vivo* animal models. For instance, chronic subcutaneous injection of TCDD to hamster results in formation cutaneous SCC (31). In addition, application of 7,12-Dimethylbenz[*a*]anthracene (DMBA), a member of the PAH family that is typically found in cigarette smoke, to murine skin causes lesions that are histologically similar to benign papilloma to SCC (32, 33). Whole-exome sequencing analysis has been conducted in this murine model of DMBA-induced SCC to investigate its mutational landscape (34). As a result, the majority of DMBA-induced SCC possesses mutations in oncogenes including *Hras*, *Kras*, and *Rras2*. These mutations in human SCCs are similar to those in head and neck, esophageal, lung, and cervical SCC (34–36). In addition to SCC, the development of melanoma is also accelerated by the application of DMBA in some genetically engineered mouse models of melanoma (37).

In these models of PAH-induced skin carcinogenesis, AHR plays a considerable role. Chronic topical application of organic extracts of airborne particulate matter causes SCCs in a half of AHR $^{+/+}$ mice but none of AHR$^{-/-}$ mice (11). Benzo[*a*]pyrene, another PAH contained in PM from cigarettes or air pollutants, can also induce SCC following subcutaneous or topical application to wild-type mice. This carcinogenic property of benzo[*a*]pyrene is attenuated when applied to *Ahr*-deficient mice (38). In the case of DMBA-induced carcinogenesis, the mice possessing the 375A allele of *Ahr*, encoding the high-affinity ligand-binding receptor, develop skin cancers, but the mice possessing the 375V allele, encoding the low-affinity one do not (39); in contrast, there is another report demonstrating no significant differences in carcinogenesis between *Ahr*$^{+/+}$ mice and *Ahr*$^{-/-}$ mice by topical application of DMBA (40). Taken together, these results suggest that AHR activation promotes tumor induction of PAH-induced skin carcinogenesis.

Several studies investigated the mechanism of PAHs-induced carcinogenesis and revealed that AHR-dependent induction of CYP1A1/CYP1B1 expression likely plays a key role (38). In general, CYP1A1 and CYP1B1 enzymes facilitate removal of AHR ligands by degrading them to metabolites with decreased activity and increasing their water solubility (41). In contrast, in the case of carcinogenic PAHs, the same metabolic reaction results in the metabolic activation of PAHs. For instance, CYP1B1-mediated metabolism of DMBA results in the synthesis of DMBA-trans-3,4-diol, which is highly electrophilic and causes damages to DNA (42). Moreover, CYP1A1, CYP1B1 and epoxide hydrolase-mediated metabolism of benzo[*a*]pyrene results in the synthesis of highly electrophilic benzo[*a*]pyrene-7,8-diol-9,10-epoxide (43).

Regarding the mechanism of dioxins-induced carcinogenesis and its dependency of AHR, they remain largely unknown, as dioxins are not generally metabolized to be directly genotoxic and there is lack of related articles.

MAINTENANCE OF SKIN CANCER VIA AHR ACTIVATION

In addition to the carcinogenic role of AHR activation, AHR also greatly contributes to the maintenance of various skin cancers. In non-cutaneous tumors, AHR is an established factor that induces suppression of the anti-tumor immune response, resulting in the escape of tumor cells from immune-mediated cell death (44). Furthermore, AHR affects multiple aspects of cancer biology, including cell survival and proliferation (45). Recent findings show that AHR modulates anti-tumor immunity and proliferative signals in skin cancers. In the following sections, we introduce recent findings regarding how AHR contributes to the maintenance of skin cancers, mainly focusing on melanoma.

Melanoma

Melanoma is believed to be derived from malignant transformation of melanocytes, which are pigment-producing cells that generally reside in skin (46). Studies investigating the melanocytes of *Ahr*-deficient mice indicated that AHR is essential for proliferation of melanocytes (47). In addition, some reports using melanoma cell lines indicate that AHR activation attenuates tumorigenicity (48, 49); in contrast, others reported that AHR activation promotes tumorigenicity of melanoma (50, 51). These observations suggest the contribution of the AHR system to the biology of melanoma, the details of which have been revealed in recent reports.

In the clinical setting, therapy for melanoma is based on the staging system, which scores clinical and pathological risk factors, including tumor thickness, mitotic rate, and presence of ulceration and metastases (52). In the past, once a melanoma was scored as high grade, patients were considered to have an extremely high mortality rate due to resistance to chemotherapy (53). However, recent development of molecular targeted therapies against the oncogene or checkpoint inhibitors has drastically improved the prognosis of patients with advanced melanoma (54). This improvement indicates the critical importance of BRAF and checkpoint molecules in the maintenance of melanoma. Surprisingly, recent findings have revealed a significant role for AHR in modulating the effect of these critical molecules.

The BRAF V600E mutation is the most prevalent mutation and is present in approximately half of patients with advanced melanoma (55). Specific inhibitors of mutated BRAF have achieved high response rates and improved overall survival (56). Meanwhile, the efficacy of BRAF inhibitors is transient due to acquired resistance, which usually appears within a year after the time of response and results in relapse of melanoma (57, 58). One mechanism of the induction of resistance to BRAF inhibitors is upregulation of genes related to resistance to BRAF inhibitors, including AXL receptor tyrosine kinase (*AXL*), *EGFR*, and neuropilin 1 (*NRP1*) (59, 60). Recently, Corre et al. demonstrated that in a subset of melanoma cells, AHR is constitutively activated, which drives expression of these genes that are related to resistance to BRAF inhibitors (12). In addition, they also reported that co-administration of AHR antagonists with BRAF inhibitors maintains at least partial sensitivity to BRAF inhibitors in melanoma cells.

Melanoma is a solid tumor with a high mutational burden, which induces the generation of neo-antigens and the infiltration of cytotoxic T cells (CTLs) that recognize neo-antigens (61, 62). The level of mutational burden is correlated with that of transcripts related to cytolytic activity of local immune infiltrates (63). To evade the anti-tumor immune response, melanoma cells express molecules associated with checkpoint pathways. Approximately 40% of melanoma biospecimens express programmed death-ligand 1 (PD-L1), one of the molecules associated with the checkpoint pathway (64). When PD-L1 expressed on melanoma cells binds to the PD-1 receptor expressed on CTLs, CTLs become dysfunctional, and melanoma cells escape immune-mediated cell lysis (65, 66). As mentioned, PD-1 blockade by checkpoint inhibitors significantly improves overall survival and progression-free survival compared with classical chemotherapy in patients with advanced melanoma (67). These findings imply the importance of elucidating how melanoma cells upregulate the expression of PD-1 on CTLs. Liu et al. found that tumor-repopulating cells, a subpopulation of cancer cells having stem cell-like property that are tumorigenic and can grow in soft 3D matrices, produce kynurenine, a known AHR ligand of tryptophan metabolism, by type I IFN-induced expression of indolamine 2,3-dioxygenase. Then kynurenine activates AHR in tumor-repopulating cells, which enters them into dormancy, the condition resistant to immune-therapies (68, 69). In addition, released kynurenine is taken up by surrounding CTLs and upregulates PD-1 expression on CTLs in an AHR-dependent manner (13). This finding tells us that the AHR system may be a significant modulator of PD-1-mediated suppression of the anti-melanoma immune response.

Other Cutaneous Carcinomas

Several reports have suggested possible links between the AHR system and tumor biology in Merkel cell carcinoma (MCC) and extramammary Paget's disease (EMPD).

MCC is a rare and aggressive neuroendocrine skin cancer, and ~80% of patients are infected with merkel cell polyomavirus. Univariate analysis of clinical specimens revealed that a longer overall survival is achieved in the group with lower expression of tryptophan 2,3-dioxygenase 2 (TDO2) and AHR in cells surrounding the tumor (70). As TDO2 is an enzyme in the tryptophan-kynurenine metabolic pathway, the TDO2-AHR axis may play a significant role in the pathophysiology of MCC.

Another study of EMPD, an adenocarcinoma of apocrine origin, reported that the epidermis adjacent to EMPD lesions expresses CYP1A1 and CCL20, an interleukin-17-related chemokine. Malassezia yeast, which are often pathogenic in apocrine lesions, produce a metabolite that activates AHR and induces the Th17 immune response. Thus, a possible link may be present between Malassezia metabolite-induced AHR activation and the Th17-skewed tumor immune response in EMPD (71).

CONCLUDING REMARKS

As summarized above, AHR was recently found to be a key modulator of UVR- and carcinogenic chemical-induced skin carcinogenesis. In addition, this molecule is associated with the efficacy of BRAF inhibitors and checkpoint inhibitors, which are core therapeutic drugs in melanoma. Taken together, these data underscore the importance of the AHR system in carcinogenesis and maintenance of skin cancers, especially SCC and melanoma. This means that the AHR system is a putative target, particularly for chemoprevention and cancer chemotherapy of skin cancer. The emergence of research investigating the effect of AHR antagonists for various skin cancers is promising and eagerly awaited.

AUTHOR CONTRIBUTIONS

TH wrote the manuscript. TF and SA supervised and reviewed this work.

REFERENCES

1. Guy GP, Machlin SR, Ekwueme DU, Yabroff KR. Prevalence and costs of skin cancer treatment in the U.S., 2002–2006 and 2007–2011. *Am J Prev Med.* (2015) 48:183–87. doi: 10.1016/j.amepre.2014.08.036
2. Leiter U, Eigentler T, Garbe C. Epidemiology of skin cancer. *Adv Exp Med Biol.* (2014) 810:120–40. doi: 10.1007/978-1-4939-0437-2_7
3. Elias PM, Choi EH. Interactions among stratum corneum defensive functions. *Exp Dermatol.* (2005) 14:719–26. doi: 10.1111/j.1600-0625.2005.00363.x
4. Zegarska B, Pietkun K, Zegarski W, Bolibok P, Wiśniewski M, Roszek K, et al. Air pollution, UV irradiation and skin carcinogenesis: what we know, where we stand and what is likely to happen in the future? *Postep dermatologii i Alergol.* (2017) 34:6–14. doi: 10.5114/ada.2017.65616
5. Hahn ME, Karchner SI, Shapiro MA, Perera SA. Molecular evolution of two vertebrate aryl hydrocarbon (dioxin) receptors (AHR1 and AHR2) and the PAS family. *Proc Natl Acad Sci USA.* (1997) 94:13743–8. doi: 10.1073/pnas.94.25.13743
6. Fujii-Kuriyama Y, Mimura J. Molecular mechanisms of AhR functions in the regulation of cytochrome P450 genes. *Biochem Biophys Res Commun.* (2005) 338:311–7. doi: 10.1016/j.bbrc.2005.08.162
7. Safe S, Cheng Y, Jin UH. The aryl hydrocarbon receptor (AhR) as a drug target for cancer chemotherapy. *Curr Opin Toxicol.* (2017) 2:24–9. doi: 10.1016/j.cotox.2017.01.012
8. Chahal HS, Lin Y, Ransohoff KJ, Hinds DA, Wu W, Dai HJ, et al. Genome-wide association study identifies novel susceptibility loci for cutaneous squamous cell carcinoma. *Nat Commun.* (2016) 7:12048. doi: 10.1038/ncomms12048
9. Lv JW, Zheng ZQ, Wang ZX, Zhou GQ, Chen L, Mao YP, et al. Pan-cancer genomic analyses reveal prognostic and immunogenic features of the tumor melatonergic microenvironment across 14 solid cancer types. *J Pineal Res.* (2019) 66:1–13. doi: 10.1111/jpi.12557
10. Pollet M, Shaik S, Mescher M, Frauenstein K, Tigges J, Braun SA, et al. The AHR represses nucleotide excision repair and apoptosis and contributes to UV-induced skin carcinogenesis. *Cell Death Differ.* (2018) 25:1823–36. doi: 10.1038/s41418-018-0160-1
11. Matsumoto Y, Ide F, Kishi R, Akutagawa T, Sakai S, Nakamura M, et al. Aryl hydrocarbon receptor plays a significant role in mediating airborne particulate-induced carcinogenesis in mice. *Environ Sci Technol.* (2007) 41:3775–80. doi: 10.1021/es062793g
12. Corre S, Tardif N, Mouchet N, Leclair HM, Boussemart L, Gautron A, et al. Sustained activation of the Aryl hydrocarbon Receptor transcription factor promotes resistance to BRAF-inhibitors in melanoma. *Nat Commun.* (2018) 9: doi: 10.1038/s41467-018-06951-2
13. Liu Y, Liang X, Dong W, Fang Y, Lv J, Zhang T, et al. Tumor-repopulating cells induce PD-1 expression in CD8+ T cells by transferring kynurenine and AhR activation. *Cancer Cell.* (2018) 33:480-494.e7. doi: 10.1016/j.ccell.2018.02.005
14. Vitaliano PP, Urbach F. The relative importance of risk factors in nonmelanoma carcinoma. *Arch Dermatol.* (1980) 116:454–6.
15. Cadet J, Sage E, Douki T. Ultraviolet radiation-mediated damage to cellular DNA. *Mutat Res.* (2005) 571:3–17. doi: 10.1016/j.mrfmmm.2004.09.012
16. Roos WP, Thomas AD, Kaina B. DNA damage and the balance between survival and death in cancer biology. *Nat Rev Cancer.* (2016) 16:20–33. doi: 10.1038/nrc.2015.2

17. DiGiovanna JJ, Kraemer KH. Shining a light on xeroderma pigmentosum. *J Invest Dermatol.* (2012) 132:785–96. doi: 10.1038/jid.2011.426

18. Garibyan L, Fisher DE. How sunlight causes melanoma. *Curr Oncol Rep.* (2010) 12:319–26. doi: 10.1007/s11912-010-0119-y

19. Fritsche E, Schäfer C, Calles C, Bernsmann T, Bernshausen T, Wurm M, et al. Lightening up the UV response by identification of the arylhydrocarbon receptor as a cytoplasmatic target for ultraviolet B radiation. *Proc Natl Acad Sci USA.* (2007) 104:8851–6. doi: 10.1073/pnas.0701764104

20. Frauenstein K, Sydlik U, Tigges J, Majora M, Wiek C, Hanenberg H, et al. Evidence for a novel anti-apoptotic pathway in human keratinocytes involving the aryl hydrocarbon receptor, E2F1, and checkpoint kinase 1. *Cell Death Differ.* (2013) 20:1425–34. doi: 10.1038/cdd.2013.102

21. Muthusamy V, Piva TJ. The UV response of the skin: a review of the MAPK, NFkappaB and TNFalpha signal transduction pathways. *Arch Dermatol Res.* (2010) 302:5–17. doi: 10.1007/s00403-009-0994-y

22. Smith KJ, Boyer JA, Muku GE, Murray IA, Gowda K, Desai D, et al. Editor's highlight: Ah receptor activation potentiates neutrophil chemoattractant (C-X-C Motif) ligand 5 expression in keratinocytes and skin. *Toxicol Sci.* (2017) 160:83–94. doi: 10.1093/toxsci/kfx160

23. Tanaka Y, Uchi H, Hashimoto-Hachiya A, Furue M. Tryptophan photoproduct FICZ upregulates IL1A, IL1B, and IL6 expression via oxidative stress in keratinocytes. *Oxid Med Cell Longev.* (2018) 2018:9298052. doi: 10.1155/2018/9298052

24. Buckman SY, Gresham A, Hale P, Hruza G, Anast J, Masferrer J, Pentland AP. COX-2 expression is induced by UVB exposure in human skin: implications for the development of skin cancer. *Carcinogenesis.* (1998) 19:723–9.

25. Loomis D, Grosse Y, Lauby-Secretan B, Ghissassi F El, Bouvard V, Benbrahim-Tallaa L, et al. The carcinogenicity of outdoor air pollution. *Lancet Oncol.* (2013) 14:1262–3. doi: 10.1016/s1470-2045(13)70487-x

26. Burnett RT1, Pope CA III, Ezzati M, Olives C, Lim SS, Mehta S, et al. An integrated risk function for estimating the global burden of disease attributable to ambient fine particulate matter exposure. *Environ Health Perspect.* (2014) 122:397–403. doi: 10.1289/ehp.1307049

27. Harrison RM, Smith DJT, Kibble AJ. What is responsible for the carcinogenicity of PM2.5? *Occup Environ Med.* (2004) 61:799–805. doi: 10.1136/oem.2003.010504

28. Sanders CL, Skinner C, Gelman RA. Percutaneous absorption of 7, 10 14C-benzo[a]pyrene and 7, 12 14C-dimethylbenz[a]anthracene in mice. *J Environ Pathol Toxicol Oncol.* (1984) 7:25–34.

29. Kao J, Patterson FK, Hall J. Skin penetration and metabolism of topically applied chemicals in six mammalian species, including man: an *in vitro* study with benzo[a]pyrene and testosterone. *Toxicol Appl Pharmacol.* (1985) 81:502–16. doi: 10.1016/0041-008X(85)90421-1

30. Chu I, Dick D, Bronaugh R, Tryphonas L. Skin reservoir formation and bioavailability of dermally administered chemicals in hairless guinea pigs. *Food Chem Toxicol.* (1996) 34:267–76. doi: 10.1016/0278-6915(95)00112-3

31. Rao MS, Subbarao V, Prasad JD, Scarpelli DG. Carcinogenicity of 2,3,7,8-tetrachlorodibenzo-p-dioxin in the Syrian golden hamster. *Carcinogenesis.* (1988) 9:1677–9. doi: 10.1093/carcin/9.9.1677

32. Melendez-Colon VJ, Luch A, Seidel A, Baird WM. Cancer initiation by polycyclic aromatic hydrocarbons results from formation of stable DNA adducts rather than apurinic sites. *Carcinogenesis.* (1999) 20:1885–91.

33. Huang PY, Balmain A. Modeling cutaneous squamous carcinoma development in the mouse. *Cold Spring Harb Perspect Med.* (2014) 4:a013623. doi: 10.1101/cshperspect.a013623

34. Nassar D, Latil M, Boeckx B, Lambrechts D, Blanpain C. Genomic landscape of carcinogen-induced and genetically induced mouse skin squamous cell carcinoma. *Nat Med.* (2015) 21:946–54. doi: 10.1038/nm.3878

35. McCreery MQ, Halliwill KD, Chin D, Delrosario R, Hirst G, Vuong P, et al. Evolution of metastasis revealed by mutational landscapes of chemically induced skin cancers. *Nat Med.* (2015) 21:1514–20. doi: 10.1038/nm.3979

36. Ginos MA, Page GP, Michalowicz BS, Patel KJ, Volker SE, Pambuccian SE, et al. Identification of a gene expression signature associated with recurrent disease in squamous cell carcinoma of the head and neck. *Cancer Res.* (2004) 64:55–63. doi: 10.1158/0008-5472.CAN-03-2144

37. Tormo D, Ferrer A, Gaffal E, Wenzel J, Basner-Tschakarjan E, Steitz J, et al. Rapid growth of invasive metastatic melanoma in carcinogen treated hepatocyte growth factor/scatter factor-transgenic mice carrying

an oncogenic CDK4 mutation. *Am J Pathol.* (2006) 169:665–72. doi: 10.2353/ajpath.2006.060017

38. Shimizu Y, Nakatsuru Y, Ichinose M, Takahashi Y, Kume H, Mimura J, Fujii-Kuriyama Y, Ishikawa T. Benzo[a]pyrene carcinogenicity is lost in mice lacking the aryl hydrocarbon receptor. *Proc Natl Acad Sci USA.* (2000) 97:779–82. doi: 10.1073/pnas.97.2.779

39. De Souza VRC, Cabrera WK, Galvan A, Ribeiro OG, De Franco M, Vorraro F, et al. Aryl hydrocarbon receptor polymorphism modulates DMBA-induced inflammation and carcinogenesis in phenotypically selected mice. *Int J Cancer.* (2009) 124:1478–82. doi: 10.1002/ijc.24066

40. Ide F, Suka N, Kitada M, Sakashita H, Kusama K, Ishikawa T. Skin and salivary gland carcinogenicity of 7,12-dimethylbenz[a]anthracene is equivalent in the presence or absence of aryl hydrocarbon receptor. *Cancer Lett.* (2004) 214:35–41. doi: 10.1016/j.canlet.2004.04.014

41. Guengerich FP. Cytochrome p450 and chemical toxicology. *Chem Res Toxicol.* (2008) 21:70–83. doi: 10.1021/tx700079z

42. Kleiner HE, Vulimiri SV, Reed MJ, Uberecken A, DiGiovanni J. Role of cytochrome P450 1a1 and 1b1 in the metabolic activation of 7,12-dimethylbenz[a]anthracene and the effects of naturally occurring furanocoumarins on skin tumor initiation. *Chem Res Toxicol.* (2002) 15:226–35. doi: 10.1021/tx010151v

43. Shimada T. Xenobiotic-metabolizing enzymes involved in activation and detoxification of carcinogenic polycyclic aromatic hydrocarbons. *Drug Metab Pharmacokinet.* (2006) 21:257–76. doi: 10.2133/dmpk.21.257

44. Xue P, Fu J, Zhou Y. The aryl hydrocarbon receptor and tumor immunity. *Front Immunol.* (2018) 9:286. doi: 10.3389/fimmu.2018.00286

45. Feng S, Cao Z, Wang X. Role of aryl hydrocarbon receptor in cancer. *Biochim Biophys Acta.* (2013) 1836:197–210. doi: 10.1016/j.bbcan.2013.05.001

46. Lin JY, Fisher DE. Melanocyte biology and skin pigmentation. *Nature.* (2007) 445:843–50. doi: 10.1038/nature05660

47. Jux B, Kadow S, Luecke S, Rannug A, Krutmann J, Esser C. The aryl hydrocarbon receptor mediates UVB radiation-induced skin tanning. *J Invest Dermatol.* (2011) 131:203–10. doi: 10.1038/jid.2010.269

48. O'Donnell EF, Kopparapu PR, Koch DC, Jang HS, Phillips JL, Tanguay RL, et al. The Aryl hydrocarbon receptor mediates leflunomide-induced growth inhibition of melanoma cells. *PLoS ONE.* (2012) 7: doi: 10.1371/journal.pone.0040926

49. Contador-Troca M, Alvarez-Barrientos A, Barrasa E, Rico-Leo EM, Catalina-Fernández I, Menacho-Márquez M, et al. The dioxin receptor has tumor suppressor activity in melanoma growth and metastasis. *Carcinogenesis.* (2013) 34:2683–93. doi: 10.1093/carcin/bgt248

50. Villano CM, Murphy KA, Akintobi A, White LA. 2,3,7,8-tetrachlorodibenzo-p-dioxin (TCDD) induces matrix metalloproteinase (MMP) expression and invasion in A2058 melanoma cells. *Toxicol Appl Pharmacol.* (2006) 210:212–24. doi: 10.1016/j.taap.2005.05.001

51. Barretina J, Caponigro G, Stransky N, Venkatesan K, Margolin AA, Kim S, et al. The Cancer Cell Line Encyclopedia enables predictive modelling of anticancer drug sensitivity. *Nature.* (2012) 483:603–7. doi: 10.1038/nature11003

52. Coit DG, Thompson JA, Algazi A, Andtbacka R, Bichakjian CK, Carson WE, et al. Melanoma, Version 2.2016, NCCN clinical practice guidelines in oncology. *J Natl Compr Canc Netw.* (2016) 14:450–73. doi: 10.6004/jnccn.2016.0051

53. Miller AJ, Mihm MC. Melanoma. *N Engl J Med.* (2006) 355:51–65. doi: 10.1056/NEJMra052166

54. Luther C, Swami U, Zhang J, Milhem M, Zakharia Y. Advanced stage melanoma therapies: detailing the present and exploring the future. *Crit Rev Oncol Hematol.* (2019) 133:99–111. doi: 10.1016/j.critrevonc.2018.11.002

55. Colombino M, Capone M, Lissia A, Cossu A, Rubino C, De Giorgi V, et al. BRAF/NRAS mutation frequencies among primary tumors and metastases in patients with melanoma. *J Clin Oncol.* (2012) 30:2522–9. doi: 10.1200/JCO.2011.41.2452

56. Chapman PB, Hauschild A, Robert C, Haanen JB, Ascierto P, Larkin J, et al. Improved survival with vemurafenib in melanoma with BRAF V600E mutation. *N Engl J Med.* (2011) 364:2507–16. doi: 10.1056/NEJMoa1103782

57. Hauschild A, Grob JJ, Demidov LV, Jouary T, Gutzmer R, Millward M, et al. Dabrafenib in BRAF-mutated metastatic melanoma: a multicentre,

open-label, phase 3 randomised controlled trial. *Lancet.* (2012) 380:358–65. doi: 10.1016/S0140-6736(12)60868-X

58. Long GV, Weber JS, Infante JR, Kim KB, Daud A, Gonzalez R, et al. Overall survival and durable responses in patients with BRAF V600-mutant metastatic melanoma receiving dabrafenib combined with trametinib. *J Clin Oncol.* (2016) 34:871–8. doi: 10.1200/JCO.2015.62.9345

59. Müller J, Krijgsman O, Tsoi J, Robert L, Hugo W, Song C, et al. Low MITF/AXL ratio predicts early resistance to multiple targeted drugs in melanoma. *Nat Commun.* (2014) 5:5712. doi: 10.1038/ncomms6712

60. Kong X, Kuilman T, Shahrabi A, Boshuizen J, Kemper K, Song JY, et al. Cancer drug addiction is relayed by an ERK2-dependent phenotype switch. *Nature.* (2017) 550:270–4. doi: 10.1038/nature24037

61. Alexandrov LB, Nik-Zainal S, Wedge DC, Aparicio SAJR, Behjati S, Biankin AV, et al. Signatures of mutational processes in human cancer. *Nature.* (2013) 500:415–21. doi: 10.1038/nature12477

62. Efremova M, Finotello F, Rieder D, Trajanoski Z. Neoantigens generated by individual mutations and their role in cancer immunity and immunotherapy. *Front Immunol.* (2017) 8:1–8. doi: 10.3389/fimmu.2017.01679

63. Rooney MS, Shukla SA, Wu CJ, Getz G, Hacohen N. Molecular and genetic properties of tumors associated with local immune cytolytic activity. *Cell.* (2015) 160:48–61. doi: 10.1016/j.cell.2014.12.033

64. Rodić N, Anders RA, Eshleman JR, Lin MT, Xu H, Kim JH, et al. PD-L1 expression in melanocytic lesions does not correlate with the BRAF V600E mutation. *Cancer Immunol Res.* (2015) 3:110–5. doi: 10.1158/2326-6066.CIR-14-0145

65. Dong H, Strome SE, Salomao DR, Tamura H, Hirano F, Flies DB, et al. Tumor-associated B7-H1 promotes T-cell apoptosis: a potential mechanism of immune evasion. *Nat Med.* (2002) 8:793–800. doi: 10.1038/nm730

66. Hirano F, Kaneko K, Tamura H, Dong H, Wang S, Ichikawa M, et al. Blockade of B7-H1 and PD-1 by monoclonal antibodies potentiates cancer therapeutic immunity. *Cancer Res.* (2005) 65:1089–96.

67. Robert C, Long GV, Brady B, Dutriaux C, Maio M, Mortier L, et al. Nivolumab in previously untreated melanoma without BRAF mutation. *N Engl J Med.* (2015) 372:320–30. doi: 10.1056/NEJMoa1412082

68. Liu Y, Liang X, Yin X, Lv J, Tang K, Ma J, et al. Blockade of IDO-kynurenine-AhR metabolic circuitry abrogates IFN-γ-induced immunologic dormancy of tumor-repopulating cells. *Nat Commun.* (2017) 8:15207. doi: 10.1038/ncomms15207

69. Liu Y, Lv J, Liu J, Liang X, Jin X, Xie J, et al. STAT3/p53 pathway activation disrupts IFN-β-induced dormancy in tumor-repopulating cells. *J Clin Invest.* (2018) 128:1057–73. doi: 10.1172/JCI96329

70. Wardhani LO, Matsushita M, Iwasaki T, Kuwamoto S, Nonaka D, Nagata K, Expression of the IDO1/TDO2-AhR pathway in tumor cells or the tumor microenvironment is associated with Merkel cell polyomavirus status and prognosis in Merkel cell carcinoma. *Hum Pathol.* (2019) 84:52–61. doi: 10.1016/j.humpath.2018.09.003

71. Sato Y, Fujimura T, Tanita K, Lyu C, Matsushita S, Fujisawa Y, et al. Malassezia-derived aryl hydrocarbon receptor ligands enhance the CCL20/ Th17/soluble CD163 pathogenic axis in extra-mammary Paget's disease. *Exp Dermatol.* (2019) 28:933–39. doi: 10.1111/exd.13944

Biomarkers for Immune Checkpoint Inhibitors in Melanoma

8

Shigehisa Kitano[1,2]*, Takayuki Nakayama[1] and Makiko Yamashita[1]

[1] Department of Experimental Therapeutics, National Cancer Center Hospital, Tokyo, Japan, [2] Division of Cancer Immunotherapy, Exploratory Oncology Research and Clinical Trial Center, National Cancer Center, Tokyo, Japan

*Correspondence:
Shigehisa Kitano
skitano@ncc.go.jp

Immune checkpoint inhibitors have now become a standard therapy for malignant melanoma. However, as immunotherapies are effective in only a limited number of patients, biomarker development remains one of the most important clinical challenges. Biomarkers predicting clinical benefit facilitate appropriate selection of individualized treatments for patients and maximize clinical benefits. Many biomarkers derived from tumors and peripheral blood components have recently been reported, mainly in retrospective settings. This review summarizes the recent findings of biomarker studies for predicting the clinical benefits of immunotherapies in melanoma patients. Taking into account the complex interactions between the immune system and various cancers, it would be difficult for only one biomarker to predict clinical benefits in all patients. Many efforts to discover candidate biomarkers are currently ongoing. In the future, verification, by means of a prospective study, may allow some of these candidates to be combined into a scoring system based on bioinformatics technology.

Keywords: biomarker, immune checkpoint inhibitor, malignant melanoma, cytotoxic T-lymphocyte-associated antigen 4, programmed death-1

INTRODUCTION

In recent years, immune checkpoint inhibitors have increasingly been applied to the clinical development of cancer immunotherapy. For malignant melanoma, ipilimumab, a humanized monoclonal antibody (mAb) that blocks cytotoxic T-lymphocyte-associated antigen 4 (CTLA-4) and nivolumab, as well as pembrolizumab, a humanized mAb that blocks programmed death-1 (PD-1) on primed T cells, have been approved and are now used as standard therapies. Several clinical trials have investigated new agents, alone and in combination, for use in the treatment of advanced malignant melanoma. However, immunotherapies are effective in only a limited number of patients and severe immune-related adverse events (irAEs) develop in some patients. Biomarkers predicting clinical benefit support appropriate the selection of individualized treatments for patients and maximize clinical benefits. Thus, one of the most important tasks for advancing this form of therapy is to identify "baseline (pretreatment)" biomarkers predicting responses or toxicities. In general, biomarkers are mainly divided into two functional categories, "prognostic" and "predictive." A prognostic biomarker can be defined based on the effects of patient or tumor biology on the patient's clinical outcome. This includes patients at high risk for disease relapse who may thus derive benefit from earlier treatments. On the other hand, a predictive biomarker is defined by the effects of treatment, including tumor response and improvements in overall survival (OS), disease-free survival (DFS), and progression-free survival (PFS). Many biomarker candidates have been identified, to date, in retrospective settings. This review summarizes recent findings of biomarker studies designed to identify means of predicting the clinical benefits of immunotherapies in melanoma patients, focusing on three categories: tumor tissue, peripheral blood, and others (**Table 1**).

TABLE 1 | Biomarkers for metastatic melanoma patients treated with immune checkpoint inhibitor therapy.

Tumor (microenvironment)	Reference
Immunohistochemistry (IHC)	
Programmed death-ligand 1 (PD-L1) expression on tumor cells	(1–4)
PD-L1 expression on immune cells	(5–7)
Programmed death-1 expression on T cells	(25)
Infiltration of CD8+ cells	(37–41)
Infiltration of CD4+ cells	(40)
Regulatory T cells (Tregs)	(29, 30)
Myeloid-derived suppressor cells (MDSC)	(31–35)
Tumor-associated macrophages (M2)	(36)
Gene profiling (expression/mutation/amplification)	
Tumor mutation burden	(9–14)
Number of somatic mutations (non-synonymous mutations)	(10, 11, 15–19)
Activation of IFN-γ signaling	(21, 22)
Amplification of WNT/β-catenine signaling	(23)
Janus kinase (JAK) 1/JAK2 loss-of-function mutations	(25, 26)
Peripheral blood	
Number of lymphocytes	(42, 43)
Number of Tregs	(38, 44, 45)
Number of MDSCs	(46–50)
Number of proliferating CD8+ T cells	(52–57)
Number of memory CD4+ T cells	(58–60)
Concentrations of cytokines (e.g., IL-6, IL-8, IL-10, and TGF-β)	(62–64)
Concentration of VEGF	(66)
PD-L1 expression on circulating tumor cells	(8)
Soluble PD-L1	(67)
Others	
Microbiome	(68–70)
Fatty acids	(71)
Vitiligo and rash	(72–75)

BIOMARKERS IN TUMOR TISSUE

PD-L1 Expression on Tumor Cells

Programmed death-ligand 1 (PD-L1) expression has been investigated as a potential biomarker for PD-1 or the PD-L1 inhibitor. In phase I trials, PD-L1 expression on tumor cells correlated with the response to anti-PD-1 antibody (1). Given these promising results, several companies developed PD-L1 companion diagnostic tests for anti-PD-1/PD-L1 antibody and patients with PD-L1-positive tumors were considered to be good candidates for anti-PD-1/PD-L1 antibody treatment. In fact, the U.S. Food and Drug Administration has approved pembrolizumab, an anti-PD-1 antibody, for the treatment of PD-L1-positive non-small cell lung cancer (NSCLC) and gastric cancer. However, there are several problems while using PD-L1 expression as a biomarker for immunotherapy. First, PD-L1 expression levels show heterogeneity within tumors (2). Second, PD-L1 is a dynamic marker that can be affected by treatment and local inflammation (3). Third, the optimal threshold level of PD-L1 expression remains uncertain (4). In fact, some PD-L1 negative patients also derive benefit from treatment with an anti-PD-1/PD-L1 inhibitor.

Interestingly, PD-L1 expression on tumor infiltrating immune cells may be more predictive of responsiveness to anti-PD-1 antibody than the level of PD-L1 expression by the tumor (5). Furthermore, while PD-L1 expression on tumor cells did not tend to be related to the response rate in melanoma patients

treated with anti-PD-1 antibody (nivolumab) and anti-CTLA-4-antibody (ipilimumab), there was a correlation with a good response in non-small lung cancer patients treated with these drugs (6, 7). On the other hand, Schott et al. reported that PD-L1 expression on "circulating" tumor cells might also be a potential biomarker (8). They suggested circulating tumor cells to possibly be precursors of metastatic disease, with PD-L1 expression allowing stratification according to the anticipated response to therapy. Further study is needed to determine the clinical significance of PD-LI expression.

Genes: Mutation-Burden and Gene-Expression

Melanoma is characterized by having one of the highest mutation burdens of any cancer (9, 10). These somatic mutations generate immunogenic-neoantigens recognized as tumor-antigens, possibly triggering effective anti-tumor immune responses (11–13). Genomic analysis revealed that a high mutational load at baseline may predict better survival but not treatment responses (13), and the mutation burden after PD-1 therapy was reportedly decreased in melanoma patients who responded to treatment (14).

Genes harboring significant mutations included *BRAF*, *CDKN2A*, *NRAS*, *PTEN*, and *TP53* in cutaneous melanoma, *BRAF*, *NRAS*, *NF1*, and *KIT* in acral melanoma (hands and feet), and *SF3B1* in mucosal melanoma (internal body surfaces) (15–17). The *BRAF* mutation was the most common, being detected in approximately half of metastatic melanoma patients. In the current treatment of melanoma, only *BRAF* V600 mutations are regarded as being molecular markers applicable to treatment decision-making strategies (10, 18). Several studies of CTLA-4 and PD-1 therapy have revealed that *BRAF* V600E mutations do not correlate with either the response to CTLA-4 therapy or the resulting OS, whereas the correlation with the response of melanomas to PD-1 therapy was significant (11, 19). On the other hand, inactivation of *CDKN2A* and/or *PTEN* is regarded as an important mechanism underlying resistance and/or durable responses to BRAF-inhibitor-based therapy, but is not currently taken into consideration in the clinical decision-making process (10).

Previous sequence studies, such as The Cancer Genome Atlas study, used exome and low-pass whole-genome sequencing (WGS). In 2017, Hayward et al. reported the first large, high-coverage WGS study of melanomas (cutaneous, acral, and mucosal subtypes), including analysis of the non-coding region. Their report showed that the number of mutations in the non-coding region was detected as a number equivalent to that in the coding region, and that the most common mutations in the non-coding region were in the *TERT* promoter upstream from the initiation codon (69% of all melanomas and 86% of cutaneous melanomas) (17). Moreover, Ishida et al. preliminarily reported a correlation between HLA-A*26 alleles and the response to anti-PD-1 (nivolumab) therapy in Japanese patients with metastatic melanoma (20). HLA accounts for some of the individual differences in antigen-specific immune responses, and might provide useful information for devising individualized immunotherapeutic regimens. The associations of these new findings with clinical responses to immunotherapies merit further investigation.

On the other hand, there have been several investigations of the gene expressions on tumor tissues, for their value in predicting responses to immune checkpoint inhibitors. Immunohistochemistry and gene profiling assays have suggested the presence of a "T-cell-inflamed tumor microenvironment," with an abundance of chemokines and an IFN-γ signature, to correlate with the clinical efficacy of immune checkpoint inhibitors in melanoma patients (21, 22). Numerous studies have revealed the molecular mechanisms underlying lack of T-cell infiltration and resistance of melanomas to immune checkpoint therapy, such as the melanoma-intrinsic active WNT/β-catenin-signaling pathway (23) and enrichment for mutations in PTEN (24), loss-of-function mutations in Janus kinase (JAK1)/JAK2 (which are involved in IFNγ signaling), and β2 microglobulin (an MHC class I subunit) (25, 26).

Tumor Infiltrating Lymphocytes (TILs)

Tumor infiltrating lymphocytes, such as T cells, macrophages, and various types of immune suppressive cells, are considered to be the most important players in the regulation of anti-tumor immune responses. Several studies have demonstrated an increase in the TIL number to correlate with good clinical responses and a higher survival rate of patients with melanoma and various other cancers (27, 28).

In melanoma patients, immune suppressive cells, such as regulatory T cells (Tregs) (29, 30), monocytic myeloid-derived suppressor cells (m-MDSCs) (31–35), and tumor-associated (activated) macrophages (TAM; M2) (36), were reportedly increased in number and thereby inhibited effector T cells, resulting in an increase in tumor growth.

In contrast, a number of investigators have reported the quantity of infiltrating CD8+CD45RO+ effector memory T cells to be clearly associated with longer DFS and OS, for many cancer types including melanoma (37–39). Recently, Wei et al. comprehensively profiled the effects of CTLA-4/PD-1-targeted immunotherapy on tumor infiltrating immune cells. Their study revealed that PD-1 blockade and CTLA-4 blockade both led to a subset of exhausted-like CD8+ T cells (CD45RO+PD-1+T-bet+EOMES+). They also showed that CTLA-4 blockade induced the expansion of an ICOS+ Th1-like CD4 effector population (CD45RO+PD-1loTBET+ and CD69+) in melanoma patients. These observations suggested that these two immunotherapies target specific subsets of exhausted-like CD8+ T cells, but drive different cellular mechanisms to induce tumor rejection (40). Moreover, Canale et al. described high expression of CD39 on CD8+ infiltrating T cells as being increased in melanoma lesions. CD39 is the immunosuppressive enzyme termed ATP ectonucleotidase, and CD39highCD8+ T cells reportedly exhibit features of cellular exhaustion, such as reduced production of tumor necrosis factor and interleukin (IL)-2, as well as expressions of co-inhibitory receptors (41).

BIOMARKERS IN PERIFERAL BLOOD

Peripheral Blood Mononuclear Cells (PBMCs)

Blood biomarkers have most frequently been analyzed for correlations with clinical responses to immunotherapies. Baseline and/or post-treatment changes in absolute counts of white blood cells, lymphocytes, eosinophils, neutrophils, and monocytes, as well as ratios of neutrophils or monocytes to lymphocytes may both be promising and routinely available blood markers that have shown associations with responses to immune checkpoint inhibitors (11, 42, 43).

Recently, several studies have raised the possibility of circulating immune cells as predictive biomarkers for immune checkpoint inhibitors. The frequency of circulating Tregs is reportedly associated with disease progression and poor patient survival for many carcinomas treated with immunotherapy (38, 44, 45). Numerous studies have found that high levels of circulating m-MDSCs in various forms of cancer, including melanoma, correlate with poor survival (46–48). In patients treated with anti-PD-1 antibody, m-MDSCs were reported to be a blood cytology marker showing significant correlations with all outcome parameters (49, 50). However, human MDSCs have yet to be clearly characterized both biologically and phenotypically. A very recent study demonstrated that the frequency of CD14+CD16-HLA-DRhi monocytes predicts both PFS and OS of melanoma patients treated with anti-PD-1 antibody, based on analysis employing high-dimensional single-cell mass cytometry (51). This CD14+ population including MDSCs might be useful as a predictive and/or prognostic biomarker for cancer patients receiving immunotherapy, but further investigation is needed to clarify the phenotype and biological characteristics of this diverse population of cells.

On the other hand, several studies examining circulating T cells have shown the involvement of CD8+ T cells, such as the proliferating (Ki67+) CD8+ effector-like T cells, in NSCLC patients receiving PD-1-therapy (52), and neoantigen-specific circulating CD8+ T cells in melanoma (53, 54). The latter are CD8+ T cells expressing PD-1. In addition, two complementary reports showed that CD28, a member of the same family as PD-1 (including CTLA-4 and ICOS), expressed on CD8+ T cells is a key molecule in PD-1-targeted therapy (55). Hui et al. showed that "CD28 is the primary target of PD-1 signaling," using a cell-free membrane reconstitution system. Their report revealed that PD-1 was phosphorylated in response to PD-L1 ligation, thereby preferentially inducing dephosphorylation of CD28 (but not the T cell receptor), resulting in the inhibition of T cell proliferation (56). On the other hand, Kamphorst et al. found that, in lung cancer patients, proliferating Ki67+PD-1+CD8+ T cells were increased in peripheral blood, and subsequently activated (CD38+, HLA-DR+) and mostly expressed CD28 (57), implying that CD28 signaling is associated with rescue of the exhausted CD8+ T cells in PD-1 targeted therapies. These findings are reasonable and it is interesting that CD28, belonging to the same family as PD-1, is a key molecule in PD-1-targeted therapy, although its applicability as a predictive/prognostic biomarker in melanoma patients is as yet unclear. Moreover, whether other family members, including CTLA-4 and ICOS, have similar features in immune checkpoint therapy, remains unknown. Elucidating these issues might reveal novel useful biomarkers for use alone and/or in combination with PD-1-targeted therapy. Another interesting, and potentially important, finding of these studies is that proliferating CD8+

effector-like T cells were reportedly increased following PD-1-targeted therapy.

Several recent studies, focusing on circulating CD4+ T cells, found that increases in central memory CD4+ T cells (CD27+, FAS−, CD45RA−, and CCR7+) (58), and IL-9-producing CD4+ T helper (Th9) cells (59), correlated with good clinical responses of melanoma patients to anti-PD-1 therapy. Moreover, in lung cancer patients treated with nivolumab, the frequencies of CD62L^{low}CD4+ T cells and Tregs (CD25+Foxp3+CD4+) in pretreatment PBMC were reported to correlate significantly with clinical responses (60). Their ASCO presentation outlined the major differences in pre-existing immunity, among patients showing a partial response, stable disease, or progressive disease, in response to anti-PD-1 Ab, as reflected by the status of CD4+ T cells, i.e., the balance between primed effector and Tregs. These recent reports raised the possibility that, in peripheral blood, not only T cell exhaustion but also activation of effector CD8+ T cells and increases in memory T cells appear to be highly important, and not only phenotyping markers but also functional molecules can serve important roles as prognostic and/or predictive factors for immune checkpoint inhibitors. Although peripheral blood analysis may provide valuable insights into the responses of cancer patients to immune checkpoint inhibitors, more investigation is needed before these biomarkers can be applied in clinical settings.

OTHERS

Soluble Factors (Serum/Circulating Factors)

Lactate dehydrogenase was frequently investigated in previous studies and showed significant correlations with OS and PFS, whereas there were no correlations with responses to treatments (61). Recently, several studies have revealed that serum cytokine levels to correlate with responses to immune checkpoint inhibitors. Sanmamed et al. showed serum IL-8 levels to be highly correlated with tumor burden changes in metastatic melanoma and NSCLC patients during treatment with anti-PD-1/anti-CTLA-4 therapy (62, 63), and Yamazaki et al. reported that pretreatment serum IFN-γ, IL-6, and IL-10 levels were significantly higher in those with tumor progression among patients with advanced melanoma given nivolumab (64). In addition, in patients with metastatic melanoma receiving nivolumab, the activity of soluble CD73, which is an enzyme that hydrolyzes extracellular AMP to adenosine, in blood was shown to be significantly associated with clinical outcomes (65). Moreover, Frankhauser et al., studying metastatic melanoma patients, reported gene expression of vascular endothelial growth factor-C (VEGF-C) to correlate markedly with both CCL21 and T cell inflammation, and that serum VEGF-C concentrations were associated with both T cell activation/expansion and clinical responses to checkpoint blockade (66).

Soluble PD-L1 (sPD-L1)

Pretreatment sPD-L1 levels reportedly correlate with progression of advanced melanoma treated with anti-CTLA-4 or anti-PD-1 antibody. Although changes in circulating sPD-L1 in the early phase after starting treatment did not distinguish responders from non-responders, patients who had increased circulating sPD-L1 after 5 months of treatment tended to show partial responses (67). The biology of sPD-L1 remains unclear and merits further research.

Microbiome

A vast number of microbes colonize the human body. This colonization is associated with many diseases, including various malignancies. During the past decade, the advent of metagenomic sequencing that combines next-generation DNA sequencing technologies with computational analyses has allowed us to analyze the relationships between the microbiome and various cancers. Recent studies have suggested that the gut microbiome may affect the efficacy of immune checkpoint inhibitors and, consequently, that changing the gut microbiome of a mouse or even a human patient might make tumors more responsive to immune checkpoint inhibitors. This possibility was first evaluated using preclinical models. Vétizou et al. showed that the efficacy of anti-CTLA-4 therapy was diminished in a germ-free mouse model. In addition, the use of broad-spectrum antibiotics to eliminate gut microbiota altered the anti-tumor effect of anti-CTLA-4 therapy (68). Sivan et al. reported that *Bifidobacterium* counts decreased in parallel with the anti-tumor effects of anti-PD-L1 therapy in a mouse model (69). Furthermore, Gopalakrishnan et al. indicated that anti-PD-1 immunotherapy in melanoma patients may be modulated by the gut microbiome. These researchers reported significantly higher alpha diversity and a relative abundance of Ruminococcaceae bacteria in the gut microbiome of responders (70). These findings indicated that specific organisms comprising the gut microbiome enhanced anti-tumor responses in patients treated with immune checkpoint inhibitors. Although the gut microbiome is a potential predictive marker of immunotherapy, a larger prospective study is needed to confirm these results.

Fatty Acids

Kim et al. investigated cellular metabolome and lipidome alterations related to melanoma metastasis. Their analysis showed a progressive increase in phosphatidylinositol species with saturated and monounsaturated fatty acyl chains, as the metastatic potential of the melanoma cells rose, highlighting these lipids as possible biomarkers (71).

Vitiligo and Rash

Immune checkpoint inhibitors have a rather unique adverse event profile, generally described as irAEs, which are most commonly observed in the skin, the gastrointestinal tract, the lungs, the liver, endocrine system, and other organs. Cutaneous irAEs are much more common adverse events in patients with melanoma than in those with other solid tumors. Although vitiligo is attributed to an autoantibody to melanocytes, the etiology of vitiligo is not understood in detail. Vitiligo occurrence has long been speculated to be related to tumor shrinkage in melanoma patients (72). Vitiligo develops in 13–26% of patients treated with nivolumab (73, 74), though grade III/IV disease is rare.

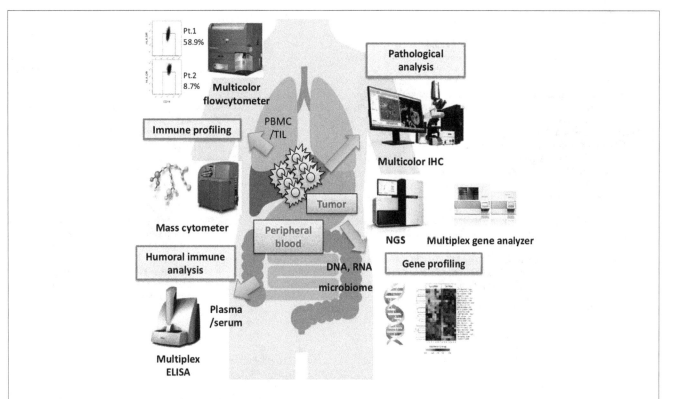

FIGURE 1 | Various assay systems for identifying biomarkers. Several biomarkers derived from the tumor microenvironment, peripheral blood biology, and other factors have been proposed as distinct biomarkers of responses to immune checkpoint blockade therapy. Recently, there have been innovative advancements in assay technology that have made it possible to comprehensively profile the biology and phenotype of the tumor-microenvironment, peripheral blood, and other factors. It would be very difficult, however, for a single biomarker to predict clinical responses and/or serve as a patient selection criterion, though multifactorial biomarkers including these and other novel findings might have great value for predicting clinical responses and/or patient prognosis.

Recent studies have shown vitiligo and rash to be associated with a significant OS improvement in metastatic melanoma patients treated with immune checkpoint inhibitors (73–75). Furthermore, Nakamura et al. suggested that the occurrence of vitiligo might not be regarded as an early marker of good clinical response because the mean time to vitiligo occurrence was approximately 5 months after starting nivolumab (73). The onset times of vitiligo vary considerably depending on the type of drug administered and patient features. Thus, when we use cutaneous irAEs as a biomarker for immune checkpoint inhibitors, we should take into consideration the characteristics of each drug.

CONCLUSION

Numerous candidate biomarkers are currently the focus of research, based mainly on retrospective analyses. Most notably, tumor mutation burden, intratumoral or immune cell expressions of PD-L1, and CD8+ T cell infiltration into the tumor have been documented in several cohorts. For example, not only melanoma but also lung carcinoma, one of the carcinomas which also has a high mutation burden, shows good clinical responses to PD-1/PD-L1 therapy. In lung carcinoma, mutation burden, TIL accumulation, and/or PD-L1 expression on tumor cells correlated with good clinical responses. However, renal cell carcinoma is also reportedly responsive to PD-1 therapy,

despite having a low mutation burden, while TIL accumulation and PD-L1 expression did not correlate with treatment effectiveness. These observations suggest that these factors are not always applicable to predicting clinical benefits. Taking into account the complex interactions between the immune system and malignancies *via* cell surface molecules, such as immune checkpoint molecules, humoral factors, including proteins, cytokines, and so on, it is not unreasonable to speculate that a single biomarker would not allow clinical benefits to be predicted in all patients. In the near future, by applying bioinformatics technology, several biomarkers might be combined to produce a useful scoring system, depending on the type of cancer, the stage, individual treatments, and the timing of intervention. Recent advancements in assay technology, such as mass cytometry (CyTOF), multicolor IHC, multiplex gene analyzer, and so on (**Figure 1**), have the potential to provide an abundance of biological and/or phenotypical observations in a range of environments. Now is the time to discover the candidate biomarkers which might comprise such a future scoring system. Finally, needless to say, a prospective study on a large patient population is essential.

AUTHOR CONTRIBUTIONS

SK: conception/design of the manuscript. SK, TN, and MY: writing of the manuscript.

REFERENCES

1. Topalian SL, Hodi FS, Brahmer JR, Gettinger SN, Smith DC, McDermott DF, et al. Safety, activity, and immune correlates of anti-PD-1 antibody in cancer. *N Engl J Med* (2012) 366:2443–54. doi:10.1056/NEJMoa1200690

2. McLaughlin J, Han G, Schalper KA, Carvajal-Hausdorf D, Pelekanou V, Rehman J, et al. Quantitative assessment of the heterogeneity of PD-L1 expression in non-small-cell lung cancer. *JAMA Oncol* (2016) 2:46–54. doi:10.1001/jamaoncol.2015.3638

3. Vilain RE, Menzies AM, Wilmott JS, Kakavand H, Madore J, Guminski A, et al. Dynamic changes in PD-L1 expression and immune infiltrates early during treatment predict response to PD-1 blockade in melanoma. *Clin Cancer Res* (2017) 23:5024–33. doi:10.1158/1078-0432.CCR-16-0698

4. Hutarew G. PD-L1 testing, fit for routine evaluation? From a pathologist's point of view. *Memo* (2016) 9:201–6. doi:10.1007/s12254-016-0292-2

5. Herbst RS, Soria JC, Kowanetz M, Fine GD, Hamid O, Gordon MS, et al. Predictive correlates of response to the anti-PD-L1 antibody MPDL3280A in cancer patients. *Nature* (2014) 515:563–7. doi:10.1038/nature14011

6. Larkin J, Chiarion-Sileni V, Gonzalez R, Grob JJ, Cowey CL, Lao CD, et al. Combined nivolumab and ipilimumab or monotherapy in untreated melanoma. *N Engl J Med* (2015) 373:23–34. doi:10.1056/NEJMoa1504030

7. Hellmann MD, Gettinger SN, Goldman J, Brahmer J, Borghaei H, Chow LQ, et al. Safety and efficacy of first-line (1L) nivolumab (nivo; N) and ipilimumab (ipi; I) in advanced (adv) NSCLC. *J Clin Oncol* (2016) 34:abstr3001.

8. Schott DS, Pizon M, Pachmann U, Pachmann K. Sensitive detection of PD-L1 expression on circulating epithelial tumor cells (CETCs) could be a potential biomarker to select patients for treatment with PD-1/PD-L1 inhibitors in early and metastatic solid tumors. *Oncotarget* (2017) 8:72755–72. doi:10.18632/oncotarget.20346

9. Alexandrov LB, Nik-Zainal S, Wedge DC, Aparicio SA, Behjati S, Biankin AV, et al. Signatures of mutational processes in human cancer. *Nature* (2013) 500:415–21. doi:10.1038/nature12477

10. Luke JJ, Flaherty KT, Ribas A, Long GV. Targeted agents and immunotherapies: optimizing outcomes in melanoma. *Nat Rev Clin Oncol* (2017) 14:463–82. doi:10.1038/nrclinonc.2017.43

11. Jessurun CAC, Vos JAM, Limpens J, Luiten RM. Biomarkers for response of melanoma patients to immune checkpoint inhibitors: a systematic review. *Front Oncol* (2017) 7:233. doi:10.3389/fonc.2017.00233

12. van Rooij N, van Buuren MM, Philips D, Velds A, Toebes M, Heemskerk B, et al. Tumor exome analysis reveals neoantigen-specific T-cell reactivity in an ipilimumab-responsive melanoma. *J Clin Oncol* (2013) 31:e439–42. doi:10.1200/JCO.2012.47.7521

13. Hugo W, Zaretsky JM, Sun L, Song C, Moreno BH, Hu-Lieskovan S, et al. Genomic and transcriptomic features of response to anti-PD-1 therapy in metastatic melanoma. *Cell* (2016) 165:35–44. doi:10.1016/j.cell.2016.02.065

14. Riaz N, Havel JJ, Makarov V, Desrichard A, Urba WJ, Sims JS, et al. Tumor and microenvironment evolution during immunotherapy with nivolumab. *Cell* (2017) 171:934–49.e15. doi:10.1016/j.cell.2017.09.028

15. Kamb A, Gruis NA, Weaver-Feldhaus J, Liu Q, Harshman K, Tavtigian SV, et al. A cell cycle regulator potentially involved in genesis of many tumor types. *Science* (1994) 264:436–40. doi:10.1126/science.8153634

16. Albino AP, Le Strange R, Oliff AI, Furth ME, Old LJ. Transforming ras genes from human melanoma: a manifestation of tumour heterogeneity? *Nature* (1984) 308:69–72. doi:10.1038/308069a0

17. Hayward NK, Wilmott JS, Waddell N, Johansson PA, Field MA, Nones K, et al. Whole-genome landscapes of major melanoma subtypes. *Nature* (2017) 545:175–80. doi:10.1038/nature22071

18. Davies H, Bignell GR, Cox C, Stephens P, Edkins S, Clegg S, et al. Mutations of the BRAF gene in human cancer. *Nature* (2002) 417:949–54. doi:10.1038/nature00766

19. Mangana J, Cheng PF, Schindler K, Weide B, Held U, Frauchiger AL, et al. Analysis of BRAF and NRAS mutation status in advanced melanoma patients treated with anti-CTLA-4 antibodies: association with overall survival? *PLoS One* (2015) 10:e0139438. doi:10.1371/journal.pone.0139438

20. Ishida Y, Otsuka A, Tanaka H, Levesque MP, Dummer R, Kabashima K. HLA-A*26 is correlated with response to nivolumab in Japanese melanoma patients. *J Invest Dermatol* (2017) 137:2443–4. doi:10.1016/j.jid.2017.06.023

21. Gajewski TF, Schreiber H, Fu YX. Innate and adaptive immune cells in the tumor microenvironment. *Nat Immunol* (2013) 14:1014–22. doi:10.1038/ni.2703

22. Spranger S, Luke JJ, Bao R, Zha Y, Hernandez KM, Li Y, et al. Density of immunogenic antigens does not explain the presence or absence of the T-cell-inflamed tumor microenvironment in melanoma. *Proc Natl Acad Sci U S A* (2016) 113:E7759–68. doi:10.1073/pnas.1609376113

23. Spranger S, Bao R, Gajewski TF. Melanoma-intrinsic beta-catenin signalling prevents anti-tumour immunity. *Nature* (2015) 523:231–5. doi:10.1038/nature14404

24. Peng W, Chen JQ, Liu C, Malu S, Creasy C, Tetzlaff MT, et al. Loss of PTEN promotes resistance to T cell-mediated immunotherapy. *Cancer Discov* (2016) 6:202–16. doi:10.1158/2159-8290.CD-15-0283

25. Zaretsky JM, Garcia-Diaz A, Shin DS, Escuin-Ordinas H, Hugo W, Hu-Lieskovan S, et al. Mutations associated with acquired resistance to PD-1 blockade in melanoma. *N Engl J Med* (2016) 375:819–29. doi:10.1056/NEJMoa1604958

26. Shin DS, Zaretsky JM, Escuin-Ordinas H, Garcia-Diaz A, Hu-Lieskovan S, Kalbasi A, et al. Primary resistance to PD-1 blockade mediated by JAK1/2 mutations. *Cancer Discov* (2017) 7:188–201. doi:10.1158/2159-8290.CD-16-1223

27. Nishino M, Ramaiya NH, Hatabu H, Hodi FS. Monitoring immune-checkpoint blockade: response evaluation and biomarker development. *Nat Rev Clin Oncol* (2017) 14:655–68. doi:10.1038/nrclinonc.2017.88

28. Tumeh PC, Harview CL, Yearley JH, Shintaku IP, Taylor EJ, Robert L, et al. PD-1 blockade induces responses by inhibiting adaptive immune resistance. *Nature* (2014) 515:568–71. doi:10.1038/nature13954

29. Jandus C, Bioley G, Speiser DE, Romero P. Selective accumulation of differentiated FOXP3(+) CD4 (+) T cells in metastatic tumor lesions from melanoma patients compared to peripheral blood. *Cancer Immunol Immunother* (2008) 57:1795–805. doi:10.1007/s00262-008-0507-4

30. Ouyang Z, Wu H, Li L, Luo Y, Li X, Huang G. Regulatory T cells in the immunotherapy of melanoma. *Tumour Biol* (2016) 37:77–85. doi:10.1007/s13277-015-4315-0

31. Kumar V, Patel S, Tcyganov E, Gabrilovich DI. The nature of myeloid-derived suppressor cells in the tumor microenvironment. *Trends Immunol* (2016) 37:208–20. doi:10.1016/j.it.2016.01.004

32. Umansky V, Sevko A. Melanoma-induced immunosuppression and its neutralization. *Semin Cancer Biol* (2012) 22:319–26. doi:10.1016/j.semcancer.2012.02.003

33. De Sanctis F, Solito S, Ugel S, Molon B, Bronte V, Marigo I. MDSCs in cancer: conceiving new prognostic and therapeutic targets. *Biochim Biophys Acta* (2016) 1865:35–48. doi:10.1016/j.bbcan.2015.08.001

34. Parker KH, Beury DW, Ostrand-Rosenberg S. Myeloid-derived suppressor cells: critical cells driving immune suppression in the tumor microenvironment. *Adv Cancer Res* (2015) 128:95–139. doi:10.1016/bs.acr.2015.04.002

35. Blattner C, Fleming V, Weber R, Himmelhan B, Altevogt P, Gebhardt C, et al. CCR5(+) myeloid-derived suppressor cells are enriched and activated in melanoma lesions. *Cancer Res* (2018) 78:157–67. doi:10.1158/0008-5472.CAN-17-0348

36. Pollard JW. Tumour-educated macrophages promote tumour progression and metastasis. *Nat Rev Cancer* (2004) 4:71–8. doi:10.1038/nrc1256

37. Fridman WH, Pages F, Sautes-Fridman C, Galon J. The immune contexture in human tumours: impact on clinical outcome. *Nat Rev Cancer* (2012) 12:298–306. doi:10.1038/nrc3245

38. Tarhini AA, Edington H, Butterfield LH, Lin Y, Shuai Y, Tawbi H, et al. Immune monitoring of the circulation and the tumor microenvironment in patients with regionally advanced melanoma receiving neoadjuvant ipilimumab. *PLoS One* (2014) 9:e87705. doi:10.1371/journal.pone.0087705

39. Tietze JK, Angelova D, Heppt MV, Reinholz M, Murphy WJ, Spannagl M, et al. The proportion of circulating CD45RO(+)CD8(+) memory T cells is correlated with clinical response in melanoma patients treated with ipilimumab. *Eur J Cancer* (2017) 75:268–79. doi:10.1016/j.ejca.2016.12.031

40. Wei SC, Levine JH, Cogdill AP, Zhao Y, Anang NAS, Andrews MC, et al. Distinct cellular mechanisms underlie anti-CTLA-4 and anti-PD-1 checkpoint blockade. *Cell* (2017) 170:1120–33.e17. doi:10.1016/j.cell.2017.07.024

41. Canale FP, Ramello MC, Nunez N, Furlan CLA, Bossio SN, Serran MG, et al. CD39 expression defines cell exhaustion in tumor-infiltrating CD8(+) T cells. *Cancer Res* (2018) 78:115–28. doi:10.1158/0008-5472.CAN-16-2684

42. Ferrucci PF, Gandini S, Cocorocchio E, Pala L, Baldini F, Mosconi M, et al. Baseline relative eosinophil count as a predictive biomarker for ipilimumab treatment in advanced melanoma. *Oncotarget* (2017) 8:79809–15. doi:10.18632/oncotarget.19748

43. Jacquelot N, Roberti MP, Enot DP, Rusakiewicz S, Ternes N, Jegou S, et al. Predictors of responses to immune checkpoint blockade in advanced melanoma. *Nat Commun* (2017) 8:592. doi:10.1038/s41467-017-00608-2

44. Retseck J, VanderWeele R, Lin HM, Lin Y, Butterfield LH, Tarhini AA. Phenotypic and functional testing of circulating regulatory T cells in advanced melanoma patients treated with neoadjuvant ipilimumab. *J Immunother Cancer* (2016) 4:38. doi:10.1186/s40425-016-0141-1

45. Ward-Hartstonge KA, Kemp RA. Regulatory T-cell heterogeneity and the cancer immune response. *Clin Transl Immunology* (2017) 6:e154. doi:10.1038/cti.2017.43

46. Meyer C, Cagnon L, Costa-Nunes CM, Baumgaertner P, Montandon N, Leyvraz L, et al. Frequencies of circulating MDSC correlate with clinical outcome of melanoma patients treated with ipilimumab. *Cancer Immunol Immunother* (2014) 63:247–57. doi:10.1007/s00262-013-1508-5

47. Kitano S, Postow MA, Ziegler CG, Kuk D, Panageas KS, Cortez C, et al. Computational algorithm-driven evaluation of monocytic myeloid-derived suppressor cell frequency for prediction of clinical outcomes. *Cancer Immunol Res* (2014) 2:812–21. doi:10.1158/2326-6066.CIR-14-0013

48. Gebhardt C, Sevko A, Jiang H, Lichtenberger R, Reith M, Tarnanidis K, et al. Myeloid cells and related chronic inflammatory factors as novel predictive markers in melanoma treatment with ipilimumab. *Clin Cancer Res* (2015) 21:5453–9. doi:10.1158/1078-0432.CCR-15-0676

49. Gibney GT, Kudchadkar RR, DeConti RC, Thebeau MS, Czupryn MP, Tetteh L, et al. Safety, correlative markers, and clinical results of adjuvant nivolumab in combination with vaccine in resected high-risk metastatic melanoma. *Clin Cancer Res* (2015) 21:712–20. doi:10.1158/1078-0432.CCR-14-2468

50. Weber J, Gibney G, Kudchadkar R, Yu B, Cheng P, Martinez AJ, et al. Phase I/II study of metastatic melanoma patients treated with nivolumab who had progressed after ipilimumab. *Cancer Immunol Res* (2016) 4:345–53. doi:10.1158/2326-6066.CIR-15-0193

51. Krieg C, Nowicka M, Guglietta S, Schindler S, Hartmann FJ, Weber LM, et al. High-dimensional single-cell analysis predicts response to anti-PD-1 immunotherapy. *Nat Med* (2018) 24(2):144–53. doi:10.1038/nm.4466

52. Kamphorst AO, Pillai RN, Yang S, Nasti TH, Akondy RS, Wieland A, et al. Proliferation of PD-1 + CD8 T cells in peripheral blood after PD-1-targeted therapy in lung cancer patients. *Proc Natl Acad Sci U S A* (2017) 114:4993–8. doi:10.1073/pnas.1705327114

53. Gros A, Parkhurst MR, Tran E, Pasetto A, Robbins PF, Ilyas S, et al. Prospective identification of neoantigen-specific lymphocytes in the peripheral blood of melanoma patients. *Nat Med* (2016) 22:433–8. doi:10.1038/nm.4051

54. McGranahan N, Furness AJ, Rosenthal R, Ramskov S, Lyngaa R, Saini SK, et al. Clonal neoantigens elicit T cell immunoreactivity and sensitivity to immune checkpoint blockade. *Science* (2016) 351:1463–9. doi:10.1126/science.aaf1490

55. Krueger J, Rudd CE. Two strings in one bow: PD-1 negatively regulates via co-receptor CD28 on T cells. *Immunity* (2017) 46:529–31. doi:10.1016/j.immuni.2017.04.003

56. Hui E, Cheung J, Zhu J, Su X, Taylor MJ, Wallweber HA, et al. T cell costimulatory receptor CD28 is a primary target for PD-1-mediated inhibition. *Science* (2017) 355:1428–33. doi:10.1126/science.aaf1292

57. Kamphorst AO, Wieland A, Nasti T, Yang S, Zhang R, Barber DL, et al. Rescue of exhausted CD8 T cells by PD-1-targeted therapies is CD28-dependent. *Science* (2017) 355:1423–7. doi:10.1126/science.aaf0683

58. Takeuchi Y, Tanemura A, Tada Y, Katayama I, Kumanogoh A, Nishikawa H. Clinical response to PD-1 blockade correlates with a sub-fraction of peripheral central memory CD4 + T cells in patients with malignant melanoma. *Int Immunol* (2018) 30:13–22. doi:10.1093/intimm/dxx073

59. Nonomura Y, Otsuka A, Nakashima C, Seidel JA, Kitoh A, Dainichi T, et al. Peripheral blood Th9 cells are a possible pharmacodynamic biomarker of nivolumab treatment efficacy in metastatic melanoma patients. *Oncoimmunology* (2016) 5:e1248327. doi:10.1080/2162402X.2016.1248327

60. Kagamu H, Yamaguchi O, Shiono A, Mouri A, Miyauchi S, Utsugi H, et al. CD4 + T cells in PBMC to predict the outcome of anti-PD-1 therapy. *J Clin Oncol* (2017) 35:abstr11525.

61. Weide B, Martens A, Hassel JC, Berking C, Postow MA, Bisschop K, et al. Baseline biomarkers for outcome of melanoma patients treated with pembrolizumab. *Clin Cancer Res* (2016) 22:5487–96. doi:10.1158/1078-0432.CCR-16-0127

62. Sanmamed MF, Carranza-Rua O, Alfaro C, Onate C, Martin-Algarra S, Perez G, et al. Serum interleukin-8 reflects tumor burden and treatment response across malignancies of multiple tissue origins. *Clin Cancer Res* (2014) 20:5697–707. doi:10.1158/1078-0432.CCR-13-3203

63. Sanmamed MF, Perez-Gracia JL, Schalper KA, Fusco JP, Gonzalez A, Rodriguez-Ruiz ME, et al. Changes in serum interleukin-8 (IL-8) levels reflect and predict response to anti-PD-1 treatment in melanoma and non-small-cell lung cancer patients. *Ann Oncol* (2017) 28:1988–95. doi:10.1093/annonc/mdx190

64. Yamazaki N, Kiyohara Y, Uhara H, Iizuka H, Uehara J, Otsuka F, et al. Cytokine biomarkers to predict antitumor responses to nivolumab suggested in a phase 2 study for advanced melanoma. *Cancer Sci* (2017) 108:1022–31. doi:10.1111/cas.13226

65. Morello S, Capone M, Sorrentino C, Giannarelli D, Madonna G, Mallardo D, et al. Soluble CD73 as biomarker in patients with metastatic melanoma patients treated with nivolumab. *J Transl Med* (2017) 15:244. doi:10.1186/s12967-017-1348-8

66. Fankhauser M, Broggi MAS, Potin L, Bordry N, Jeanbart L, Lund AW, et al. Tumor lymphangiogenesis promotes T cell infiltration and potentiates immunotherapy in melanoma. *Sci Transl Med* (2017) 9:eaal4712. doi:10.1126/scitranslmed.aal4712

67. Zhou J, Mahoney KM, Giobbie-Hurder A, Zhao F, Lee S, Liao X, et al. Soluble PD-L1 as a biomarker in malignant melanoma treated with checkpoint blockade. *Cancer Immunol Res* (2017) 5:480–92. doi:10.1158/2326-6066.CIR-16-0329

68. Vetizou M, Pitt JM, Daillere R, Lepage P, Waldschmitt N, Flament C, et al. Anticancer immunotherapy by CTLA-4 blockade relies on the gut microbiota. *Science* (2015) 350:1079–84. doi:10.1126/science.aad1329

69. Sivan A, Corrales L, Hubert N, Williams JB, Aquino-Michaels K, Earley ZM, et al. Commensal *Bifidobacterium* promotes antitumor immunity and facilitates anti-PD-L1 efficacy. *Science* (2015) 350:1084–9. doi:10.1126/science.aac4255

70. Gopalakrishnan V, Spencer CN, Nezi L, Reuben A, Andrews MC, Karpinets TV, et al. Gut microbiome modulates response to anti-PD-1 immunotherapy in melanoma patients. *Science* (2018) 359:97–103. doi:10.1126/science.aan4236

71. Kim HY, Lee H, Kim SH, Jin H, Bae J, Choi HK. Discovery of potential biomarkers in human melanoma cells with different metastatic potential by metabolic and lipidomic profiling. *Sci Rep* (2017) 7:8864. doi:10.1038/s41598-017-08433-9

72. Richards JM, Mehta N, Ramming K, Skosey P. Sequential chemoimmunotherapy in the treatment of metastatic melanoma. *J Clin Oncol* (1992) 10:1338–43. doi:10.1200/JCO.1992.10.8.1338

73. Nakamura Y, Tanaka R, Asami Y, Teramoto Y, Imamura T, Sato S, et al. Correlation between vitiligo occurrence and clinical benefit in advanced melanoma patients treated with nivolumab: a multi-institutional retrospective study. *J Dermatol* (2017) 44:117–22. doi:10.1111/1346-8138.13520

74. Freeman-Keller M, Kim Y, Cronin H, Richards A, Gibney G, Weber JS. Nivolumab in resected and unresectable metastatic melanoma: characteristics of immune-related adverse events and association with outcomes. *Clin Cancer Res* (2016) 22:886–94. doi:10.1158/1078-0432.CCR-15-1136

75. Nakamura Y, Kitano S, Takahashi A, Tsutsumida A, Namikawa K, Tanese K, et al. Nivolumab for advanced melanoma: pretreatment prognostic factors and early outcome markers during therapy. *Oncotarget* (2016) 7:77404–15. doi:10.18632/oncotarget.12677

9

Immune Cell Infiltration of the Primary Tumor, Not PD-L1 Status, is Associated with Improved Response to Checkpoint Inhibition in Metastatic Melanoma

Christiane Kümpers[1], Mladen Jokic[1], Ozan Haase[2], Anne Offermann[1], Wenzel Vogel[1], Victoria Grätz[2], Ewan A. Langan[2,3], Sven Perner[1†] and Patrick Terheyden[2*†]

[1] Pathology of the University Hospital Schleswig-Holstein, Luebeck and Research Center Borstel, Leibniz Lung Center, Luebeck, Germany, [2] Department of Dermatology, University of Luebeck, Luebeck, Germany, [3] Department of Dermatological Sciences, University of Manchester, Manchester, United Kingdom

*Correspondence:
Patrick Terheyden
Patrick.Terheyden@uksh.de

† These authors have contributed equally to this work

Immune checkpoint inhibition has resulted in dramatic improvements in overall and relapse-free survival in patients with metastatic melanoma. The most commonly used immune checkpoint inhibitors are monoclonal antibodies targeting programmed cell death protein 1 and cytotoxic T-lymphocyte-associated protein 4. Unfortunately, a significant subset of patients fail to respond to these therapies, which has resulted in intense research efforts to identify the factors which are associated with treatment response. To this end, we investigated immune cell infiltration in primary melanomas and melanoma metastases, in addition to tumor cell PD-L1 expression, to determine whether these factors are associated with an improved outcome after immune checkpoint inhibition. Indeed, the extent of the immune cell infiltration in the primary melanoma, measured by the Immunoscore, was associated with a significantly improved response to immune checkpoint inhibition in terms of increased overall survival. However, the Immunoscore did not predict which patients would respond to treatment. The Immunoscore was significantly reduced in metastases when compared to primary melanomas. In contrast, PD-L1 expression, exhaustively tested using four commercially available anti-PD-L1 clones, did not differ significantly between primary tumors and melanoma metastases and was not associated treatment response. Whilst replication in larger, prospective studies is required, our data demonstrates the relevance of immune cell infiltration in the primary melanoma as a novel marker of improved overall survival in response to immune checkpoint inhibition.

Keywords: melanoma, PD-L1, immunoscore, checkpoint inhibition, lymphocyte, metastases, checkpoint inhibitor therapy

INTRODUCTION

Although melanoma is highly refractory to treatment with conventional chemotherapy, the advent of immune checkpoint inhibition has dramatically improved the clinical outcome in metastatic disease (1). Immune checkpoint inhibition in melanoma relies on the use of antibodies blocking either the programmed cell death protein 1 (PD-1), for example Nivolumab and Pembrolizumab, preventing melanoma tumor cells from escaping toxic T-cell action, or antibodies targeting the cytotoxic T-lymphocyte-associated protein 4 (CTLA-4), namely Ipilimumab, leading to prolonged T-cell activation and resulting in clonal expansion and enlarged T-cell repertoire. Whilst immune checkpoint inhibition has been associated with impressive long-term response rates, there remains a subset of patients who either fail to respond to therapy (primary resistance), or lose the initial response (secondary resistance) during treatment (2).

Therefore, current research efforts are focused on identifying factors associated with treatment response in order to individually tailor treatment (3). For example, an increased tumor mutational load is associated with improved outcome under checkpoint inhibition, potentially via the induction of immune cells which differentially recognize tumor- from normal cells (4, 5). On the other hand, melanoma can express a specific mutational profile which is able to induce an innate anti-PD1 resistance (IPRES) phenotype, rendering the melanoma effectively unresponsive to immune checkpoint inhibition (6).

The expression of programmed cell death ligand 1 (PD-L1) in melanoma is perhaps the most intensively studied marker of response to treatment with checkpoint inhibition (7, 8). In a comprehensive review of biomarkers for response of melanoma to checkpoint inhibition, Jessurun et al. found a significant correlation between tumor PD-1 and PD-L1 expression and response to checkpoint inhibition in five out of eight analyses. Interestingly, there was no significant correlation with progression-free survival. Whilst divergent methodology may make comparison of these studies difficult, it is clear that overall response, progression-free survival and overall survival are not synonymous, and were correctly reported separately. Moreover, prognostic markers are not necessarily predictive markers of response to treatment (8).

Ultimately, whilst PD-L1 status has been shown to correlate with response to treatment with anti-PD-1 antibodies in metastatic melanoma in some studies (9, 10), the expression of PD-L1 *per se* has not emerged as a predictive marker for treatment response, potentially due to its crucial role in engaging PD-1, a dominant negative regulator of anti-tumor T cell effector function (1, 9, 11). In the clinical setting, PD-L1 expression cannot be relied upon as a predictive marker of treatment response, given that not all tumors expressing PD-L1 respond to PD- inhibitors (12) and melanomas with little or no PD-L1 expression may still respond to checkpoint inhibition.

In contrast, pre-existing tumor immune cell infiltration is considered to be an important factor determining successful immune checkpoint inhibition and consequently treatment response (13). Melanoma is recognized as a tumor that is often infiltrated with immune cells; the grade of tumor-infiltrating lymphocytes being an independent predictor of survival irrespective of the treatment type (14–17). Given the immunogenic nature of melanoma (18), as well as the poor prognosis associated with metastatic disease, we sought to objectively determine the immune cell infiltration (Immunoscore) and PD-L1 status of both primary tumors and metastases in a retrospective cohort based study of patients with metastatic melanoma, treated with anti-CTLA-4 and/or anti-PD-1 antibodies. The Immunoscore captures the number und distribution of tumor-infiltrating lymphocytes and was first described by Clark et al. (19) The grade of tumor-infiltrating lymphocytes is defined as either brisk, nonbrisk or absent. Given the range of commercially available anti-PD-L1 antibodies, we also investigated antibody specificity before utilizing the optimal antibody for the immunohistochemical staining. Finally, we addressed the question of whether immune cell infiltration and/or PD-L1 status of primary melanomas and metastases were associated with the clinical response, specifically in terms of overall survival, to immune checkpoint inhibition.

MATERIALS AND METHODS
Study Population/Case Selection
The patient cohort comprised 32 patients (25 male, 7 female), who were diagnosed with metastatic melanoma and treated with checkpoint inhibitors at the Department of Dermatology, University of Luebeck. Patients underwent treatment with CTLA-4-inhibition (Ipilimumab) and/or anti-PD1-therapy (Nivolumab or (Pembrolizumab). 2 Patients were treated with Ipilimumab monotherapy. 12 patients were treated with Nivolumab ($n = 6$) or Pembrolizumab ($n = 6$). 11 patients received Ipilimumab prior to anti-PD-1-therapy, 4 patients received Ipilimumab prior to combined therapy with Ipilimumab and a PD-1-inhibitor and 3 patients initially received combination therapy with Ipilimumab and a PD1-inhibitor followed by a PD-1-inhibitor (**Table 1**).

The median age at time of diagnosis was 64 years. Nine patients remained alive at the last follow up point. Tissue blocks were retrieved from the archive, having been initially obtained between 2006 and 2016.

Out of the 32 patients, we retrieved primary tumor tissue from 22 patients, while from 10 patients only metastatic tissue was available. From a total of 22 patients for whom primary tumor samples were available, corresponding metastatic tissue was available from 19 cases. Out of the 19 patients with primary and metastatic lesions, 15 had metastatic lesions obtained prior to initiation of anti-PD-1-therapy (matched pairs). Up to 9 metastases (distant and/or lymph node) were available per patient.

Primary tumors, as well as lymph node and distant metastases, obtained before and after immune checkpoint inhibitor therapy were analyzed separately. The "tumor groups" were classified as follows (i) primary tumors (22 patients), (ii) distant metastases obtained pre-treatment (15 patients), (iii) lymph node metastases obtained pre-treatment (12 patients), (iv) distant metastases obtained during treatment (7 patients) and (v) lymph node metastases obtained during treatment (1 patient).

Baseline characteristics of the cohort including sex, age at diagnose, vital status at last follow up, treatment, overall survival, progression free survival, interval between diagnose and first dose checkpoint inhibitor, composition of FFPE material and the Immunoscore of primary tumors and metastases were recorded (**Table 1**). Observation time was the interval from the date of diagnosis to the date of last follow-up or death. Overall survival and progression-free survival ranged from 31 to 3,527

TABLE 1 | Patients' baseline characteristics.

SEX	
male	25
female	7
AGE AT DIAGNOSIS (YEARS)	
mean	64
range	32-91
VITAL STATUS AT LAST FOLLOW UP	
alive	9
dead	23
IMMUNE CHECKPOINT INHIBITOR THERAPY	
Ipilimumab mono	2
Nivolumab mono	6
Pembrolizumab mono	6
first Ipilimumab, afterwards PD-1-Inhibitor	11
first Ipilimumab, afterwards combinated therapy	4
first combinated therapy, afterwards PD-1-Inhibitor	3
OVERALL SURVIVAL (DAYS)	
mean	1272
range	31-3527
PROGRESSION FREE SURVIVAL	
mean	194
range	3-1310
INTERVAL BETWEEN DIAGNOSE AND FIRST DOSE OF PD-1-INHIBITOR (DAYS)	
mean	862
range	14-3425
BRAF-MUTATION STATUS	
wildtype	20
mutation	12
COMPOSITION OF FFPE MATERIAL	
cases with tissue from primary tumor and metastases	19
cases with tissue solely from primary tumors	3
cases with tissue solely from metastases	10
number of all metastases samples	88
number of naive metastases	54
number of metastasespost anti-PD1-therapy	20
number of metastases post Ipilimumab	14
TIL GRADE IN PRIMARY TUMORS	
non-brisk	9 (41%)
brisk	13 (59%)
TIL GRADE IN PRIMARY METASTASES	
non-brisk	37 (68,5%)
brisk	17 (31,5%)
TIL GRADE IN RELAPSED METASTASES (AFTER ANTI-PD1-THERAPY)	
non-brisk	16 (80%)
brisk	4 (20%)

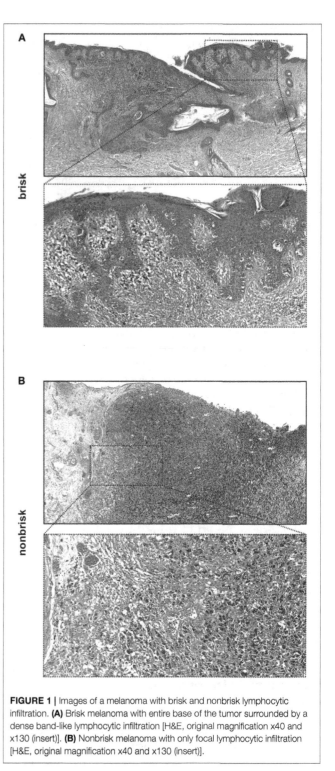

FIGURE 1 | Images of a melanoma with brisk and nonbrisk lymphocytic infiltration. **(A)** Brisk melanoma with entire base of the tumor surrounded by a dense band-like lymphocytic infiltration [H&E, original magnification x40 and x130 (insert)]. **(B)** Nonbrisk melanoma with only focal lymphocytic infiltration [H&E, original magnification x40 and x130 (insert)].

days (mean 1272 days) and from 3 to 1,310 days (mean 194 days), respectively.

Ethical approval for using human material in this study was obtained from the Internal Review Board of University of Luebeck (17–186). All data were anonymized before included to this retrospective study cohort.

Histopathological Analysis

Formalin-fixed paraffin-embedded (FFPE) tissue blocks were retrieved from the archives of the Department of Pathology of the University Hospital Schleswig-Holstein, Campus Luebeck and Research Center Borstel, Leibniz Lung Center, Site Luebeck, the Clinic for Dermatology of the University Hospital Schleswig-Holstein, Campus Luebeck. Tissue microarrays (TMA) were constructed from metastatic samples in triplicates of 0.6 mm diameter cores. A tumor sample was included for further investigation if at least two cores were evaluable. Values of protein expression generated by Immunohistochemistry (IHC) for all examined cores of a patient sample were recorded as a mean value. The TMA included 74 samples of metastatic lesions from 24 patients. Tissue from 14 metastases (from 9 patients) was too small for TMA and therefore investigated as a whole section. All primary tumors were investigated as a whole section due to the small tumor size in most cases. Evaluation of protein expression by IHC was performed by two independent pathologists (CK, SP) who were blinded to the clinico-pathological data.

Immunohistochemical Analysis

Immunohistochemical (IHC) staining was performed using the Ventana Discovery (Ventana Medical System) automated staining system. In brief, slides were incubated at room temperature with the following primary antibodies (dilution, clone, company): anti-PD-L1 (1: 50, E1L3N, Cell Signaling), anti-PD-L1 (RTU, SP263, Roche), anti-PD-L1 (RTU, SP 142, Roche), anti-PD-L1 (1:100, 28.8, Abcam), anti-PD-L2 (1:100, OTI6C3, Acris), anti-PD-1 (RTU, NAT105, Roche), anti-CD8 (RTU, SP57, Roche), anti-CD4 (RTU, SP35, Roche), anti-CD56 (RTU, MRQ-42, Roche), anti-FoxP3 (1:100, 236A/E7, Thermo Fisher) and anti-CTLA4 (1:100, BNI3, Abcam). Expression of PD-L1 and PD-L2 was investigated on tumor and immune cells. CD8, CD4, CD56, FoxP3, CTLA-4, and PD1 staining were used to further characterize the lymphocytes.

Scoring of Tumor Infiltrating Lymphocytes

The Immunoscore was investigated according to criteria formulated by Clark et al (19). In brief, lymphocytes were classified as brisk if they diffusely infiltrated the entire invasive component and were interposed between melanoma cells or if they were present alongside the entire base of tumor. Lymphocytes were classified as nonbrisk if they focally infiltrated the tumor and were not present along the entire tumor base. If no lymphocytes were present or if lymphocytes did not infiltrate the tumor, they were classified as absent.

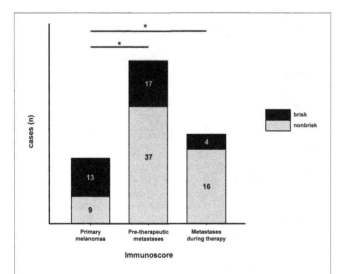

FIGURE 2 | Distribution of brisk vs. nonbrisk infiltration in primary melanomas, pre-therapeutic metastases and metastases which developed during anti-PD-1-therapy. Number of brisk cases is indicated in black and of nonbrisk cases in gray fields. Statistical significance between investigated groups was determined by Fischer's exact test (*p < 0.05).

Immunoscore dynamics

Patient ID	Primary tumors	Pre-therapeutic metastases
Patient ID 1	nonbrisk	nonbrisk
Patient ID 20	nonbrisk	nonbrisk
Patient ID 24	brisk	brisk
Patient ID 26	brisk	brisk
Patient ID 28	brisk	brisk
Patient ID 30	brisk	brisk
Patient ID 16	nonbrisk	brisk
Patient ID 23	nonbrisk	brisk
Patient ID 39	nonbrisk	brisk
Patient ID 2	brisk	nonbrisk
Patient ID 9	brisk	nonbrisk
Patient ID 15	brisk	nonbrisk
Patient ID 31	brisk	nonbrisk
Patient ID 33	brisk	nonbrisk
Patient ID 34	brisk	nonbrisk

FIGURE 3 | Immunoscore dynamics between primary melanomas and pre-therapeutic metastases in the same patient. Top down: No change in Immunoscore was seen in 6 patients, increased Immunoscore in metastases was seen in 3 patients, and a decreased Immunoscore in metastases was seen in 6 patients. Patient identification numbers are denoted besides.

Lymphocytes were morphologically identified by H&E while subtyping of the lymphocytic infiltrate was performed by staining for CD8, CD4, CD56, FoxP, CTLA-4, PD1, PD-L1, and PD-L2.

Quantification of Lymphocytic Subtypes

Percentage of lymphocytes positive for CD8, CD4, CD56, Fox P3, CTLA-4, and PD-1 was calculated according to the total number of tumor infiltrating lymphocytes in a sample. Additionally, we determined ratios of CD4- and CD8-positive lymphocytes. Geographical associations of lymphocytic subtypes and tumor cells could not be investigated due to TMA used for the majority of samples. PD-L2 was evaluated as described below for PD-L1 immunohistochemistry.

Quantification of PD-L1 Expression

In order to determine the most specific PD-L1 expression pattern, we evaluated IHC obtained using four well-established anti-PD-L1 clones (E1L3N, cell signaling; SP263, Roche; SP142, Roche; 28.8, Abcam). Thereafter, PD-L1 staining in tumor cells was considered positive if staining was membranous, regardless of intensity. Tumors were defined as positive if they contained ≥5% PD-L1 positive tumor cells. Expression of PD-L1 in tumor infiltrating lymphocytes was evaluated by measuring the area of PD-L1 positive lymphocytes from the whole tumor area (20).

Statistical Analysis

Fisher's exact test was used to assess the differences in the distribution of brisk vs. nonbrisk lymphocytes between primary melanomas and metastases (including those present prior to initiation of treatment and those which developed during treatment.

Kaplan-Meier curves were used to determine overall survival and progression-free survival depending on the Immunoscore, PD-L1/PD-L2 expression of tumor and immune cells, the different lymphocytic subtypes and CD4/CD8-ratio. Data were statistically proved by log-rank tests.

T-tests were used to compare the mean expression between patients with or without progression during anti-PD1-therapy. Statistical tests were performed within the same tumor groups (primary tumors, lymph node metastases and distant metastases before and after checkpoint-inhibitor therapy).

All statistical analyses were performed using SPSS 2.0. p levels <0.05 were considered significant.

RESULTS

Immune Infiltration Is Significantly Increased in Primary Melanoma When Compared to That Seen in Metastases

We first determined the Immunoscore based on lymphocytic infiltration, classifying the tumors into absent, brisk and nonbrisk groups (**Figure 1**). We assessed the Immunoscore in a total of 22 samples of primary melanomas; 13 (59.1%) were classified as brisk and 9 (40.9%) samples were classified as nonbrisk. We additionally analyzed 88 metastases out of

TABLE 2 | Immunscore and PD-L1 expression before and after anti-PD1 therapy.

Patient ID	Pre-therapeutic tissue	n	PD-L1 expression (mean%)	Immunoscore	Metastases during therapy	n	PD-L1 expression (mean %)	Immunoscore
6	primary tumor	1	5	2	distant metastases	1	0	2
8	primary tumor	1	20	2	lymphe node metastases	3	60	2
9	distant metastases	1	<1	1	distant metastases	6	<1	1
11	satellite metastases	2	2	2	distant metastases	1	10	1
13	not available	X	X	X	distant metastases	1	15	1
14	distant metastases	1	20	1	distant metastases	1	30	1
21	lymphe node metastases	1	25	2	lymphe node- and distant metastases	7	0	1

TABLE 3 | Immunscore and PD-L1 expression before and after anti CTLA-4 therapy.

Patient ID	Pre-therapeutic tissue	n	PD-L1 expression (mean%)	Immunoscore	Metastases during therapy	n	PD-L1 expression (mean %)	Immunoscore
2	lymph node- and distant metastases	3	15	1	distant metastases	2	35	1
3	primary tumor	1	0	1	distant metastases	1	<1	1
4	lymphe node metastases	2	30	1	distant metastases	1	0	1
9	distant metastases	1	<1	1	distant metastases	1	2	1
12	not available	X	X	X	distant metastases	8	<1	1
21	lymphe node metastases	1	25	2	distant metastases	1	15	1

which 54 were obtained before treatment and 20 were obtained post treatment with anti-PD-1-therapy. Seventeen (31.5%) pre-therapeutic metastases (metastases present before any treatment) were classified as brisk and 37 (68.5%) as nonbrisk. In the cohort of metastases which developed during treatment, 4 (20%) were classified as brisk while 16 (80%) were classified as nonbrisk (**Figure 2**). The remaining metastases (n = 14) that were obtained after initial Ipilimumab therapy in patients that had not undergone Nivolumab/Pembrolizumab therapy were not included in the Immunoscoring.

In order to investigate the differential distribution of lymphocytic infiltration we compared brisk status in primary melanomas (prior to anti-tumor therapy) vs. pre-therapeutic metastases as well as between primary melanomas and metastases which developed during anti-PD-1-therapy. Immune infiltration was not only significantly increased in primary melanomas when compared to pre-therapeutic metastases ($p = 0.0381$), but also increased when immune infiltration in the primary melanomas was compared to that in metastases developed during treatment ($p = 0.0135$; **Figure 2**).

Next, we compared the Immunoscore in primary melanomas to that in pre-therapeutic metastases in the same patient (intra-individual immune cell infiltration). In 40% of cases there was no difference in the Immunoscore (6/15 patients). Whilst there was an increased metastatic Immunoscore in 20% of cases (3/15), in the remaining 40% (6/15) there

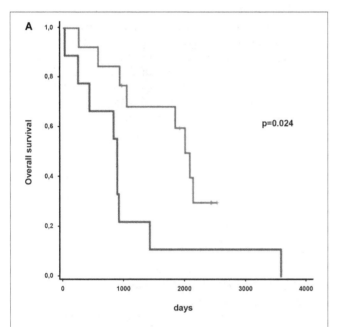

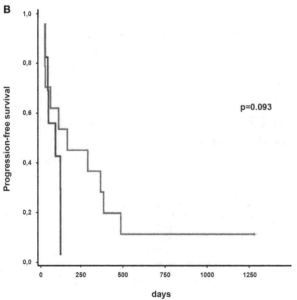

FIGURE 4 | Survival of melanoma patients treated with immune-checkpoint inhibitors depending on immune infiltration of primary tumors classified as brisk or nonbrisk. **(A)** Kaplan-Meier curves indicating overall survival of brisk (in blue) and nonbrisk (in red) primary tumors from melanoma patients. Survival groups were compared by log-rank test. *p*-values are indicated. **(B)** Kaplan-Meier curves indicating progression-free survival of brisk (in blue) and nonbrisk (in red) primary tumors from melanoma patients. Survival groups were compared by log-rank test. p values are indicated.

TABLE 4 | Association between BRAF status und immunoscore.

BRAF-status		Immunoscore		
		Nonbrisk	Brisk	Total
Wildtype	n	4	10	14
Mutation	n	5	3	8
Total	n	9	13	22
				$p = 0.187$

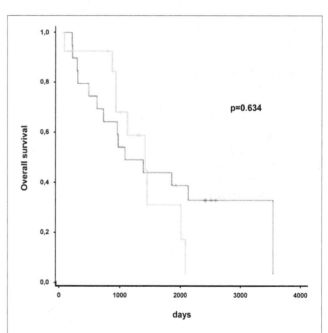

FIGURE 5 | BRAF mutation status in patients undergoing immune checkpoint therapy was not significantly associated with overall survival. Green line represents patients with BRAF mutation, blue line indicates patients without BRAF mutation.

was increased Immunoscore in the primary melanoma when compared to that in the pre-therapeutic metastases (**Figure 3** and **Tables 2**, **3**). Due to low number of metastases which developed during checkpoint therapy, we were not able compare Immunoscores from pre-therapeutic metastases to the Immunscore in metastases which developed during checkpoint therapy in the same patient.

The Immunoscore Is Associated With Improved Overall Survival During Checkpoint Therapy

Next, we aimed to determine whether the Immunoscore was associated with overall survival in melanoma. This was chosen as the most clinically significant parameter. We observed a statistically significant increase in overall survival in patients with a brisk lymphocytic infiltrate compared to patients with a nonbrisk infiltrate of their primary tumors ($p = 0.024$; **Figure 4A**). 5 year-survival rate for patients with a brisk tumor infiltrate and a nonbrisk infiltrate was 59.8 and 11.1%, respectively. Concordantly, we observed a trend in increased progression-free survival progression free survival of patients with a brisk lymphocytic tumor-infiltrate compared to patients with a nonbrisk infiltrate ($p = 0.093$; **Figure 4B**).

An association between the Immunoscore and survival rates could be demonstrated when evaluating primary melanomas, but there was no association between the Immunoscore in metastases and survival. Moreover, subtyping lymphocytic infiltrate using CD8, CD4, CD56, FoxP3, CTLA-4, PD-1, PD-L1, or PD-L2 expression did not lead to significant associations with overall survival (data not shown).

The Impact of BRAF Mutation Status on Clinical Outcome

We further evaluated the association of BRAF mutations with clinical outcome. BRAF mutation status was investigated in context of diagnostic work-up and not specifically for the current study. 20 (62.5%) out of 32 patients showed wt BRAF and 12 (37.5%) harbored mutations in the BRAF gene. Out of these 12 cases, 10 had the V600E mutation, 1 exhibited the D594V mutation and a further patient had the L597Q mutation. There was no association between BRAF status and either overall survival or progression-free in our melanoma cohort. We also observed no association between BRAF status and Immunoscore and/or PD-L1 status (**Table 4** and **Figure 5**).

The PD-L1 Antibody Clone SP263 Demonstrated the Highest Immunohistochemical Specificity

In order to determine the optimal protocol for determining PD-L1 expression in melanoma, we tested four distinct anti-PD-L1 clones, namely SP263, 28.8, E1L3N, and SP142 in 22 primary melanomas and 88 metastases. Two metastases were excluded from the results due to exhaustion of tissue material during the immunohistochemical staining. We observed strikingly different staining patterns as representatively shown in **Figure 6**. The

percentage of PD-L1 positive tumor cells in the same investigated sample varied from 100% (clone SP263) to 0% (clone SP142). Using clone 28.8 and E1L3N, 60 and 20% respectively of tumor cells were PD-L1 positive. When comparing PD-L1 expression in primary tumors vs. metastases using the four antibody clones the results were also divergent. Specifically, in 22 cases of primary tumors, half (n = 11) were interpreted as PD-L1 positive by using clone SP263 (**Table 5**). On the other hand, by using clones 28.8, E1L3N and SP142, we observed 3 (13.6%), 3 (13.6%), and 1 (4.5%) positive cases, respectively. Mean PD-L1 expression value of positive tumor cells for clone SP263 was 11.5%, for clone 28.8 was 3.63%, for clone E1L3N was 3.75% and for SP142 was 2.27%. Expression range reached from 0 to 100 positive tumor cells for clone SP263, from 0 to 40 for clone 28.8, from 0 to 70 for clone E1L3N und 0-50 for clone SP142. When investigating metastases for PD-L1 expression, we observed a similar pattern. By using clone SP263, we observed 27 (31.4%) positive cases while for clones 28.8, E1L3N and SP142, we observed 11 (12.8%), 4 (4.7%), and 4 (4.7%), respectively. Mean PD-L1 expression value of positive tumor cells for clone SP263 was 12.9%, for clone 28.8 was 5.3%, for clone E1L3N was 1.7% and for SP142 was 1.1%. Expression range reached from 0 to 100 positive tumor cells for clone SP263, from 0 to 95 for clone 28.8, from 0-80 for clone E1L3N und 0-40 for clone SP142.

Overall, clone SP263 showed highest specificity and the strongest staining intensity of PD-L1 in both primary tumors and metastases. Conversely, clones 28.8 and E1L3N showed weaker staining intensity with a discrete staining of the cell membranes while clone 28.8 showed additional granular background staining. Clone SP142 showed the weakest staining intensity as well as the lowest frequency of positive tumor cells. These observations supported the use of clone SP263 for further investigations.

PD-L1 Expression Is Not Associated With Overall Survival

Given that the immune infiltration was significantly higher in primary melanomas when compared to pre-therapeutic metastases, we next sought to determine intra-individual PD-L1 expression in primary melanomas and untreated metastases. We were able to evaluate PD-L1 expression in primary melanomas and untreated metastases in 13 out of 15 patients. There was no difference in PD-L1 expression in 3 (23.1%) cases, PD-L1 was upregulated in metastases in 7 (53.8%) cases, and higher PD-L1 expression in primary tumors, when compared to metastases obtained before immunotherapy, was present in 3 cases (23.1%) (**Figure 7**).

There was no correlation between PD-L1 expression and overall survival of melanoma patients treated with immune checkpoint inhibitors.

We also investigated any possible association between PD-L1 expression and the Immunoscore but observed no statistically significant difference in PD-L1 status between the brisk and nonbrisk groups.

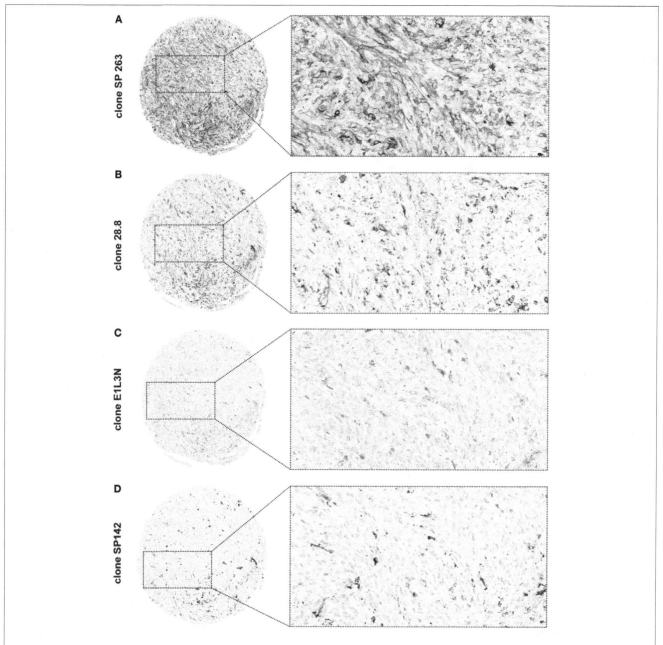

FIGURE 6 | PD-L1 expression using different anti-PD-L1 clones demonstrated on the same tumor core [original magnification x84 and x300 (insert)]. **(A)** Clone SP263 stains the highest proportion of tumor cells and shows the strongest expression. **(B)** Clone 28.8. shows weaker expression and additionally a granular background. **(C)** Clone E1L3N shows weak expression with a discreet staining of cell membranes. **(D)** Clone SP142 shows the weakest expression (black pigment accord to melanin pigment).

DISCUSSION

The treatment of metastatic melanoma continues to represent a major clinical challenge, not only due to the aggressive nature of the disease, but also due to the potentially life-threatening side-effects associated with immunotherapy. However, the development of immuno checkpoint inhibitors has markedly increased our therapeutic armamentarium and translated into impressive improvements in overall survival. Unfortunately, a significant proportion of patients still fail to respond to treatment. In order to determine which patients may respond best to checkpoint inhibition we retrospectively analyzed immune cell infiltration and PD-L1 status in a cohort of melanoma treated with CTLA-4 and/or anti-PD-1 inhibitors. Increased tumor immune infiltration in primary melanomas (measured by the Immunoscore) prior to immune checkpoint inhibition was associated with

TABLE 5 | PD-L1 expression using different anti-PD-L1 clones.

	Mean PD-L1 expression	Range	Number of positive cases	Number of negative cases	Positive cases (%)	Negative cases (%)
Primary tumors (n = 22)						
SP263	11.5	0–100	11	11	50	50
Abcam 28.8	3.63	0–40	3	19	13.6	86.4
E1L3N	3.75	0–70	3	19	13.6	86.4
SP142	2.27	0–50	1	21	4.5	95.5
Metastases (n = 86)						
SP263	12.9	0–100	27	59	31.4	68.6
Abcam 28.8	5.3	0–95	11	75	12.8	87.2
E1L3N	1.7	0–80	4	82	4.7	95.3
SP142	1.1	0–40	4	82	4.7	95.3

improved overall patient survival (**Figure 4**). Interestingly, increased recruitment of cytotoxic CD8+ lymphocytes alone was not observed in the favorable "brisk" setting (data not shown). Furthermore, no significant difference was observed in the number of CD4+ helper cells between the brisk and nonbrisk groups and consequently no difference was observed in CD4+/CD8+ ratio between two settings (data not shown).

However, the long-term benefit of immune checkpoint inhibition was evidenced by increased overall survival in patients that harbored highly infiltrated primary melanomas. It is important to bear in mind that response, overall survival and progression-free survival are independent parameters. For example, response may vary over time, especially in the context of acquired resistance and progression-free survival does not necessarily equate with improved overall survival (see **Supplementary Table 1**). Furthermore, there is an important and recognized difference between predictors of treatment response and prognostic markers (8). In this context, the Immunoscore represents a novel prognostic marker of treatment response, but is not a suitable stand-alone parameter to predict which patients will clinically benefit from checkpoint inhibition.

In contrast to previous studies (1, 17), we did not find an association between CD8+ cell infiltration with response to checkpoint inhibition in melanoma patients. In fact, Madonna et al. (21) reported low densities of CD8+ lymphocytes at the tumor periphery and an association with response to Ipilimumab. PD-L1 status was not a predictive marker for survival or treatment response.

Whilst the reason for the divergent results in terms of CD8+ infiltration is unclear, it is important to draw attention to the methodological differences between the studies. For example, Tumeh et al. (13) investigated patients who underwent PD-1 (Pembrolizumab) monotherapy, albeit in three difference dosing schedules, and Madonna et al examined patients treated with Ipilimumab. Our "real world" cohort was more heterogeneous in terms of treatment modality (PD-1/CTLA4 monotherapy vs. PD-1/CTLA4 combined therapy) which may have influenced CD8+ cell infiltration. Large, prospective studies would be required to

determine the extent to which CD8+ cell infiltration in treatment type dependent. Moreover, it would be interesting to determine the extent to which PD-L1 expression on peripheral T cells correlates with intratumoural T cell PD-L1 expression, given the association between circulating T cell PD-L1 expression and response to checkpoint inhibition (22, 23). We cannot exclude that the Immunoscore reflects a pre-existing anti-melanoma T cell response. However, this would be difficult to experimentally and/or clinically confirm or refute given that we do not have a patient cohort remain untreated. In any case, given that the Immunoscore in metastases was *not* associated with improved overall survival in our study, such pre-existing anti-melanoma T cell responses would have been limited to the primary tumor.

Next, we investigated BRAF mutation status in the context of absent, brisk and non-brisk Immunoscores in primary tumors and overall survival. BRAF status was not predictive for overall survival of melanoma patients during immune checkpoint therapy. The frequency of BRAF mutation in our cohort was similar to previous melanoma cohorts (24). Whilst there is conflicting data regarding the effect of BRAF status on treatment outcome during checkpoint immunotherapy, our study is in line with studies showing that Nivolumab treatment efficacy irrespective of BRAF status (25). It is currently unclear whether initial therapy with BRAF/MEK inhibitors followed by immune checkpoint therapy, or vice versa, translates to improved overall rates of survival for patients with the BRAF mutation.

Nevertheless, our study highlights the utility of the Immunoscore, a robust and readily available scoring tool, which is associated with overall survival in patients with metastatic melanoma undergoing immune checkpoint therapy.

We also aimed to clarify whether the pattern of tumor immune cell infiltration differs between primary melanoma, untreated metastases and metastases which developed during treatment with immune checkpoint inhibition. Due to more aggressive nature of metastastic melanoma, we expected to observe an increased immune-cell infiltration in primary melanomas when compared to that in metastases. Indeed, the pattern of immune-cell infiltration was dramatically different between primary

PD-L1 expression dynamics

	Primary tumors	Pre-therapeutic metastases
Patient ID 1	0%	0%
Patient ID 20	100%	100%
Patient ID 9	0%	<1%
Patient ID 2	0%	15%
Patient ID 16	10%	50%
Patient ID 23	0%	15%
Patient ID 24	0%	2%
Patient ID 28	0%	60%
Patient ID 31	0%	10%
Patient ID 39	0%	50%
Patient ID 30	5%	0%
Patient ID 33	2%	0%
Patient ID 34	10%	1%

FIGURE 7 | PD-L1 melanoma expression dynamics between primary melanomas and pre-therapeutic metastases in the same patient. Top down: No change in PD-L1 expression was seen in 3 patients, higher PD-L1 expression in metastases was seen in 7 patients and lower PD-L1 expression in metastases was seen in 3 patients. PD-L1 expression (clone SP 263) is reported as percentage of PD-L1 positive tumor cells from all tumor cells. In case of more than one metastasis, mean value is stated. Patient identification numbers are denoted besides. For patients with identification number 15 and 26 evaluation of PD-L1 expression was not possible.

Theoretically, both immune cell tumor infiltration and expression of PD-L1 on tumor cells are required for successful anti-PD-1 and anti-PD-L1 checkpoint therapy. Therefore, we further investigated the correlation of tumor PD-L1 status in the context of the brisk and nonbrisk group as well as alone on the survival of melanoma patients after anti-PD-1 immunotherapy. We found no significant correlations in either setting (9). We also observed no correlation of PD-L1 expression dynamics in matching primary melanomas and corresponding metastases of the same patient. Again, it is important to note (i) the variations in immune-checkpoint inhibitor treatment regiments (single vs. combined anti-CTLA-4 and anti-PD-1/PD-L1 vs. sequential combined anti-CTLA-4 and anti-PD-1/PD-L1 immuno-checkpoint inhibition), (ii) the various antibodies used to detect tumor PD-L1 status, (iii) the tumor type (predominantly cutaneous melanoma as opposed to mucosal and/or acral) and (iv) the small size of metastases when taking our data into account. We could demonstrate that PD-L1 expression was heavily dependent on the PD-L1 antibody clone which was used, perhaps partially explaining the, at times, confounding effect of PD-L1 expression reported in the literature (**Figure 6** and **Table 5**). Based on our data, we selected and employed the most specific clone (263) and the overall level of melanoma PD-L1 expression in our study was similar to that reported in the literature (26, 27).

In conclusion, the results of our study suggest that total tumor immune infiltration, not PD-L1 status, is important for predicting the survival of melanoma patients undergoing checkpoint inhibitor therapy. However, this may be specific to our cohort where many melanoma patients were pretreated with Ipilimumab prior to administering Nivolumab/Pembrolizumab (see **Supplementary Table 1**). Whilst our results require replication in a large, prospective study, they provide evidence that the Immunoscore, a validated and easy to use tool, which does not require laborious and potentially erroneous cell counting, is a novel marker for survival in melanoma patients treated with immune checkpoint therapy. Provided that our findings can be replicated in larger, prospective studies, the Immunscore may represent an inexpensive, simple and robust tool which can be rapidly incorporated into routine clinico-pathological practice.

AUTHOR CONTRIBUTIONS

PT, SP, and CK: planned the research project. CK, MJ, AO, and WV: performed the pathological staining and data analysis. CK, MJ, EL, OH, VG, SP, and PT: wrote and/or revised the manuscript.

melanomas and both metastases subgroups, in line with our hypothesis (**Figure 2**). We then sought to compare the Immunoscore from primary tumors and metastases in individual patients. Although we observed generally a lower Immunoscore in untreated metastases, there was no reduction in tumor immune cell infiltration when comparing the primary melanoma to the metastases in every patient, probably due to the heterogenous nature of these tumors (**Figure 3**).

REFERENCES

1. Ribas A, Wolchok JD. Cancer immunotherapy using checkpoint blockade. *Science.* (2018) 359:1350–5. doi: 10.1126/science.aar4060
2. Gide TN, Wilmott JS, Scolyer RA, Long GV. Primary and acquired resistance to immune checkpoint inhibitors in metastatic melanoma. *Clin Cancer Res.* (2018) 24:1260–70. doi: 10.1158/1078-0432.CCR-17-2267
3. Tarhini A, Kudchadkar RR. Predictive and on-treatment monitoring biomarkers in advanced melanoma:Moving toward personalized medicine. *Cancer Treat Rev.* (2018) 71:8–18. doi: 10.1016/j.ctrv.2018.09.005
4. Blank CU, Haanen JB, Ribas A, Schumacher TN. CANCER IMMUNOLOGY. The "cancer immunogram." *Science.* (2016) 352:658–60. doi: 10.1126/science.aaf2834
5. Schumacher TN, Schreiber RD. Neoantigens in cancer immunotherapy. *Science.* (2015) 348:69–74. doi: 10.1126/science.aaa4971
6. Hugo W, Zaretsky JM, Sun L, Song C, Moreno BH, Hu-Lieskovan S, et al. Genomic and transcriptomic features of response to anti-PD-1 therapy in metastatic melanoma. *Cell.* (2016) 165:35–44. doi: 10.1016/j.cell.2016.02.065
7. Carbognin L, Pilotto S, Milella M, Vaccaro V, Brunelli M, Caliò A, et al. Differential activity of nivolumab, pembrolizumab and MPDL3280A according to the tumor expression of programmed Death-Ligand-1 (PD-L1): sensitivity analysis of trials in melanoma, lung and genitourinary cancers. *PLoS ONE.* (2015) 10:e0130142. doi: 10.1371/journal.pone.0130142
8. Jessurun CAC, Vos JAM, Limpens J, Luiten RM. Biomarkers for response of melanoma patients to immune checkpoint inhibitors: a systematic review. *Front Oncol.* (2017) 7:233. doi: 10.3389/fonc.2017.00233
9. Wolchok JD, Chiarion-Sileni V, Gonzalez R, Rutkowski P, Grob JJ, Cowey CL, et al. Overall survival with combined nivolumab and ipilimumab in advanced melanoma. *N Engl J Med.* (2017) 377:1345–56. doi: 10.1056/NEJMoa1709684
10. Buder-Bakhaya K, Hassel JC. Biomarkers for clinical benefit of immune checkpoint inhibitor treatment-a review from the melanoma perspective and beyond. *Front Immunol.* (2018) 9:1474. doi: 10.3389/fimmu.2018.01474
11. Robert C, Long GV, Brady B, Dutriaux C, Maio M, Mortier L, et al. Nivolumab in previously untreated melanoma without BRAF mutation. *N Engl J Med.* (2015) 372:320–30. doi: 10.1056/NEJMoa1412082
12. Aguiar PN Jr, Santoro IL, Tadokoro H, de Lima Lopes G, Filardi BA, Oliveira P, et al. The role of PD-L1 expression as a predictive biomarker in advanced non-small-cell lung cancer:a network meta-analysis. *Immunotherapy.* (2016) 8:479–88. doi: 10.2217/imt-2015-0002
13. Tumeh PC, Harview CL, Yearley JH, Shintaku IP, Taylor EJ, Robert L, et al. PD-1 blockade induces responses by inhibiting adaptive immune resistance. *Nature.* (2014) 515:568–71. doi: 10.1038/nature13954
14. Azimi F, Scolyer RA, Rumcheva P, Moncrieff M, Murali R, McCarthy SW, et al. Tumor-infiltrating lymphocyte grade is an independent predictor of sentinel lymph node status and survival in patients with cutaneous melanoma. *J Clin Oncol.* (2012) 30:2678–83. doi: 10.1200/JCO.2011.37.8539
15. Thomas NE, Busam KJ, From L, Kricker A, Armstrong BK, Anton-Culver H, et al. Tumor-infiltrating lymphocyte grade in primary melanomas is independently associated with melanoma-specific survival in the population-based genes, environment and melanoma study. *J Clin Oncol.* (2013) 31:4252–9. doi: 10.1200/JCO.2013.51.3002
16. Kluger HM, Zito CR, Barr ML, Baine MK, Chiang VL, Sznol M, et al. Characterization of PD-L1 expression and associated t-cell infiltrates in metastatic melanoma samples from variable anatomic sites. *Clin Cancer Res.* (2015) 21:3052–60. doi: 10.1158/1078-0432.CCR-14-3073
17. Madore J, Vilain RE, Menzies AM, Kakavand H, Wilmott JS, Hyman J, et al. PD-L1 expression in melanoma shows marked heterogeneity within and between patients:implications for anti-PD-1/PD-L1 clinical trials. *Pigment Cell Melanoma Res.* (2015) 28:245–53. doi: 10.1111/pcmr.12340
18. Daud AI, Wolchok JD, Robert C, Hwu WJ, Weber JS, Ribas A, et al. Programmed death-ligand 1 expression and response to the anti-programmed death 1 antibody pembrolizumab in melanoma. *J Clin Oncol.* (2016) 34:4102–9. doi: 10.1200/JCO.2016.67.2477
19. Clark WH Jr, Elder DE, Guerry D IV, Braitman LE, Trock BJ, Schultz D, et al. Model predicting survival in stage I melanoma based on tumor progression. *J Natl Cancer Inst.* (1989) 81:1893–904. doi: 10.1093/jnci/81.24.1893
20. Scheel AH, Dietel M, Heukamp LC, Jöhrens K, Kirchner T, Reu S, et al. [Predictive PD-L1 immunohistochemistry for non-small cell lung cancer:Current state of the art and experiences of the first German harmonization study]. *Pathologe.* (2016) 37:557–67. doi: 10.1007/s00292-016-0189-1
21. Madonna G, Ballesteros-Merino C, Feng Z, Bifulco C, Capone M, Giannarelli D, et al. PD-L1 expression with immune-infiltrate evaluation and outcome prediction in melanoma patients treated with ipilimumab. *Oncoimmunology.* (2018) 7:e1405206. doi: 10.1080/2162402X.2017.1405206
22. Takeuchi Y, Tanemura A, Tada Y, Katayama I, Kumanogoh A, Nishikawa H. Clinical response to PD-1 blockade correlates with a sub-fraction of peripheral central memory CD4+ T cells in patients with malignant melanoma. *Int Immunol.* (2018) 30:13–22. doi: 10.1093/intimm/dxx073
23. Jacquelot N, Roberti MP, Enot DP, Rusakiewicz S, Ternès N, Jegou S, et al. Predictors of responses to immune checkpoint blockade in advanced melanoma. *Nat Commun.* (2017) 8:592. doi: 10.1038/s41467-017-00608-2
24. Robert C, Schachter J, Long GV, Arance A, Grob JJ, Mortier L, et al. Pembrolizumab versus Ipilimumab in advanced melanoma. *N Engl J Med.* (2015) 372:2521–32. doi: 10.1056/NEJMoa1503093
25. Larkin J, Lao CD, Urba WJ, McDermott DF, Horak C, Jiang J, et al. Efficacy and safety of nivolumab in patients with BRAF V600 mutant and BRAF wild-type advanced melanoma:a pooled analysis of 4 clinical trials. *JAMA Oncol.* (2015) 1:433–40. doi: 10.1001/jamaoncol.2015.1184
26. Wolchok JD, Kluger H, Callahan MK, Postow MA, Rizvi NA, Lesokhin AM, et al. Nivolumab plus ipilimumab in advanced melanoma. *N Engl J Med.* (2013) 369:122–33. doi: 10.1056/NEJMoa1302369
27. Morrison C, Pabla S, Conroy JM, Nesline MK, Glenn ST, Dressman D, et al. Predicting response to checkpoint inhibitors in melanoma beyond PD-L1 and mutational burden. *J Immunother Cancer.* (2018) 6:32. doi: 10.1186/s40425-018-0344-8

10

New Therapies and Immunological Findings in Cutaneous T-Cell Lymphoma

Kazuyasu Fujii*

Department of Dermatology, Kagoshima University Graduate School of Medical and Dental Sciences, Kagoshima, Japan

*Correspondence:
Kazuyasu Fujii
kazfujii@m2.kufm.kagoshima-u.ac.jp

Primary cutaneous lymphomas comprise a group of lymphatic malignancies that occur primarily in the skin. They represent the second most common form of extranodal non-Hodgkin's lymphoma and are characterized by heterogeneous clinical, histological, immunological, and molecular features. The most common type is mycosis fungoides and its leukemic variant, Sézary syndrome. Both diseases are considered T-helper cell type 2 (Th2) diseases. Not only the tumor cells but also the tumor microenvironment can promote Th2 differentiation, which is beneficial for the tumor cells because a Th1 environment enhances antitumor immune responses. This Th2-dominant milieu also underlies the infectious susceptibility of the patients. Many components, such as tumor-associated macrophages, cancer-associated fibroblasts, and dendritic cells, as well as humoral factors, such as chemokines and cytokines, establish the tumor microenvironment and can modify tumor cell migration and proliferation. Multiagent chemotherapy often induces immunosuppression, resulting in an increased risk of serious infection and poor tolerance. Therefore, overtreatment should be avoided for these types of lymphomas. Interferons have been shown to increase the time to next treatment to a greater degree than has chemotherapy. The pathogenesis and prognosis of cutaneous T-cell lymphoma (CTCL) differ markedly among the subtypes. In some aggressive subtypes of CTCLs, such as primary cutaneous gamma/delta T-cell lymphoma and primary cutaneous CD8+ aggressive epidermotropic cytotoxic T-cell lymphoma, hematopoietic stem cell transplantation should be considered, whereas overtreatment should be avoided with other, favorable subtypes. Therefore, a solid understanding of the pathogenesis and immunological background of cutaneous lymphoma is required to better treat patients who are inflicted with this disease. This review summarizes the current knowledge in the field to attempt to achieve this objective.

Keywords: cutaneous T-cell lymphoma, mycosis fungoides, Sézary syndrome, primary cutaneous CD30+ T-cell lymphoproliferative disorders, adult T-cell leukemia/lymphoma

OVERVIEW OF CUTANEOUS T-CELL LYMPHOMAS (CTCLs)

Non-Hodgkin lymphomas can occur at extranodal sites in approximately 27% of cases, with the gastrointestinal tract and skin being the first and second most common sites of extranodal involvement (1). Most nodal non-Hodgkin lymphomas are B-cell derived, which is in contrast to the approximately 75–05% of primary cutaneous lymphomas that are T-cell derived (2–6). The incidence of CTCLs has been increasing (7); consequently, 4–8 people per million currently suffer from these cancers (8, 9). CTCL represents a series of skin-based neoplasms of T-cell origin,

TABLE 1 | List of primary CTCLs.

Study group	Frequency, %			Disease-specific 5-year survival[2], %
	DACLG[2]	SEER16[5]	JSCS[6]	
Mycosis fungoides	61.5	54.1	51.7	88
Sézary syndrome	3.5	1.2	2.3	24
Primary cutaneous CD30[+] T-cell lymphoproliferative disorders	26.0	14.4	14.3	
Lymphomatoid papulosis	16.1		4.5	100
Primary cutaneous anaplastic large-cell lymphoma	9.9		9.4	95
Adult T-cell leukemia/lymphoma[a]		0.1	20.0	
Subcutaneous panniculitis-like T-cell lymphoma	1.2	0.8	2.3	82
Primary cutaneous gamma/delta T-cell lymphoma	0.9		0.3	NR
Primary cutaneous CD4[+] small/medium T-cell lymphoproliferative disorder[b]	2.7		1.7	75
Hydroa vacciniforme-like lymphoproliferative disorder[b]				
Primary cutaneous acral CD8[+] T-cell lymphoma[b]				
Primary cutaneous CD8[+] aggressive epidermotropic cytotoxic T-cell lymphoma	1.0		0.4	18
Peripheral T-cell lymphoma, NOS[a]	3.2	29.4	6.9	16
Total no. of CTCL	1,469	2,750	1,451	

NR, not reached; CTCL, cutaneous T-cell lymphoma.
[a]A portion of these diseases is considered as primary CTCL.
[b]Provisional entity in World Health Organization classification (2016).

predominantly comprised of peripheral CD4[+] T-cells. There are 12 distinct CTCL subtypes (**Table 1**), with mycosis fungoides (MF) being the most common (10). Primary cutaneous CD30[+] T-cell lymphoproliferative disorders are the second most common, except in some countries in the Pacific where adult T-cell leukemia/lymphoma (ATL) ranks second (6, 11).

MF/SÉZARY SYNDROME (SS)

Mycosis fungoides and SS constitute the most common types of primary CTCLs. MF is characterized by erythematous patches, plaques, or tumors on the skin (**Figure 1**), with the involvement of lymph nodes, blood, and viscera also possible. MF can mimic benign inflammatory skin disorders, such as atopic dermatitis or psoriasis; thus, it is not unusual for MF to remain undiagnosed for years. Although MF is typically an indolent disorder, the disease may progress toward or exhibit *de novo* more advanced forms including tumors and erythroderma (>80% of the body surface area showing patches/plaques without overt leukemia). This can lead to lymph node or organ involvement, accompanied by increased morbidity and mortality. Patients are classified as having either early-stage (patches/plaques) or advanced-stage (tumors, erythroderma, lymph node, and/or visceral involvement) (12, 13). SS is the leukemic form of the disease, in which erythroderma is accompanied by measurable levels of malignant lymphocytes with cerebriform nuclei [i.e., Sézary cells (SC)] in the blood. Typical SC counts would be ≥1,000/μL, with a CD4/CD8 ratio of ≥10 and a loss of one or more T-cell antigens (CD4[+]CD7[−] > 30% or CD4[+]CD26[−] > 40%). Furthermore, CD30 expression is associated with a significantly reduced disease-specific survival and is often associated with histologically detectable large cell transformation, hallmarking a more aggressive clinical course (14).

In the past, SS has been considered a leukemic and aggressive variant of MF. However, a recent study determined that MF and SS arose from distinct T-cell subsets: SS from central memory

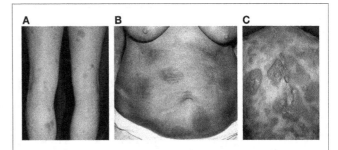

FIGURE 1 | Clinical findings of mycosis fungoides/Sézary syndrome. **(A)** Patches, **(B)** plaques, **(C)** and nodules on the plaque. Written informed consent was obtained from each patient.

T-cells and MF from skin-resident effector memory T-cells (15). CD158k/killer cell immunoglobulin-like receptor 3DL2 represents a specific marker for the evaluation of SC (16); in particular, CD4[+] CD158k[+] lymphocytes in blood from patients with SS correspond to the malignant clonal cell population (17). In addition, immunohistological finding of CD158k in affected skin is reported to distinguish SS from MF (18). Clonal malignant T-cells from the blood of patients with SS coexpress the lymph node homing molecules C–C motif chemokine receptor 7 (CCR7)/CD197 and CD62L/L-selectin, as well as the CD27 differentiation marker, a characteristic of central memory T-cells. This is consistent with the clinical presentation of peripheral blood disease, lymphadenopathy, and diffuse erythroderma of the skin. In contrast, T-cells from MF skin lesions do not express CCR7, L-selectin, and CD27, but strongly express CCR4 and cutaneous lymphocyte antigen (CLA)/CD162, characteristics of skin-resident effector memory T-cells. This difference in the putative origins between SS (central memory T-cell-derived) and MF (tissue-resident memory-derived) can explain their distinct clinical behaviors; central memory T-cells are long-lived, apoptosis-resistant cells that can be found in the peripheral blood, lymph nodes, and skin, whereas skin-resident memory T-cells remain in the skin and do not enter the general circulation. That MF and SS are derived from different T-cell precursors is also supported by comparative genomic hybridization and gene-expression profiling, demonstrating that the CTCL genotypes are distinct (19, 20). Overall, MF is characterized by gains on chromosomes 1 and 7 and losses on chromosome 9, whereas SS is characterized by gains on chromosomes 8 and 17 and losses on chromosome 10. A multiplatform genomic analysis of patients with SS detected (1) activating *CCR4* and caspase recruitment domain-containing protein 11 (*CARD11*) mutations in nearly one-third of patients; (2) deletion of zinc finger E-box binding homeobox 1 (*ZEB1*), encoding a transcriptional repressor essential for T-cell differentiation, in over one-half of patients; and (3) overexpression of interleukin 32 (IL-32) and interleukin-2 receptor subunit gamma in nearly all patients (21).

ROLES OF CHEMOKINES IN DEVELOPMENT OF SKIN PATHOLOGY

Malignant T-cells are suggested exhibit phenotypes of mature CD4+ memory T-cells, along with type 2 or 17 (Th2 or Th17 (22)) T-helper cell phenotypes, or be comprised of FOXP3 regulatory T-cells (Treg) (23, 24). Many chemokines are also reportedly expressed in the affected skin of patients with CTCL, suggesting that chemokine–receptor interactions play important roles in disease progression (25). Chemokine receptor expression on tumor cells in MF varies with disease stage. In the patch and plaque stages of MF, most infiltrating cells express CXC chemokine receptor (CXCR) 3/CD183 in the affected skin (26). CXCR3 binds three distinct ligands, namely CXC chemokine ligand (CXCL) 9/monokine induced by gamma interferon (MIG), interferon-gamma-inducible protein-10 (CXCL10/IP-10), and interferon-inducible T cell alpha chemoattractant (CXCL11/ITAC)/IP-9; all are expressed in the affected skin in the patch and plaque stages of MF (27–29). Various cell types express these chemokines including keratinocytes, dermal fibroblasts, and Langerhans cells. In the early stages of MF, expression of CXCL9, CXCL10, and CXCR3 is believed to be important for recruitment and accumulation of tumor cells in the skin (25, 28). However, later in the tumor stage, the tumor cells increase in size and tend to express CCR4 instead of CXCR3 (30). The expression levels of CXCL9 and CXCL10 also tend to be lower in the affected skin of patients with MF during the tumor stage than during the patch and plaque stages (31). Moreover, CCR6/CD196 and its ligand CCL20/macrophage inflammatory protein (MIP)-3α are upregulated in advanced CTCL (32). Tumor MF cells exhibit high levels of CCR7 (33), which is considered to be associated with loss of epidermotropism and migration to peripheral lymph nodes, which constitutively synthesize the CCR7 ligands, CCL19 and 21 (34). CCR7 is also expressed at high levels in SC (35), as mentioned in Section "MF/Sézary syndrome (SS)".

Circulating SC and skin-infiltrating cells in SS also express CCR4 (30, 35, 36). CCR4-expressing T-cells were found in CTCL lesions along with high expression of two CCR4 ligands, namely CC chemokine ligand (CCL) 17/thymus and activation-regulated chemokine and CCL22/macrophage-derived chemokine (30). CCL17 is expressed by endothelial cells and keratinocytes in the affected skin of patients with MF and SS (30, 37). During the

tumor stage of MF, serum CCL17 levels are much higher than those during the patch/plaque stages (37), suggesting the importance of CCL17–CCR4 interactions in tumor cell trafficking to the skin of these patients. CCL22 is expressed by dendritic-like cells and keratinocytes (30, 37). Serum CCL22 levels are significantly higher in patients with MF than in healthy controls or patients with psoriasis vulgaris (37).

CC chemokine ligand 27/cutaneous T cell attracting chemokine is a CCR10 ligand that is constitutively produced by activated keratinocytes in various diseases (38). CCR10 is expressed on the tumor cells of MF and SS (35, 39). Strong immunostaining of CCL27 has been observed in the affected skin of patients with MF compared to that of unaffected individuals (39, 40). Serum CCL27 levels and the number of circulating CCR10+ CD4+ cells are both increased in patients with MF compared to that of control patients (39). Therefore, CCR10–CCL27 interactions may also contribute to the migration of lymphoma cells to the affected skin in MF and SS. In addition to CCR4 and CCR10, expression of the receptor for CXCL12/stromal cell-derived factor 1, CXCR4, is observed in SC (36). CXCL12 is a chemoattractant for CXCR4-positive cells and is strongly expressed in the affected skin of patients with MF (41) and SS (36). Therefore, CXCL12–CXCR4 interactions may also facilitate the recruitment of lymphoma cells to the skin.

Th2-DOMINANT MICROENVIRONMENT

As the microenvironment in early-stage MF consists of non-malignant Th1 cells and CD8+ tumor-infiltrating T cells, MF and SS are considered Th2-type diseases, which are frequently accompanied by eosinophilia and high serum levels of IgE. In the early 1990s, peripheral blood mononuclear cells in patients with SS and non-leukemic CTCL were reported to be Th2 dominant (42, 43). In 1994, mRNA for Th2 cytokine was detected in the skin of patients with MF (44). T-cell clones from patients with SS were identified thereafter to have Th2-like properties (45). However, in the early stages of MF, affected skin and peripheral blood T-cells express a profile of Th1 cytokines (46, 47). The Th2 phenotype appears to be caused by leukemic T-cells, as culturing benign T-cells away from malignant clones reduces Th2 and enhances Th1 responses (48). The Th2-dominant microenvironment is advantageous for tumor cells, because interferon (IFN)-γ-producing Th1 cells enhance immune responses against the tumor. Indeed, IFN-γ has been shown to be effective for CTCL treatment (49, 50). Adenoviral-mediated gene therapies that increase expression of IFN-γ have also been used successfully in CTCL (51–53). CTCL cells can inhibit T-cell proliferation and suppress dendritic cell (DC) maturation by secretion of Th2 cytokines (54). Skin and nasal colonization with *Staphylococcus aureus* is common in patients with MF/SS; in particular, a Th2-dominant microenvironment may underlie this susceptibility to infection (55). Infections of *S. aureus* and sepsis also frequently occur in patients with CTCL (56). Accordingly, the major cause of death in patients with erythrodermic MF and SS is intravenous line sepsis, with *S. aureus* often being the causative microorganism (57).

In early-stage MF, signal transducers and activators of transcription (STAT) 4, the activation of which is required for Th1 differentiation, are overexpressed by IL-12 signaling *via* JAK2/TYK2 (58). In later stages, IL-2 and IL-15 signaling *via* JAK1 and JAK3 kinases activates STAT5, which increases the expression of oncogenic miR-155 (59) and subsequently inhibits STAT4 expression (60), resulting in a switch from Th1 to Th2 phenotype in malignant T cells. Downregulation of STAT4 is also induced by deficiencies in IL-12 expression (58, 61) and lack of the IL-12R β2 chain (58). During this switch, the expression of STAT6 is often upregulated in CTCL (60). STAT5 activation is seen in both early and late stages. Specifically, in the late stage, constitutive STAT5 activation is induced by cytokine-independent JAK1/JAK3 signaling (59). In the advanced stage, such constitutive STAT3 activation, which increases survival and resistance to apoptosis and promotes Th2 and Th17 phenotypes, is induced by an IL-21 autocrine signaling loop (62), the presence of IL-7 and IL-15 in the microenvironment (63), and/or constitutive cytokine-independent activation of JAK1 and JAK3 signaling (64, 65). Moreover, GATA3, a transcriptional regulator of Th2-cells, is overexpressed in SC *via* proteasome dysregulation (66).

CANCER-ASSOCIATED FIBROBLASTS

Fibroblasts are crucial components of the tumor microenvironment, promoting the growth and invasion of cancer cells through various mechanisms (67). The fibroblasts in the affected skin of patients with advanced CTCL promote a Th2-dominant microenvironment by augmenting Th2 and attenuating Th1 immune responses. Increased expression of CCL26/eotaxin-3 is observed in the dermal fibroblasts, keratinocytes, and endothelial cells of the affected skin of patients with advanced MF (68). In addition, serum CCL26 and CCL11/eotaxin-1 levels were shown to be higher in patients with CTCL than in healthy control patients, which correlated with serum soluble interleukin-2 receptor (sIL-2R) levels. However, CCR3/CD193, a receptor for CCL26 and other ligands, is not expressed on lymphoma cells in MF or SS (69). Because mRNA for CCR3 is detected in affected skin (68) and CCR3 is expressed on eosinophils and subpopulations of Th2 cells (70, 71), CCL26 and CCL11 are believed to support the Th2-dominant microenvironment in MF and SS disease lesions (25).

Periostin constitutes an extracellular matrix protein that is expressed in several cancers (72); it is prominent in the stromal area during the patch and plaque stages of MF, but decreases during the tumor stage (73). Fibroblasts are reportedly the source of periostin in MF (74). IL-4 and IL-13 can induce periostin secretion by dermal fibroblasts, periostin mediates thymic stromal protein (TSLP) production by keratinocytes, and TSLP subsequently activates immature myeloid DCs, which modulate Th2 immune responses *via* CCL17 production (75). Serum (76) and plasma (77) TSLP levels are increased in patients with CTCL, suggesting that TSLP contributes to the Th2-dominant microenvironment in MF lesions. TSLP also induces the growth of CTCL cells (74). Therefore, periostin can directly stimulate the growth of CTCL tumor cells in addition to inducing a Th2-dominant environment in CTCL tumors.

Expression of herpesvirus entry mediator (HVEM)/CD270, a member of the tumor necrosis factor-receptor superfamily, on dermal fibroblasts in the affected skin of patients with MF

and SS is decreased as the disease progresses. In addition, low HVEM expression on dermal fibroblasts in the affected skin of patients with advanced CTCL attenuates the expression of Th1 chemokines, resulting in Th2-dominant microenvironments. This occurs because the interaction between HVEM and tumor necrosis factor superfamily member 14 (also termed LIGHT)/CD258 on dermal fibroblasts increases the secretion of CXCL9–11, which are chemokines that recruit CXCR3-positive Th1 cells (29).

TUMOR-ASSOCIATED MACROPHAGES (TAMs)

Macrophages constitute a major component of the leukocyte infiltrate in the tumor microenvironment (78), in which they are termed TAMs. TAMs usually comprise polarized M2 macrophages that contribute to an immune-suppressive environment and promote tumor cell growth (79). CD163 is recognized as a marker for TAMs. As with many malignancies (80), the presence of M2 macrophages in the affected skin of patients with MF has been correlated with patient prognosis (81, 82), and the presence of M2 macrophages has been correlated with lymph node staging (83); this suggests that TAMs play a significant role in MF pathogenesis. Serum sCD163 levels in patients with CTCL are significantly higher than those in normal controls and they significantly correlate with serum sIL-2R levels. TAMs are believed to play a role in the formation of CTCL by secreting various chemokines (73, 82, 84). Periostin-stimulated macrophages produce CXCL5 and CXCL10 (73), which correlates with MF tumor formation in a xenograft CTCL mouse model (84). CCL18/alternative macrophage activation-associated CC chemokine 1/MIP-4 is secreted by M2 macrophages (85) and binds to its receptor (i.e., CCR8) on Th2 cells (86). The expression of CCR8 on MF or SS tumor cells has not been reported, although the mRNA expression of CCR8 is known to be upregulated in patients with SS (21). TAMs are known to express CCL18 in the skin of patients with CTCL (87, 88). Serum CCL18 levels were significantly higher in patients with CTCL than in healthy controls, and these levels significantly correlated with modified severity-weighted assessment scores, serum sIL-2R, lactate dehydrogenase, Th2 cytokines, and chemokines (88). Furthermore, high serum levels of CCL18 were associated with poor patient prognosis (88). In the affected skin of patients with MF/SS, TAMs highly express CD30, which is the target of the anti-CD30 antibody–drug conjugate, brentuximab vedotin (89).

DENDRITIC CELLS

Dendritic cells are antigen-presenting cells with a unique capacity to induce primary immune responses (90). By secreting Th2 cytokines, CTCL cells can suppress the maturation of DCs (54). Notably, IL-10 downregulates DC functions and may promote tolerance by skin DCs, rather than immune defense (91). Immature DCs can induce tolerance by presenting antigens to T-cells without appropriate costimulation. A significant increase in various DC subsets is seen in the affected dermis of patients with MF/SS, with the majority being immature CD209/

DC-specific ICAM-3 grabbing non-integrin (DC-SIGN)-positive DCs. Increases in CD208/DC-lysosome-associated membrane glycoprotein-positive DCs (i.e., mature DCs) and CD303/blood dendritic cell antigen 2-positive DCs (i.e., plasmacytoid DCs) are also observed, but the numbers of cells expressing CD208 or CD303 are few, suggesting that many DCs in the dermis of CTCL lesions are immature. Increased number of immature DCs in CTCL lesions may be important for immunological tolerance against malignant T-cells (92). However, some CD208-positive, mature DCs may attempt to mount an immune response against the cancer cells, as mature CD208-positive DCs are elevated in the skin draining lymph nodes of patients with MF (83).

OTHER KEY PLAYERS

The keratinocytes in the affected skin of patients with MF/SS release multiple chemokines including CCL17, CCL26, CCL27, CXCL9, and CXCL10, which help to attract T-cells to the epidermis, as mentioned above. Nerve growth factor (NGF) expression is also elevated in the affected skin of patients with SS, which stimulates the sprouting of nerve fibers. NGF is associated with the severity of pruritus in atopic dermatitis (93), and serum NGF levels are elevated in patients with SS (94). The enhanced expression of NGF is supposedly associated with pruritus in SS.

Mast cells also serve as critical stimulators of the tumor microenvironment (95). Patients with CTCL have increased number of mast cells in their affected skin and this correlates with disease progression (96). Moreover, in a model of cutaneous lymphoma, tumor growth in mast cell-deficient mice was significantly decreased. Therefore, mast cells represent key players in the development of CTCL.

Th22 cells, which produce IL-22 but not IFN-γ, IL-4, or IL-17, express CCR6, CCR4, and CCR10, thus enhancing skin infiltration. IL-22 mediates host defenses against bacterial infection (97). The affected skin of patients with MF/SS expresses high levels of IL-22 and low levels of IL-17 (32). A case of SS reportedly also had high IL-22 expression that was modulated by systemic bacterial infections (98). The serum levels of IL-22 and IL-22-induced CCL20 are increased in patients with MF/SS and are associated with disease severity (32); this suggests an important role of IL-22 in establishing the tumor microenvironment in MF and SS.

Myeloid-derived suppressor cells (MDSCs) are also recognized as key players in tumor immune escape mechanisms (99). The progression from early patch/plaque lesions to tumors in MF is related to an increase in MDSCs (100). Therefore, MDSCs play a role in MF progression by decreasing antitumor immune responses.

T-cell exhaustion *via* immune checkpoints also constitutes an important factor underlying tumor survival. The expression levels of PD-1 (101, 102), PD-L1 (102), CTLA-4 (103), and ICOS (104) have been described at different stages of the disease, suggesting a role for immune checkpoint inhibitor therapies.

TREATMENT

There is currently no cure for CTCL, thus treatment is aimed primarily at improving symptoms and quality of life and maintaining

remission. Therapies are tailored to the individual patient, based on age, performance status, extent of disease burden, rate of disease progression, and prior treatments (105). A typical MF progression starts at the patch and plaque stage and then advances to dermal-based tumors over many years. Effective immune control in the initial disease stages can slow disease progression. Hughes et al. reported that chemotherapy shortens the median time until the next treatment in patients with MF/SS (106). Multiagent chemotherapy often induces immunosuppression, which leads to an increased risk of infection and poor tolerance (107). Therefore, chemotherapy should be limited until all other options are exhausted. In comparison, IFN and histone deacetylase inhibitors afford greater times to next treatment than those from chemotherapy.

Both IFN-α and IFN-γ represent effective clinical treatments for CTCLs, including MF, *via* their cytotoxic and immunological effects on tumor-associated T-cells (108–110). A meta-analysis suggested that the overall response rate (ORR) to IFN-α was 70% (109). In all stages of MF, IFN-α achieves a superior time to next treatment compared to that of chemotherapy (106). IFN-γ shifts the Th2-dominant tumor microenvironment to a Th1 environment, as mentioned above. IFN-α2a and IFN-γ have been shown to decrease the expression and production of CCL17 and CCL18 and increase those of CXCL10 and CXCL11. Furthermore, subcutaneous administration of IFN-α increased the number of CXCL11-producing cells in the affected skin of patients with advanced MF (111).

Toll-like receptor (TLR) agonists induce anticancer effects by stimulating the innate immune system. Imiquimod is a topical immunomodulator that stimulates Th1 responses by activating TLR7 on plasmacytoid DCs, which leads to the production of IFN-α, IL-12, and tumor necrosis factor-α (112). The effectiveness of topical imiquimod has been reported in early-stage (113–115), folliculotropic, and tumor-stage MF (116). Resiquimod, a TLR7/8 agonist, is also effective for early-stage MF (117). TLR8 is expressed by myeloid-derived DCs, which are the most abundant DCs in human skin. Resiquimod, but not imiquimod, potently activates these cells (118).

The acetylation of histones plays a critical role in gene expression regulation (119). Histone acetylation and deacetylation control gene transcription and are mediated by histone acetyltransferases and deacetylases, respectively. Histone deacetylase inhibitors enhance the acetylation of histones and non-histone proteins and can induce apoptosis (120). Histone deacetylase inhibitors are potential therapeutic agents for the treatment of lymphoid neoplasms (121–124). Pruritus relief has also been reported with these inhibitors (121, 122, 124–126), supposedly through the reduction in the levels of IL-31-expressing T-cells (127).

Brentuximab vedotin (mentioned above) is an antibody-drug conjugate, in which an anti-CD30 monoclonal antibody is linked with the anti-tubulin agent, monomethyl auristatin E (128). Brentuximab vedotin is effective in the treatment of CD30-positive relapsed/refractory Hodgkin's lymphoma (129) and anaplastic large cell lymphoma (130). In a phase II study for MF/SS with variable CD30 expression levels, an ORR of 70% was observed with brentuximab vedotin (127). In addition, a significant improvement in objective response was observed in a randomized, phase III clinical trial (131).

Mogamulizumab, a defucosylated humanized anti-CCR4 antibody that was first approved for relapsed ATL, as described in further detail in Section "Adult T-cell leukemia/lymphoma," is also effective for CTCL including MF/SS (132, 133), and approved for relapsed or refractory CCR4-positive CTCL. In addition, an anti-CD158k monoclonal antibody, IPH4102, has also recently been developed (134), for which clinical studies in CTCL are ongoing (135). Lenalidomide (136), bortezomib (137), and immune checkpoint blockade are also under investigation.

PRIMARY CUTANEOUS CD30⁺ T-CELL LYMPHOPROLIFERATIVE DISORDERS

Primary cutaneous CD30⁺ T-cell lymphoproliferative disorders (PC CD30⁺ T-LPD) constitute the second most common form of CTCL, representing approximately 30% of all cutaneous lymphomas (2). They comprise a spectrum of diseases from lymphomatoid papulosis (LyP) to primary cutaneous anaplastic large-cell lymphoma (PCALCL) (138). The expression of CD30, a cytokine receptor belonging to the tumor necrosis factor receptor superfamily, by atypical T-cells is the common immunophenotype of this disorder.

Primary cutaneous anaplastic large-cell lymphoma is characterized by large T-cells with prominent nuclear pleomorphisms along with CD30 expression by more than 75% of the tumor cells (2). A single tumor or a group of firm nodules is seen clinically (**Figure 2**). PCALCL was established as a distinct form of ALCL because its clinical course, phenotype, and genotype are significantly different from those of systemic ALCL, including ALK-positive and ALK-negative forms (139–141). Moreover, IFN regulatory factor-4 translocations are reported to be specific for PCALCL (142). In contrast to that of systemic ALCL, the prognosis of PCALCL is reportedly excellent (143), with the exception of cases in Japan that appear to have a less favorable prognosis (144). PCALCL arising on the legs tends to produce poorer outcomes (145). The typical histology of PCALCL is a

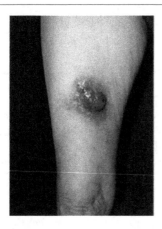

FIGURE 2 | Clinical findings of primary cutaneous CD30⁺ T-cell lymphoma. Eroded tumor is seen on the right thigh. Written informed consent was obtained from the patient.

circumscribed nodular infiltrate of cohesively arranged large lymphoid cells that extends into the deep dermis or hypodermis. Neutrophil-rich and eosinophil-rich variants have been noted and appear to be associated with immunodeficiency (146). The abundant infiltration of neutrophils can be explained by the release of IL-8, a potent neutrophil chemoattractant, from the tumor cells (147).

The tumor cells in PCALCL possess an activated T-cell phenotype and express CD2, CD4, and CD45RO, with a loss of CD2 and CD5 occurring variably. CD3 may be lacking or expressed at lower levels owing to genetic alterations in the T-cell receptor (TCR) coding regions on chromosome 1 in the tumor cells (148). Additionally, CD25/IL-2R, CD71, human leukocyte antigen–antigen D related, and CLA/CD162, as well as cytotoxic proteins, such as T-cell intracellular antigen 1 (TIA-1), granzyme B, and perforin, are expressed in half of PCALCL cases. PCALCL is often negative for epithelial membrane antigen, which differentiates it from systemic ALCL. Numerous quantities of TAMs are also present.

As opposed to MF/SS, the tumor cells of PCALCL express CCR3. CCL11, a CCR3 ligand, is also expressed by PCALCL cells and is detected in the connective tissue cells in the tumor. The CCR3⁺ tumor cells abundantly express IL-4 but not IFN-γ (69). The expression of both CCL11 and CCR3 on the tumor cells can lead to homotypic aggregation, which can be observed as cohesive clusters of tumor cells, a characteristic finding in ALCL (149). As CCR3 is also expressed on eosinophils and subpopulations of Th2 cells (70, 71), CCR3⁺ cells secreting CCL11 and IL-4 may produce a Th2-dominant microenvironment, which is suitable for tumor growth.

Lymphomatoid papulosis was first described by the dermatologist, Warren L. Macaulay, as a chronic recurrent, self-regressing papulonodular skin eruption with histologic features of a malignant lymphoma (138). Five histological variants (types A to E) are recognized as original variants in the updated World Health Organization classification of 2016 (10). LyP type A is the most common subtype, accounting for 75% of LyP cases (150). Type A is characterized by wedge-shaped dermal infiltrates with scattered large CD30⁺ cells. Histiocytes, eosinophils, and neutrophils comprise the background inflammatory cells. Type B shows epidermotropic infiltrates of small to medium-sized lymphocytes with variable CD30 expression and atypical chromatin-dense nuclei. Type C shows nodular cohesive infiltrates of large CD30⁺ pleomorphic or anaplastic lymphocytes. Type D shows epidermotropic infiltrates of atypical, small to medium-sized pleomorphic CD8⁺ cytotoxic cells (151). Type E shows angioinvasive infiltrates of mainly medium-sized pleomorphic CD30⁺ cells (152). Vascular occlusion by atypical lymphocytes and/or thrombi, hemorrhage, ulceration, and extensive necrosis are observed. LyP can persist for years or decades, but is not life-threatening (143, 153). However, some patients with LyP can develop secondary lymphoid neoplasms, in particular MF, Hodgkin's lymphoma, and cutaneous or nodal CD30⁺ ALCL (140, 146, 154). Surgical excision or radiation therapy is the recommended therapy for solitary or grouped lesion(s) of PCALCL, whereas methotrexate is the most prescribed therapy for multifocal lesions (138). The brentuximab vedotin (128) has been granted breakthrough therapy designation; in addition, bexarotene, a retinoid X receptor-specific agonist, has also been shown to be effective for both PCALCL (ORR: 50%) and LyP (ORR: 60%) in clinical trials (155). HDAC inhibitors (156), crizotinib, an ALK inhibitor (157), and anti-PD-1 are under investigation.

ADULT T-CELL LEUKEMIA/LYMPHOMA

Adult T-cell leukemia/lymphoma is a distinct T-cell malignancy caused by human T-lymphotropic virus type I (HTLV-1). HTLV-I infections are endemic in many parts of the world including southwest Japan, the Caribbean basin, and parts of central Africa and South America. Neoplastic T-cells are usually CD4+CD25+CCR4+ (158). The general characteristics of ATL are lymphadenopathy, hepatosplenomegaly, hypercalcemia, abnormal peripheral blood lymphocytes with multilobulated nuclei, and skin lesions (**Figure 3**).

There are four clinical subtypes of ATL (159): acute, lymphoma, chronic, and smoldering, based on peripheral blood involvement, organ complications, and laboratory examinations. Patients with ATL can be stratified into two groups: aggressive, which consists of the acute, lymphoma, and unfavorable chronic types, and indolent, which consists of the favorable chronic and smoldering types. The chronic type is separated into the favorable and unfavorable subgroups according to significant prognostic factors. This stratification is important for treatment selection, with most patients with aggressive ATL being given systemic chemotherapy, whereas those with indolent ATL are given topical therapy or are placed on observation.

Cutaneous involvement is frequently observed in patients with ATL at 30–70% (160, 161), regardless of ATL subtype. Cutaneous manifestation in the smoldering type of ATL has been suggested to reflect poor prognosis (162), and cutaneous ATL was recently proposed to include the lymphoma type as an extranodal variant (163). The majority of skin lesions are caused by the direct invasion of ATL tumor cells, forming various types of eruptions (164). In addition to these primary invasive lesions, patients with ATL may present with secondary inflammatory or infectious lesions (165). Compared to those of peripheral blood tumor cells, skin-infiltrating ATL tumor cells exhibit enhanced characteristics, such as increased expression of chemokine receptors. The interaction between chemokines and chemokine receptors drives T-cell migration and activation, which plays a critical role in the pathogenesis of various neoplastic and inflammatory disorders. ATL cells produce several chemokines including CCL3/MIP-1α, CCL4/MIP-1β (166), CCL2/monocyte chemoattractant protein-1 (MCP-1) (167), and CCL1/I-309 (168), as well as several chemokine receptors, including CCR4 (158, 169), CCR7 (170), and CCR8/CDw198 (168). Overexpression of chemokine CCL1 and its receptor, CCR8, contributes to autocrine anti-apoptotic effects ATL cells (168). Increased CCR7 expression is associated with lymphoid organ infiltration (170).

Adult T-cell leukemia/lymphoma cells not only express CCR4 but also its ligands, CCL17 and CCL22 (171). Neoplastic T-cells that highly express the Th2 chemokine receptor, CCR4, are found in the peripheral blood and affected skin of patients with ATL. In CTCL, extravasation of lymphoma cells into the skin is mediated by CCL17 and CCL22 released from epidermal cells (30). In contrast, one of the major sources of CCL17 in the affected skin of patients with ATL is the tumor cell itself (171). Moreover, CCL17 and CCL22 can also attract CCR4-expressing Treg cells, which may further suppress cytotoxic T-cells and prevent tumor immunosurveillance of the ATL cells (165). As ATL cells share the CD4+CD25+CCR4+ phenotype with Treg cells, ATL cells have been postulated as being Treg cells. In addition to CD25 and CCR4, ATL cells express CTLA-4 and FoxP3, both of which are expressed in Treg cells (172, 173). However, whether ATL cells can function as Treg cells is controversial because tumor cells possess very limited regulatory ability (174).

Th17 cells play an important role in cutaneous innate immunity. Th17-derived cytokines stimulate keratinocytes to produce antimicrobial peptides (175). ATL tumor cells can reduce the number and/or function of Th17 cells. Studies have shown that cellular immune responses are greatly impaired in patients with ATL, and ATL cells have been shown to secrete immunosuppressive cytokines such as IL-10 and transforming growth factor-β1 *in vitro*. In particular, ATL cells, as well as Treg or Th2 cells residing in the blood, produce IL-10, thereby suppressing Th17 activity (176). IL-17 enhances the synthesis of various antimicrobial peptides, such as human β-defensin 2, LL-37 (177), and S100A7, in keratinocytes. These peptides are active against fungi, such as those causing ringworm (178). More than 60% of patients with

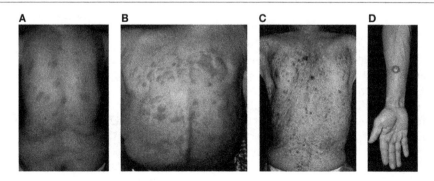

FIGURE 3 | Clinical findings of adult T-cell lymphoma/leukemia **(A)** Patch, **(B)** plaque, **(C)** multiple nodulotumoral lesion, and **(D)** tumor. Written informed consent was obtained from each patient.

ATL have tinea pedis/unguium/corporis, candidiasis, or other cutaneous fungal infections (165). Other skin infections may occur in these patients in addition to superficial fungal infections. It has been reported that scabies is sometimes superimposed on the skin lesions of patients with ATL (179).

Programmed cell death (PD)-1/CD279 constitutes a cell surface receptor that suppresses the immune system. PD-1 expression on HTLV-1-specific cytotoxic T-cells is dramatically upregulated in HTLV-1 carriers and patients with ATL (180). PD-1 is expressed at high levels on CD4$^+$ neoplastic and non-neoplastic cells, but not on CD8$^+$ cells (181). Because normal CD4$^+$ T-cells can be infected with HTLV-1, they can sometimes express PD-1, leading to immunosuppression. Moreover, it is noteworthy that PD-L1 is expressed in ATL cells (181). Expression of both PD-1 and PD-L1 by the ATL cells suggests a self-destructive state of the tumor cells. However, it may be more important that the PD-L1 expressed by the tumor cells suppresses the function of PD-1-expressing normal CD4$^+$ T-cells, resulting in immune evasion. Of note, 25% of patients with ATL have structural variations in the 3'-region of the gene for PD-L1, which leads to marked elevations of aberrant *PDL1* transcripts (182).

The fact that the tumor cells express CCR4 provides a therapeutic strategy for ATL. The anti-CCR4 monoclonal antibody mogamulizumab markedly enhances antibody-dependent cellular cytotoxicity and has been approved for the treatment of patients with CCR4-positive ATL, peripheral T-cell lymphoma, and CTCL. In a phase II trial of patients with relapsed CCR4-positive ATL, the ORR was 50%, with a complete response rate of 30% (183). Mogamulizumab is more effective against the peripheral blood tumor cells than those in the skin and lymph nodes. Cutaneous adverse reactions (CARs) are frequently observed during treatment (183, 184) and are supposedly indicative of favorable prognoses in ATL (185); a reduction in Treg by mogamulizumab is believed to induce CARs (186, 187). Recently, pretransplantation mogamulizumab has been reported to increase the risk of severe acute graft-versus-host disease (188, 189), and non-relapse mortality is significantly higher in patients with pretransplantation mogamulizumab. Therefore, mogamulizumab should be carefully considered and monitored for patients with ATL who are eligible for allogeneic hematopoietic stem-cell transplantation.

PANNICULITIS-LIKE T-CELL LYMPHOMA

Subcutaneous panniculitis-like T-cell lymphoma (SPTCL) with α/β phenotype and SPTCL with γ/δ phenotype have been recognized as unique entities, considering their clinical, histological, and immunological characteristics (2, 190, 191). The term SPTCL is now used exclusively for cases with the α/β T-cell phenotype, whereas those of the γ/δ T-cell phenotype have been reclassified as primary cutaneous gamma/delta T-cell lymphoma (PCGD-TCL) (2). The differential diagnosis of these two diseases is important, as each has a different prognosis and therapeutic strategy. In addition, both entities should be differentiated from other types of malignant lymphoma with preferential subcutaneous involvement and from other forms of lobular panniculitis, especially lupus panniculitis (192, 193).

SUBCUTANEOUS PANNICULITIS-LIKE T-CELL LYMPHOMA

Patients with SPTCL present clinically with multiple nodules or deeply seated plaques without ulceration. The skin lesions usually involve the legs, arms, and trunk. Systemic symptoms, such as pyrexia, fatigue, and weight loss, and laboratory abnormalities, including cytopenia and elevated liver function tests, are commonly observed. Hemophagocytic syndrome (HPS) is observed in <20% of patients (194). Dissemination to extracutaneous sites rarely occurs. As many as 20% of patients have associated autoimmune disease, which is commonly systemic lupus erythematosus (194).

The histopathological findings in SPTCL are dense, nodular, or diffuse subcutaneous infiltrates with a pattern similar to lobular panniculitis. The epidermis is not typically involved. The rimming of individual fat cells by neoplastic T-cells is a curious finding, although it is not diagnostic (193). The neoplastic T-cells are interspersed with small reactive lymphocytes and many histiocytes, whereas other inflammatory cells, including neutrophils and eosinophils, as well as the plasma cells and plasmacytoid DCs that are common in lupus panniculitis (195, 196), are usually lacking (193). High-throughput sequencing of the TCR genes can assist in the diagnosis of SPTCL (192). The neoplastic cells have a mature CD3$^+$CD4$^-$CD8$^+$ T-cell phenotype and express cytotoxic proteins, such as granzyme B, TIA-1, and perforin (194). Although the exact mechanisms that neoplastic cells utilize to migrate into the hypodermis are still mostly unknown, CCR5 expression on neoplastic cells and its ligands, CCL3, CCL4, and CCL5, which can be secreted from immunologically activated adipocytes, may contribute to the pathogenesis of SPTCL (197, 198).

The differential diagnosis of SPTCL includes both PCGD-TCL and lupus panniculitis. Differentiation is critical because PCGD-TCL with panniculitis-like features generally has a poor prognosis and requires systemic chemotherapy. In contrast, SPTCL has an excellent prognosis, especially in the cases without HPS (194). Both SPTCL and PCGD-TCL have nodular skin lesions with panniculitis-like features and rimming of fat cells. In contrast to that of SPTCL, PCGD-TCL involves ulceration of the hypodermis, dermis, and/or epidermis (194). Expression of βF1, but not TCRγ/δ or CD56, is useful to differentiate between SPTCL and PCGD-TCL.

Multiagent chemotherapy is not recommended as a first-line treatment for SPTCL without HPS. Systemic corticosteroids or other immunosuppressive agents, such as cyclosporine or methotrexate, are preferred, which is also the case with relapsing disease (199–201). Oral bexarotene has also shown good response rates (202).

PRIMARY CUTANEOUS GAMMA/DELTA T-CELL LYMPHOMA

Primary cutaneous gamma/delta T-cell lymphoma is a lymphoma composed of a clonal proliferation of mature, activated γ/δ T-cells with a cytotoxic phenotype. Most patients present with deep dermal or subcutaneous plaques or tumors, either with or without epidermal ulceration and necrosis (194, 203, 204). The skin lesions are often generalized and involve the extremities. Some patients may present with a single tumor, or scaly patches/plaques, clinically resembling early-stage MF (204). The involvement of mucosal and other extranodal sites is frequently noted, although lymph nodes, spleen, and bone marrow are rarely involved (204, 205). Most patients present with systemic symptoms including B symptoms. PCGD-TCL is frequently accompanied by HPS, particularly in patients with panniculitis-like tumors (194, 203). Chronic antigenic stimulation has been hypothesized to be involved in the pathogenesis of PCGD-TCL (206). PCGD-TCL is also associated with opportunistic infections in patients with congenital or acquired immunosuppression and autoimmunity (207–209).

The lymphoid infiltrates have a variable histological pattern and may be epidermotropic, dermal, and/or subcutaneous (203, 204). In contrast to that of SPTCL, a pure panniculitic pattern is rarely observed (204), and variable patterns can be found in skin biopsies obtained from different sites or different parts of the same biopsy (190, 203, 204). Lichenoid or vascular interface dermatitis-like patterns of epidermal infiltration may occur, which may be associated with intraepidermal vesiculation and necrosis (204). Panniculitis-like lesions may show the rimming of fat cells observed in SPTCL. Angiocentricity, angiodestruction, and tissue necrosis may be seen. Hemophagocytosis may be present, especially in cases with HPS. The tumor cells have a characteristic phenotype of TCR γ/δ+, βF1−, CD3+, CD2+, CD5−, and CD56+, with a strong expression of cytotoxic proteins. PCGD-TCL with subcutaneous panniculitis-like infiltrate preferentially derives from the V2 subtype (205). PCGD-TCL is resistant to multiagent chemotherapy. The effectiveness of hematopoietic stem cell transplantation has been reported in some patients with PCGD-TCL (204, 210, 211).

PRIMARY CUTANEOUS CD4+ SMALL/MEDIUM T-CELL LYMPHOPROLIFERATIVE DISORDER

Primary cutaneous small/medium-sized T-cell lymphoma (PCSM-TCL) has recently been reclassified as primary cutaneous small/medium-sized T-cell lymphoproliferative disorder (PCSM-TCLPD) because of its indolent behavior and uncertain malignancy (10). PCSM-TCL was originally associated with a favorable 5-year survival rate of 60–80% (2). However, fatal outcomes have not been documented in subsequent reports (212, 213).

Primary cutaneous small/medium-sized T-cell lymphoproliferative disorder characteristically presents with a single lesion on the head, neck, or upper arms, but rarely presents as multiple papules, plaques, or tumors (212, 214). Histopathologically, PCSM-TCLPD is characterized by many small- to medium-sized CD3+CD4+CD8− T-cells, with a small number of large CD4+ pleomorphic T-cells and variable admixtures of CD8+ T-cells, B-cells, histiocytes, plasma cells, and eosinophils (2).

The few, large pleomorphic CD4+ T-cells in PCSM-TCLPD express PD-1, BCL6, and CXCL13 (215), all of which are expressed on a particular germinal center T-cell subset, termed follicular helper T (TFH) cells. TFH cells are important in germinal center formation and plasma cell development. The expression of PD-1, BCL6, and CXCL13 by these large CD4+ T-cells suggests that PCSM-TCLPD originates from TFH cells (215). PD-1 is typically expressed by atypical cells in PCSM-TCL and pseudo-T-cell lymphomas (216). The clinical presentation, pathological features, and immunohistochemical findings of PCSM-TCLPD are very similar to those of pseudo-T-cell lymphomas (217, 218). The demonstration of a T-cell clone and loss of pan-T-cell antigens are useful diagnostic criteria for PCSM-TCL (218). The staining pattern for nuclear factor of activated T-cells, cytoplasmic 1 is also reported to be useful for the differential diagnosis between PCSM-TCLPD and pseudo-T-cell lymphomas (219), where NFAT1c nuclear staining indicates PCSM-TCLPD and cytoplasmic staining indicates pseudo-T-cell lymphoma. The cytoplasmic staining pattern is also seen in MF, ALCL, and LyP. The clinical behavior of PCSM-TCLPD is almost always indolent, with most patients showing localized disease. Treatment with local therapies, such as excision or radiation therapy, is often curative (214, 220, 221).

HYDROA VACCINIFORME-LIKE LYMPHOPROLIFERATIVE DISORDER (HVLL)

Typical hydroa vacciniforme (HV) is characterized by light-induced herpetiform vesiculopapules on the sun-exposed areas. The eruptions form crusts and then heal to leave varicelliform scars. Systemic symptoms are absent, and the disease usually improves spontaneously in adolescence and young adulthood (222). Routine laboratory tests are normal. Since the first report in 1986 (223), peculiar HV-like eruptions have been recognized in children mainly from Asia and Central and South America. HVLL was included for the first time in the 2008 World Health Organization classification of tumors of hematopoietic and lymphoid tissues (224). HVLL is defined as an Epstein–Barr virus (EBV)-positive CTCL that occurs in children and less often in young adults (225). Unlike typical HV, HVLL eruptions become more severe with age, presenting with marked facial edema and vesiclopapules followed by ulceration and crusting. Systemic symptoms, including high-grade fever and liver damage, are usually present. Hepatosplenomegaly and lymphadenopathy are frequently observed during the acute phase. The lesions are associated with EBV infection and frequently possess monoclonal rearrangements of the TCR genes (226, 227). Although the skin lesions are not limited to sun-exposed areas, there is an increased occurrence during the summer. Most cases have a CD8+ T-cell phenotype (228), whereas a small number of cases have been reported to have a natural killer-cell phenotype (229, 230). Regardless of cell-type derivation, the lymphoid cells are positive for cytotoxic markers, such as granzyme B and TIA-1 (231).

SEVERE MOSQUITO BITE ALLERGY

An associated cutaneous disorder is a severe allergy/hypersensitivity to mosquito bites (232). It is defined as an EBV+ NK-cell lymphoproliferation that is characterized by high fever, ulcers, skin necrosis, and deep scarring, with the potential to progress into overt NK/T-cell lymphoma or aggressive NK-cell leukemia in the protracted clinical course (233). Severe mosquito bite allergy was included for the first time in the 2017 World Health Organization classification of tumors of hematopoietic and lymphoid tissues (234).

PRIMARY CUTANEOUS ACRAL CD8⁺ T-CELL LYMPHOMA

Primary cutaneous acral CD8⁺ T-cell lymphoma is characterized as a solitary, slow-growing nodule without prior patches or plaques (235), but with precedence of bilateral, symmetrical disease and recurrent disease (236). Most cases appear on the ear, although other peripheral locations, such as the nose, hands, and feet, have been noted (237).

Primary cutaneous acral CD8⁺ T-cell lymphoma and PCSM-TCLPD are often indistinguishable morphologically. Moreover, the overt clinical features of both diseases are similar, such as targeting adults, a preference for the face and neck, solitary tumors without ulceration, and an indolent behavior. However, T follicular markers, such as CD10, Bcl-6, PD-1, and CXCL13, which are expressed on neoplastic cells of PCSM-TCLPD, are negative in primary cutaneous acral CD8⁺ T-cell lymphoma (236). Granzyme B expression is also typically negative in the latter (238). The clinical course for primary cutaneous acral CD8⁺ T-cell lymphoma is invariably indolent; cutaneous relapse may occur, but there have been no reports of progression to extracutaneous sites, and overtreatment should be avoided (238). Localized therapy, such as topical steroids, radiotherapy, and surgical excision, or careful monitoring, is preferred. IFN,

psoralen-ultraviolet A phototherapy, and methotrexate have been used for patients with multifocal cutaneous disease (238).

PRIMARY CUTANEOUS CD8⁺ AGGRESSIVE EPIDERMOTROPIC CYTOTOXIC T-CELL LYMPHOMA

Primary cutaneous CD8⁺ aggressive epidermotropic cytotoxic T-cell lymphoma (PCAETCL) is characterized by disseminated, rapidly developing papules, plaques, and nodules with central ulceration or necrosis. PCAETCL may spread to other visceral organs including the lungs, testes, central nervous system, and oral mucosa (239–241); it carries an overall poor prognosis. However, the lymph nodes are rarely involved. Histological findings demonstrate prominent epidermotropism, with necrotic keratinocytes and ulceration (240). Dermal infiltrates consist of atypical lymphocytes, often extending into the deep dermis and subcutaneous fat. Adnexal invasion is frequently observed (242). Blistering, angiocentricity, angioinvasion, riming of adipocytes, and destruction of adnexal structures may be seen (240). Cells invariably demonstrate CD8⁺CD4⁻ phenotypes and usually express CD3, β-F1, and TIA-1. CD45RA is expressed in the majority of cases (239). T-cell clonality is usually demonstrated. Conventional therapies for CTCL are ineffective and multiagent chemotherapies have unsatisfactory outcomes (240). Hematopoietic stem cell transplantation is a reasonable treatment choice for PCAETCL (243).

AUTHOR CONTRIBUTIONS

The author confirms being the sole contributor of this work and approved it for publication.

REFERENCES

1. Groves FD, Linet MS, Travis LB, Devesa SS. Cancer surveillance series: non-Hodgkin's lymphoma incidence by histologic subtype in the United States from 1978 through 1995. *J Natl Cancer Inst* (2000) 92:1240–51. doi:10.1093/jnci/92.15.1240
2. Willemze R, Jaffe ES, Burg G, Cerroni L, Berti E, Swerdlow SH, et al. WHO-EORTC classification for cutaneous lymphomas. *Blood* (2005) 105:3768–85. doi:10.1182/blood-2004-09-3502
3. Criscione VD, Weinstock MA. Incidence of cutaneous T-cell lymphoma in the United States, 1973-2002. *Arch Dermatol* (2007) 143:854–9. doi:10.1001/archderm.143.7.854
4. Assaf C, Gellrich S, Steinhoff M, Nashan D, Weisse F, Dippel E, et al. Cutaneous lymphomas in Germany: an analysis of the central cutaneous lymphoma registry of the German society of dermatology (DDG). *J Dtsch Dermatol Ges* (2007) 5:662–8. doi:10.1111/j.1610-0387.2007.06337.x
5. Bradford PT, Devesa SS, Anderson WF, Toro JR. Cutaneous lymphoma incidence patterns in the United States: a population-based study of 3884 cases. *Blood* (2009) 113:5064–73. doi:10.1182/blood-2008-10-184168
6. Hamada T, Iwatsuki K. Cutaneous lymphoma in Japan: a nationwide study of 1733 patients. *J Dermatol* (2014) 41:3–10. doi:10.1111/1346-8138.12299
7. Weinstock MA, Horm JW. Mycosis fungoides in the United States. Increasing incidence and descriptive epidemiology. *JAMA* (1988) 260:42–6. doi:10.1001/jama.1988.03410010050033
8. Holterhues C, Vries E, Louwman MW, Koljenovic S, Nijsten T. Incidence and trends of cutaneous malignancies in the Netherlands, 1989-2005. *J Invest Dermatol* (2010) 130:1807–12. doi:10.1038/jid.2010.58
9. Sokolowska-Wojdylo M, Olek-Hrab K, Ruckemann-Dziurdzinska K. Primary cutaneous lymphomas: diagnosis and treatment. *Postepy Dermatol Alergol* (2015) 32:368–83. doi:10.5114/pdia.2015.54749
10. Swerdlow SH, Campo E, Pileri SA, Harris NL, Stein H, Siebert R, et al. The 2016 revision of the World Health Organization classification of lymphoid neoplasms. *Blood* (2016) 127:2375–90. doi:10.1182/blood-2016-01-643569
11. Ruiz R, Morante Z, Mantilla R, Mas L, Casanova L, Gomez HL. Primary cutaneous T-cell lymphoma: experience from the Peruvian National Cancer Institute. *An Bras Dermatol* (2017) 92:649–54. doi:10.1590/abd1806-4841.20176825
12. Olsen E, Vonderheid E, Pimpinelli N, Willemze R, Kim Y, Knobler R, et al. Revisions to the staging and classification of mycosis fungoides and Sezary syndrome: a proposal of the International Society for Cutaneous Lymphomas (ISCL) and the cutaneous lymphoma task force of the European Organization of Research and Treatment of Cancer (EORTC). *Blood* (2007) 110:1713–22. doi:10.1182/blood-2007-03-055749
13. Agar NS, Wedgeworth E, Crichton S, Mitchell TJ, Cox M, Ferreira S, et al. Survival outcomes and prognostic factors in mycosis fungoides/Sezary syndrome: validation of the revised International Society for Cutaneous Lymphomas/European Organisation for Research and treatment of cancer staging proposal. *J Clin Oncol* (2010) 28:4730–9. doi:10.1200/JCO.2009.27.7665
14. Benner MF, Jansen PM, Vermeer MH, Willemze R. Prognostic factors in transformed mycosis fungoides: a retrospective analysis of 100 cases. *Blood* (2012) 119(7):1643–9. doi:10.1182/blood-2011-08-376319
15. Campbell JJ, Clark RA, Watanabe R, Kupper TS. Sezary syndrome and mycosis fungoides arise from distinct T-cell subsets: a biologic rationale

for their distinct clinical behaviors. *Blood* (2010) 116:767–71. doi:10.1182/blood-2009-11-251926

16. Bagot M, Moretta A, Sivori S, Biassoni R, Cantoni C, Bottino C, et al. CD4(+) cutaneous T-cell lymphoma cells express the p140-killer cell immunoglobulin-like receptor. *Blood* (2001) 97(5):1388–91. doi:10.1182/blood.V97.5.1388

17. Poszepczynska-Guigne E, Schiavon V, D'Incan M, Echchakir H, Musette P, Ortonne N, et al. CD158k/KIR3DL2 is a new phenotypic marker of Sezary cells: relevance for the diagnosis and follow-up of Sezary syndrome. *J Invest Dermatol* (2004) 122(3):820–3. doi:10.1111/j.0022-202X.2004.22326.x

18. Wechsler J, Bagot M, Nikolova M, Parolini S, Martin-Garcia N, Boumsell L, et al. Killer cell immunoglobulin-like receptor expression delineates in situ Sezary syndrome lymphocytes. *J Pathol* (2003) 199(1):77–83. doi:10.1002/path.1251

19. van Doorn R, van Kester MS, Dijkman R, Vermeer MH, Mulder AA, Szuhai K, et al. Oncogenomic analysis of mycosis fungoides reveals major differences with Sezary syndrome. *Blood* (2009) 113:127–36. doi:10.1182/blood-2008-04-153031

20. Laharanne E, Oumouhou N, Bonnet F, Carlotti M, Gentil C, Chevret E, et al. Genome-wide analysis of cutaneous T-cell lymphomas identifies three clinically relevant classes. *J Invest Dermatol* (2010) 130:1707–18. doi:10.1038/jid.2010.8

21. Wang L, Ni X, Covington KR, Yang BY, Shiu J, Zhang X, et al. Genomic profiling of Sezary syndrome identifies alterations of key T cell signaling and differentiation genes. *Nat Genet* (2015) 47:1426–34. doi:10.1038/ng.3444

22. Krejsgaard T, Ralfkiaer U, Clasen-Linde E, Eriksen KW, Kopp KL, Bonefeld CM, et al. Malignant cutaneous T-cell lymphoma cells express IL-17 utilizing the Jak3/Stat3 signaling pathway. *J Invest Dermatol* (2011) 131(6):1331–8. doi:10.1038/jid.2011.27

23. Berger CL, Tigelaar R, Cohen J, Mariwalla K, Trinh J, Wang N, et al. Cutaneous T-cell lymphoma: malignant proliferation of T-regulatory cells. *Blood* (2005) 105(4):1640–7. doi:10.1182/blood-2004-06-2181

24. Heid JB, Schmidt A, Oberle N, Goerdt S, Krammer PH, Suri-Payer E, et al. FOXP3+CD25− tumor cells with regulatory function in Sezary syndrome. *J Invest Dermatol* (2009) 129(12):2875–85. doi:10.1038/jid.2009.175

25. Sugaya M. Chemokines and cutaneous lymphoma. *J Dermatol Sci* (2010) 59:81–5. doi:10.1016/j.jdermsci.2010.05.005

26. Lu D, Duvic M, Medeiros LJ, Luthra R, Dorfman DM, Jones D. The T-cell chemokine receptor CXCR3 is expressed highly in low-grade mycosis fungoides. *Am J Clin Pathol* (2001) 115:413–21. doi:10.1309/3N7P-J84L-JQ9K-G89R

27. Sarris AH, Esgleyes-Ribot T, Crow M, Broxmeyer HE, Karasavvas N, Pugh W, et al. Cytokine loops involving interferon-gamma and IP-10, a cytokine chemotactic for CD4+ lymphocytes: an explanation for the epidermotropism of cutaneous T-cell lymphoma? *Blood* (1995) 86:651–8.

28. Tensen CP, Vermeer MH, van der Stoop PM, van Beek P, Scheper RJ, Boorsma DM, et al. Epidermal interferon-gamma inducible protein-10 (IP-10) and monokine induced by gamma-interferon (Mig) but not IL-8 mRNA expression is associated with epidermotropism in cutaneous T cell lymphomas. *J Invest Dermatol* (1998) 111:222–6. doi:10.1046/j.1523-1747.1998.00263.x

29. Miyagaki T, Sugaya M, Suga H, Morimura S, Ohmatsu H, Fujita H, et al. Low herpesvirus entry mediator (HVEM) expression on dermal fibroblasts contributes to a Th2-dominant microenvironment in advanced cutaneous T-cell lymphoma. *J Invest Dermatol* (2012) 132:1280–9. doi:10.1038/jid.2011.470

30. Ferenczi K, Fuhlbrigge RC, Pinkus J, Pinkus GS, Kupper TS. Increased CCR4 expression in cutaneous T cell lymphoma. *J Invest Dermatol* (2002) 119:1405–10. doi:10.1046/j.1523-1747.2002.19610.x

31. Miyagaki T, Sugaya M. Immunological milieu in mycosis fungoides and Sezary syndrome. *J Dermatol* (2014) 41:11–8. doi:10.1111/1346-8138.12305

32. Miyagaki T, Sugaya M, Suga H, Kamata M, Ohmatsu H, Fujita H, et al. IL-22, but not IL-17, dominant environment in cutaneous T-cell lymphoma. *Clin Cancer Res* (2011) 17(24):7529–38. doi:10.1158/1078-0432.CCR-11-1192

33. Kallinich T, Muche JM, Qin S, Sterry W, Audring H, Kroczek RA. Chemokine receptor expression on neoplastic and reactive T cells in the skin at different stages of mycosis fungoides. *J Invest Dermatol* (2003) 121(5):1045–52. doi:10.1046/j.1523-1747.2003.12555.x

34. Wu XS, Lonsdorf AS, Hwang ST. Cutaneous T-cell lymphoma: roles for chemokines and chemokine receptors. *J Invest Dermatol* (2009) 129(5):1115–9. doi:10.1038/jid.2009.45

35. Sokolowska-Wojdylo M, Wenzel J, Gaffal E, Lenz J, Speuser P, Erdmann S, et al. Circulating clonal CLA(+) and CD4(+) T cells in Sezary syndrome

express the skin-homing chemokine receptors CCR4 and CCR10 as well as the lymph node-homing chemokine receptor CCR7. *Br J Dermatol* (2005) 152:258–64. doi:10.1111/j.1365-2133.2004.06325.x

36. Narducci MG, Scala E, Bresin A, Caprini E, Picchio MC, Remotti D, et al. Skin homing of Sezary cells involves SDF-1-CXCR4 signaling and down-regulation of CD26/dipeptidylpeptidase IV. *Blood* (2006) 107:1108–15. doi:10.1182/blood-2005-04-1492

37. Kakinuma T, Sugaya M, Nakamura K, Kaneko F, Wakugawa M, Matsushima K, et al. Thymus and activation-regulated chemokine (TARC/CCL17) in mycosis fungoides: serum TARC levels reflect the disease activity of mycosis fungoides. *J Am Acad Dermatol* (2003) 48:23–30. doi:10.1067/mjd.2003.132

38. Morales J, Homey B, Vicari AP, Hudak S, Oldham E, Hedrick J, et al. CTACK, a skin-associated chemokine that preferentially attracts skin-homing memory T cells. *Proc Natl Acad Sci U S A* (1999) 96:14470–5. doi:10.1073/pnas.96.25.14470

39. Fujita Y, Abe R, Sasaki M, Honda A, Furuichi M, Asano Y, et al. Presence of circulating CCR10+ T cells and elevated serum CTACK/CCL27 in the early stage of mycosis fungoides. *Clin Cancer Res* (2006) 12:2670–5. doi:10.1158/1078-0432.CCR-05-1513

40. Goteri G, Rupoli S, Campanati A, Zizzi A, Picardi P, Cardelli M, et al. Serum and tissue CTACK/CCL27 chemokine levels in early mycosis fungoides may be correlated with disease-free survival following treatment with interferon alfa and psoralen plus ultraviolet A therapy. *Br J Dermatol* (2012) 166:948–52. doi:10.1111/j.1365-2133.2012.10818.x

41. Maj J, Jankowska-Konsur AM, Halon A, Wozniak Z, Plomer-Niezgoda E, Reich A. Expression of CXCR4 and CXCL12 and their correlations to the cell proliferation and angiogenesis in mycosis fungoides. *Postepy Dermatol Alergol* (2015) 32:437–42. doi:10.5114/pdia.2015.48034

42. Vowels BR, Cassin M, Vonderheid EC, Rook AH. Aberrant cytokine production by Sezary syndrome patients: cytokine secretion pattern resembles murine Th2 cells. *J Invest Dermatol* (1992) 99:90–4. doi:10.1111/1523-1747.ep12611877

43. Dummer R, Kohl O, Gillessen J, Kagi M, Burg G. Peripheral blood mononuclear cells in patients with nonleukemic cutaneous T-cell lymphoma. Reduced proliferation and preferential secretion of a T helper-2-like cytokine pattern on stimulation. *Arch Dermatol* (1993) 129:433–6. doi:10.1001/archderm.1993.01680250045005

44. Vowels BR, Lessin SR, Cassin M, Jaworsky C, Benoit B, Wolfe JT, et al. Th2 cytokine mRNA expression in skin in cutaneous T-cell lymphoma. *J Invest Dermatol* (1994) 103:669–73. doi:10.1111/1523-1747.ep12398454

45. Dummer R, Heald PW, Nestle FO, Ludwig E, Laine E, Hemmi S, et al. Sezary syndrome T-cell clones display T-helper 2 cytokines and express the accessory factor-1 (interferon-gamma receptor beta-chain). *Blood* (1996) 88:1383–9.

46. Asadullah K, Haeussler A, Sterry W, Docke WD, Volk HD. Interferon gamma and tumor necrosis factor alpha mRNA expression in mycosis fungoides progression. *Blood* (1996) 88:757–8.

47. Asadullah K, Docke WD, Haeussler A, Sterry W, Volk HD. Progression of mycosis fungoides is associated with increasing cutaneous expression of interleukin-10 mRNA. *J Invest Dermatol* (1996) 107:833–7. doi:10.1111/1523-1747.ep12330869

48. Guenova E, Watanabe R, Teague JE, Desimone JA, Jiang Y, Dowlatshahi M, et al. TH2 cytokines from malignant cells suppress TH1 responses and enforce a global TH2 bias in leukemic cutaneous T-cell lymphoma. *Clin Cancer Res* (2013) 19:3755–63. doi:10.1158/1078-0432.CCR-12-3488

49. Kaplan EH, Rosen ST, Norris DB, Roenigk HH Jr., Saks SR, Bunn PA Jr. Phase II study of recombinant human interferon gamma for treatment of cutaneous T-cell lymphoma. *J Natl Cancer Inst* (1990) 82:208–12. doi:10.1093/jnci/82.3.208

50. Sugaya M, Tokura Y, Hamada T, Tsuboi R, Moroi Y, Nakahara T, et al. Phase II study of i.v. interferon-gamma in Japanese patients with mycosis fungoides. *J Dermatol* (2014) 41:50–6. doi:10.1111/1346-8138.12341

51. Dummer R, Hassel JC, Fellenberg F, Eichmuller S, Maier T, Slos P, et al. Adenovirus-mediated intralesional interferon-gamma gene transfer induces tumor regressions in cutaneous lymphomas. *Blood* (2004) 104:1631–8. doi:10.1182/blood-2004-01-0360

52. Urosevic M, Fujii K, Calmels B, Laine E, Kobert N, Acres B, et al. Type I IFN innate immune response to adenovirus-mediated IFN-gamma gene transfer contributes to the regression of cutaneous lymphomas. *J Clin Invest* (2007) 117:2834–46. doi:10.1172/JCI32077

53. Dummer R, Eichmuller S, Gellrich S, Assaf C, Dreno B, Schiller M, et al. Phase II clinical trial of intratumoral application of TG1042 (adenovirus-interferon-gamma) in patients with advanced cutaneous T-cell lymphomas and multilesional cutaneous B-cell lymphomas. *Mol Ther* (2010) 18:1244–7. doi:10.1038/mt.2010.52

54. Thumann P, Luftl M, Moc I, Bagot M, Bensussan A, Schuler G, et al. Interaction of cutaneous lymphoma cells with reactive T cells and dendritic cells: implications for dendritic cell-based immunotherapy. *Br J Dermatol* (2003) 149:1128–42. doi:10.1111/j.1365-2133.2003.05674.x

55. Talpur R, Bassett R, Duvic M. Prevalence and treatment of *Staphylococcus aureus* colonization in patients with mycosis fungoides and Sezary syndrome. *Br J Dermatol* (2008) 159:105–12. doi:10.1111/j.1365-2133.2008.08612.x

56. Tsambiras PE, Patel S, Greene JN, Sandin RL, Vincent AL. Infectious complications of cutaneous t-cell lymphoma. *Cancer Control* (2001) 8:185–8. doi:10.1177/107327480100800213

57. Talpur R, Singh L, Daulat S, Liu P, Seyfer S, Trynosky T, et al. Long-term outcomes of 1,263 patients with mycosis fungoides and Sezary syndrome from 1982 to 2009. *Clin Cancer Res* (2012) 18:5051–60. doi:10.1158/1078-0432.CCR-12-0604

58. Showe LC, Fox FE, Williams D, Au K, Niu Z, Rook AH. Depressed IL-12-mediated signal transduction in T cells from patients with Sezary syndrome is associated with the absence of IL-12 receptor beta 2 mRNA and highly reduced levels of STAT4. *J Immunol* (1999) 163(7):4073–9.

59. Kopp KL, Ralfkiaer U, Gjerdrum LM, Helvad R, Pedersen IH, Litman T, et al. STAT5-mediated expression of oncogenic miR-155 in cutaneous T-cell lymphoma. *Cell Cycle* (2013) 12(12):1939–47. doi:10.4161/cc.24987

60. Netchiporouk E, Litvinov IV, Moreau L, Gilbert M, Sasseville D, Duvic M. Deregulation in STAT signaling is important for cutaneous T-cell lymphoma (CTCL) pathogenesis and cancer progression. *Cell Cycle* (2014) 13(21):3331–5. doi:10.4161/15384101.2014.965061

61. Rook AH, Kubin M, Fox FE, Niu Z, Cassin M, Vowels BR, et al. The potential therapeutic role of interleukin-12 in cutaneous T-cell lymphoma. *Ann N Y Acad Sci* (1996) 795:310–8. doi:10.1111/j.1749-6632.1996.tb52680.x

62. van der Fits L, Out-Luiting JJ, van Leeuwen MA, Samsom JN, Willemze R, Tensen CP, et al. Autocrine IL-21 stimulation is involved in the maintenance of constitutive STAT3 activation in Sezary syndrome. *J Invest Dermatol* (2012) 132(2):440–7. doi:10.1038/jid.2011.293

63. Qin JZ, Kamarashev J, Zhang CL, Dummer R, Burg G, Dobbeling U. Constitutive and interleukin-7- and interleukin-15-stimulated DNA binding of STAT and novel factors in cutaneous T cell lymphoma cells. *J Invest Dermatol* (2001) 117(3):583–9. doi:10.1046/j.0022-202x.2001.01436.x

64. Nielsen M, Kaestel CG, Eriksen KW, Woetmann A, Stokkedal T, Kaltoft K, et al. Inhibition of constitutively activated Stat3 correlates with altered Bcl-2/Bax expression and induction of apoptosis in mycosis fungoides tumor cells. *Leukemia* (1999) 13(5):735–8. doi:10.1038/sj.leu.2401415

65. van Kester MS, Out-Luiting JJ, von dem Borne PA, Willemze R, Tensen CP, Vermeer MH. Cucurbitacin I inhibits Stat3 and induces apoptosis in Sezary cells. *J Invest Dermatol* (2008) 128(7):1691–5. doi:10.1038/sj.jid.5701246

66. Gibson HM, Mishra A, Chan DV, Hake TS, Porcu P, Wong HK. Impaired proteasome function activates GATA3 in T cells and upregulates CTLA-4: relevance for Sezary syndrome. *J Invest Dermatol* (2013) 133(1):249–57. doi:10.1038/jid.2012.265

67. Liotta LA, Kohn EC. The microenvironment of the tumour-host interface. *Nature* (2001) 411:375–9. doi:10.1038/35077241

68. Miyagaki T, Sugaya M, Fujita H, Ohmatsu H, Kakinuma T, Kadono T, et al. Eotaxins and CCR3 interaction regulates the Th2 environment of cutaneous T-cell lymphoma. *J Invest Dermatol* (2010) 130:2304–11. doi:10.1038/jid.2010.128

69. Kleinhans M, Tun-Kyi A, Gilliet M, Kadin ME, Dummer R, Burg G, et al. Functional expression of the eotaxin receptor CCR3 in CD30+ cutaneous T-cell lymphoma. *Blood* (2003) 101:1487–93. doi:10.1182/blood-2002-02-0475

70. Sallusto F, Mackay CR, Lanzavecchia A. Selective expression of the eotaxin receptor CCR3 by human T helper 2 cells. *Science* (1997) 277:2005–7. doi:10.1126/science.277.5334.2005

71. Forssmann U, Uguccioni M, Loetscher P, Dahinden CA, Langen H, Thelen M, et al. Eotaxin-2, a novel CC chemokine that is selective for the chemokine receptor CCR3, and acts like eotaxin on human eosinophil and basophil leukocytes. *J Exp Med* (1997) 185:2171–6. doi:10.1084/jem.185.12.2171

72. Kikuchi Y, Kunita A, Iwata C, Komura D, Nishiyama T, Shimazu K, et al. The niche component periostin is produced by cancer-associated fibroblasts, supporting growth of gastric cancer through ERK activation. *Am J Pathol* (2014) 184:859–70. doi:10.1016/j.ajpath.2013.11.012

73. Furudate S, Fujimura T, Kakizaki A, Kambayashi Y, Asano M, Watabe A, et al. The possible interaction between periostin expressed by cancer stroma and tumor-associated macrophages in developing mycosis fungoides. *Exp Dermatol* (2016) 25:107–12. doi:10.1111/exd.12873

74. Takahashi N, Sugaya M, Suga H, Oka T, Kawaguchi M, Miyagaki T, et al. Thymic stromal chemokine TSLP Acts through Th2 cytokine production to induce cutaneous T-cell lymphoma. *Cancer Res* (2016) 76:6241–52. doi:10.1158/0008-5472.CAN-16-0992

75. Soumelis V, Reche PA, Kanzler H, Yuan W, Edward G, Homey B, et al. Human epithelial cells trigger dendritic cell mediated allergic inflammation by producing TSLP. *Nat Immunol* (2002) 3:673–80. doi:10.1038/ni805

76. Miyagaki T, Sugaya M, Fujita H, Saeki H, Tamaki K. Increased serum thymic stromal lymphopoietin levels in patients with cutaneous T cell lymphoma. *Clin Exp Dermatol* (2009) 34:539–40. doi:10.1111/j.1365-2230.2008.02990.x

77. Tuzova M, Richmond J, Wolpowitz D, Curiel-Lewandrowski C, Chaney K, Kupper T, et al. CCR4+T cell recruitment to the skin in mycosis fungoides: potential contributions by thymic stromal lymphopoietin and interleukin-16. *Leuk Lymphoma* (2015) 56:440–9. doi:10.3109/10428194.2014.919634

78. Mantovani A, Bottazzi B, Colotta F, Sozzani S, Ruco L. The origin and function of tumor-associated macrophages. *Immunol Today* (1992) 13:265–70. doi:10.1016/0167-5699(92)90008-U

79. Hao NB, Lu MH, Fan YH, Cao YL, Zhang ZR, Yang SM. Macrophages in tumor microenvironments and the progression of tumors. *Clin Dev Immunol* (2012) 2012:948098. doi:10.1155/2012/948098

80. Bingle L, Brown NJ, Lewis CE. The role of tumour-associated macrophages in tumour progression: implications for new anticancer therapies. *J Pathol* (2002) 196:254–65. doi:10.1002/path.1027

81. Sugaya M, Miyagaki T, Ohmatsu H, Suga H, Kai H, Kamata M, et al. Association of the numbers of CD163(+) cells in lesional skin and serum levels of soluble CD163 with disease progression of cutaneous T cell lymphoma. *J Dermatol Sci* (2012) 68:45–51. doi:10.1016/j.jdermsci.2012.07.007

82. Assaf C, Hwang ST. Mac attack: macrophages as key drivers of cutaneous T-cell lymphoma pathogenesis. *Exp Dermatol* (2016) 25:105–6. doi:10.1111/exd.12894

83. Tada K, Hamada T, Asagoe K, Umemura H, Mizuno-Ikeda K, Aoyama Y, et al. Increase of DC-LAMP+ mature dendritic cell subsets in dermatopathic lymphadenitis of mycosis fungoides. *Eur J Dermatol* (2014) 24:670–5. doi:10.1684/ejd.2014.2437

84. Wu X, Schulte BC, Zhou Y, Haribhai D, Mackinnon AC, Plaza JA, et al. Depletion of M2-like tumor-associated macrophages delays cutaneous T-cell lymphoma development in vivo. *J Invest Dermatol* (2014) 134:2814–22. doi:10.1038/jid.2014.206

85. Kodelja V, Muller C, Politz O, Hakij N, Orfanos CE, Goerdt S. Alternative macrophage activation-associated CC-chemokine-1, a novel structural homologue of macrophage inflammatory protein-1 alpha with a Th2-associated expression pattern. *J Immunol* (1998) 160:1411–8.

86. Islam SA, Ling MF, Leung J, Shreffler WG, Luster AD. Identification of human CCR8 as a CCL18 receptor. *J Exp Med* (2013) 210:1889–98. doi:10.1084/jem.20130240

87. Gunther C, Zimmermann N, Berndt N, Grosser M, Stein A, Koch A, et al. Up-regulation of the chemokine CCL18 by macrophages is a potential immunomodulatory pathway in cutaneous T-cell lymphoma. *Am J Pathol* (2011) 179:1434–42. doi:10.1016/j.ajpath.2011.05.040

88. Miyagaki T, Sugaya M, Suga H, Ohmatsu H, Fujita H, Asano Y, et al. Increased CCL18 expression in patients with cutaneous T-cell lymphoma: association with disease severity and prognosis. *J Eur Acad Dermatol Venereol* (2013) 27:e60–7. doi:10.1111/j.1468-3083.2012.04495.x

89. Kim YH, Tavallaee M, Sundram U, Salva KA, Wood GS, Li S, et al. Phase II investigator-initiated study of brentuximab vedotin in mycosis fungoides and Sezary syndrome with variable CD30 expression level: a multi-institution collaborative project. *J Clin Oncol* (2015) 33:3750–8. doi:10.1200/JCO.2014.60.3969

90. Bancherau J, Steinman RM. Dendritic cells and the control of immunity. *Nature* (1998) 392:245–52. doi:10.1038/32588

91. Luftl M, Feng A, Licha E, Schuler G. Dendritic cells and apoptosis in mycosis fungoides. *Br J Dermatol* (2002) 147:1171–9. doi:10.1046/j.1365-2133.2002.04994.x

92. Schlapbach C, Ochsenbein A, Kaelin U, Hassan AS, Hunger RE, Yawalkar N. High numbers of DC-SIGN+ dendritic cells in lesional skin of cutaneous T-cell lymphoma. *J Am Acad Dermatol* (2010) 62:995–1004. doi:10.1016/j.jaad.2009.06.082

93. Yamaguchi J, Aihara M, Kobayashi Y, Kambara T, Ikezawa Z. Quantitative analysis of nerve growth factor (NGF) in the atopic dermatitis and psoriasis horny layer and effect of treatment on NGF in atopic dermatitis. *J Dermatol Sci* (2009) 53:48–54. doi:10.1016/j.jdermsci.2008.08.011

94. Suga H, Sugaya M, Miyagaki T, Ohmatsu H, Fujita H, Kagami S, et al. Association of nerve growth factor, chemokine (C-C motif) ligands and immunoglobulin E with pruritus in cutaneous T-cell lymphoma. *Acta Derm Venereol* (2013) 93:144–9. doi:10.2340/00015555-1428

95. Ribatti D, Crivellato E. Mast cells, angiogenesis and cancer. *Adv Exp Med Biol* (2011) 716:270–88. doi:10.1007/978-1-4419-9533-9_14

96. Rabenhorst A, Schlaak M, Heukamp LC, Forster A, Theurich S, von Bergwelt-Baildon M, et al. Mast cells play a protumorigenic role in primary cutaneous lymphoma. *Blood* (2012) 120:2042–54. doi:10.1182/blood-2012-03-415638

97. Zheng Y, Valdez PA, Danilenko DM, Hu Y, Sa SM, Gong Q, et al. Interleukin-22 mediates early host defense against attaching and effacing bacterial pathogens. *Nat Med* (2008) 14:282–9. doi:10.1038/nm1720

98. Shimauchi T, Sasada K, Kito Y, Mori T, Hata M, Fujiyama T, et al. CD8+ Sezary syndrome with interleukin-22 production modulated by bacterial sepsis. *Br J Dermatol* (2013) 168:881–3. doi:10.1111/bjd.12051

99. Gabrilovich DI, Nagaraj S. Myeloid-derived suppressor cells as regulators of the immune system. *Nat Rev Immunol* (2009) 9:162–74. doi:10.1038/nri2506

100. Pileri A, Agostinelli C, Sessa M, Quaglino P, Santucci M, Tomasini C, et al. Langerhans, plasmacytoid dendritic and myeloid-derived suppressor cell levels in mycosis fungoides vary according to the stage of the disease. *Virchows Arch* (2017) 470:575–82. doi:10.1007/s00428-017-2107-1

101. Samimi S, Benoit B, Evans K, Wherry EJ, Showe L, Wysocka M, et al. Increased programmed death-1 expression on CD4+ T cells in cutaneous T-cell lymphoma: implications for immune suppression. *Arch Dermatol* (2010) 146(12):1382–8. doi:10.1001/archdermatol.2010.200

102. Kantekure K, Yang Y, Raghunath P, Schaffer A, Woetmann A, Zhang Q, et al. Expression patterns of the immunosuppressive proteins PD-1/CD279 and PD-L1/CD274 at different stages of cutaneous T-cell lymphoma/mycosis fungoides. *Am J Dermatopathol* (2012) 34(1):126–8. doi:10.1097/DAD.0b013e31821c35cb

103. Wong HK, Wilson AJ, Gibson HM, Hafner MS, Hedgcock CJ, Berger CL, et al. Increased expression of CTLA-4 in malignant T-cells from patients with mycosis fungoides – cutaneous T cell lymphoma. *J Invest Dermatol* (2006) 126(1):212–9. doi:10.1038/sj.jid.5700029

104. Bosisio FM, Cerroni L. Expression of T-follicular helper markers in sequential biopsies of progressive mycosis fungoides and other primary cutaneous T-cell lymphomas. *Am J Dermatopathol* (2015) 37(2):115–21. doi:10.1097/DAD.0000000000000258

105. Wilcox RA. Cutaneous T-cell lymphoma: 2017 update on diagnosis, risk-stratification, and management. *Am J Hematol* (2017) 92:1085–102. doi:10.1002/ajh.24876

106. Hughes CF, Khot A, McCormack C, Lade S, Westerman DA, Twigger R, et al. Lack of durable disease control with chemotherapy for mycosis fungoides and Sezary syndrome: a comparative study of systemic therapy. *Blood* (2015) 125:71–81. doi:10.1182/blood-2014-07-588236

107. Akilov OE, Geskin L. Therapeutic advances in cutaneous T-cell lymphoma. *Skin Therapy Lett* (2011) 16:1–5.

108. Olsen EA, Rosen ST, Vollmer RT, Variakojis D, Roenigk HH Jr., Diab N, et al. Interferon alfa-2a in the treatment of cutaneous T cell lymphoma. *J Am Acad Dermatol* (1989) 20:395–407. doi:10.1016/S0190-9622(89)70049-9

109. Suchin KR, Cucchiara AJ, Gottlieb SL, Wolfe JT, DeNardo BJ, Macey WH, et al. Treatment of cutaneous T-cell lymphoma with combined immunomodulatory therapy: a 14-year experience at a single institution. *Arch Dermatol* (2002) 138:1054–60. doi:10.1001/archderm.138.8.1054

110. Pichardo DA, Querfeld C, Guitart J, Kuzel TM, Rosen ST. Cutaneous T-cell lymphoma: a paradigm for biological therapies. *Leuk Lymphoma* (2004) 45:1755–65. doi:10.1080/10428190410001693560

111. Furudate S, Fujimura T, Kakizaki A, Hidaka T, Asano M, Aiba S. Tumor-associated M2 macrophages in mycosis fungoides acquire immunomodulatory function by interferon alpha and interferon gamma. *J Dermatol Sci* (2016) 83:182–9. doi:10.1016/j.jdermsci.2016.05.004

112. Sauder DN. Immunomodulatory and pharmacologic properties of imiquimod. *J Am Acad Dermatol* (2000) 43(1 Pt 2):S6–11. doi:10.1067/mjd.2000.107808

113. Suchin KR, Junkins-Hopkins JM, Rook AH. Treatment of stage IA cutaneous T-Cell lymphoma with topical application of the immune response modifier imiquimod. *Arch Dermatol* (2002) 138:1137–9. doi:10.1001/archderm.138.9.1137

114. Dummer R, Urosevic M, Kempf W, Kazakov D, Burg G. Imiquimod induces complete clearance of a PUVA-resistant plaque in mycosis fungoides. *Dermatology* (2003) 207:116–8. doi:10.1159/000070962

115. Coors EA, Schuler G, Von Den Driesch P. Topical imiquimod as treatment for different kinds of cutaneous lymphoma. *Eur J Dermatol* (2006) 16:391–3.

116. Gordon MC, Sluzevich JC, Jambusaria-Pahlajani A. Clearance of folliculotropic and tumor mycosis fungoides with topical 5% imiquimod. *JAAD Case Rep* (2015) 1:348–50. doi:10.1016/j.jdcr.2015.08.007

117. Rook AH, Gelfand JM, Wysocka M, Troxel AB, Benoit B, Surber C, et al. Topical resiquimod can induce disease regression and enhance T-cell effector functions in cutaneous T-cell lymphoma. *Blood* (2015) 126:1452–61. doi:10.1182/blood-2015-02-630335

118. Gorden KB, Gorski KS, Gibson SJ, Kedl RM, Kieper WC, Qiu X, et al. Synthetic TLR agonists reveal functional differences between human TLR7 and TLR8. *J Immunol* (2005) 174:1259–68. doi:10.4049/jimmunol.174.3.1259

119. Marks P, Rifkind RA, Richon VM, Breslow R, Miller T, Kelly WK. Histone deacetylases and cancer: causes and therapies. *Nat Rev Cancer* (2001) 1:194–202. doi:10.1038/35106079

120. Marks PA, Jiang X. Histone deacetylase inhibitors in programmed cell death and cancer therapy. *Cell Cycle* (2005) 4:549–51. doi:10.4161/cc.4.4.1564

121. Olsen EA, Kim YH, Kuzel TM, Pacheco TR, Foss FM, Parker S, et al. Phase IIb multicenter trial of vorinostat in patients with persistent, progressive, or treatment refractory cutaneous T-cell lymphoma. *J Clin Oncol* (2007) 25:3109–15. doi:10.1200/JCO.2006.10.2434

122. Duvic M, Talpur R, Ni X, Zhang C, Hazarika P, Kelly C, et al. Phase 2 trial of oral vorinostat (suberoylanilide hydroxamic acid, SAHA) for refractory cutaneous T-cell lymphoma (CTCL). *Blood* (2007) 109:31–9. doi:10.1182/blood-2006-06-025999

123. Piekarz RL, Frye R, Turner M, Wright JJ, Allen SL, Kirschbaum MH, et al. Phase II multi-institutional trial of the histone deacetylase inhibitor romidepsin as monotherapy for patients with cutaneous T-cell lymphoma. *J Clin Oncol* (2009) 27:5410–7. doi:10.1200/JCO.2008.21.6150

124. Whittaker SJ, Demierre MF, Kim EJ, Rook AH, Lerner A, Duvic M, et al. Final results from a multicenter, international, pivotal study of romidepsin in refractory cutaneous T-cell lymphoma. *J Clin Oncol* (2010) 28:4485–91. doi:10.1200/JCO.2010.28.9066

125. Wada H, Tsuboi R, Kato Y, Sugaya M, Tobinai K, Hamada T, et al. Phase I and pharmacokinetic study of the oral histone deacetylase inhibitor vorinostat in Japanese patients with relapsed or refractory cutaneous T-cell lymphoma. *J Dermatol* (2012) 39:823–8. doi:10.1111/j.1346-8138.2012.01554.x

126. Kim YH, Demierre MF, Kim EJ, Lerner A, Rook AH, Duvic M, et al. Clinically meaningful reduction in pruritus in patients with cutaneous T-cell lymphoma treated with romidepsin. *Leuk Lymphoma* (2013) 54:284–9. doi:10.3109/10428194.2012.711829

127. Cedeno-Laurent F, Singer EM, Wysocka M, Benoit BM, Vittorio CC, Kim EJ, et al. Improved pruritus correlates with lower levels of IL-31 in CTCL patients under different therapeutic modalities. *Clin Immunol* (2015) 158:1–7. doi:10.1016/j.clim.2015.02.014

128. Francisco JA, Cerveny CG, Meyer DL, Mixan BJ, Klussman K, Chace DF, et al. cAC10-vcMMAE, an anti-CD30-monomethyl auristatin E conjugate with potent and selective antitumor activity. *Blood* (2003) 102:1458–65. doi:10.1182/blood-2003-01-0039

129. Younes A, Gopal AK, Smith SE, Ansell SM, Rosenblatt JD, Savage KJ, et al. Results of a pivotal phase II study of brentuximab vedotin for patients with relapsed or refractory Hodgkin's lymphoma. *J Clin Oncol* (2012) 30:2183–9. doi:10.1200/JCO.2011.38.0410

130. Forero-Torres A, Fanale M, Advani R, Bartlett NL, Rosenblatt JD, Kennedy DA, et al. Brentuximab vedotin in transplant-naive patients with relapsed or

refractory Hodgkin lymphoma: analysis of two phase I studies. *Oncologist* (2012) 17:1073–80. doi:10.1634/theoncologist.2012-0133

131. Prince HM, Kim YH, Horwitz SM, Dummer R, Scarisbrick J, Quaglino P, et al. Brentuximab vedotin or physician's choice in CD30-positive cutaneous T-cell lymphoma (ALCANZA): an international, open-label, randomised, phase 3, multicentre trial. *Lancet* (2017) 390:555–66. doi:10.1016/S0140-6736(17)31266-7

132. Ogura M, Ishida T, Hatake K, Taniwaki M, Ando K, Tobinai K, et al. Multicenter phase II study of mogamulizumab (KW-0761), a defucosylated anti-cc chemokine receptor 4 antibody, in patients with relapsed peripheral T-cell lymphoma and cutaneous T-cell lymphoma. *J Clin Oncol* (2014) 32(11):1157–63. doi:10.1200/JCO.2013.52.0924

133. Duvic M, Pinter-Brown LC, Foss FM, Sokol L, Jorgensen JL, Challagundla P, et al. Phase 1/2 study of mogamulizumab, a defucosylated anti-CCR4 antibody, in previously treated patients with cutaneous T-cell lymphoma. *Blood* (2015) 125(12):1883–9. doi:10.1182/blood-2014-09-600924

134. Sicard H, Bonnafous C, Morel A, Bagot M, Bensussan A, Marie-Cardine A. A novel targeted immunotherapy for CTCL is on its way: anti-KIR3DL2 mAb IPH4102 is potent and safe in non-clinical studies. *Oncoimmunology* (2015) 4(9):e1022306. doi:10.1080/2162402X.2015.1022306

135. Bagot M. New targeted treatments for cutaneous T-cell Lymphomas. *Indian J Dermatol* (2017) 62(2):142–5. doi:10.4103/ijd.IJD_73_17

136. Querfeld C, Rosen ST, Guitart J, Duvic M, Kim YH, Dusza SW, et al. Results of an open-label multicenter phase 2 trial of lenalidomide monotherapy in refractory mycosis fungoides and Sezary syndrome. *Blood* (2014) 123(8):1159–66. doi:10.1182/blood-2013-09-525915

137. Zinzani PL, Musuraca G, Tani M, Stefoni V, Marchi E, Fina M, et al. Phase II trial of proteasome inhibitor bortezomib in patients with relapsed or refractory cutaneous T-cell lymphoma. *J Clin Oncol* (2007) 25(27):4293–7. doi:10.1200/JCO.2007.11.4207

138. Kempf W, Pfaltz K, Vermeer MH, Cozzio A, Ortiz-Romero PL, Bagot M, et al. EORTC, ISCL, and USCLC consensus recommendations for the treatment of primary cutaneous CD30-positive lymphoproliferative disorders: lymphomatoid papulosis and primary cutaneous anaplastic large-cell lymphoma. *Blood* (2011) 118:4024–35. doi:10.1182/blood-2011-05-351346

139. Stein H, Foss HD, Durkop H, Marafioti T, Delsol G, Pulford K, et al. CD30(+) anaplastic large cell lymphoma: a review of its histopathologic, genetic, and clinical features. *Blood* (2000) 96:3681–95.

140. Kadin ME, Carpenter C. Systemic and primary cutaneous anaplastic large cell lymphomas. *Semin Hematol* (2003) 40:244–56. doi:10.1016/S0037-1963(03)00138-0

141. Fornari A, Piva R, Chiarle R, Novero D, Inghirami G. Anaplastic large cell lymphoma: one or more entities among T-cell lymphoma? *Hematol Oncol* (2009) 27:161–70. doi:10.1002/hon.897

142. Wada DA, Law ME, Hsi ED, Dicaudo DJ, Ma L, Lim MS, et al. Specificity of IRF4 translocations for primary cutaneous anaplastic large cell lymphoma: a multicenter study of 204 skin biopsies. *Mod Pathol* (2011) 24(4):596–605. doi:10.1038/modpathol.2010.225

143. Bekkenk MW, Geelen FA, van Voorst Vader PC, Heule F, Geerts ML, van Vloten WA, et al. Primary and secondary cutaneous CD30(+) lymphoproliferative disorders: a report from the Dutch Cutaneous Lymphoma Group on the long-term follow-up data of 219 patients and guidelines for diagnosis and treatment. *Blood* (2000) 95:3653–61.

144. Fujita A, Hamada T, Iwatsuki K. Retrospective analysis of 133 patients with cutaneous lymphomas from a single Japanese medical center between 1995 and 2008. *J Dermatol* (2011) 38:524–30. doi:10.1111/j.1346-8138.2010.01049.x

145. Lee WJ, Moon IJ, Lee SH, Won CH, Chang SE, Choi JH, et al. Cutaneous anaplastic large-cell lymphoma (ALCL): A comparative clinical feature and survival outcome analysis of 52 cases according to primary tumor site. *J Am Acad Dermatol* (2016) 74:1135–43. doi:10.1016/j.jaad.2015.12.053

146. Kempf W. A new era for cutaneous CD30-positive T-cell lymphoproliferative disorders. *Semin Diagn Pathol* (2017) 34:22–35. doi:10.1053/j.semdp.2016.11.005

147. Burg G, Kempf W, Kazakov DV, Dummer R, Frosch PJ, Lange-Ionescu S, et al. Pyogenic lymphoma of the skin: a peculiar variant of primary cutaneous neutrophil-rich CD30+ anaplastic large-cell lymphoma. Clinicopathological study of four cases and review of the literature. *Br J Dermatol* (2003) 148:580–6. doi:10.1046/j.1365-2133.2003.05248.x

148. Geissinger E, Sadler P, Roth S, Grieb T, Puppe B, Muller N, et al. Disturbed expression of the T-cell receptor/CD3 complex and associated signaling molecules in CD30+ T-cell lymphoproliferations. *Haematologica* (2010) 95:1697–704. doi:10.3324/haematol.2009.021428

149. Kadin ME. Primary Ki-1-positive anaplastic large-cell lymphoma: a distinct clinicopathologic entity. *Ann Oncol* (1994) 5(Suppl 1):25–30. doi:10.1093/annonc/5.suppl_1.S25

150. El Shabrawi-Caelen L, Kerl H, Cerroni L. Lymphomatoid papulosis: reappraisal of clinicopathologic presentation and classification into subtypes A, B, and C. *Arch Dermatol* (2004) 140:441–7. doi:10.1001/archderm.140.4.441

151. Saggini A, Gulia A, Argenyi Z, Fink-Puches R, Lissia A, Magana M, et al. A variant of lymphomatoid papulosis simulating primary cutaneous aggressive epidermotropic CD8+ cytotoxic T-cell lymphoma. Description of 9 cases. *Am J Surg Pathol* (2010) 34:1168–75. doi:10.1097/PAS.0b013e3181e75356

152. Kempf W, Kazakov DV, Scharer L, Rutten A, Mentzel T, Paredes BE, et al. Angioinvasive lymphomatoid papulosis: a new variant simulating aggressive lymphomas. *Am J Surg Pathol* (2013) 37:1–13. doi:10.1097/PAS.0b013e3182648596

153. Paulli M, Berti E, Rosso R, Boveri E, Kindl S, Klersy C, et al. CD30/Ki-1-positive lymphoproliferative disorders of the skin – clinicopathologic correlation and statistical analysis of 86 cases: a multicentric study from the European Organization for Research and Treatment of Cancer Cutaneous Lymphoma Project Group. *J Clin Oncol* (1995) 13:1343–54. doi:10.1200/JCO.1995.13.6.1343

154. Zackheim HS, Jones C, Leboit PE, Kashani-Sabet M, McCalmont TH, Zehnder J. Lymphomatoid papulosis associated with mycosis fungoides: a study of 21 patients including analyses for clonality. *J Am Acad Dermatol* (2003) 49:620–3. doi:10.1067/S0190-9622(03)01577-9

155. Weichenthal M, Goldinger S, Wehkamp U, Beyer M, Stein A, Tsianakas A, et al. Response of rare variants of cutaneous T cell lymphoma (CTCL) to treatment with bexarotene. A prospective German DeCOG trial. *Blood* (2013) 122:4379.

156. Foss F, Advani R, Duvic M, Hymes KB, Intragumtornchai T, Lekhakula A, et al. A Phase II trial of Belinostat (PXD101) in patients with relapsed or refractory peripheral or cutaneous T-cell lymphoma. *Br J Haematol* (2015) 168(6):811–9. doi:10.1111/bjh.13222

157. Lamant L, Pileri S, Sabattini E, Brugieres L, Jaffe ES, Delsol G. Cutaneous presentation of ALK-positive anaplastic large cell lymphoma following insect bites: evidence for an association in five cases. *Haematologica* (2010) 95(3):449–55. doi:10.3324/haematol.2009.015024

158. Yoshie O, Fujisawa R, Nakayama T, Harasawa H, Tago H, Izawa D, et al. Frequent expression of CCR4 in adult T-cell leukemia and human T-cell leukemia virus type 1-transformed T cells. *Blood* (2002) 99:1505–11. doi:10.1182/blood.V99.5.1505

159. Shimoyama M. Diagnostic criteria and classification of clinical subtypes of adult T-cell leukaemia-lymphoma. A report from the Lymphoma Study Group (1984-87). *Br J Haematol* (1991) 79:428–37. doi:10.1111/j.1365-2141.1991.tb08051.x

160. Nosaka K, Iwanaga M, Imaizumi Y, Ishitsuka K, Ishizawa K, Ishida Y, et al. Epidemiological and clinical features of adult T-cell leukemia-lymphoma in Japan, 2010-2011: a nationwide survey. *Cancer Sci* (2017) 108:2478–86. doi:10.1111/cas.13398

161. Bittencourt AL, Barbosa HS, Vieira MD, Farre L. Adult T-cell leukemia/lymphoma (ATL) presenting in the skin: clinical, histological and immunohistochemical features of 52 cases. *Acta Oncol* (2009) 48:598–604. doi:10.1080/02841860802657235

162. Setoyama M, Katahira Y, Kanzaki T. Clinicopathologic analysis of 124 cases of adult T-cell leukemia/lymphoma with cutaneous manifestations: the smouldering type with skin manifestations has a poorer prognosis than previously thought. *J Dermatol* (1999) 26:785–90. doi:10.1111/j.1346-8138.1999.tb02093.x

163. Tsukasaki K, Imaizumi Y, Tokura Y, Ohshima K, Kawai K, Utsunomiya A, et al. Meeting report on the possible proposal of an extranodal primary cutaneous variant in the lymphoma type of adult T-cell leukemia-lymphoma. *J Dermatol* (2014) 41:26–8. doi:10.1111/1346-8138.12374

164. Sawada Y, Hino R, Hama K, Ohmori S, Fueki H, Yamada S, et al. Type of skin eruption is an independent prognostic indicator for adult T-cell leukemia/lymphoma. *Blood* (2011) 117:3961–7. doi:10.1182/blood-2010-11-316794

165. Tokura Y, Sawada Y, Shimauchi T. Skin manifestations of adult T-cell leukemia/lymphoma: clinical, cytological and immunological features. *J Dermatol* (2014) 41:19–25. doi:10.1111/1346-8138.12328

166. Tanaka Y, Mine S, Figdor CG, Wake A, Hirano H, Tsukada J, et al. Constitutive chemokine production results in activation of leukocyte function-associated antigen-1 on adult T-cell leukemia cells. *Blood* (1998) 91:3909–19.

167. Mori N, Ueda A, Ikeda S, Yamasaki Y, Yamada Y, Tomonaga M, et al. Human T-cell leukemia virus type I tax activates transcription of the human monocyte chemoattractant protein-1 gene through two nuclear factor-kappaB sites. *Cancer Res* (2000) 60:4939–45.

168. Ruckes T, Saul D, Van Snick J, Hermine O, Grassmann R. Autocrine antiapoptotic stimulation of cultured adult T-cell leukemia cells by overexpression of the chemokine I-309. *Blood* (2001) 98:1150–9. doi:10.1182/blood. V98.4.1150

169. Ishida T, Utsunomiya A, Iida S, Inagaki H, Takatsuka Y, Kusumoto S, et al. Clinical significance of CCR4 expression in adult T-cell leukemia/lymphoma: its close association with skin involvement and unfavorable outcome. *Clin Cancer Res* (2003) 9(10 Pt 1):3625–34.

170. Hasegawa H, Nomura T, Kohno M, Tateishi N, Suzuki Y, Maeda N, et al. Increased chemokine receptor CCR7/EBI1 expression enhances the infiltration of lymphoid organs by adult T-cell leukemia cells. *Blood* (2000) 95:30–8.

171. Shimauchi T, Imai S, Hino R, Tokura Y. Production of thymus and activation-regulated chemokine and macrophage-derived chemokine by CCR4+ adult T-cell leukemia cells. *Clin Cancer Res* (2005) 11:2427–35. doi:10.1158/1078-0432.CCR-04-0491

172. Karube K, Ohshima K, Tsuchiya T, Yamaguchi T, Kawano R, Suzumiya J, et al. Expression of FoxP3, a key molecule in CD4CD25 regulatory T cells, in adult T-cell leukaemia/lymphoma cells. *Br J Haematol* (2004) 126:81–4. doi:10.1111/j.1365-2141.2004.04999.x

173. Kohno T, Yamada Y, Akamatsu N, Kamihira S, Imaizumi Y, Tomonaga M, et al. Possible origin of adult T-cell leukemia/lymphoma cells from human T lymphotropic virus type-1-infected regulatory T cells. *Cancer Sci* (2005) 96:527–33. doi:10.1111/j.1349-7006.2005.00080.x

174. Shimauchi T, Kabashima K, Tokura Y. Adult T-cell leukemia/lymphoma cells from blood and skin tumors express cytotoxic T lymphocyte-associated antigen-4 and Foxp3 but lack suppressor activity toward autologous CD8+ T cells. *Cancer Sci* (2008) 99:98–106. doi:10.1111/j.1349-7006.2007.00646.x

175. Eyerich K, Pennino D, Scarponi C, Foerster S, Nasorri F, Behrendt H, et al. IL-17 in atopic eczema: linking allergen-specific adaptive and microbial-triggered innate immune response. *J Allergy Clin Immunol* (2009) 123:59–66e4. doi:10.1016/j.jaci.2008.10.031

176. Sawada Y, Nakamura M, Kabashima-Kubo R, Shimauchi T, Kobayashi M, Tokura Y. Defective epidermal innate immunity and resultant superficial dermatophytosis in adult T-cell leukemia/lymphoma. *Clin Cancer Res* (2012) 18:3772–9. doi:10.1158/1078-0432.CCR-12-0292

177. Peric M, Koglin S, Kim SM, Morizane S, Besch R, Prinz JC, et al. IL-17A enhances vitamin D3-induced expression of cathelicidin antimicrobial peptide in human keratinocytes. *J Immunol* (2008) 181:8504–12. doi:10.4049/jimmunol.181.12.8504

178. Sawada Y, Nakamura M, Kabashima-Kubo R, Shimauchi T, Kobayashi M, Tokura Y. Defective epidermal induction of S100A7/psoriasin associated with low frequencies of skin-infiltrating Th17 cells in dermatophytosis-prone adult T cell leukemia/lymphoma. *Clin Immunol* (2013) 148:1–3. doi:10.1016/j.clim.2013.03.013

179. Kabashima R, Kabashima K, Hino R, Shimauchi T, Tokura Y. Scabies superimposed on skin lesions of adult T-cell leukemia/lymphoma: case report and literature review. *Int J Dermatol* (2008) 47:1168–71. doi:10.1111/j. 1365-4632.2008.03707.x

180. Kozako T, Yoshimitsu M, Fujiwara H, Masamoto I, Horai S, White Y, et al. PD-1/PD-L1 expression in human T-cell leukemia virus type 1 carriers and adult T-cell leukemia/lymphoma patients. *Leukemia* (2009) 23:375–82. doi:10.1038/leu.2008.272

181. Shimauchi T, Kabashima K, Nakashima D, Sugita K, Yamada Y, Hino R, et al. Augmented expression of programmed death-1 in both neoplastic and non-neoplastic CD4+ T-cells in adult T-cell leukemia/lymphoma. *Int J Cancer* (2007) 121:2585–90. doi:10.1002/ijc.23042

182. Kataoka K, Shiraishi Y, Takeda Y, Sakata S, Matsumoto M, Nagano S, et al. Aberrant PD-L1 expression through 3'-UTR disruption in multiple cancers. *Nature* (2016) 534:402–6. doi:10.1038/nature18294

183. Ishida T, Joh T, Uike N, Yamamoto K, Utsunomiya A, Yoshida S, et al. Defucosylated anti-CCR4 monoclonal antibody (KW-0761) for relapsed adult T-cell leukemia-lymphoma: a multicenter phase II study. *J Clin Oncol* (2012) 30:837–42. doi:10.1200/JCO.2011.37.3472

184. Tokunaga M, Yonekura K, Nakamura D, Haraguchi K, Tabuchi T, Fujino S, et al. Clinical significance of cutaneous adverse reaction to mogamulizumab in relapsed or refractory adult T-cell leukaemia-lymphoma. *Br J Haematol* (2018) 181:539–42. doi:10.1111/bjh.14634

185. Yonekura K, Tokunaga M, Kawakami N, Takeda K, Kanzaki T, Nakano N, et al. Cutaneous adverse reaction to mogamulizumab may indicate favourable prognosis in adult T-cell leukaemia-lymphoma. *Acta Derm Venereol* (2016) 96:1000–2. doi:10.2340/00015555-2421

186. Ishida T, Ito A, Sato F, Kusumoto S, Iida S, Inagaki H, et al. Stevens-Johnson syndrome associated with mogamulizumab treatment of adult T-cell leukemia/ lymphoma. *Cancer Sci* (2013) 104:647–50. doi:10.1111/cas.12116

187. Yonekura K, Kanzaki T, Gunshin K, Kawakami N, Takatsuka Y, Nakano N, et al. Effect of anti-CCR4 monoclonal antibody (mogamulizumab) on adult T-cell leukemia-lymphoma: cutaneous adverse reactions may predict the prognosis. *J Dermatol* (2014) 41:239–44. doi:10.1111/1346-8138.12419

188. Fuji S, Inoue Y, Utsunomiya A, Moriuchi Y, Uchimaru K, Choi I, et al. Pretransplantation Anti-CCR4 antibody mogamulizumab against adult T-cell leukemia/lymphoma is associated with significantly increased risks of severe and corticosteroid-refractory graft-versus-host disease, nonrelapse mortality, and overall mortality. *J Clin Oncol* (2016) 34:3426–33. doi:10.1200/JCO.2016.67.8250

189. Sugio T, Kato K, Aoki T, Ohta T, Saito N, Yoshida S, et al. Mogamulizumab treatment prior to allogeneic hematopoietic stem cell transplantation induces severe acute graft-versus-host disease. *Biol Blood Marrow Transplant* (2016) 22:1608–14. doi:10.1016/j.bbmt.2016.05.017

190. Salhany KE, Macon WR, Choi JK, Elenitsas R, Lessin SR, Felgar RE, et al. Subcutaneous panniculitis-like T-cell lymphoma: clinicopathologic, immunophenotypic, and genotypic analysis of alpha/beta and gamma/delta subtypes. *Am J Surg Pathol* (1998) 22:881–93. doi:10.1097/00000478-199807000-00010

191. Massone C, Chott A, Metze D, Kerl K, Citarella L, Vale E, et al. Subcutaneous, blastic natural killer (NK), NK/T-cell, and other cytotoxic lymphomas of the skin: a morphologic, immunophenotypic, and molecular study of 50 patients. *Am J Surg Pathol* (2004) 28:719–35. doi:10.1097/01.pas.0000126719.71954.4f

192. LeBlanc RE, Tavallaee M, Kim YH, Kim J. Useful parameters for distinguishing subcutaneous panniculitis-like T-cell lymphoma from lupus erythematosus panniculitis. *Am J Surg Pathol* (2016) 40:745–54. doi:10.1097/PAS.0000000000000596

193. Willemze R. Cutaneous lymphomas with a panniculitic presentation. *Semin Diagn Pathol* (2017) 34:36–43. doi:10.1053/j.semdp.2016.11.009

194. Willemze R, Jansen PM, Cerroni L, Berti E, Santucci M, Assaf C, et al. Subcutaneous panniculitis-like T-cell lymphoma: definition, classification, and prognostic factors: an EORTC Cutaneous Lymphoma Group Study of 83 cases. *Blood* (2008) 111:838–45. doi:10.1182/blood-2007-04-087288

195. Massone C, Kodama K, Salmhofer W, Abe R, Shimizu H, Parodi A, et al. Lupus erythematosus panniculitis (lupus profundus): clinical, histopathological, and molecular analysis of nine cases. *J Cutan Pathol* (2005) 32:396–404. doi:10.1111/j.0303-6987.2005.00351.x

196. Liau JY, Chuang SS, Chu CY, Ku WH, Tsai JH, Shih TF. The presence of clusters of plasmacytoid dendritic cells is a helpful feature for differentiating lupus panniculitis from subcutaneous panniculitis-like T-cell lymphoma. *Histopathology* (2013) 62:1057–66. doi:10.1111/his.12105

197. Honda Y, Otsuka A, Nonomura Y, Kaku Y, Dainichi T, Miyachi Y, et al. CCR5 and CXCR3 expression in a case of subcutaneous panniculitis-like T-cell lymphoma. *J Eur Acad Dermatol Venereol* (2016) 30:1413–5. doi:10.1111/jdv.13258

198. Kitayama N, Otsuka A, Honda Y, Matsumura Y, Honda T, Kabashima K. CCR4 and CCR5 expression in a case of subcutaneous panniculitis-like T-cell lymphoma. *Eur J Dermatol* (2017) 27:414–5. doi:10.1684/ejd.2017.3016

199. Guenova E, Schanz S, Hoetzenecker W, DeSimone JA, Mehra T, Voykov B, et al. Systemic corticosteroids for subcutaneous panniculitis-like T-cell lymphoma. *Br J Dermatol* (2014) 171:891–4. doi:10.1111/bjd.13053

200. Rojnuckarin P, Nakorn TN, Assanasen T, Wannakrairot P. Intragumtorichial T. Cyclosporin in subcutaneous panniculitis-like T-cell lymphoma. *Leuk Lymphoma* (2007) 48:560–3. doi:10.1080/10428190601078456

201. Mizutani S, Kuroda J, Shimura Y, Kobayashi T, Tsutsumi Y, Yamashita M, et al. Cyclosporine A for chemotherapy-resistant subcutaneous panniculitis-like T cell lymphoma with hemophagocytic syndrome. *Acta Haematol* (2011) 126:8–12. doi:10.1159/000323565

202. Mehta N, Wayne AS, Kim YH, Hale GA, Alvarado CS, Myskowski P, et al. Bexarotene is active against subcutaneous panniculitis-like T-cell lymphoma in adult and pediatric populations. *Clin Lymphoma Myeloma Leuk* (2012) 12:20–5. doi:10.1016/j.clml.2011.06.016

203. Toro JR, Liewehr DJ, Pabby N, Sorbara L, Raffeld M, Steinberg SM, et al. Gamma-delta T-cell phenotype is associated with significantly decreased survival in cutaneous T-cell lymphoma. *Blood* (2003) 101:3407–12. doi:10.1182/blood-2002-05-1597

204. Guitart J, Weisenburger DD, Subtil A, Kim E, Wood G, Duvic M, et al. Cutaneous gammadelta T-cell lymphomas: a spectrum of presentations with overlap with other cytotoxic lymphomas. *Am J Surg Pathol* (2012) 36:1656–65. doi:10.1097/PAS.0b013e31826a5038

205. Przybylski GK, Wu H, Macon WR, Finan J, Leonard DG, Felgar RE, et al. Hepatosplenic and subcutaneous panniculitis-like gamma/delta T cell lymphomas are derived from different Vdelta subsets of gamma/delta T lymphocytes. *J Mol Diagn* (2000) 2:11–9. doi:10.1016/S1525-1578(10)60610-1

206. Tripodo C, Iannitto E, Florena AM, Pucillo CE, Piccaluga PP, Franco V, et al. Gamma-delta T-cell lymphomas. *Nat Rev Clin Oncol* (2009) 6:707–17. doi:10.1038/nrclinonc.2009.169

207. Arnulf B, Copie-Bergman C, Delfau-Larue MH, Lavergne-Slove A, Bosq J, Wechsler J, et al. Nonhepatosplenic gammadelta T-cell lymphoma: a subset of cytotoxic lymphomas with mucosal or skin localization. *Blood* (1998) 91:1723–31.

208. Toro JR, Beaty M, Sorbara L, Turner ML, White J, Kingma DW, et al. Gamma delta T-cell lymphoma of the skin: a clinical, microscopic, and molecular study. *Arch Dermatol* (2000) 136:1024–32. doi:10.1001/archderm.136.8.1024

209. Koens L, Senff NJ, Vermeer MH, Ronday HK, Willemze R, Jansen PM. Cutaneous gamma/delta T-cell lymphoma during treatment with etanercept for rheumatoid arthritis. *Acta Derm Venereol* (2009) 89:653–4. doi:10.2340/00015555-0728

210. Alaibac M, Berti E, Pigozzi B, Chiarion V, Aversa S, Marino F, et al. High-dose chemotherapy with autologous blood stem cell transplantation for aggressive subcutaneous panniculitis-like T-cell lymphoma. *J Am Acad Dermatol* (2005) 52(5 Suppl 1):S121–3. doi:10.1016/j.jaad.2004.05.042

211. Gibson JF, Alpdogan O, Subtil A, Girardi M, Wilson LD, Roberts K, et al. Hematopoietic stem cell transplantation for primary cutaneous gammadelta T-cell lymphoma and refractory subcutaneous panniculitis-like T-cell lymphoma. *J Am Acad Dermatol* (2015) 72:1010.e–5.e. doi:10.1016/j.jaad.2015.01.003

212. Beltraminelli H, Leinweber B, Kerl H, Cerroni L. Primary cutaneous CD4+ small-/medium-sized pleomorphic T-cell lymphoma: a cutaneous nodular proliferation of pleomorphic T lymphocytes of undetermined significance? A study of 136 cases. *Am J Dermatopathol* (2009) 31:317–22. doi:10.1097/DAD.0b013e31819f19bb

213. Baum CL, Link BK, Neppalli VT, Swick BL, Liu V. Reappraisal of the provisional entity primary cutaneous CD4+ small/medium pleomorphic T-cell lymphoma: a series of 10 adult and pediatric patients and review of the literature. *J Am Acad Dermatol* (2011) 65:739–48. doi:10.1016/j.jaad.2010.07.028

214. Grogg KL, Jung S, Erickson LA, McClure RF, Dogan A. Primary cutaneous CD4-positive small/medium-sized pleomorphic T-cell lymphoma: a clonal T-cell lymphoproliferative disorder with indolent behavior. *Mod Pathol* (2008) 21:708–15. doi:10.1038/modpathol.2008.40

215. Rodriguez Pinilla SM, Roncador G, Rodriguez-Peralto JL, Mollejo M, Garcia JF, Montes-Moreno S, et al. Primary cutaneous CD4+ small/medium-sized pleomorphic T-cell lymphoma expresses follicular T-cell markers. *Am J Surg Pathol* (2009) 33:81–90. doi:10.1097/PAS.0b013e31818e52fe

216. Cetinozman F, Jansen PM, Willemze R. Expression of programmed death-1 in primary cutaneous CD4-positive small/medium-sized pleomorphic T-cell lymphoma, cutaneous pseudo-T-cell lymphoma, and other types of cutaneous T-cell lymphoma. *Am J Surg Pathol* (2012) 36:109–16. doi:10.1097/PAS.0b013e318230df87

217. Rijlaarsdam JU, Willemze R. Cutaneous pseudolymphomas: classification and differential diagnosis. *Semin Dermatol* (1994) 13:187–96.

218. Bakels V, van Oostveen JW, van der Putte SC, Meijer CJ, Willemze R. Immunophenotyping and gene rearrangement analysis provide additional criteria to differentiate between cutaneous T-cell lymphomas and pseudo-T-cell lymphomas. *Am J Pathol* (1997) 150:1941–9.

219. Magro CM, Momtahen S. Differential NFATc1 expression in primary cutaneous CD4+ small/medium-sized pleomorphic T-cell lymphoma and other forms of cutaneous T-cell lymphoma and pseudolymphoma. *Am J Dermatopathol* (2017) 39:95–103. doi:10.1097/DAD.0000000000000597

220. Garcia-Herrera A, Colomo L, Camos M, Carreras J, Balague O, Martinez A, et al. Primary cutaneous small/medium CD4+ T-cell lymphomas: a heterogeneous group of tumors with different clinicopathologic features and outcome. *J Clin Oncol* (2008) 26:3364–71. doi:10.1200/JCO.2008.16.1307

221. Williams VL, Torres-Cabala CA, Duvic M. Primary cutaneous small- to medium-sized CD4+ pleomorphic T-cell lymphoma: a retrospective case series and review of the provisional cutaneous lymphoma category. *Am J Clin Dermatol* (2011) 12:389–401. doi:10.2165/11590390-000000000-00000

222. Goldgeier MH, Nordlund JJ, Lucky AW, Sibrack LA, McCarthy MJ, McGuire J. Hydroa vacciniforme: diagnosis and therapy. *Arch Dermatol* (1982) 118:588–91. doi:10.1001/archderm.118.8.588

223. Oono T, Arata J, Masuda T, Ohtsuki Y. Coexistence of hydroa vacciniforme and malignant lymphoma. *Arch Dermatol* (1986) 122:1306–9. doi:10.1001/archderm.122.11.1306

224. Quintanilla-Martinez L, Ridaura C, Nagl F, Saez-de-Ocariz M, Duran-McKinster C, Ruiz-Maldonado R, et al. Hydroa vacciniforme-like lymphoma: a chronic EBV+ lymphoproliferative disorder with risk to develop a systemic lymphoma. *Blood* (2013) 122:3101–10. doi:10.1182/blood-2013-05-502203

225. Cho KH, Kim CW, Heo DS, Lee DS, Choi WW, Rim JH, et al. Epstein-Barr virus-associated peripheral T-cell lymphoma in adults with hydroa vacciniforme-like lesions. *Clin Exp Dermatol* (2001) 26:242–7. doi:10.1046/j.1365-2230.2001.00805.x

226. Magana M, Sangueza P, Gil-Beristain J, Sanchez-Sosa S, Salgado A, Ramon G, et al. Angiocentric cutaneous T-cell lymphoma of childhood (hydroa-like lymphoma): a distinctive type of cutaneous T-cell lymphoma. *J Am Acad Dermatol* (1998) 38:574–9. doi:10.1016/S0190-9622(98)70120-3

227. Iwatsuki K, Xu Z, Takata M, Iguchi M, Ohtsuka M, Akiba H, et al. The association of latent Epstein-Barr virus infection with hydroa vacciniforme. *Br J Dermatol* (1999) 140:715–21. doi:10.1046/j.1365-2133.1999.02777.x

228. Barrionuevo C, Anderson VM, Zevallos-Giampietri E, Zaharia M, Misad O, Bravo F, et al. Hydroa-like cutaneous T-cell lymphoma: a clinicopathologic and molecular genetic study of 16 pediatric cases from Peru. *Appl Immunohistochem Mol Morphol* (2002) 10:7–14. doi:10.1097/00129039-200203000-00002

229. Kawa K, Okamura T, Yagi K, Takeuchi M, Nakayama M, Inoue M. Mosquito allergy and Epstein-Barr virus-associated T/natural killer-cell lymphoproliferative disease. *Blood* (2001) 98:3173–4. doi:10.1182/blood.V98.10.3173

230. Iwatsuki K, Satoh M, Yamamoto T, Oono T, Morizane S, Ohtsuka M, et al. Pathogenic link between hydroa vacciniforme and Epstein-Barr virus-associated hematologic disorders. *Arch Dermatol* (2006) 142:587–95. doi:10.1001/archderm.142.5.587

231. Wu YH, Chen HC, Hsiao PF, Tu MI, Lin YC, Wang TY. Hydroa vacciniforme-like Epstein-Barr virus-associated monoclonal T-lymphoproliferative disorder in a child. *Int J Dermatol* (2007) 46:1081–6. doi:10.1111/j.1365-4632.2007.03102.x

232. Tokura Y, Tamura Y, Takigawa M, Koide M, Satoh T, Sakamoto T, et al. Severe hypersensitivity to mosquito bites associated with natural killer cell lymphocytosis. *Arch Dermatol* (1990) 126:362–8. doi:10.1001/archderm.126.3.362

233. Kimura H, Ito Y, Kawabe S, Gotoh K, Takahashi Y, Kojima S, et al. EBV-associated T/NK-cell lymphoproliferative diseases in nonimmunocompromised hosts: prospective analysis of 108 cases. *Blood* (2012) 119:673–86. doi:10.1182/blood-2011-10-381921

234. Quintanilla-Martinez L, Ko YH, Kimura H, Jaffe ES. EBV-positive T-cell and NK-cell lymphoproliferative diseases of childhood. In: Swerdlow SH, Campo E, Harris NL, Jaffe ES, Pileri SA, Stein H, et al. editors. *WHO Classification of Tumours of Haematopoietic and Lymphoid Tissues*. Lyon: International Agency for Research on Cancer (2017). p. 355–63.

235. Kempf W, Kazakov DV, Cozzio A, Kamarashev J, Kerl K, Plaza T, et al. Primary cutaneous CD8(+) small- to medium-sized lymphoproliferative disorder in extrafacial sites: clinicopathologic features and concept on their classification. *Am J Dermatopathol* (2013) 35:159–66. doi:10.1097/DAD.0b013e31825c3a33

236. Greenblatt D, Ally M, Child F, Scarisbrick J, Whittaker S, Morris S, et al. Indolent CD8(+) lymphoid proliferation of acral sites: a clinicopathologic study of six patients with some atypical features. *J Cutan Pathol* (2013) 40:248–58. doi:10.1111/cup.12045

237. Hathuc VM, Hristov AC, Smith LB. Primary cutaneous acral CD8(+) T-cell lymphoma. *Arch Pathol Lab Med* (2017) 141:1469–75. doi:10.5858/arpa.2017-0230-RA

238. Kluk J, Kai A, Koch D, Taibjee SM, O'Connor S, Persic M, et al. Indolent CD8-positive lymphoid proliferation of acral sites: three further cases of a rare entity and an update on a unique patient. *J Cutan Pathol* (2016) 43:125–36. doi:10.1111/cup.12633

239. Berti E, Tomasini D, Vermeer MH, Meijer CJ, Alessi E, Willemze R. Primary cutaneous CD8-positive epidermotropic cytotoxic T cell lymphomas. A distinct clinicopathological entity with an aggressive clinical behavior. *Am J Pathol* (1999) 155:483–92. doi:10.1016/S0002-9440(10)65144-9

240. Nofal A, Abdel-Mawla MY, Assaf M, Salah E. Primary cutaneous aggressive epidermotropic CD8+ T-cell lymphoma: proposed diagnostic criteria and therapeutic evaluation. *J Am Acad Dermatol* (2012) 67:748–59. doi:10.1016/j.jaad.2011.07.043

241. Robson A, Assaf C, Bagot M, Burg G, Calonje E, Castillo C, et al. Aggressive epidermotropic cutaneous CD8+ lymphoma: a cutaneous lymphoma with distinct clinical and pathological features. Report of an EORTC cutaneous lymphoma task force workshop. *Histopathology* (2015) 67:425–41. doi:10.1111/his.12371

242. Guitart J, Martinez-Escala ME, Subtil A, Duvic M, Pulitzer MP, Olsen EA, et al. Primary cutaneous aggressive epidermotropic cytotoxic T-cell lymphomas: reappraisal of a provisional entity in the 2016 WHO classification of cutaneous lymphomas. *Mod Pathol* (2017) 30:761–72. doi:10.1038/modpathol.2016.240

243. Liu V, Cutler CS, Young AZ. Case records of the Massachusetts general hospital. Case 38-2007. A 44-year-old woman with generalized, painful, ulcerated skin lesions. *N Engl J Med* (2007) 357:2496–505. doi:10.1056/NEJMcpc0706687

11

Association of Baseline Serum Levels of CXCL5 With the Efficacy of Nivolumab in Advanced Melanoma

Taku Fujimura[1*†], Yota Sato[1†], Kayo Tanita[1], Chunbing Lyu[1], Yumi Kambayashi[1], Ryo Amagai[1], Atsushi Otsuka[2], Yasuhiro Fujisawa[3], Koji Yoshino[4], Shigeto Matsushita[5], Hiroshi Uchi[6], Yuki Yamamoto[7], Hiroo Hata[8], Takeru Funakoshi[9], Yumi Nonomura[2], Ryota Tanaka[3], Hisako Okuhira[7], Naoko Wada[6], Akira Hashimoto[1] and Setsuya Aiba[1]

[1] Department of Dermatology, Tohoku University Graduate School of Medicine, Sendai, Japan, [2] Department of Dermatology, Kyoto University Graduate School of Medicine, Kyoto, Japan, [3] Department of Dermatology, University of Tsukuba, Tsukuba, Japan, [4] Department of Dermatology, Tokyo Metropolitan Cancer and Infectious Disease Center Komagome Hospital, Tokyo, Japan, [5] Department of Dermato-Oncology/Dermatology, National Hospital Organization Kagoshima Medical Center, Kagoshima, Japan, [6] Department of Dermatology, Kyushu University Graduate School of Medicine, Fukuoka, Japan, [7] Department of Dermatology, Wakayama Medical University, Wakayama, Japan, [8] Department of Dermatology, Hokkaido University Graduate School of Medicine, Sapporo, Japan, [9] Department of Dermatology, Keio University School of Medicine, Tokyo, Japan

*Correspondence:
Taku Fujimura
tfujimura1@mac.com

[†] These authors have contributed equally to this work

Anti-programmed cell death protein 1 (PD1) antibodies are in wide use for the treatment of various cancers. PD1 antibody-based immunotherapy, co-administration of nivolumab and ipilimumab, is one of the optimal immunotherapies, especially in advanced melanoma with high tumor mutation burden. Since this combined therapy leads to a high frequency of serious immune-related adverse events (irAEs) in patients with advanced melanoma, biomarkers are needed to evaluate nivolumab efficacy to avoid serious irAEs caused by ipilimumab. This study analyzed baseline serum levels of CXCL5, CXCL10, and CCL22 in 46 cases of advanced cutaneous melanoma treated with nivolumab. Baseline serum levels of CXCL5 were significantly higher in responders than in non-responders. In contrast, there were no significant differences in baseline serum levels of CXCL10 and CCL22 between responders and non-responders. These results suggest that baseline serum levels of CXCL5 may be useful as a biomarker for identifying patients with advanced cutaneous melanoma most likely to benefit from anti-melanoma immunotherapy.

Keywords: baseline levels of CXCL5, melanoma, nivolumab, prediction of efficacy, nivolumab and ipilimumab combined therapy

INTRODUCTION

Anti-programmed cell death protein 1 (PD-1) antibodies such as nivolumab and pembrolizumab are in wide use for the treatment of various cancers, including advanced melanoma (1, 2), but cost-effective analyses of their use are sometimes controversial (3). Therefore, biomarkers for the evaluation of the efficacy of anti-PD1 antibody therapy are needed. Previous clinical studies suggested that the efficacy of nivolumab monotherapy is ~40% in the Caucasian population (2, 4), which contains a high ratio of superficial spreading melanoma (SSM) with high levels of tumor mutation burden (TMB) (5). In contrast, in the Japanese population, there is a high ratio of acral lentiginous melanoma (ALM) and mucosal melanoma (6), which have low levels of TMB (5). The efficacies of nivolumab and pembrolizumab in Japan have been reported to be 34.1% and 24.1%, respectively (7, 8), suggesting that another drug that could enhance the anti-tumor immune response in melanoma is needed.

Ipilimumab is a fully humanized immunoglobulin (Ig)G1 monoclonal antibody that blocks cytotoxic T-lymphocyte antigen (CTLA-4) and is one of the promising drugs that enhance the anti-tumor immune response for patients with advanced melanoma with or without BRAF gene mutation in combination with nivolumab (1, 4, 9). Indeed, the efficacy of this combination therapy for advanced melanoma has been reported to be 57.8% (4), and, therefore, combination therapy with nivolumab and ipilimumab is recommended by the NCCN guideline for cutaneous melanoma as a first-line therapy (10). This combination therapy achieves a high efficacy rate even for the treatment of brain metastases of melanoma (11). In addition, Blank et al. reported that the efficacy of co-administration of nivolumab and ipilimumab does not parallel TMB (12). In addition to co-administration of nivolumab and ipilimumab, sequential administration of nivolumab and ipilimumab with a planned switch leads to high efficacy in the treatment of advanced melanoma (4, 9). On the other hand, both co-administration of nivolumab and ipilimumab and sequential administration of nivolumab and ipilimumab with a planned switch lead to a high frequency of serious immune-related adverse events (irAEs), such as hepatitis, colitis, polyneuropathy, etc., in patients with advanced melanoma (1, 4, 11). Therefore, determining the efficacy of nivolumab monotherapy before starting first-line immune therapy for melanoma is important.

CXCL5 is a chemokine that can recruit not only neutrophils, but also CXCR2+ myeloid-derived suppressor cells (MDSCs) and CXCR2+ monocytes that can be precursors of tumor-associated macrophages (TAMs) (13–15). Indeed, Soler-Cardona et al. reported that CXCL5-overexpressing melanomas had significantly increased lymph node metastases of melanoma (15) caused by the recruitment of immunosuppressive PD-L1-expressing neutrophils, leading to interference with systemic activation of the anti-tumor immune system using poly (I: C) (14). In another report, the recruitment of CXCR2-expressing MDSCs played significant roles in the development of colitis-associated colon cancer (13). These reports suggested the production of CXCL5 in the cancer stroma of melanoma.

In addition to autoimmune-related chemokines, chronic inflammatory chemotactic factors such as CXCL10 are also important for the recruitment of immunosuppressive cells such as regulatory T cells (Tregs) and MDSCs. Jiang et al. reported that, compared to patients with stable disease, advanced melanoma patients had increased levels of IL-1β and CXCL10 in the serum associated with accumulation of monocytic (Mo)-MDSCs and Tregs in peripheral blood, which correlated with the progression-free survival of these patients (16). In addition, other reports also suggested that serum CXCL10 levels were correlated with disease activity in advanced melanomas (17) and angiosarcomas (10). These reports suggested that serum CXCL10 levels may represent disease activity in advanced melanoma.

Not only MDSCs, but Tregs are also important for tumor progression in melanoma (19, 20). Indeed, Johansenn et al. previously reported that Tregs at the tumor sites were correlated with tumor progression in melanoma (20). More recently, Ha et al. reported the significance of high CTLA4 expression for Tregs, leading to selective depletion of Tregs in melanoma, which might be an important tool in designing cancer immunotherapy (21). In addition, as described above, the reduction of CCL22 by TAMs decreases Tregs in the tumor site, which enhances the therapeutic effects of immune therapy in the mouse melanoma model (22). Taken together, these reports suggest that serum CCL22 may be correlated with the efficacy of immune therapy.

From the above findings, in this report, the baseline serum levels of TAM-associated chemokines were investigated in 46 advanced melanoma patients treated with nivolumab.

PATIENTS AND METHODS

Ethics Statement for Human Experiments
The protocol for this human study was approved by the ethics committee of Tohoku University Graduate School of Medicine, Sendai, Japan (Permit No: 2017-1-064). All methods were performed in accordance with the relevant guidelines and regulations. All patients provided their written, informed consent.

Patients
Data from patients treated with nivolumab were collected from eight institutes in Japan. Patients were eligible if they had unresectable stage III melanoma, or if the patients had stage IV melanoma with accessible cutaneous, subcutaneous, and/or nodal lesions (staging was performed according to the AJCC Staging Manual, 7th edition, 2011). All patients received 2 mg/kg of nivolumab followed by a 3-week rest period or 3 mg/kg of nivolumab followed by 2 weeks of rest, both of which are approved dosing schedules in Japan. Serum was obtained from patients before the administration of nivolumab. The response to nivolumab was assessed according to Response Evaluation Criteria In Solid Tumors.

Baseline Serum Levels of CXCL5 and CXCL10
Before nivolumab administration, the serum was stored, and serum levels of CXCL5, CXCL10, and CCL22 were then analyzed by enzyme-linked immunoassay (ELISA) according to the protocol provided by the manufacturer (R&D Systems, Minneapolis, MN).

Statistical Methods
Receiver operating characteristic (ROC) curves were used to calculate cut-off values for serum levels of CXCL5, CXCL10, and CCL22 and areas under the curves (AUCs). Cut-offs were determined using Youden's index 12 (sensitivity + specificity −1) to determine the point of the maximum index value (23). ROC curves were established to evaluate serum levels of CXCL5 and CXCL10 in patients administered nivolumab. All statistical analyses were performed using JMP version 14.1 software (SAS

TABLE 1 | Characteristics and serum levels of CXCL5, CXCL10, and CCL22 in patients with cutaneous melanoma.

	Age (y)	Sex	Location	Efficacy	CXCL5 (pg/ml)	CXCL10 (pg/ml)	CCL22 (pg/ml)
1	51–60	M	Trunk	SD	226.9	69.31	290.9
2	31–40	F	Extremities	PD	307.7	212.8	814.6
3	61–70	F	Vagina	PD	237.6	117.9	611.2
4	61–70	M	Extremities	PR	497.5	144.4	314.6
5	61–70	M	Extremities	PR	332.6	72.13	401.5
6	81–90	F	Extremities	PR	434.8	355.5	977.3
7	61–70	M	Trunk	PD	862.1	113.0	891.5
8	81–90	F	Extremities	PD	433.9	186.1	1340
9	71–80	M	Head and neck	SD	461.3	97.21	615.7
10	81–90	F	Trunk	PD	314.9	74.89	637.2
11	91–100	M	Extremities	PD	423.4	122.2	582.6
12	71–80	M	Extremities	SD	471.9	84.24	1031
13	61–70	M	Extremities	PD	222.6	202.5	448.7
14	61–70	F	Vagina	SD	667.8	322.7	548.3
15	71–80	M	Trunk	PR	502.8	358.7	603.8
16	71–80	F	Extremities	PR	408.6	550.1	523.0
17	81–90	F	Unknown	SD	940	266.1	701.2
18	71–90	M	Nasal cavity	SD	332.5	188.1	840.2
19	61–70	M	Nasal cavity	PD	162.9	1001	788.0
20	61–70	M	Paranasal	PD	292.1	247.1	678.2
21	61–70	F	Vagina	PD	292.4	368.2	497.1
22	61–70	F	Vagina	PD	271.6	386.9	475.7
23	51–60	F	Conjunctiva	SD	380.9	336.7	355.5
24	81–90	M	Digestive duct	PD	237.4	208.1	438.3
25	61–70	F	Digestive duct	SD	5026	336.8	987.9
26	61–70	F	Trunk	PD	474.3	245.3	84.71
27	71–80	M	Extremities	PD	494.1	116.7	630.4
28	51–60	F	Head and neck	PD	370.5	93.53	983.2
29	31–40	M	Trunk	SD	501.8	97.59	857.8
30	31–40	F	Extremities	PR	407	138.7	963.1
31	71–80	M	Extremities	SD	529.6	108.4	637.7
32	31–40	M	Extremities	PD	687.1	147.1	845.1
33	71–80	F	Extremities	SD	544.7	104.6	935.6
34	71–80	M	Head and neck	PD	701.3	77.79	918.5
35	41–50	M	Extremities	PD	655.4	432.3	617.5
36	71–80	F	Extremities	PR	465.3	184.8	1065
37	61–70	M	Trunk	PR	555.2	105.7	915.5
38	41–50	M	Head and neck	SD	740.9	65.85	830.3
39	41–50	M	Extremities	PD	723.8	54.08	944.6
40	61–70	F	Head and neck	SD	410.7	62.46	470.7
41	71–80	F	Extremities	PR	1196	71.03	606.1
42	61–70	M	Digestive duct	PR	564	190.4	498.5
43	61–70	F	Palate	PR	1600	51.84	619.5
44	51–60	F	Extremities	CR	687.3	80.09	701.3
45	61–70	M	Paranasal	CR	1142	192	211.3
46	61–70	F	Vagina	CR	4939	68.73	573

Changes of CXCL5, CXCL10, and CCL22 serum levels in each patient (n = 46) before the administration of nivolumab were examined by ELISA. Data for each donor represent the means of duplicate assays.
CR, complete response.
PR, partial response.
SD, stable disease.
PD, progress disease.

Institute, Tokyo, Japan). For a single comparison of two groups, the Mann-Whitney U-test was used. The level of significance was set at $p < 0.05$.

RESULTS

Patients

Data were collected from 46 melanoma patients treated with nivolumab (**Table 1**). The mean patient age was 67 years (range, 33–93 years). Of the patients with melanoma, 58.7% were males, and 41.3% were females. The most common primary tumor site was the extremities (41.3%), followed by mucosal origin (30.4%), trunk (15.2%), head and neck (10.9%), and unknown origin (2.2%).

Efficacy and Adverse Events (AEs) of Nivolumab 3 Months After First Administration

In patients with advanced melanoma, complete response (CR) was seen in 3 patients (6.5%; 95% confidence interval [CI], 0–13.0%), partial response (PR) was seen in 11 patients (23.9%; 95%CI, 0–47.8%), stable disease (SD) was seen in 13 patients (28.3%; 95%CI, 0–56.6%), and progressive disease (PD) was seen in 25 patients (41.3%; 95%CI, 0–82.6%). The objective response rate 3 months after first administration was thus 30.4% (95%CI, 0–60.8%). Tumor responses of individual patients are listed in **Table 1**. The incidence of AEs was 41.3% (Grade 4: 2.2%, Grade 3: 19.6%, Grade 2: 17.4%, Grade 1: 2.2%) (**Table 2**).

Serum Levels of CXCL5, CXCL10, and CCL22

To determine whether baseline serum levels of CXCL5, CXCL10, and CCL22 may be associated with early response in melanoma patients treated with nivolumab, their levels were evaluated in 46 patients with advanced melanoma treated using nivolumab. Increases in baseline serum CXCL5 and efficacy 3 months after the first administration of nivolumab in each patient are shown in **Table 1**. The threshold value of CXCL5 at baseline to distinguish responders from non-responders was 497.5 pg/ml. The sensitivity and specificity of the baseline serum CXCL5 in advanced melanoma were 70.6 and 69.0%, respectively ($p = 0.0016$; **Figure 1A**). High baseline serum levels of CXCL5 were correlated with objective response to nivolumab in patients with advanced melanoma (**Figure 1B**). On the other hand, there were no significant relationships between serum levels of CXCL10 (**Figure 2A**) and CCL22 (**Figure 3A**) and the objective response to nivolumab in patients with advanced melanoma (CXCL10: $p = 0.674$, CCL22: $p = 0.360$). The threshold values of CXCL10 and CCL22 at baseline to distinguish responders from non-responders were 336.8 and 619.5 pg/ml, respectively. There were no significant differences in serum CXCL10 and CCL22 levels in patients with objective response and non-responding patients (**Figures 2B**, **3B**). Baseline serum CXCL5, CXCL10, and CCL22 levels in each patient are shown in **Table 1**. There were no significant relationships between serum levels

of CXCL5 ($p = 0.0703$), CXCL10 ($p = 0.1748$), and CCL22 ($p = 0.2207$) and irAEs in patients with nivolumab-treated advanced melanoma.

TABLE 2 | Immune-related adverse events in patients with cutaneous melanoma.

	Adverse events	Grade
1	N.A.	N.A.
2	N.A.	N.A.
3	N.A.	N.A.
4	Bursitis	3
5	Hypophisitis	4
6	Radiation dermatitis	3
7	N.A.	N.A.
8	Thyroid dysfunction	2
9	N.A.	N.A.
10	N.A.	N.A.
11	N.A.	N.A.
12	N.A.	N.A.
13	Thyroid dysfunction	2
14	Thyroid dysfunction	2
15	Psoriasiform dermatitis	3
16	N.A.	N.A.
17	CIDP	3
18	N.A.	N.A.
19	Psoriasiform dermatitis	3
20	N.A.	N.A.
21	N.A.	N.A.
22	N.A.	N.A.
23	N.A.	N.A.
24	N.A.	N.A.
25	Rheumarthritis	3
26	Hypophisitis	2
27	N.A.	N.A.
28	Diarrhea	2
29	Abdominal pain	2
30	Hypophisitis	1
31	N.A.	N.A.
32	Diarrhea	2
33	N.A.	N.A.
34	N.A.	N.A.
35	N.A.	N.A.
36	N.A.	N.A.
37	N.A.	N.A.
38	N.A.	N.A.
39	Diarrhea	2
40	N.A.	N.A.
41	N.A.	N.A.
42	N.A.	N.A.
43	Hypophisitis	3
44	IDDM	3
45	N.A.	N.A.
46	IDDM	3

CIDP, chronic inflammatory demyelinating polyneuropathy.
IDDM, insulin dependent diabetes mellitus.

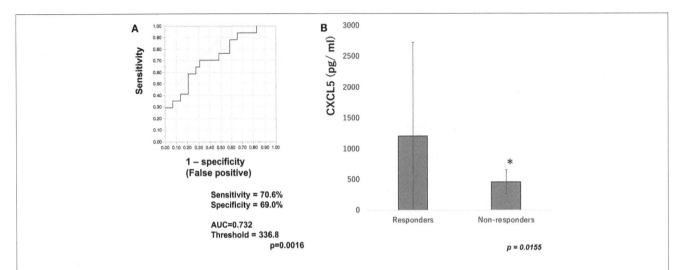

FIGURE 1 | Serum levels of CXCL5 and the ROC curve in melanoma. The ROC curve was used to calculate cut-offs for CXCL5 serum levels and the AUC. Cut-offs were determined to distinguish responders from non-responders using Youden's index **(A)**. Mean serum levels of CXCL5 in responders ($n = 16$) and non-responders ($n = 30$) at day 0 **(B)**. *$p < 0.05$ (n.s, not significant).

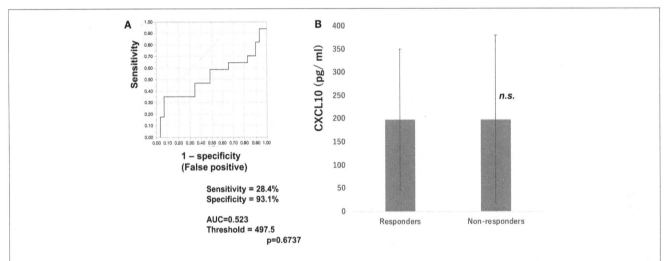

FIGURE 2 | Serum levels of CXCL10 and the ROC curve in melanoma. The ROC curve was used to calculate cut-offs for CXCL10 serum levels and the AUC. Cut-offs were determined to distinguish responders from non-responders using Youden's index **(A)**. Mean serum levels of CXCL10 in responders ($n = 16$) and non-responders ($n = 30$) at day 0 **(B)**. (n.s, not significant).

DISCUSSION

As previously reported, increased levels of soluble(s) CD163 at 6 weeks could predict the efficacy of nivolumab monotherapy 2–3 months after its first administration for the treatment of advanced cutaneous melanoma (24). Indeed, the sensitivity and specificity of serum sCD163 for the prediction of efficacy of nivolumab in cutaneous melanoma were 84.6 and 87.0%, respectively ($p = 0.0030$). Moreover, the absolute serum levels of sCD163 (baseline levels of sCD163 compared with day 42) were significantly increased in advanced melanoma patients who developed irAEs (24). This report concludes that the absolute serum levels of sCD163 are useful for the prediction of irAEs in melanoma patients, especially in

combination with the absolute value of CXCL5 (25). Since serum sCD163 and CXCL5 are, at least in part, derived from CD163+ TAMs that are activated by periostin (24, 26), and chemokine profiles from TAMs are determined by the stimulation of stromal factors (27), spontaneously produced TAM-related factors could be detected in serum from melanoma patients (17, 25, 27). Notably, CD163+ M2 macrophages could be activated by periostin, leading to the production of characteristic chemokines, such as CXCL5, CXCL10, and CCL22, (28) that are correlated with recruitment of both immunosuppressive cells and immune-reactive anti-tumor cells (25). On the other hand, PD-1 expression is a key factor in maintaining TAMs as M2-polarized, and blockade of PD-1/PD-L1 leads to conversion of TAMs into

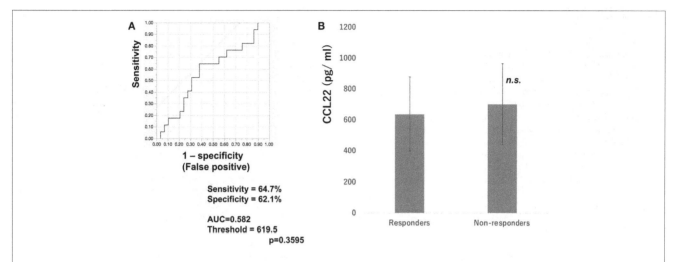

FIGURE 3 | Serum levels of CCL22 and the ROC curve in melanoma. The ROC curve was used to calculate cut-offs for CCL22 serum levels and the AUC. Cut-offs were determined to distinguish responders from non-responders using Youden's index **(A)**. Mean serum levels of CCL22 in responders ($n = 16$) and non-responders ($n = 30$) at day 0 **(B)**. (n.s, not significant).

M1-polarized activated macrophages (29). Since CD163+ TAMs are activated by anti-PD1 antibody (29), the TAM-related chemokines such as sCD163 and CXCL5 are important to evaluate the recruitment of anti-PD1 antibody in the tumor microenvironment.

From the above findings, in this report, we hypothesized that baseline serum levels of TAM-related chemokines, CXCL5, CXCL10, and CCL22, might be correlated with the efficacy of nivolumab in patients with advanced melanomas. To prove this hypothesis, serum levels of CXCL5, CXCL10, and CCL22 were analyzed in 46 cases of advanced melanoma treated with nivolumab. Baseline serum levels of CXCL5 were significantly increased in the response group compared to the non-response group in melanoma. In contrast, no significant differences in baseline serum levels of CXCL10 and CCL22 were seen between the nivolumab response and non-response groups. This discrepancy might be caused by the different sources of CXCL10 and CCL22, such as dendritic cells and endothelial cells that express lower levels of PD1 (29), leading to no effect of anti-PD1 antibody on the production of these chemokines in melanoma patients. Since CXCL5 is also reported as a biomarker for various T helper 17 cell-mediated autoimmune disorders (30–32), the high serum levels of CXCL5 might be correlated with the anti-tumor immune response of anti-PD1 antibody that could also induce autoimmune-like responses such as interstitial pneumonia, autoimmune-like colitis, and hepatitis (33). Taken together, CXCL5 may represent a predictive biomarker for evaluating the efficacy of nivolumab 3 months after its first administration for advanced melanoma. The present study suggested that CXCL5 may be a useful biomarker for the selection of those melanoma patients most likely to benefit from anti-melanoma immunotherapy using nivolumab and ipilimumab combined therapy. Because this was a pilot study, future independent studies with larger patient cohorts are needed to confirm the present findings.

ETHICS STATEMENT

The protocol for this human study was approved by the ethics committee of Tohoku University Graduate School of Medicine, Sendai, Japan (Permit No: 2017-1-064). All methods were performed in accordance with the relevant guidelines and regulations. All patients provided their written, informed consent.

AUTHOR CONTRIBUTIONS

TFuj designed the research study. YS, TFuj, KT, CL, and YK gathered and analyzed the ELISA data. TFuj, YK, RA, AO, YF, KY, SM, HU, YY, HH, TFun, YN, RT, HO, NW and AH treated the patients and acquired the clinical data and samples. TFuj wrote the manuscript. TFuj and SA supervised the study.

REFERENCES

1. Wolchok JD, Chiarion-Sileni V, Gonzalez R, Rutkowski P, Grob JJ, Cowey CL, et al. Overall survival with combined nivolumab and ipilimumab in advanced melanoma. *N Engl J Med.* (2017) 377:1345–56. doi: 10.1056/NEJMoa1709684

2. Robert C, Long GV, Brady B, Dutriaux C, Maio M, Mortier L, et al. Nivolumab in previously untreated melanoma without BRAF mutation. *N Engl J Med.* (2015) 372:320–30. doi: 10.1056/NEJMoa1412082

3. Tarhini A, Benedict A, McDermott D, Rao S, Ambavane A, Gupte-Singh K, et al. Sequential treatment approaches in the management of BRAF wild-type advanced melanoma: a cost-effectiveness analysis. *Immunotherapy.* (2018) 10:1241–52. doi: 10.2217/imt-2018-0085

4. Larkin J, Chiarion-Sileni V, Gonzalez R, Grob JJ, Cowey CL, Lao CD, et al. Combined nivolumab and ipilimumab or monotherapy in untreated melanoma. *N Engl J Med.* (2015) 373:23–34. doi: 10.1056/NEJMoa1504030

5. Hayward NK, Wilmott JS, Waddell N, Johansson PA, Field MA, Nones K, et al. Whole-genome landscapes of major melanoma subtypes. *Nature.* (2017) 545:175–80. doi: 10.1038/nature22071

6. Ishihara K, Saida T, Yamamoto A. Japanese Skin Cancer Society Prognosis and Statistical Investigation Committee. Updated statistical data for malignant melanoma in Japan. *Int J Clin Oncol.* (2001) 6:109–16. doi: 10.1007/PL00012091

7. Yamazaki N, Kiyohara Y, Uhara H, Uehara J, Fujimoto M, Takenouchi T, et al. Efficacy and safety of nivolumab in Japanese patients with previously untreated advanced melanoma: a phase II study. *Cancer Sci.* (2017) 108:1223–30. doi: 10.1111/cas.13241

8. Yamazaki N, Takenouchi T, Fujimoto M, Ihn H, Uchi H, Inozume T, et al. Phase 1b study of pembrolizumab (MK-3475; anti-PD-1 monoclonal antibody) in Japanese patients with advanced melanoma (KEYNOTE-041). *Cancer Chemother Pharmacol.* (2017) 79:651–60. doi: 10.1007/s00280-016-3237-x

9. Weber JS, Gibney G, Sullivan RJ, Sosman JA, Slingluff CL Jr, Lawrence DP, et al. Sequential administration of nivolumab and ipilimumab with a planned switch in patients with advanced melanoma (CheckMate 064): an open-label, randomised, phase 2 trial. *Lancet Oncol.* (2016) 17:943–55. doi: 10.1016/S1470-2045(16)30126-7

10. NCCN. *Clinical Practice Guidelines in Oncology (NCCN Guidelines®) Melanoma Version* 2. (2019). Available online at: https://www.nccn.org/professionals/physician_gls/pdf/cutaneous_melanoma.pdf (accessed March 12, 2019).

11. Tawbi HA, Forsyth PA, Algazi A, Hamid O, Hodi FS, Moschos SJ, et al. Combined nivolumab and ipilimumab in melanoma metastatic to the brain. *N Engl J Med.* (2018) 379:722–30. doi: 10.1056/NEJMoa1805453

12. Blank CU, Rozeman EA, Fanchi LF, Sikorska K, van de Wiel B, Kvistborg P, et al. Neoadjuvant versus adjuvant ipilimumab plus nivolumab in macroscopic stage III melanoma. *Nat Med.* (2018) 24:1655–61. doi: 10.1038/s41591-018-0198-0

13. Katoh H, Wang D, Daikoku T, Sun H, Dey SK, Dubois RN, et al. CXCR2-expressing myeloid-derived suppressor cells are essential to promote colitis-associated tumorigenesis. *Cancer Cell.* (2013) 24:631–44. doi: 10.1016/j.ccr.2013.10.009

14. Forsthuber A, Lipp K, Andersen L, Ebersberger S, Graña-Castro, Ellmeier W, et al. CXCL5 as regulator of neutrophil function in cutaneous melanoma. *J Invest Dermatol.* (2019) 139:186–94. doi: 10.1016/j.jid.2018.07.006

15. Soler-Cardona A, Forsthuber A, Lipp K, Ebersberger S, Heinz M, Schossleitner K, et al. CXCL5 facilitates melanoma cell-neutrophil interaction and lymph node metastasis. *J Invest Dermatol.* (2018) 138:1627–35. doi: 10.1016/j.jid.2018.01.035

16. Jiang H, Gebhardt C, Umansky L, Beckhove P, Schulze TJ, Utikal J, et al. Elevated chronic inflammatory factors and myeloid-derived suppressor cells indicate poor prognosis in advanced melanoma patients. *Int J Cancer.* (2015) 136:2352–60. doi: 10.1002/ijc.29297

17. Sato Y, Fujimura T, Kambayashi Y, Tanita K, Tono H, Hashimoto A, et al. Two cases of dabrafenib and trametinib therapy-failed advanced melanoma successfully controlled by nivolumab monotherapy. *J Dermatol.* (2018) 45:1105–8. doi: 10.1111/1346-8138.14508

18. Fujimura T, Sato Y, Kambayashi Y, Tanita K, Tsukada A, Terui T, et al. Three patients with advanced cutaneous angiosarcoma treated with eribulin: investigation of serum soluble CD163 and chemokine (C-X-C motif) ligand 10 as possible biomarkers predicting the biological behaviour of angiosarcoma. *Br J Dermatol.* (2018) 179:1392–5. doi: 10.1111/bjd.16676

19. Weber R, Fleming V, Hu X, Nagibin V, Groth C, Altevogt P, et al. Myeloid-derived suppressor cells hinder the anti-cancer activity of immune checkpoint inhibitors. *Front Immunol.* (2018) 9:1310. doi: 10.3389/fimmu.2018.01310

20. Johansen LL, Lock-Andersen J, Hviid TV. The pathophysiological impact of HLA class Ia and HLA-G expression and regulatory T cells in malignant melanoma: a review. *J Immunol Res.* (2016) 2016:6829283. doi: 10.1155/2016/6829283

21. Ha D, Tanaka A, Kibayashi T, Tanemura A, Sugiyama D, Wing JB, et al. Differential control of human Treg and effector T cells in tumor immunity by Fc-engineered anti-CTLA-4 antibody. *Proc Natl Acad Sci USA.* (2019) 116:609–18. doi: 10.1073/pnas.1812186116

22. Kakizaki A, Fujimura T, Furudate S, Kambayashi Y, Yamauchi T, Yagita H, et al. Immunomodulatory effect of peritumoral administration of interferon-beta on melanoma through tumor-associated macrophages. *Oncoimmunology.* (2015) 4:e1047584. doi: 10.1080/2162402X.2015.1047584

23. Youden WJ. Index for rating diagnostic tests. *Cancer.* (1950) 3:32–5.

24. Fujimura T, Sato Y, Tanita K, Kambayashi Y, Otsuka A, Fujisawa Y, et al. Serum level of soluble CD163 may be a predictive marker of the effectiveness of nivolumab in patients with advanced cutaneous melanoma. *Front Oncol.* (2018) 8:530. doi: 10.3389/fonc.2018.00530

25. Fujimura T, Sato Y, Tanita K, Kambayashi Y, Otsuka A, Fujisawa Y, et al. Serum soluble CD163 and CXCL5 could be predictive markers for immune related adverse event in patients with advanced melanoma treated with nivolumab. *Oncotarget.* (2018) 9:15542–51. doi: 10.18632/oncotarget.24509

26. Jensen TO, Schmidt H, Møller HJ, Høyer M, Maniecki MB, Sjoegren P, et al. Macrophage markers in serum and tumor have prognostic impact in American Joint Committee on Cancer stage I/II melanoma. *J Clin Oncol.* (2009) 27:3330–37. doi: 10.1200/JCO.2008.19.9919

27. Fujimura T, Kambayashi Y, Fujisawa Y, Hidaka T, Aiba S. Tumor-associated macrophages: therapeutic targets for skin cancer. *Front Oncol.* (2018) 8:3. doi: 10.3389/fonc.2018.00003

28. Furudate S, Fujimura T, Kakizaki A, Kambayashi Y, Asano M, Watabe A, et al. The possible interaction between periostin expressed by cancer stroma and tumor-associated macrophages in developing mycosis fungoides. *Exp Dermatol.* (2016) 25:107–12. doi: 10.1111/exd.12873

29. Gordon SR, Maute RL, Dulken BW, Hutter G, George BM, McCracken MN, et al. PD-1 expression by tumour-associated macrophages inhibits phagocytosis and tumour immunity. *Nature.* (2017) 545:495–9. doi: 10.1038/nature22396

30. Rumble JM, Huber AK, Krishnamoorthy G, Srinivasan A, Giles DA, Zhang X, et al. Neutrophil-related factors as biomarkers in EAE and MS. *J Exp Med.* (2015) 212:23–35. doi: 10.1084/jem.20141015

31. Buckland J. Rheumatoid arthritis: citrullination alters the inflammatory properties of chemokines in inflammatory arthritis. *Nat Rev Rheumatol.* (2014) 10:446. doi: 10.1038/nrrheum.2014.112

32. Fujimura T, Kakizaki A, Furudate S, Aiba S. A possible interaction between periostin and CD163+ skin-resident macrophages in pemphigus vulgaris and bullous pemphigoid. *Exp Dermatol.* (2017) 26:1193–8. doi: 10.1111/exd.13157

33. Spain L, Diem S, Larkin J. Management of toxicities of immune checkpoint inhibitors. *Cancer Treat Rev.* (2016) 44:51–60. doi: 10.1016/j.ctrv.2016.02.001

12

Melanoma Immunotherapy: Next-Generation Biomarkers

Sabrina A. Hogan[1,2], Mitchell P. Levesque[1,2] and Phil F. Cheng[1,2]*

[1] Department of Dermatology, UniversitätsSpital Zürich, Gloriastrasse, Zurich, Switzerland, [2] Faculty of Medicine, Universität Zürich, Zürich, Switzerland

*Correspondence:
Phil F. Cheng
phil.cheng@usz.ch

The recent emergence of cancer immunotherapies initiated a significant shift in the clinical management of metastatic melanoma. Prior to 2011, melanoma patients only had palliative treatment solutions which offered little to no survival benefit. In 2018, with immunotherapy, melanoma patients can now contemplate durable or even complete remission. Treatment with novel immune checkpoint inhibitors, anti-cytotoxic T-lymphocyte protein 4 and anti-programmed cell death protein 1, clearly result in superior median and long-term survivals compared to standard chemotherapy; however, more than half of the patients do not respond to immune checkpoint blockade. Currently, clinicians do not have any effective way to stratify melanoma patients for immunotherapies. Research is now focusing on identifying biomarkers which could predict a patient's response prior treatment initiation (or very early during treatment course), in order to maximize therapeutic efficacy, avoid unnecessary costs, and undesirable heavy side effects for the patient. Given the rapid developments in this field and the translational potential for some of the biomarkers, we will summarize the current state of biomarker research for immunotherapy in melanoma, with an emphasis on omics technologies such as next-generation sequencing and mass cytometry (CyTOF).

Keywords: melanoma, immunotherapy, biomarkers, next-generation sequencing, review literature as topic

Immunotherapy has revolutionized the management of metastatic melanoma. Prior to 2011, the median survival for metastatic melanoma was 9 months, compared to greater than 18 months in 2017 (1). Patients now benefit from novel immune checkpoint inhibitors (ICIs), anti-cytotoxic T-lymphocyte protein 4 (CTLA-4) and anti-programmed cell death protein 1 (PD-1). From the latest survival data of the Checkmate 067 trial, progression-free survival (PFS) for ipilimumab is 2.9 months, for nivolumab 6.9 months, and for the combination of nivolumab and ipilimumab 11.5 months. Overall survival (OS) of the ipilimumab group was 19.9 and 37.6 months for the nivolumab group. Median OS was not reached in the combination nivolumab and ipilimumab group with a minimum follow-up time of 36 months (2–6). Although OS is extended, not all patients benefit from immunotherapy. Response rates for ipilimumab range from 11% to 19% (4, 5) and for pembrolizumab or nivolumab from 33% to 44% (2, 6, 7). These new ICIs clearly show superior median and long-term survivals compared to standard chemotherapy; however, more than half of the patients do not respond to immune checkpoint blockade. Currently, there are no clinically approved biomarkers to aid in patient selection in melanoma. In this review, we seek to delineate the current state of biomarker research for immunotherapy in melanoma, with an emphasis on omics technologies such as next-generation sequencing (NGS) and mass cytometry (CyTOF). Given the urgent clinical need for such biomarkers, we decided to focus on human studies only, which we think are more clinically relevant.

IMMUNE CHECKPOINTS

CTLA-4 and PD-1 are two immune checkpoints regulating immune homeostasis. CTLA-4 is a negative regulator of T-cell priming that acts to control naïve T-cell activation by competing with the co-stimulatory molecule CD28 for binding to shared ligands CD80 and CD86 on antigen-presenting cells (APCs) in the lymph node (8). Ipilimumab, a monoclonal antibody against CTLA-4, was the first agent approved for the treatment of unresectable or metastatic melanoma that showed an OS benefit in a randomized phase III trial (4). PD-1 is a T-cell exhaustion marker which is upregulated by T-cells upon activation during priming or expansion and binds to one of two ligands: programmed cell death 1-ligand 1 (PD-L1) and -ligand 2 (PD-L2) (9–11). Pembrolizumab and nivolumab are monoclonal antibodies against PD-1 that have both shown OS benefit in randomized phase III trials and are approved for the treatment of metastatic melanoma (2, 7). Furthermore, nivolumab and pembrolizumab have both improved OS compared with ipilimumab in metastatic melanoma patients that are naïve to both agents. Combination therapy with ipilimumab and nivolumab has demonstrated additional clinical activity with objective response rates ranging from 50% to 60% and improved OS compared to ipilimumab alone. Although ipilimumab, nivolumab, and pembrolizumab have significantly improved the survival of melanoma patients, there are major toxicities associated with the use of these drugs [reviewed in Ref. (12)]. Grade 3 and higher adverse events are seen in about 20% of patients treated with ipilimumab, in 15% of patients treated with nivolumab, and in 50% of patients treated with the combination of both drugs (6). As these therapies result in objective responses for only a subset of patients, there is a crucial need to identify biomarkers that can potentially predict the efficacy of anti-CTLA-4 or anti-PD-1 treatment or identify a specific subset of patients who may benefit from immunotherapy. A summary of current potential biomarkers for immunotherapies in metastatic melanoma patients is listed in **Figure 1**.

CLINICAL BIOMARKERS

Approved markers for melanoma monitoring have not substantially evolved over the past decade. Clinicians have mainly used the TNM staging system as a diagnostic and prognostic indicator. In 2009, lactate dehydrogenase (LDH) was shown to be an independent predictor of survival in melanoma and was therefore added to the AJCC guidelines (13). Accelerated metabolism in cancer cells requires increased glycolysis that creates a high amount of LDH as a byproduct, which is therefore a robust proxy to assess tumor burden (14). It is the only accepted serum biomarker with prognostic value for OS in melanoma (15). In the context of immunotherapies, elevated LDH is a negative prognostic marker for patients treated with ipilimumab (16) and with pembrolizumab (17, 18). However, subgroup analysis of anti-PD-1 treated cohorts recently pointed out that LDH level is not correlated with the duration of response (KEYNOTE-006). Indeed, once patients show response to the treatment, the LDH level is not associated with the duration of the remission period.

As described by Diem et al. in a study specifically assessing the role of LDH as a marker for anti-PD-1 therapy, LDH is nevertheless a useful marker to monitor disease progression and help treatment decisions (19).

Another well-known marker to monitor melanoma is S100, which is a good indicator of advanced clinical disease stage (20). S100 was shown to be predictive of response to anti-CTLA-4 (16). However, similar to LDH, S100 seems to mainly be a proxy of disease stage, able to highlight very ill patients who are more unlikely to respond to the treatment due to the high tumor burden of the disease, but not actually able to predict response to immunotherapies. The same is true for the number of organs involved, which was another potential marker, proposed by Diem et al., to stratify patients prior to anti-CTLA-4 therapy (21).

C-reactive protein (CRP) was described as a negative prognostic factor for anti-CTLA-4 treatment (22). Unlike LDH and S100, CRP is directly related to immune response. However, it is a general marker of inflammation and is not specific to melanoma, ergo, an increase in CRP levels may also be the result of any other ongoing infection (23). For anti-PD-1 therapy, intra-tumoral PD-L1 expression, evaluated by immunohistochemistry, has been assessed as a predictive biomarker. The results have been inconclusive due to a lack of standards for PD-L1 "positivity". Different antibodies and different evaluation criteria have been used for PD-L1 expression in clinical trials. Some studies have used a >5% cutoff (Checkmate-066 and Checkmate-067), whereas others have used >1% cutoff (KEYNOTE-006). In the Checkmate-066 trial, both PD-L1 negative and positive patients had better outcomes than chemotherapy-treated patients, suggesting that PD-L1 status was not a relevant stratification marker (2). More research will be needed to standardize the assessment of PD-L1 expression for it to become a biomarker for anti-PD-1 therapy in melanoma. Blood markers which hold the most potential toward predicting response to immunotherapies are immune cell populations. Indeed, they are either themselves part of or directly influencing the immune response against the tumor. The different findings related to blood cytology as a biomarker for immunotherapy in melanoma are summarized in **Figure 1**. Briefly, for anti-CTLA-4 treatment, absolute neutrophil count, absolute lymphocyte count, neutrophil to lymphocyte ratio, absolute eosinophil count, relative lymphocyte count (RLC), absolute monocyte count, antibodies against NY-ESO1, T-regulatory cell count, and myeloid-derived suppressor cell (MDSC) count have been described as predictive biomarkers. In anti-PD-1-treated patients, RLC, relative eosinophil count (REC), and MDSC count seem to hold some predictive potential prior to treatment initiation. In addition, increased serum levels of TGFβ and increased frequency of Th9 cells in the peripheral blood were detected in responders to nivolumab prior to therapy initiation (24). Unfortunately, most of the studies were performed on small cohorts and the results have not been verified in larger prospective trials (25). Although guidelines have been published about how to best perform biomarker studies (26), most research groups have different evaluation criteria. In this review, we sought to document the most relevant biomarkers associated with immunotherapy outcome in melanoma patients. For a systematic review of clinical biomarkers, see Ref. (18).

Technique

CyTOF · TCR profiling · NGS · Serum, Blood markers

BLOOD

Drug	# patients	Markers	Correlation	Outcome	Method / Threshold	Reference
Anti-PD1	4	↑CD4+ and CD4+CD8+ T-cells after 6-13 weeks of treatment; ↑Central Memory T-cell after 6-13 weeks of treatment	+	Response	High dimentional clustering viSNE and SPADE	Takeuchi et al 2017
Anti-PD1	20	↑CD4+ and CD8+ T-cells; ↑Classical monocytes frequency	+	Response	High dimentional clustering FlowSOM	Krieg et al. 2018
Anti-PD1	9	↑CD8+ expressig IL-2	+	Response	High dimentional clustering SPADE	Hiniker et al. 2016
Anti-CTLA4 + Anti-PD1	9	↑Transitional Memory T-cells frequency	+	Response	DVS Cytobank software	Das et al. 2015
Various	28	↑APC-like population frequency (+); ↑MDSC-like population frequency (-); Even abundance of MDSC- and APC-like cells (+); ↓Early differentiated CD4 correlate with (-); ↑Highly cytotoxic NK cell population (+)		Overall survival	Matrix boolean analysis	Wistuba-Hamprecht et al. 2017
Anti-PD1	12	↓TCR richness and evenness	-	Response	Multiplex PCR - CDR3 TCRβ-VJ	Postow et al. 2015
Anti-CTLA4	21	↑Frequency of clonotypes maintained overtime; ↓Decrease in the number of clones overtime	+	Overall survival	NGS - CDR3 TCRβ-VDJ	Cha et al. 2014
Anti-CTLA4	21	↑TCR repertoire diversity after 30-60d of treatment; ↑TCR repertoire richness and diversity after 30-60d of treatment	+	Response / Toxicity	NGS - CDR3 TCRβ-V	Robert et al. 2014
Anti-CTLA4	360	15 gene classifier (ADAM17, CDK2, CDKN2A, DPP4, ERBB2, HLA-DRA, ICOS, ITGA4, LARGE, MYC, NAB2, NRAS, RHOC, TGFBI, TIMP1)	+	Overall survival and response	qPCR	Friedlander et al 2017
Anti-PD1	512	↓Lactate dehydrogenase (LDH)	+	Overall survival	LDH ratio >2.5	Weide et al. 2016; Diem et al. 2016
Anti-PD1	88	↑Myeloid derived supressor cells (MDSC)	-	Overall survival / PFS	12.60%	Weber et al. 2016
Anti-PD1	512	↓Relative lymphocyte counts (RLC)	+	Overall survival	17.50%	Weide et al. 2016
Anti-PD1	512	↓Relative eosinophils counts (REC)	+	Overall survival	1.50%	Weide et al. 2016
Anti-PD1	46	↓TGFβ in serum	+	Response		Nonomura et al. 2016
Anti-PD1	46	↑Th9 early during treatment	+	Response		Nonomura et al. 2016
	311	↓Lactate dehydrogenase (LDH)		Response	2x ULN	Wolchok et al. 2016
Anti-CTLA4	200	↓Lactate dehydrogenase (LDH)	+	Overall survival	ULN	Martens et al. 2016
	134	↓Lactate dehydrogenase (LDH) during treatment		Overall survival	Continuous variable	Diem et al. 2015
Anti-CTLA4	100	↑absolute lymphocyte count (ALC)	+	PFS	1×10^9	Alexander et al. 2014
	95	↑absolute lymphocyte count (ALC) during treatment		Response		Simeone et al. 2014
Anti-CTLA4	720	↑Absolute neutrophil count (ANC)	-	Overall survival / PFS	7500	Ferrucci et al. 2016
Anti-CTLA4	200	↑Absolute eosinophil count (AEC)	+	Overall survival	50/µg	Martens et al. 2016; Weide et al. 2016
Anti-CTLA4	200	↑Relative lymphocyte counts (RLC)	+	Overall survival / PFS	10.50%	Martens et al. 2016
Anti-CTLA4	720	↑Derived neutrophil-to-lymphocyte ratio (dNLR)	-	Overall survival	3	Ferrucci et al. 2016
	58	↑Neutrophil-to-lymphocyte ratio (NLR)		PFS	4	Zaragoza et al. 2016
Anti-CTLA4	200	↑Absolute monocyte count (AMC)	+	Overall survival	650/µl	Martens et al. 2016
	134	↑Number of organs involved	-	Overall survival	Continuous variable	Diem et al. 2015
Anti-CTLA4	113	↑S100	-	Overall survival	1x ULN	Kelderman et al. 2014
Anti-CTLA4	120	↑C-reactive protein during treatment		Response	5 mg/mL	Simeone et al. 2014
Anti-CTLA4	68	↓Myeloid derived supressor cells (MDSC)	+	Overall survival	Flow Cytometry	Kitano et al. 2014
Anti-CTLA4	120	↓T-regulatory cells (Treg)	+	Response	0.50%	Simeone et al. 2014
	200	↓T-regulatory cells (Treg)		Overall survival	1.50%	Martens et al. 2016
Anti-CTLA4	144	↑Circulating antibodies against NY-ESO-1; ↑NY-ESO-1 specific CD8+ T-cells	+	Response / Overall survival	Titer > 100 / Continuous variable	Yuan et al. 2011

TUMOR

TCR profiling · NGS · IHC markers

Drug	# patients	Markers	Correlation	Outcome	Method / Threshold	Reference
Anti-PD1	46	↑Clonal TCR repertoire	+	Response	NGS - CDR3 TCRβ-VJ	Tumeh et al. 2014
Anti-PD1	8	↑TCR repertoire clonality under prior anti-CTLA4	+	Response	NGS - CDR3 TCRβ-VJ	Roh et al. 2017
	56	↑TCR repertoire clonality at baseline				
Anti-PD1	10	↓TCR repertoire diversity index	+	Response	NGS - CDR3 TCRβ-VDJ	Inoue et al. 2016
Anti-PD1	34	↓TCR evenness in ipi-naive, ↑TCR richness in ipi-progressive	+	Response	NGS - CDR3 TCRβ-VJ	Riaz et al. 2017
Anti-PD1	68 pre- 41 pre- and post-therapy	↑Mutational load in ipi-N; ↓Mutational load and neoantigen load during therapy	+	Overall survival / Response	WES	Riaz et al.2017
	45	Immune signature (T-cell activation and lymphocyte aggregation)		Response	RNAseq	
Anti-PD1	65	↑Mutational load and LRP1B mutation	+	Overall survival	Targeted Panel Seq	Johnson et al. 2016
Anti-PD1	38 / 28	BRCA2 mutation, IPRES gene signature	+	Response	WES / RNAseq	Hugo et al. 2016
Anti-PD1	30	↑Burden of copy number loss	-	Response	WES	Roh et al. 2017
Anti-CTLA4	174	SERPINB3 or SERPINB4 mutation	+	Overall survival	WES	Riaz et al 2016
Anti-CTLA4	64	↑Mutational load	+	Overall survival	WES	Snyder et al. 2014
Anti-CTLA4	110 / 40	↑Mutational load, neoantigen load, cytolytic gene expression	+	Overall survival	WES / RNAseq	Van Allen et al. 2015
Anti-CTLA4	110 / 64	↑Aneuploidy	-	Response / Overall survival / Overall survival	WES	Davoli et al. 2017
Anti-PD1	24	↑CD8+, CD3+ and CD45RO+; ↑CD4, CD8, CD3+, CD45RO+, PD-L1, PD1, LAG-3, FoxP3, GranzB early on treatment	+	Response	Immunohistochemistry	Chen et al. 2016
Anti-PD1	41	↑PD-L1 expression	+	Response	Immunohistochemistry (≥ 5%)	Taube et al. 2014
Anti-PD1	210 / 549	↑PD-L1 expression	+	Overall survival and PFS	Immunohistochemistry (≥ 5%) / Immunohistochemistry (≥ 1%)	Robert et al. 2014; Robert et al. 2015
Anti-PD1	35	↓Indoleamine 2,3-dioxygenase (IDO)	+	Response	Immunohistochemistry	Hamid et al. 2011
Anti-PD1	46	↑T-cell infiltration in the tumor	+	Response	Immunohistochemistry	Tumeh et al. 2014
Anti-CTLA4	24	↑CD8+ T-cells early during treatment	+	Response	Immunohistochemistry	Chen et al. 2016
Anti-CTLA4	27	↑T-cell infiltration in the tumor at 4 weeks	+	Response	Immunohistochemistry	Hamid et al. 2011
Anti-CTLA4	45	↑Expression of immune related genes (CCL4, CCL5, CXCL9, CXCL10, CXCL11, IFN-γ, IDO1, GBP1, MHC II molecules, GBP1)	+	Response	Affymetrix gene expression analysis	Ji et al. 2012

FIGURE 1 | Summary of the biomarker studies performed on peripheral blood and tumor on anti-CTLA4 and anti-PD1 treatment.

BIOMARKERS FROM NEXT-GENERATION SEQUENCING

Whole exome (WES) and RNA sequencing (RNAseq) are powerful tools for evaluating the genomic landscape of a tumor. WES only captures the exonic gene regions, so it enriches for mutations in coding regions, while RNAseq can provide the entire transcriptome of a sample and is useful for establishing gene signatures for specific cohorts within a patient group. In terms of immunotherapy, WES has been useful in determining mutational load and discovering neoantigens in melanoma tumors (27). Melanoma has one of the highest mutation rates of all cancers (28–30) and has a high probability for neoantigen generation. Neoantigens are the result of somatic mutations which translate into a mutated protein that is detected and presented by APCs. Neoantigens are an attractive target for immunotherapy as they are only expressed by the tumor and not by the normal tissue. Many studies have utilized WES and RNAseq to evaluate the mutation profile and gene expression changes in patients treated with anti-CTLA-4 and anti-PD-1, with the aim to find biomarkers to predict response.

Snyder et al. performed WES on 64 patients treated with anti-CTLA-4 (31). This study was the first to associate mutational burden to clinical benefit and they also defined a neoantigen signature associated with clinical benefit. They concluded that, although patients with high mutation burden are more likely to respond to anti-CTLA-4, the types of neoantigen the patient expresses will ultimately determine their response. Van Allen et al. performed WES on 110 patients and RNAseq on 40 patients treated with anti-CTLA-4 (32). They could confirm that mutational load is associated with clinical benefit to anti-CTLA-4 treatment. Neoantigen load was also measured and this parameter was also significantly associated with response; however, they could not detect the neoantigen signature seen in the study performed by Snyder and colleagues. They concluded that clinically beneficial neoantigens are most likely private events (specific to each individual) and recurrent neoantigens (consistent in the general population) are quite rare. Van Allen and colleagues also analyzed the transcriptome in a subset of these patients and found that expression of cytolytic markers, such as granzyme A and perforin, were beneficial for response. Expression of CTLA-4 and PD-L2 was also associated with clinical benefit. Riaz et al. performed WES on 174 patients treated with anti-CTLA-4 therapy (33). They discovered 48 patients with mutations in SERPINB3 or SERPIN4 and observed that those patients were more likely to be responders. Patients with SERPINB3 or SERPINB4 mutations also had higher mutational loads. Friedlander et al. performed a quantitative polymerase chain reaction (PCR) study on peripheral blood from 360 patients receiving anti-CTLA-4 therapy (34). From a panel of 169 genes, they established a 15 gene signature that was predictive and prognostic for response and 1-year OS to anti-CTLA-4 treatment. The 15 genes are ITGA4, LARGE, CDK2, TIMP1, DPP4, NRAS, ERBB2, NAB2, ADAM17, RHOC, TGFB1, CDKN2A, HLADRA, MYC, and ICOS.

In order to elucidate resistance mechanisms and biomarkers of response to treatment, Hugo et al. used WES (38 patients) and RNAseq (28 patients) on a set of melanoma patients treated with anti-PD-1 (35). Mutational load did not have a significant association to response to anti-PD-1 therapy and neoantigen load was not significantly correlated with response either. Nonetheless, mutational load was associated with OS suggesting that other factors influence response to anti-PD-1 and survival. BRCA2 mutations occurred in 30% of the responders to anti-PD-1. RNAseq analysis uncovered a co-enrichment of 26 gene signatures in 9 of the 13 non-responding patients, which the authors termed innate anti-PD-1 resistance (IPRES) signature. They validated the IPRES signature on three other datasets and found over-representation in anti-PD-1 non-responding samples.

In a small study of four patients treated with anti-PD-1, Zaretsky et al. used WES on patients that developed new lesions under anti-PD-1 therapy. They discovered that the progressive tumors acquired JAK1, JAK2, or B2M loss of function mutations. JAK1 and JAK2 mutations cause insensitivity to interferon gamma-induced arrest and B2M mutations led to a loss of MHC class 1 expression (36). In a follow-up study, Shin et al. performed WES on 23 patients before anti-PD-1 treatment (37). In their cohort, mutational load had no association to response and one of the non-responders had a loss of function mutation in JAK1. This study confirms the role of JAK1 as a marker for innate and adaptive resistance to anti-PD-1, although it might be a rare occurrence.

Roh et al. performed WES on sequential biopsies of patients treated with anti-CTLA-4 and then anti-PD-1. Thirty patients had WES at baseline, 3 on anti-CTLA-4 treatment, 25 at anti-CTLA-4 progression, 18 on anti-PD-1 treatment, and 12 at anti-PD-1 progression. Overall, they found that mutation burden was not associated with response, but high copy number loss was associated with poor response (38). In the regions with recurrent copy number loss, PTEN was one of the notable tumor suppressor genes suggesting that it could be a driver of resistance mechanisms to immunotherapy. Another study also observed that PTEN loss was associated with resistance to anti-CTLA-4 therapy (39).

Johnson et al. performed targeted panel sequencing on 65 patients treated with anti-PD-1 therapy. In their cohort, mutational load was associated with response to anti-PD-1 and patients with high mutational load (>23.1 mutations/MB) had longer PFS and OS compared to the intermediate mutational load group (3.3–23.1 mutations/MB) and the low mutation load (<3.3 mutations/MB) group. They observed more frequent BRCA2 mutations in responders than in non-responders (5/32 vs. 2/33). LRP1B mutations were significantly enriched in the responder group (11/32) compared to the non-responder group (1/33). LRP1B mutated patients also had a higher mutational load compared to LRP1B wild-type patients.

Riaz et al. performed WES on 68 patients treated with anti-PD-1 that had previously progressed on anti-CTLA-4 therapy (35 patients) or were naïve to anti-CTLA-4 (33 patients). Mutational load was associated with clinical benefit in the anti-CTLA-4-naïve group, but not the anti-CTLA-4-resistant group. No single gene mutations were significantly associated with response or resistance to therapy. Decreased mutational and neoantigen load during therapy was associated with response in both anti-CTLA-4-naïve and anti-CTLA-4-resistant groups. RNAseq analysis of the pretreatment samples showed an enrichment in T-cell activation and lymphocyte aggregation pathways. These signatures indicate an immunologically active tumor, or "hot tumor," and all patients with complete response or partial response in the anti-CTLA-4-resistant group had the "hot tumor" signature, although not all responders in the anti-CTLA-4-naïve group had the "hot tumor" signature. Riaz et al. also investigated the early effects of anti-PD-1 treatment (29 days after start) by RNAseq and uncovered a global increase in immune checkpoint genes such as PD-1, CTLA-4, CD274 (PD-L1), ICOS, and LAG3 in all samples. For responders, the significant pathways included inflammatory response and cytokine-mediate signaling pathways.

Finally, Davoli et al. investigated the role of aneuploidy in response to immunotherapy (40). They analyzed the copy number data from 5,255 tumor/normal samples, representing 12 cancer types from The Cancer Genome Atlas project, and found that for most tumors, there was a positive correlation between aneuploidy severity and mutational load. They also found that tumors with high levels of aneuploidy showed elevated expression of cell cycle and cell proliferation markers, as well as a reduced expression of markers for cytotoxic immune cell infiltrates. Aneuploidy levels were a stronger predictor of markers of cytotoxic immune cell infiltration than tumor mutational load. To correlate aneuploidy with response to immunotherapy, they used data from Snyder et al. and Van Allen et al. (31, 32) and found in both datasets that high levels of aneuploidy correlated with poorer survival.

BIOMARKERS FROM T-CELL RECEPTOR (TCR) PROFILING

Antigen detection by T-cells is by definition dependent on tumor-specific T-cell generation and clonal amplification. In the context of immunotherapies, which aim at enhancing the recognition of the cancer cell by the immune system, there is an obvious rational basis for examining the T-cell repertoire in order to shed light on the specific mode of action of the drug and find potential biomarkers of response.

The main challenge when analyzing TCR repertoire is its immense diversity. The TCR is a heterodimer comprised of two chains $\alpha\beta$ or $\delta\gamma$. The β and δ chains, are generated by the random rearrangement of a variable region (V), a diversity region (D), and a joining region (J) with a constant region (C). The α and γ chains, consists of segments from the V, J, and C regions. Additional complexity is introduced by random addition or deletion of nucleotides at the junction sites of V, D, and J. The theoretical limit of the TCR repertoire is in the range of 10^{15}, which is several magnitudes higher than the total amount of T-cells in the body, approximately 4×10^{11} (41). The estimated number for the TCR repertoire is in the order of 10^6 to 10^8 (42). Most of the studies mainly assess the complementarity-determining region 3 (CDR3) from β chain, which is considered an acceptable proxy for estimating diversity since it is the most variable region of the receptor and that $\alpha\beta$T-cells represent about 90% of all T-cells (43). Due to the advances in NGS, it is possible now to identify each individual TCR sequence in the CDR3 region (44). Multiplex PCR is one of the widely used methods to amplify the CDR3 region. Primers for the J alleles or the constant region of the TCR α and β chains are used together with a mix of primers for all known V alleles.

A drawback of multiplex PCR is that it is limited to known V alleles. As a result, for TCR discovery experiments, other methods such as targeted enrichment—a technique where RNA baits capture the TCR receptor, usually the CDR3 region—are preferred. Since bait capture takes into account mismatches, it allows for discovery of new alleles and TCR receptors. In the context of immunotherapy, TCR repertoire analysis is useful for determining if the tumor-reactive clones have undergone activation and clonal expansion. In an adequate immune response, the tumor-specific T-cells will represent a significant proportion of the whole repertoire and therefore be assessable at the level of the whole TCR population.

In 2014, Robert et al. compared pre- to post-treatment peripheral blood mononuclear cell (PBMC) samples from melanoma patients treated with anti-CTLA-4 (45). The results from deep sequencing of the multiplex PCR for the TCR Vβ CDR3 region showed that 19 out of 21 patients had an increased number of unique clonotype (richness). There was no significant difference in the V or J segment usage and no difference in the total of unique sequences between responders and non-responders. The number of unique productive sequences in the top 25% of clones showed a particularly high increase in diversity after treatment. Those changes were not associated with peripheral lymphocyte count; however, CD8+ tumor-infiltrating cells showed a positive correlation with the TCR repertoire diversity. Finally, they showed that patients experiencing more toxicities had more diverse sequences post treatment. Overall, this study reports that anti-CTLA-4 treatment increases TCR repertoire diversity in an unspecific manner. Subsequently, the same group performed a similar study on 9 anti-PD-1-treated patients and compared the results (46). Unlike the effect of anti-CTLA-4, anti-PD-1 therapy does not increase TCR repertoire complexity, on the contrary, 4/9 samples show a decrease >15% in the absolute number of unique sequences and only one had an increase >15%. Those results suggest that the mode of action of the two drugs is considerably different.

Cha et al. shed more light on the potential mechanism of anti-CTLA-4; their study assessed the changes in TCR repertoire between baseline and 4 weeks of treatment in PBMCs from 21 melanoma patients (47). They confirmed that anti-CTLA-4 treatment induces a significant change in the clonotypes frequency compared to healthy donors. They showed that the diversification is the result of a higher gain of new clonotypes and lower loss of existing ones. The number of therapy-induced expanding clones are not different between the responders and the non-responders, which is in line with what Robert et al. described. However, patients who survived longer exhibited less clonotypic changes overtime, they maintained the most abundant clones which were present at baseline and also had fewer clones significantly decreasing in frequency. Finally, they also demonstrated that the clones expanding in response to therapy are largely non-naïve T-cells, suggesting that patients who respond to the therapy already have pre-primed T-cells in circulation before the onset of anti-CTLA-4 treatment.

In light of these findings, Postow et al. hypothesized that the shape of the TCR repertoire prior to treatment initiation may influence the likelihood of a response to the treatment (48). Twelve baseline PBMC samples from 4 responders and 8 non-responders to anti-CTLA-4 were analyzed for richness and evenness of the TCR repertoire. In this small cohort, they first showed that patients who responded to the treatment have more similar VJ usage among each other than compared to the VJ usages in the non-responders. Furthermore, low richness or evenness of the TCR repertoire was significantly associated with a poor response to anti-CTLA-4. That is, a TCR repertoire composed of less unique clones (less diverse) or skewed toward a few specific clones (very clonal) is predictive of a non-response to the treatment.

The detection of clonally expanded tumor-specific T-cell in the blood indicates that the immune system mounted an immune response against a foreign entity, which could be the tumor. However, it is not certain that the activated T-cells would be able to home to the tumor efficiently and be able to kill the cancer cells. Therefore, it is also important to assess the immune status at the tumor site.

Tumeh et al. performed a very elegant study exploiting tumor samples from melanoma patients prior and during anti-PD-1 treatment (49). By qualitative and quantitative immunohisto-chemistry, they revealed that, at baseline, patients who eventually respond to the therapy, have more CD8+ T-cells at the invasive margin of the tumor compared to non-responders. This population increases and migrates toward the center of the tumor during treatment in responders. They showed that an efficient response to anti-PD-1 therapy requires pre-existing CD8+ T-cells, which are most likely tumor specific. To confirm this theory, they sequenced the TCR Vβ region of tumor baseline samples and found that responders indeed had a more clonal TCR repertoire. On treatment, samples of responders showed significantly more clonal expansion than non-responders.

Johnson et al. used NGS to assess differences between baseline samples of responders and non-responders to anti-PD-1 therapy (50). They assessed mutational load as well as specific mutations differentially occurring in responders and non-responders. They also investigated the TCR repertoire clonality of 42 samples and did not find any association with response. However, it is important to mention that times of sample acquisition were not immediately before and after treatment. The timing was quite broad, the study allowed the inclusion of samples collected over 12 months before start of treatment and also after treatment initiation. When the analysis was performed only on samples obtained within 4 months of treatment initiation, the non-responder group was only represented by five samples, including one potential outlier. Nonetheless, they noticed a trend toward higher clonality at baseline in patients who eventually responded to the therapy.

Inoue et al. analyzed the TCR repertoire of 10 pre- and post-anti-PD-1 tumor samples (51). They noticed that the clonotypes with a read frequency >0.5% at baseline significantly increased after treatment in responders. The calculation of the diversity index highlighted a slight decrease in tumors of responders compared to non-responders, which suggests oligoclonal expansion of certain TCR clones.

More recently, Roh et al. published a complementary analysis on a cohort of patients for which they performed TCR sequencing (38). They analyzed tumor samples from melanoma patients treated sequentially with anti-CTLA-4 and anti-PD-1 via WES and TCR sequencing. The TCR clonality assay revealed that there was

no significant difference between responders and non-responders, pre- or on-treatment with anti-CTLA-4. A subpopulation of the patients (n = 8) received anti-CTLA-4 followed by anti-PD-1 after progression. All three responders to anti-CTLA-4 followed by anti-PD-1 showed an increase in TCR clonality during anti-CTLA-4 treatment. In addition, higher TCR clonality was seen in the responders prior to treatment and on treatment with anti-PD-1.

Riaz et al. investigated the evolution of melanoma tumors and their microenvironment under anti-PD-1 therapy (52). Patients who had previously progressed on anti-CTLA-4 and were naïve to anti-CTLA-4 were included in the study. They performed TCR sequencing on 34 samples pre- and 4 weeks post- anti-PD-1 treatment. There were no statistically significant differences in the baseline samples of either group. On anti-PD-1 therapy, the anti-CTLA-4-pretreated group had increased TCR richness associated with response, whereas the anti-CTLA-4-naïve group had decreased TCR evenness associated with response. In line with Roh et al., pretreatment with anti-CTLA-4 seems to increase the expansion of tumor-specific T-cell cells, which are additionally expanded during anti-PD-1 treatment.

MASS CYTOMETRY (CyTOF)

The advent of CyTOF has allowed a more comprehensible analysis of the whole immune system and will be an important asset for immune oncology (53). The basic principle of CyTOF is similar to conventional flow cytometry. The assay quantifies multiple protein expression markers at the single-cell level. In contrast to flow cytometry, the detection is not achieved by fluorophore excitation, but by stable mass isotope quantification. The transition isotope bound to the antibodies are analyzed by a time of flight mass spectrometer. CyTOF has some advantages over flow cytometry, namely, the high purity of the metal isotopes reduces background noise, eliminating spectral spillover and cellular autofluorescence associated with conventional flow cytometry. It also enables the detection of more markers in the same experiment, theoretically up to a hundred. Multiple samples can be analyzed at the same time thanks to a barcoding strategy (up to 20), and therefore reduce inter-sample variation. CyTOF has primarily been used to analyze peripheral blood from patients undergoing immunotherapy. A better characterization of the precise mode of action of those drugs is crucial to help overcoming and predicting resistance as well as contributing to optimal development of future combination therapies.

In 2015, Das et al. analyzed peripheral blood from melanoma patients undergoing immunotherapy with anti-CTLA-4, anti-PD-1, or the combination of the two (54). Samples were collected at baseline and after 3 weeks of treatment. In this early study, CyTOF was mainly used to further characterize the cell population of interest previously identified by flow cytometry. The analysis revealed that the Ki67+ cells, increasing after combination treatment, have a transitional memory T-cell-like phenotype. Additional experiments were performed using other techniques than CyTOF, which lead the authors to conclude that anti-PD-1 and anti-CTLA-4 have distinct effects on the immune system.

In the context of a clinical trial assessing the safety of combining radiotherapy and immunotherapy in melanoma patients,

Hiniker et al. analyzed baseline and follow-up PBMC samples from 9 patients (3 progressive disease, 6 complete response/partial response) (55). CyTOF analysis revealed that the level of CD8+ T-cells expressing IL-2 were higher at baseline and in the follow-up samples of responding patients. The same was true for central memory CD8+ T-cell levels. However, the cytokine production was not significantly different from the population seen in non-responding patients, thereby suggesting that the cells are not functionally different from the non-responders.

The first study to use CyTOF as a main technique for analyzing human melanoma patient samples was performed by Wistuba-Hamprecht et al. in early 2017 (56). The analysis consisted in performing CyTOF on 28 PBMC samples from stage IV melanoma patients who received different courses of treatments. A higher frequency in the APC-like population had a positive association with OS, whereas a higher frequency in the MDSC-like population showed negative association with OS. Overall, an equal abundance of MDSC- and APC-like cells is associated with better survival. The analysis of the T-cell compartment revealed that there was a clear interpatient heterogeneity in the CD4+ and CD8+ T-cell compartments compared to the other compartments which have more homogenous frequencies between patients. Only one αβT-cell population had some prognostic potential: a higher level of early differentiated CD4+ T-cell was correlated with poorer OS. In the natural killer cell compartment, a highly cytotoxic cell population tends to correlate with better OS. Finally, a comprehensive analysis of immune signatures of all the melanoma-associated phenotypes identified a specific cluster with high prognostic capacity, performing even better than LDH. This cluster is significantly associated with poor OS and represented by an overall lower diversity across all the compartments, and especially in the myeloid compartment.

Takeuchi et al. investigated the effect of immunotherapy in melanoma patients by comparing PBMCs from 4 different patients receiving anti-PD-1 (2 responders and 2 non-responders) (57). The panel was composed of 35 markers and they used high-dimensional clustering to analyze the data. The main finding in this paper is that CD4+ and CD4+CD8+ cell populations increase during therapy. CD4+CD27+FAS− central memory T-cell were shown to expand in a higher proportion in responders than in non-responders. These results were validated in a separate cohort ($n = 4$).

More recently, Krieg et al. performed a comprehensive analysis, assessing the correlation between baseline peripheral immune signature and response to anti-PD-1 in melanoma patients (58). The cohort was composed of 20 patients from whom baseline and on treatment samples were obtained. They used an optimized immune marker panel and a customized, interactive bioinformatics pipeline in order to identify potential predictive biomarkers. Three different CyTOF panels were used: one for the phenotypic characterization of lymphocytes, one to assess the T-cell functions, and the third one to characterize monocytes, which consisted of 30, 26, and 25 markers, respectively. By performing hierarchical clustering of all the samples pooled together, they identified a differential marker expression in responders compared to non-responders. Further analysis, and validation in an independent, blinded cohort by conventional flow cytometry,

revealed that, at baseline, responders had a higher frequency of classical monocytes and lower frequency of lymphocytes compared to the non-responders.

OUTLOOK

The development of high-throughput technologies such as NGS and CyTOF have allowed researchers and clinicians to evaluate hundreds to tens of thousands of genes from a bulk tumor to a single-cell level. NGS is an invaluable tool for analyzing mutations and copy number profiles, gene expression changes and gene signatures, epigenetic alterations, the TCR repertoire, and single-cell gene expression changes. The recent development of CyTOF has also allowed the analysis of many markers at a single-cell level. In the context of immunotherapy, these high dimensional datasets will enhance the discovery of novel biomarkers, prognostic markers, and resistance mechanisms.

Next-generation sequencing biomarker discovery for anti-CTLA-4 treatment have uncovered that mutational load and neoantigen load are the most informative for response and OS, but they are not perfect biomarkers as some non-responders may also present with high mutational load. Aneuploidy could also help foresee response to anti-CTLA4 since it was highlighted as an independent predictor in a multivariate Cox model which included mutational load. Copy number analysis could as well be informative as loss in chromosome 10 was shown to be a poor prognostic marker in two studies. Many of these studies also analyzed tumor samples upon progression and found no recurrent genetic mutation, which could mean that resistance to anti-CTLA-4 is patient specific. In the context of anti-PD-1 treatment, mutational load is not a clear informative marker for response. As anti-PD-1 is a relatively new therapy, no large cohort studies with over 100 patients for NGS biomarker discovery have yet been performed. There are single patient examples showing that genes involved in the JAK–STAT pathway or antigen presentation could be predictive biomarkers for anti-PD-1 treatment. Loss of function mutations in JAK1, JAK2, and B2M are negative biomarkers for response and are involved in resistance to anti-PD-1 treatment in individual cases, but these mutations do not seem to be recurrent. RNAseq analysis from several studies suggest that tumors with high immune activity are more likely to respond to anti-PD-1. To better stratify patients for anti-CTLA-4 or anti-PD-1 treatment, a combinatorial approach investigating WES, copy number variation, and RNAseq would be needed.

Overall, most studies support that anti-CTLA-4 and anti-PD-1 modulate TCR repertoire clonality upon treatment. This strengthens the notion that tumor-specific T-cell populations are affected by CTLA-4 or PD-1 inhibition. In summary, most studies support that anti-CTLA-4 induces an expansion of clones in a non-specific manner and, therefore, broadens the TCR repertoire. On the other hand, anti-PD-1 seems to favor the proliferation of fewer specific clones giving rise to a more skewed repertoire, thereby suggesting that the baseline TCR repertoire of the patients plays a role in the response to the treatment. However, for the moment, those predictions arise mainly from early on-treatment evaluations that examined the evolution of the repertoire from baseline, as we are not yet able to precisely pinpoint the tumor-specific clones that, once clonally expanded, will facilitate tumor elimination. It is also important to highlight that the mode of action of the current immunotherapies are still debated and we do not fully comprehend their overall impact on different immune cell subpopulations. As a result, it is difficult to assess the global impact of the drugs on the immune response by investigating specific mechanisms individually. This is why high-throughput techniques discussed here are powerful emerging tools, which will allow us to elucidate this problem by looking at numerous markers simultaneously. The more we increase our knowledge of exact mechanisms, the better we will be able to exploit the therapies by using them in a targeted/patient-specific manner. Interesting work by Twyman-Saint et al. combining anti-CTLA-4, anti-PD-1 and radiotherapy, underpins this assertion (59).

To our knowledge, despite the great potential held by CyTOF technology, to date, no research was published on the analysis of human melanoma tumor samples in the context of immunotherapies. One should however expect to see more forthcoming data, thanks to a novel exciting add-on technology that is starting to emerge. Indeed, a new laser system can be coupled to the CyTOF device which allows for imaging mass cytometry (60). That is, the detection of metal-labeled antibodies, as in standard CyTOF analysis, but performed on tissue sections by using multiplexed ion beam imaging. This state of the art technology will allow, not only to assess a high range of markers at the same time, but also to obtain spatial resolution and warrant a very comprehensive analysis of the cell–cell interaction in the tumor microenvironment. New developments of the system should soon facilitate the analysis of tumor samples in a similar fashion, while gaining spatial resolution to better interrogate the role of spatial interactions in immunotherapy response (with high throughput) (61).

In conclusion, the use of NGS and CyTOF has great potential to discover novel biomarkers for immunotherapy and the studies discussed above show exciting promises, but need to be further validated before clinical application. New prospective trials with large cohorts could include these technologies as a biomarker discovery platform and could validate many of these findings. In parallel, new algorithms to integrate multiple high dimensional datasets are being developed for a combinatorial biomarker approach, which could use these existing datasets as a training model. As NGS is becoming a standard service in many clinics, the development of next generation biomarkers should ultimately improve the stratification of patients for immunotherapy and thereby extend OS for these patients.

AUTHOR CONTRIBUTIONS

SH, ML, and PC conceptualized the manuscript and oversaw all aspects of its completing including writing, figure design, and literature review.

REFERENCES

1. Luke JJ, Flaherty KT, Ribas A, Long GV. Targeted agents and immunotherapies: optimizing outcomes in melanoma. *Nat Rev Clin Oncol* (2017) 14(8):463–82. doi:10.1038/nrclinonc.2017.43
2. Robert C, Long GV, Brady B, Dutriaux C, Maio M, Mortier L, et al. Nivolumab in previously untreated melanoma without BRAF mutation. *N Engl J Med* (2015) 372(4):320–30. doi:10.1056/NEJMoa1412082
3. Maio M, Grob JJ, Aamdal S, Bondarenko I, Robert C, Thomas L, et al. Five-year survival rates for treatment-naive patients with advanced melanoma who received ipilimumab plus dacarbazine in a phase III trial. *J Clin Oncol* (2015) 33(10):1191–6. doi:10.1200/JCO.2014.56.6018
4. Hodi FS, O'Day SJ, McDermott DF, Weber RW, Sosman JA, Haanen JB, et al. Improved survival with ipilimumab in patients with metastatic melanoma. *N Engl J Med* (2010) 363(8):711–23. doi:10.1056/NEJMoa1003466
5. Robert C, Thomas L, Bondarenko I, O'Day S, Weber J, Garbe C, et al. Ipilimumab plus dacarbazine for previously untreated metastatic melanoma. *N Engl J Med* (2011) 364(26):2517–26. doi:10.1056/NEJMoa1104621
6. Wolchok JD, Chiarion-Sileni V, Gonzalez R, Rutkowski P, Grob JJ, Cowey CL, et al. Overall survival with combined nivolumab and ipilimumab in advanced melanoma. *N Engl J Med* (2017) 377:1345–56. doi:10.1056/NEJMoa1709684
7. Robert C, Schachter J, Long GV, Arance A, Grob JJ, Mortier L, et al. Pembrolizumab versus ipilimumab in advanced melanoma. *N Engl J Med* (2015) 372(26):2521–32. doi:10.1056/NEJMoa1503093
8. Gardner D, Jeffery LE, Sansom DM. Understanding the CD28/CTLA-4 (CD152) pathway and its implications for costimulatory blockade. *Am J Transplant* (2014) 14(9):1985–91. doi:10.1111/ajt.12834
9. Dong H, Zhu G, Tamada K, Chen L. B7-H1, a third member of the B7 family, co-stimulates T-cell proliferation and interleukin-10 secretion. *Nat Med* (1999) 5(12):1365–9. doi:10.1038/70932
10. Latchman Y, Wood CR, Chernova T, Chaudhary D, Borde M, Chernova I, et al. PD-L2 is a second ligand for PD-1 and inhibits T cell activation. *Nat Immunol* (2001) 2(3):261–8. doi:10.1038/85330

11. Ishida Y, Agata Y, Shibahara K, Honjo T. Induced expression of PD-1, a novel member of the immunoglobulin gene superfamily, upon programmed cell death. *EMBO J* (1992) 11(11):3887–95.
12. Michot JM, Bigenwald C, Champiat S, Collins M, Carbonnel F, Postel-Vinay S, et al. Immune-related adverse events with immune checkpoint blockade: a comprehensive review. *Eur J Cancer* (2016) 54:139–48. doi:10.1016/j.ejca.2015.11.016
13. Balch CM, Gershenwald JE, Soong SJ, Thompson JF, Atkins MB, Byrd DR, et al. Final version of 2009 AJCC melanoma staging and classification. *J Clin Oncol* (2009) 27(36):6199–206. doi:10.1200/JCO.2009.23.4799
14. Fantin VR, St-Pierre J, Leder P. Attenuation of LDH-A expression uncovers a link between glycolysis, mitochondrial physiology, and tumor maintenance. *Cancer Cell* (2006) 9(6):425–34. doi:10.1016/j.ccr.2006.04.023
15. Gershenwald JE, Scolyer RA, Hess KR, Sondak VK, Long GV, Ross MI, et al. Melanoma staging: evidence-based changes in the American Joint Committee on Cancer eighth edition cancer staging manual. *CA Cancer J Clin* (2017) 67(6):472–92. doi:10.3322/caac.21409
16. Kelderman S, Heemskerk B, van Tinteren H, van den Brom RR, Hospers GA, van den Eertwegh AJ, et al. Lactate dehydrogenase as a selection criterion for ipilimumab treatment in metastatic melanoma. *Cancer Immunol Immunother* (2014) 63(5):449–58. doi:10.1007/s00262-014-1528-9
17. Nosrati A, Tsai KK, Goldinger SM, Tumeh P, Grimes B, Loo K, et al. Evaluation of clinicopathological factors in PD-1 response: derivation and validation of a prediction scale for response to PD-1 monotherapy. *Br J Cancer* (2017) 116(9):1141–7. doi:10.1038/bjc.2017.70
18. Jessurun CAC, Vos JAM, Limpens J, Luiten RM. Biomarkers for response of melanoma patients to immune checkpoint inhibitors: a systematic review. *Front Oncol* (2017) 7:233. doi:10.3389/fonc.2017.00233
19. Diem S, Kasenda B, Spain L, Martin-Liberal J, Marconcini R, Gore M, et al. Serum lactate dehydrogenase as an early marker for outcome in patients treated with anti-PD-1 therapy in metastatic melanoma. *Br J Cancer* (2016) 114(3):256–61. doi:10.1038/bjc.2015.467
20. Kaskel P, Berking C, Sander S, Volkenandt M, Peter RU, Krähn G. S-100 protein in peripheral blood: a marker for melanoma metastases: a prospective

2-center study of 570 patients with melanoma. *J Am Acad Dermatol* (1999) 41(6):962–9. doi:10.1016/S0190-9622(99)70254-9

21. Diem S, Kasenda B, Martin-Liberal J, Lee A, Chauhan D, Gore M, et al. Prognostic score for patients with advanced melanoma treated with ipilimumab. *Eur J Cancer* (2015) 51(18):2785–91. doi:10.1016/j.ejca.2015.09.007

22. Simeone E, Gentilcore G, Giannarelli D, Grimaldi AM, Caraco C, Curvietto M, et al. Immunological and biological changes during ipilimumab treatment and their potential correlation with clinical response and survival in patients with advanced melanoma. *Cancer Immunol Immunother* (2014) 63(7):675–83. doi:10.1007/s00262-014-1545-8

23. Li Z, Feng J, Sun X. Is C-reactive protein a specific marker in melanoma? *J Clin Oncol* (2015) 33(31):3673–4. doi:10.1200/JCO.2015.62.2696

24. Nonomura Y, Otsuka A, Nakashima C, Seidel JA, Kitoh A, Dainichi T, et al. Peripheral blood Th9 cells are a possible pharmacodynamic biomarker of nivolumab treatment efficacy in metastatic melanoma patients. *Oncoimmunology* (2016) 5(12):e1248327. doi:10.1080/2162402X.2016.1248327

25. Yuan J, Hegde PS, Clynes R, Foukas PG, Harari A, Kleen TO, et al. Novel technologies and emerging biomarkers for personalized cancer immunotherapy. *J Immunother Cancer* (2016) 4:3. doi:10.1186/s40425-016-0107-3

26. Altman DG, McShane LM, Sauerbrei W, Taube SE. Reporting Recommendations for tumor marker prognostic studies (REMARK): explanation and elaboration. *PLoS Med* (2012) 9(5):e1001216. doi:10.1371/journal.pmed.1001216

27. Johnson DB, Sosman JA. Therapeutic advances and treatment options in metastatic melanoma. *JAMA Oncol* (2015) 1(3):380–6. doi:10.1001/jamaoncol.2015.0565

28. Alexandrov LB, Nik-Zainal S, Wedge DC, Aparicio SA, Behjati S, Biankin AV, et al. Signatures of mutational processes in human cancer. *Nature* (2013) 500(7463):415–21. doi:10.1038/nature12477

29. Hayward NK, Wilmott JS, Waddell N, Johansson PA, Field MA, Nones K, et al. Whole-genome landscapes of major melanoma subtypes. *Nature* (2017) 545(7653):175–80. doi:10.1038/nature22071

30. Cancer Genome Atlas Network. Genomic classification of cutaneous melanoma. *Cell* (2015) 161(7):1681–96. doi:10.1016/j.cell.2015.05.044

31. Snyder A, Makarov V, Merghoub T, Yuan J, Zaretsky JM, Desrichard A, et al. Genetic basis for clinical response to CTLA-4 blockade in melanoma. *N Engl J Med* (2014) 371(23):2189–99. doi:10.1056/NEJMoa1406498

32. Van Allen EM, Miao D, Schilling B, Shukla SA, Blank C, Zimmer L, et al. Genomic correlates of response to CTLA-4 blockade in metastatic melanoma. *Science* (2015) 350(6257):207–11. doi:10.1126/science.aad0095

33. Riaz N, Havel JJ, Kendall SM, Makarov V, Walsh LA, Desrichard A, et al. Recurrent SERPINB3 and SERPINB4 mutations in patients who respond to anti-CTLA4 immunotherapy. *Nat Genet* (2016) 48(11):1327–9. doi:10.1038/ng.3677

34. Friedlander P, Wassmann K, Christenfeld AM, Fisher D, Kyi C, Kirkwood JM, et al. Whole-blood RNA transcript-based models can predict clinical response in two large independent clinical studies of patients with advanced melanoma treated with the checkpoint inhibitor, tremelimumab. *J Immunother Cancer* (2017) 5(1):67. doi:10.1186/s40425-017-0272-z

35. Hugo W, Zaretsky JM, Sun L, Song C, Moreno BH, Hu-Lieskovan S, et al. Genomic and transcriptomic features of response to anti-PD-1 therapy in metastatic melanoma. *Cell* (2016) 165(1):35–44. doi:10.1016/j.cell.2016.02.065

36. Zaretsky JM, Garcia-Diaz A, Shin DS, Escuin-Ordinas H, Hugo W, Hu-Lieskovan S, et al. Mutations associated with acquired resistance to PD-1 blockade in melanoma. *N Engl J Med* (2016) 375(9):819–29. doi:10.1056/NEJMoa1604958

37. Shin DS, Zaretsky JM, Escuin-Ordinas H, Garcia-Diaz A, Hu-Lieskovan S, Kalbasi A, et al. Primary resistance to PD-1 blockade mediated by JAK1/2 mutations. *Cancer Discov* (2017) 7(2):188–201. doi:10.1158/2159-8290.CD-16-1223

38. Roh W, Chen PL, Reuben A, Spencer CN, Prieto PA, Miller JP, et al. Integrated molecular analysis of tumor biopsies on sequential CTLA-4 and PD-1 blockade reveals markers of response and resistance. *Sci Transl Med* (2017) 9(379). doi:10.1126/scitranslmed.aah3560

39. Mohammad KS, Javelaud D, Fournier PG, Niewolna M, McKenna CR, Peng XH, et al. TGF-beta-RI kinase inhibitor SD-208 reduces the development and progression of melanoma bone metastases. *Cancer Res* (2011) 71(1):175–84. doi:10.1158/0008-5472.CAN-10-2651

40. Davoli T, Uno H, Wooten EC, Elledge SJ. Tumor aneuploidy correlates with markers of immune evasion and with reduced response to immunotherapy. *Science* (2017) 355(6322):eaaf8399. doi:10.1126/science.aaf8399

41. Jenkins MK, Chu HH, McLachlan JB, Moon JJ. On the composition of the preimmune repertoire of T cells specific for peptide-major histocompatibility complex ligands. *Annu Rev Immunol* (2010) 28:275–94. doi:10.1146/annurev-immunol-030409-101253

42. Qi Q, Liu Y, Cheng Y, Glanville J, Zhang D, Lee JY, et al. Diversity and clonal selection in the human T-cell repertoire. *Proc Natl Acad Sci U S A* (2014) 111(36):13139–44. doi:10.1073/pnas.1409155111

43. Laydon DJ, Bangham CR, Asquith B. Estimating T-cell repertoire diversity: limitations of classical estimators and a new approach. *Philos Trans R Soc Lond B Biol Sci* (2015) 370(1675):20140291. doi:10.1098/rstb.2014.0291

44. Rosati E, Dowds CM, Liaskou E, Henriksen EKK, Karlsen TH, Franke A. Overview of methodologies for T-cell receptor repertoire analysis. *BMC Biotechnol* (2017) 17(1):61. doi:10.1186/s12896-017-0379-9

45. Robert L, Tsoi J, Wang X, Emerson R, Homet B, Chodon T, et al. CTLA4 blockade broadens the peripheral T-cell receptor repertoire. *Clin Cancer Res* (2014) 20(9):2424–32. doi:10.1158/1078-0432.CCR-13-2648

46. Robert L, Harview C, Emerson R, Wang X, Mok S, Homet B, et al. Distinct immunological mechanisms of CTLA-4 and PD-1 blockade revealed by analyzing TCR usage in blood lymphocytes. *Oncoimmunology* (2014) 3:e29244. doi:10.4161/onci.29244

47. Cha E, Klinger M, Hou Y, Cummings C, Ribas A, Faham M, et al. Improved survival with T cell clonotype stability after anti-CTLA-4 treatment in cancer patients. *Sci Transl Med* (2014) 6(238):238ra70. doi:10.1126/scitranslmed.3008211

48. Postow MA, Manuel M, Wong P, Yuan J, Dong Z, Liu C, et al. Peripheral T cell receptor diversity is associated with clinical outcomes following ipilimumab treatment in metastatic melanoma. *J Immunother Cancer* (2015) 3:23. doi:10.1186/s40425-015-0070-4

49. Tumeh PC, Harview CL, Yearley JH, Shintaku IP, Taylor EJ, Robert L, et al. PD-1 blockade induces responses by inhibiting adaptive immune resistance. *Nature* (2014) 515(7528):568–71. doi:10.1038/nature13954

50. Johnson DB, Frampton GM, Rioth MJ, Yusko E, Xu Y, Guo X, et al. Targeted next generation sequencing identifies markers of response to PD-1 blockade. *Cancer Immunol Res* (2016) 4(11):959–67. doi:10.1158/2326-6066.CIR-16-0143

51. Inoue H, Park JH, Kiyotani K, Zewde M, Miyashita A, Jinnin M, et al. Intratumoral expression levels of PD-L1, GZMA, and HLA-A along with oligoclonal T cell expansion associate with response to nivolumab in metastatic melanoma. *Oncoimmunology* (2016) 5(9):e1204507. doi:10.1080/2162402X.2016.1204507

52. Riaz N, Havel JJ, Makarov V, Desrichard A, Urba WJ, Sims JS, et al. Tumor and microenvironment evolution during immunotherapy with nivolumab. *Cell* (2017) 171(4):934–949.e15. doi:10.1016/j.cell.2017.09.028

53. Chang S, Kohrt H, Maecker HT. Monitoring the immune competence of cancer patients to predict outcome. *Cancer Immunol Immunother* (2014) 63(7):713–9. doi:10.1007/s00262-014-1521-3

54. Das R, Verma R, Sznol M, Boddupalli CS, Gettinger SN, Kluger H, et al. Combination therapy with anti-CTLA-4 and anti-PD-1 leads to distinct immunologic changes in vivo. *J Immunol* (2015) 194(3):950–9. doi:10.4049/jimmunol.1401686

55. Hiniker SM, Reddy SA, Maecker HT, Subrahmanyam PB, Rosenberg-Hasson Y, Swetter SM, et al. A prospective clinical trial combining radiation therapy with systemic immunotherapy in metastatic melanoma. *Int J Radiat Oncol Biol Phys* (2016) 96(3):578–88. doi:10.1016/j.ijrobp.2016.07.005

56. Wistuba-Hamprecht K, Martens A, Weide B, Teng KW, Zelba H, Guffart E, et al. Establishing high dimensional immune signatures from peripheral blood via mass cytometry in a discovery cohort of stage IV melanoma patients. *J Immunol* (2017) 198(2):927–36. doi:10.4049/jimmunol.1600875

57. Takeuchi Y, Tanemura A, Tada Y, Katayama I, Kumanogoh A, Nishikawa H. Clinical response to PD-1 blockade correlates with a sub-fraction of peripheral central memory CD4+ T cells in patients with malignant melanoma. *Int Immunol* (2018) 30(1):13–22. doi:10.1093/intimm/dxx073

58. Krieg C, Nowicka M, Guglietta S, Schindler S, Hartmann FJ, Weber LM, et al. High-dimensional single cell analysis predicts response to anti-PD-1 immunotherapy. *Nat Med* (2018) 24(2):144–53. doi:10.1038/nm.4466

59. Twyman-Saint Victor C, Rech AJ, Maity A, Rengan R, Pauken KE, Stelekati E, et al. Radiation and dual checkpoint blockade activate non-redundant immune mechanisms in cancer. *Nature* (2015) 520(7547):373–7. doi:10.1038/nature14292

60. Schapiro D, Jackson HW, Raghuraman S, Fischer JR, Zanotelli VRT, Schulz D, et al. histoCAT: analysis of cell phenotypes and interactions in multiplex image cytometry data. *Nat Methods* (2017) 14(9):873–6. doi:10.1038/nmeth.4391

61. Di Palma S, Bodenmiller B. Unraveling cell populations in tumors by single-cell mass cytometry. *Curr Opin Biotechnol* (2015) 31:122–9. doi:10.1016/j.copbio.2014.07.004

13

Biomarkers for Immune Checkpoint Inhibitor-Mediated Tumor Response and Adverse Events

*Yoshiyuki Nakamura**

Department of Dermatology, Faculty of Medicine, University of Tsukuba, Tsukuba, Japan

*Correspondence:
Yoshiyuki Nakamura
ynakamura-tuk@umin.ac.jp

In the last decade, inhibitors targeting immune checkpoint molecules such as cytotoxic T-lymphocyte antigen 4 (CTLA-4), programmed cell death 1 (PD-1), and programmed cell death-ligand 1 (PD-L1) brought about a major paradigm shift in cancer treatment. These immune checkpoint inhibitors (ICIs) improved the overall survival of a variety of cancer such as malignant melanoma and non-small lung cancer. In addition, numerous clinical trials for additional indication of ICIs including adjuvant and neo-adjuvant therapies are also currently ongoing. Therefore, more and more patients will receive ICIs in the future. However, despite the improved outcome of the cancer treatment by ICIs, the efficacy remains still limited and tumor regression have not been obtained in many cancer patients. In addition, treatment with ICIs is also associated with substantial toxicities, described as immune-related adverse events (irAEs). Therefore, biomarkers to predict tumor response and occurrence of irAEs by the treatment with ICIs are required to avoid overtreatment of ICIs and minimize irAEs development. Whereas, numerous factors have been reported as potential biomarkers for tumor response to ICIs, factors for predicting irAE have been less reported. In this review, we show recent advances in the understanding of biomarkers for tumor response and occurrence of irAEs in cancer patients treated with ICIs.

Keywords: immune check point inhibitor, adverse event (AE), PD-1, CTLA- 4, tumor response

INTRODUCTION

The recent development of immune checkpoint inhibitors (ICIs) has led to dramatic advances in cancer therapy. Ipilimumab is a monoclonal antibody to cytotoxic T-lymphocyte antigen 4 (CTLA-4), an inhibitory receptor expressed by both conventional and regulatory T cells (Tregs) and suppresses T cell activation by competing with CD28 to bind CD80/86. Ipilimumab not only activates conventional T cells at the initial stage of maturation but also may show antibody-dependent cell-mediated lysis of the Tregs that play a vital role in suppressing the antitumor immune response (1, 2). Programmed cell death 1 (PD-1) is an inhibitory receptor expressed mainly by activated T cells and its ligand, PD-L1, is widely expressed in cell types as diverse as epithelial cells, immune cells, and cancer cells. Both anti-PD-1 antibodies (nivolumab and pembrolizumab) and anti-PD-L1 antibodies (atezolizumab, durvalumab, and avelumab) exert antitumor effects by activating previously primed T cells which have lost effector and proliferative functions (3). ICIs firstly demonstrated efficacy for patients with advanced melanoma (4–6) and subsequently in other cancers, such as non-small cell lung cancer (NSCLC) and renal cell carcinoma (7–9). A recent clinical trial revealed that adjuvant therapies with anti-PD-1 antibodies prolonged recurrence-free survival in resected high-risk melanoma (10–12). Moreover, there are currently ongoing trials for neoadjuvant therapies with anti-PD-1 antibodies in high risk resectable melanoma (11, 13). Numerous clinical trials testing additional indications of ICIs for other cancers are also ongoing (14, 15). Therefore, an ever-increasing number of patients will receive ICIs in the near future.

However, despite an improved overall survival (OS) with ICIs, the efficacy remains limited and tumor regression has not been universally achieved (16). In addition, use of ICIs may induce unique side effects, described as immune-related adverse events (irAEs). In a previous melanoma phase III clinical trial, patients who received nivolumab alone ($n = 313$), ipilimumab alone ($n = 311$) or nivolumab plus ipilimumab ($n = 313$) saw irAEs of grade 3 or 4 occurring at a rate of 21, 28, and 59%, respectively, and four patients died due to severe irAEs (16). Therefore, biomarkers to predict tumor response and irAE occurrence due to ICIs are necessary to gauge the benefits that each patient will obtain for avoiding overtreatment and minimizing irAEs. Here, we review recent advances in the understanding of biomarkers for tumor response and irAE occurrences.

Biomarkers for Tumor Response (Table 1)

Numerous factors have been reported as potential biomarkers for objective response rate (ORR), progression free survival (PFS) or OS. However, non-specific factors, which are associated with tumor responses to not only ICIs but also other therapies (such as traditional chemotherapies), can confound the use of these biomarkers. Therefore, specificity as well as correlative strength should be considered in choosing ICIs over other therapies.

Sex

Several studies have demonstrated that sex differences are associated with anti-tumor immune responses (70, 71). Although many clinical studies did not show a correlation between sex and tumor response to ICIs, meta-analyses with larger numbers of melanoma and NSCLC patients who were treated with ICIs revealed that both the PFS and OS of male patients were significantly longer than those of female patients (17). Based on a subtype analysis, sex differences in OS were greater in melanoma patients than NSCLC patients. In addition, in the anti-CTLA-4 antibodies group, the OS difference between male and female was greater than in the anti-PD-1 antibodies group. In line with this result, another study demonstrated that males were significantly associated with better ORR in melanoma patients treated with anti-PD-1 antibodies (18). Therefore, males seem to benefit more from ICIs than females do although the mechanism behind this effect has yet to be clarified.

Age

A recent preclinical study demonstrated that tumor response to anti-PD-1 antibodies in aged mice was significantly increased compared to younger mice, an effect attributed to the lower proportion of Tregs in aged mice (72). Consistent with these results, the tumor response to pembrolizumab in melanoma patients over age 60 was significantly higher than those under 60 years and the likelihood of response increased with age (72).

Similarly, Nosrati et al showed that ages older than 65 years correlated with better ORR in melanoma patients treated with anti-PD-1 antibodies (18). However, opposite results have also been reported and a meta-analysis by Nishijima et al revealed a correlation between ages younger than 75 years with better ORR in patients treated with ICIs (19). Therefore, further studies are needed to evaluate the usefulness of age as a biomarker for ICI response.

Tumor Size

Huang et al. reported that reinvigoration of exhausted CD8 T cells (T_{ex}-cell) positively correlated with tumor size and the ratio of T_{ex}-cell reinvigoration to tumor size was significantly associated with better ORR and longer OS in melanoma patients treated with pembrolizumab (73), indicating that tumor size is a predictive factor for poor response to ICI treatments. Indeed, another study demonstrated that tumor size was independently associated with OS in melanoma patients treated with pembrolizumab although it was associated with many other clinical factors (20). Therefore, early detection of metastatic lesions may be important for better response to ICIs.

Immune Cell Infiltration

Because ICIs activate the immune response to cancer, infiltration of immune cells, including T cells, into tumors may induce tumor regression following treatment. Generally, higher numbers of tumor infiltrating lymphocytes (TILs) have been a favorable prognostic factor in many types of cancers, such as melanoma and colorectal cancer (74, 75). Similarly, Tumeh et al revealed that presence of CD8[+] TILs at the invasive margin, which was associated with higher PD-1/PD-L1 expression, correlated with better tumor response in melanoma patients treated with pembrolizumab (21). An increase in CD8[+] TILs from baseline to post-treatment biopsy, specifically at the tumor center and invasive margin, has been also significantly associated with tumor regression (21). Therefore, both baseline and post-treatment TIL numbers may be important biomarkers for predicting tumor response to ICIs.

Surface Molecules and Their Related Molecules
PD-L1

Since PD-L1 is a ligand of PD-1 and serves an inhibitory signal in PD-1 expressing cells, the expression of PD-L1 in tumor environments is speculated to correlate with better response in patients treated with anti-PD-1 antibodies. Indeed, in melanoma clinical trials with anti-PD-1 antibodies, better outcomes were observed in patients with positive PD-L1 expression in tumors although the definition of positive or negative expression differed across studies (22, 23). Higher PD-L1 expression has also been associated with better outcomes in NSCLC patients treated with anti-PD-1 antibodies (24). In addition, a recent clinical trial demonstrated that combinations of nivolumab with ipilimumab showed a better OS than nivolumab monotherapy in melanoma patients with PD-L1<1%, whereas the OS was comparable between the 2 treatment groups in patients with PD-L1≥1%, suggesting that anti-PD-1 antibody efficacy is largely dependent

TABLE 1 | Biomarkers for tumor responses.

Biomarkers	Cancer type	Patient number	Treatment	Key data and clinical significance	References	Evidence level
Sex	Melanoma, NSCLC	6,096	Ipilimumab, anti-PD-1 antibodies	PFS and OS of male patients were significantly longer than those of female patients.	Wu et al. (17)	1a
Age	Melanoma	315	Anti-PD-1 antibodies	Males were significantly associated with better ORR. Ages older than 65 years correlated with better ORR.	Nosrati et al. (18)	2b
	Melanoma, prostate cancer, NSCLC, RCC	5,265	Anti-CTLA-4 antibodies, anti-PD-1 antibodies	Ages younger than 75 years correlated with better ORR.	Nishijima et al. (19)	1a
Tumor size	Melanoma	459	Pembrolizumab	Tumor size was independently associated with OS, suggesting that early detection of metastatic lesions may be important for better response to ICIs.	Joseph et al. (20)	2b
TILs	Melanoma	46	Pembrolizumab	High density of CD8+ TILs at the invasive margin correlated with better tumor response. An increase in CD8+ TILs from baseline to post-treatment was associated with tumor regression.	Tumeh et al. (21)	2b
PD L1 expression in tumors	Melanoma	277	Nivolumab after treatment with anti-CTLA-4 antibodies	Better ORR were observed in patients with positive PD-L1 expression in tumors.	Weber et al. (22)	1b
	Melanoma	451	Pembrolizumab	Better PFS and OS were observed in patients with positive PD-L1 expression in tumors.	Daud et al. (23)	2b
	NSCLC	410	Pembrolizumab + chemotherapy	Higher PD-L1 expression was associated with better PFS and OS.	Gandhi et al. (24)	1b
ICOS	Melanoma	14	Ipilimumab	Increased expression of ICOS on CD4+ T cells that is sustained for more than 12 weeks correlated with improved OS.	Carthon et al. (25)	4
TIM-3	Melanoma	67	Ipilimumab	Increased TIM-3 expression on circulating T and NK cells prior to and during treatment was associated with shorter OS.	Tallerico et al. (26)	2b
IDO	Melanoma	82	Ipilimumab	Baseline IDO expression in tumor tissue assessed by IHC correlated with better ORR.	Hamid et al. (27)	1b
	NSCLC	26	Nivolumab	IDO activity as assessed by serum kynurenine/tryptophan ratio was negatively associated with longer PFS and OS.	Botticelli et al. (28)	2b
Soluble CTLA-4	Melanoma	113	Ipilimumab	Higher serum levels of soluble CTLA-4 at baseline had both better ORR and OS.	Pistillo et al. (29)	2b
Soluble PD-L1	Melanoma	446	Ipilimumab, anti-PD-1 antibodies	Higher levels of baseline soluble PD-L1 were associated with worse response. Increases in soluble PD-1 after treatment was associated with favorable clinical responses.	Zhou et al. (30)	2b
	NSCLC	39	Nivolumab	Higher levels of baseline soluble PD-L1 were associated with shorter OS.	Okuma et al. (31)	2b
Soluble CD163	Melanoma	59	Nivolumab	Serum levels of soluble CD163 were increased after 6 weeks in responders compared to non-responders after initial treatment for cutaneous melanoma.	Fujimura et al. (32)	2b
Soluble NKG2D	Melanoma	194	Anti-CTLA-4 antibodies, anti-PD-1 antibodies	Higher levels of circulating soluble ULBP-1, soluble ULBP-2 and LDH at baseline were independent factors of shorter OS.	Maccalli et al. (33)	2b

(Continued)

TABLE 1 | Continued

Biomarkers	Cancer type	Patient number	Treatment	Key data and clinical significance	References	Evidence level
IFN-γ	Melanoma	45	Ipilimumab	The post-treatment expression levels of IFN-γ responsive genes in tumor tissues were associated with longer OS.	Ji et al. (34)	2b
	NSCLC	97	Durvalumab	High levels of pre-treatment IFN-γ expression and its related genes in tumor tissues were associated with longer OS.	Higgs et al. (35)	2b
	Melanoma	43	Atezolizumab	High expression of IFN-γ and CXCL-9 was associated with better ORR.	Herbst et al. (36)	2b
TNF-α	Melanoma	15	Nivolumab	Patients who showed complete remission, partial remission or long-term stable disease due to nivolumab response had lower serum levels of TNF-α compared to non-responders.	Tanaka et al (37)	4
Lymphocyte counts	Melanoma	209	Ipilimumab	Higher levels of relative lymphocyte counts at baseline were associated with longer OS.	Martens et al. (38)	2b
	Melanoma	50	Ipilimumab	Absolute lymphocyte counts after treatment were associated with longer OS.	Wilgenhof et al. (39)	2b
Eosinophil counts	Melanoma	98	Nivolumab	Absolute lymphocyte counts after treatment correlated with better OS.	Nakamura et al. (40)	2b
	Melanoma	209	Ipilimumab	High absolute and relative eosinophil counts at baseline were associated with a longer OS.	Martens et al. (38)	2b
	Melanoma	616	Pembrolizumab	Relative eosinophil counts at baseline were an independent factor for longer OS and better ORR.	Weide et al. (41)	2b
	Melanoma	59	Ipilimumab	Early increases in absolute eosinophil counts from baseline during treatment were an independent factor for better responses.	Gebhardt et al. (42)	2b
NLR	Melanoma	90	Nivolumab	NLR was associated with poor tumor response.	Fujisawa et al. (43)	2b
	NSCLC	175	Nivolumab	NLR was associated with poor tumor response.	Bagley et al. (44)	2b
	Melanoma	44	Anti-PD-1 antibodies	NLR was the only factor associated with both poor ORR and shorter PFS.	Nakmaura et al. (45)	2b
Tregs	Melanoma	209	Ipilimumab	High levels of circulating Tregs at baseline were associated with longer OS.	Martens et al. (38)	2b
	Melanoma	95	Ipilimumab	Decreasing levels of circulating Tregs were associated with better responses.	Simeone et al. (46)	2b
MDSC	Melanoma	92	Ipilimumab	The baseline frequency of MDSCs in blood correlated with shorter OS.	Weber et al. (47)	2b
	Melanoma	83	Nivolumab	The baseline frequency of MDSCs in blood correlated with shorter OS.	Kitano et al. (48)	2b
	Prostate cancer	28	Ipilimumab plus a cancer vaccine	The baseline frequency of circulating MDSCs correlated with shorter OS.	Santegoets et al. (49)	2b
LDH	Melanoma	73	Ipilimumab	High baseline LDH was associated with poor anti-tumor response.	Delyon et al. (50)	2b
CRP	Melanoma	95	Ipilimumab	A decrease or no change in serum levels of CRP from baseline was associated with longer OS.	Simeone et al. (46)	2b
Mutation burden	Melanoma	64	Ipilimumab	High mutation burden was associated with a longer OS.	Synder et al. (51)	2b
	Melanoma	150	Ipilimumab	High mutation burden was associated with tumor responses.	Allen et al. (52)	2b
MSI	Colorectal cancer	74	Nivolumab	A high response to anti-PD-1 antibodies in colorectal cancer with high levels of MSI compared to traditional treatments was observed.	Overman et al. (53)	2b
HLA	Melanoma	13	Nivolumab	HLA-A expression in pre-treatment was elevated in responders compared to non-responders.	Inoue et al. (54)	4

(Continued)

TABLE 1 | Continued

Biomarkers	Cancer type	Patient number	Treatment	Key data and clinical significance	References	Evidence level
T cell repertoire	Melanoma	69	Nivolumab	HLA-A26 correlated with tumor response to nivolumab in Japanese melanoma patients.	Ishida et al. (55)	2b
	Melanoma	12	Ipilimumab	Both higher richness and evenness in pre-treatment peripheral blood were associated with a better response.	Postow et al. (56)	4
Gut microbiome	Melanoma	46	Pembrolizumab	TILs with less diversity were associated with clinical response.	Tumeh et al. (21)	2b
	Melanoma	26	Ipilimumab	Patients whose baseline microbiota was enriched with *Faecalibacterium* genus and other Firmicutes showed a longer PFS and CS than those whose baseline microbiota was enriched with *Bacteroides*.	Chaput et al. (57)	2b
	Melanoma	43	Anti-PD-1 antibodies	A higher diversity of gut microbiome and relative abundance of *Ruminococcaceae* family bacteria correlated with better ORR and longer PFS.	Gopalakrishnan et al. (58)	2b
	NSCLC, RCC	100	Anti-PD-1 antibodies	The relative abundance of *Akkermansia muciniphila* was associated with better responses.	Routy et al. (59)	2b
ctDNA	Melanoma	76	Anti-PD-1 antibodies	Patients with a persistently elevated cDNA during the treatment showed a worse response and shorter PFS and OS. ctDNA may be a useful marker for differentiating pseudoprogression from true progression during immune checkpoint inhibitor treatment.	Lee et al. (60, 61)	2b
Exosomal molecules	Melanoma	44	Pembrolizumab	Lower baseline levels and increases during the treatment in exosomal PD-L1 protein correlated with tumor response.	Chen et al. (62)	2b
	Melanoma, NSCLC	26	Anti-PD-1 antibodies	Baseline exosomal PD-L1 mRNA expression was higher in responders, and exosomal PD-L1 mRNA expression in responders was decreased after treatment whereas it was stable in stabilized patients and increased in progressive disease cases.	Re et al. (63)	2b
	Melanoma	59	Ipilimumab	Increased exosomal PD-1 and CD28 levels in T cells were associated with longer PFS and OS while increased exosomal CD80 and CD86 in dendritic cells correlated with longer PFS.	Tucci et al. (64)	2b
irAE development	RCC	40	Ipilimumab	Overall irAEs were associated with tumor responses.	Yang et al. (65)	2b
	NSCLC	43	Nivolumab	Early development of all irAEs was associated with better ORR and longer PFS.	Teraoka et al. (66)	2b
	NSCLC, RCC, HNSCC, urothelial carcinoma	142	Anti-PD-1 antibodies	Only low grade irAEs were associated with better responses.	Judo et al. (67)	2b
	Melanoma	60	Ipilimumab after nivolumab	Occurrences of endocrine irAEs were associated with longer OS.	Fujisawa et al. (68)	2b
	Melanoma	5,737	Anti-CTLA-4 antibodies, anti-PD-1 antibodies	Development of vitiligo correlated with better responses.	Teuling et al. (69)	2a

NSCLC, non-small cell lung cancer; RCC, renal cell carcinoma; HNSCC, head and neck squamous cell carcinoma; ORR, overall response rate; PFS, progression free survival; OS, overall survival; TILs, tumor infiltrating lymphocytes; ICOS, inducible T cell costimulatory; IDO, indoleamine 2,3-dioxygenase; NLR, neutrophil-to-lymphocyte ratio; Tregs, regulatory T cells; MDSC, myeloid-derived suppressor cells; MSI, microsatellite instability; HLA, human leukocyte antiger; ctDNA, circulating tumor DNA; irAE, immune-related adverse event. Evidence level was evaluated based on the following criteria; 1a, systematic review/ meta-analysis of randomized controlled trials; 1b, individual randomized controlled trials; 2a, systematic review/ meta-analysis of cohort studies; 2b, individual cohort study; 3a, systematic review/meta-analysis of case-control studies; 3b, individual case-control studies; 4, case series; 5, expert opinions.

on PD-L1 expression (16). Therefore, PD-L1 expression may be a vital factor to predict tumor response to anti-PD-1 antibodies although tumor responses can be also observed in PD-L1 negative tumors. However, issues remain for accurately assessing PD-L1 expression, including different antibodies used in each study, and the low reproducibility of pathologist evaluations (76). In addition, PD-L1 expression has been reported to vary between primary tumors and metastatic sites (77). Therefore, establishing evaluative standards for tumor PD-L1 expression will enhance its usefulness as a predictive factor.

Inducible T Cell Co-stimulator (ICOS)

ICOS is a co-stimulating molecule expressed by activated conventional T cells and regulatory T cells. A previous report demonstrated that ipilimumab treatment increases expression of ICOS on conventional CD4$^+$ T cells in both blood and tumor tissue in patients with bladder cancer (78). These CD4$^+$ ICOS$^+$ T cells produced IFNγ and could recognize tumor antigens (78). In addition, increased expression of ICOS on CD4$^+$ T cells that is sustained for more than 12 weeks has been reported to correlate with improved survival in melanoma patients treated with ipilimumab (25). Thus, ICOS expression is a potential biomarker for tumor response to ICIs although further studies are needed to establish its utility.

Other Cell Surface Molecules

Pre-clinical studies using mouse models have indicated that upregulation of alternative inhibitory molecules causes resistance to anti-PD-1 antibody therapy (79). These molecules include TIM-3, LAG-3, and VISTA are therefore suggested to serve as potential target molecules for alternative checkpoint inhibitors. They could also serve as potential biomarkers for ICI response and, indeed, increased TIM-3 expression on circulating T and NK cells prior to and during treatment has been significantly associated with shorter OS in melanoma patients treated with ipilimumab (26).

Enzymes Related to Immune Response
Indoleamine 2,3-dioxygenase (IDO)

IDO is an enzyme that converts the essential amino acid l-tryptophan into kynurenine and carries an immunosuppressive effect through multiple mechanisms (80). Kynurenine, mediated by IDO, has been shown to induce T cell apoptosis (81), and IDO-induced starvation of tryptophan mediates the conversion of naïve CD4$^+$ T cells into Tregs through GCN2 kinase activation (82). A recent study demonstrated that IDO expression levels in melanoma cells were independently associated with tumor stage (83). IDO has been also reported as a predictor of anti-tumor response by ICIs. Hamid et al showed that baseline IDO expression, as well as baseline FoxP3 expression, in tumor tissue assessed by IHC significantly correlated with better ORR in melanoma patients treated with ipilimumab (27). However, on the contrary, IDO activity as assessed by serum kynurenine/tryptophan ratio has been negatively associated with longer PFS and OS in NSCLC patients treated with nivolumab (28). Therefore, through as-yet unknown mechanisms, IDO

activity may serve as a predictive marker for outcomes, which are different dependent on the assessment.

Soluble Isoform of Surface Molecules
Soluble CTLA-4 (sCTLA-4)

Soluble CTLA-4 originates from a spliced variant of an alternative transcript that lacks the transmembrane sequence (84). It can be detected in normal human serum and higher levels of sCTLA-4 have been observed in autoimmune diseases and many types of cancers (84, 85). It can bind to CD80/86 on antigen-presenting cells and block the binding of membrane-bound CTLA-4 or CD28 on T cells, thus avoiding the downregulation of the immune activation cascade (86, 87). Pistill et al. demonstrated that higher serum levels of sCTLA-4 (>200 pg/ml) at baseline had both better ORR and OS than lower sCTLA-4 serum levels (≤200 pg/ml) in melanoma patients treated with ipilimumab (29), suggesting that serum sCTLA-4 could be a biomarker for better response to ipilimumab. It is speculated that sCTLA-4 might block the binding of membrane-bound CTLA-4 to its ligand and thus result in enhanced tumor immunity in synergy with ipilimumab.

Soluble PD-L1 (sPD-L1)

Soluble PD-L1 may result from alternative variants of the PD-L1 transcripts and cytokine treatment with IFN-α, IFN-γ, or TNF-α has been shown to increase secretion of sPD-L1 as well as expression of cell surface PD-L1 in melanoma cell lines (30). It can be detected in blood and elevated levels of circulating sPD-L1 have been associated with poor prognoses in many types of cancer (88–90). Consistent with these results, higher levels of baseline sPD-L1 have been significantly associated with worse response and shorter OS in melanoma patients treated with ICIs (30, 31). Therefore, baseline sPD-L1 could represent an immune suppressive state and poor response to ICIs although the function of sPD-L1 is not fully understood. In contrast, increases in sPD-1 after treatment with ICIs have been associated with favorable clinical responses (30). Secretion of sPD-1 after ICI treatment may be caused, at least partially, by enhanced production of cytokines such as IFN-α, IFN-γ, or TNF-α due to ICI-mediated anti-tumor response because altered levels of sPD-1 after treatment of ipilimumab corresponded to changes in the circulating cytokines (30).

Soluble CD163 (sCD163)

CD163 is a member of the scavenger receptor family and is mainly expressed by macrophages/monocytes (91). Several reports have shown that CD163$^+$ M2 macrophages comprised the main population of the tumor-associated macrophages (TAMs) that play important roles for suppressing anti-tumor immune responses and serum levels of sCD163, generated by proteolytic shedding, is thought to be a marker for TAMs (91, 92). Fujimura et al. reported that serum levels of sCD163 were significantly increased after 6 weeks in responders compared to non-responders after initial treatment with nivolumab for cutaneous melanoma (32). Interestingly, such an increase was not observed in patients with mucosal melanoma although the mechanism for this phenomenon remains unclear. These results suggest that sCD163 may serve as a biomarker for patients with specific types of cancer treated with ICIs.

Soluble NKG2D Ligands (sNKG2DLs)

NKG2D is a member of the C-type lectin-like receptors and is expressed on T, NK, and NKT cells (93, 94). The binding of NKG2D with its ligands [MHC class I chain-related gene [MIC] and UL-16-binding protein [ULBP]] elicits activation signals to NK and T cells (93–95). NKG2DLs are usually absent on the surface of normal cells but are induced by various stressors (such as DNA damage) and are often overexpressed by cancer cells (93, 95, 96). Soluble NKG2DLs, generated as result of proteolytic shedding by tumor cells, can be detected in serum and their levels have been reported to correlate with tumor progression (94, 95, 97, 98). Soluble NKG2DLs suppress anti-tumor immune responses through multiple mechanisms that include the binding and subsequent endocytosis and degradation of NKG2D on NK and T cells (97, 99, 100). A multivariate analysis conducted by Maccalli et al. showed that higher levels of circulating sULBP-1, sULBP-2, and LDH at baseline were independent factors of shorter OS in melanoma patients treated with ICIs (33). Interestingly, only LDH, but not sNKG2DLs, significantly correlated with outcomes in patients treated with other therapies, such as chemotherapies and BRAF inhibitors (33), suggesting that soluble circulating sULBP-1 and sULBP-2 may be indicators that use of ICIs is more suitable than other therapies.

Cytokines and Chemokines

IFN-γ

IFN-γ is a functionally pleiotropic cytokine that modulates the expression of numerous proteins in exposed cells (101). PD-L1 expression is also upregulated mainly controlled by IFN-γ (102). IFN-γ and its targets play crucial roles in eliminating tumor cells through direct induction of cytotoxic activities as well as enhancing the Th1-related immune response (101). The post-treatment expression levels of IFN-γ responsive genes in tumor tissues were associated with better outcomes in patients treated with ipilimumab (34). Similarly, high levels of pre-treatment IFN-γ expression and its related genes in tumor tissues are associated with longer OS in NSCLC patients treated with durvalumab (35). Similar associations between high expression of IFN-γ and CXCL-9, an IFN-γ related chemokine, with better ORR was observed in melanoma patients treated with atezolizumab (36). Therefore, high expression of IFN-γ and its associated molecules in tumor tissues may be useful biomarkers that are indicative of a better anti-tumor response to ICIs.

TNF-α

TNF-α is an inflammatory cytokine produced by various cells, including immune cells and epithelial cells. It promotes tumor growth and higher serum levels of TNF-α have been reported to be associated with poor prognoses in cancer patients (103, 104). Tanaka et al. reported that melanoma patients who showed complete remission, partial remission or long-term stable disease due to nivolumab response had significantly lower serum levels of TNF-α compared to non-responders (37).

IL-6

IL-6 is produced by a broad variety of cells, including immune cell and tumor cells. It promotes tumor progression via inhibition of cancer cell apoptosis as well as promotion of angiogenesis (105). In a previous study, higher serum IL-6 was associated with shorter OS in melanoma patients treated with IL-2-based immunotherapy (106). Although association of serum IL-6 with response to ICIs has yet to be shown, CRP, whose production is mainly controlled by IL-6 (107), has been reported to be predictive of outcomes in patients treated with ICIs, which bolsters the argument of IL-6 as a potential biomarker of anti-tumor response during ICI treatment.

Blood Cell Counts

Lymphocyte Counts

Because both CTLA-4 and PD-1 are expressed mainly on lymphocytes, several reports have pointed out the association between blood lymphocyte count and tumor response to ICIs (38–40). Martens et al showed that higher levels of relative lymphocyte counts at baseline were significantly associated with longer OS in melanoma patients treated with ipilimumab (38). In another study, absolute lymphocyte counts after 2 doses of ipilimumab were associated with longer OS in melanoma patients (39). Similarly, Nakamura et al showed that absolute lymphocyte counts at week 3 and 6 after the initial administration of nivolumab significantly correlated with better OS in melanoma patients (40). These results suggest that lymphocyte counts both at baseline and after treatment with ICIs may be useful for predicting better outcomes.

Eosinophil Counts

Eosinophils also play a crucial role in tumor destruction and recruitment of T cells into the tumor environment (108). Indeed, mice with peripheral blood eosinophilia showed substantial tumor suppression (109). In addition, multiple studies have revealed a positive correlation between increased eosinophil infiltration into tumor tissues and a favorable prognosis in many cancers (110, 111). Consistent with this idea, numerous previous studies have reported that higher blood eosinophil counts correlate with favorable outcomes in patients treated with ICIs. Marten et al. demonstrated that in melanoma patients treated with ipilimumab, high absolute, and relative eosinophil counts at baseline were associated with a longer OS (38). Similarly, a multivariate study by Weide et al. demonstrated that relative eosinophil counts at baseline were an independent factor for longer OS and better ORR in melanoma patients treated with pembrolizumab (41). In addition, Gebhardt et al. reported that early increases in absolute eosinophil counts from baseline during ipilimumab treatment were an independent factor for better responses in melanoma patients (42). Therefore, eosinophil counts at both baseline and after ICI treatment may serve as biomarkers for better tumor response.

Neutrophil-to-Lymphocyte Ratio (NLR)

Fujisawa et al. showed that baseline NLR was associated with poor tumor response in melanoma patients treated with nivolumab (43). Similar findings have also been reported in melanoma patients treated with ipilimumab and NSLC patients treated with nivolumab (41, 44). In a previously published study, our multivariate analysis revealed that NLR was the only factor associated with both poor ORR and shorter PFS in melanoma patients treated with anti-PD-1 antibodies, suggesting that NLR is a strong predictive factor for poor outcome in patients treated with ICIs (45). Given that lymphocytes play vital roles in the ICI-induced immune response to tumors while neutrophilia represents the response to systemic inflammation (112), a high NLR might represent an impaired specific immune response to tumors. However, increased turnover of tumor cells causes the release of large amounts of damage-associated molecular patterns (DAMPs) from tumor debris, leading to recruitment and activation of neutrophils (113, 114). Moreover, numerous reports have also shown that NLR serves as a biomarker for poor response to other treatments, such as chemotherapies and radiation (115, 116). Therefore, the NLR might simply represent rapidly expanding tumor cell populations rather than any potential immune response mediated by ICIs.

Tregs

Tregs, a population characterized by FoxP3$^+$ CD25$^+$ CD4$^+$ T cells, significantly suppress immune responses (117), and it has been shown that their depletion effectively eradicates tumor cells via an enhanced anti-tumor immune response (118, 119). In addition to their immune suppressive function, they may be a target for antibody dependent cellular cytotoxicity (ADCC) by ipilimumab due to their high expression levels of CTLA-4 that make Tregs sentinels for ICI-mediated anti-tumor responses. Indeed, high levels of circulating Tregs at baseline have been associated with longer OS in melanoma patients treated with ipilimumab (38). In addition, decreasing or stable levels of circulating Tregs 12 weeks after initial administration of ipilimumab significantly correlated with better disease control and longer OS than increasing Treg levels. Furthermore, similar results have been obtained in another study, with decreasing levels of circulating Tregs significantly associated with better responses to ipilimumab (46). Therefore, circulating Tregs both at baseline and after treatment with ipilimumab may be useful biomarkers for anti-tumor response.

Myeloid-Derived Suppressor Cells (MDSCs)

MDSCs are a heterogeneous population of myeloid origin characterized by a failure to differentiate into granulocytes, macrophages or dendritic cells (120). They expand in tumor environments and strongly suppress the activity of immune cells, including T cells, through a variety of mechanisms such as NO production and arginase-1 overexpression. Both of these processes lead to cell cycle arrest and downregulation of the T cell receptor (120). MDSCs are defined as Lin$^-$CD14$^+$HLA$^-$DR$^{-/\text{low}}$ (120) and clinical and experimental studies have shown that high infiltration of these cells into tumor tissues are associated with poor prognosis and resistance to therapies (121, 122). MDSCs can also be detected in the blood and several studies have demonstrated that the baseline frequency of MDSCs in blood significantly correlates

with shorter OS in melanoma patients treated with ipilimumab or nivolumab (47, 48). Furthermore, in prostate cancer patients treated with ipilimumab plus a cancer vaccine, the baseline frequency of circulating MDSCs correlated with a shorter OS (49). These results suggest that the frequency of blood MDSCs also serves as a useful biomarker for ICI response.

Serum Markers
Lactate Dehydrogenase (LDH)

Generally, baseline serum LDH is an independent factor for poor prognosis in patients with advanced melanoma (123). The same applies to cases of ICI treatment and numerous reports have demonstrated that high baseline LDH was associated with poor anti-tumor response in various cancer patients who received ICI treatment (50, 124, 125). This poor outcome may simply be caused by increased turnover of tumor cells which enhances LDH release in similar fashion to a high NLR.

CRP

CRP is produced by hepatocytes and serum levels of it elevate quickly in response to most inflammation (such as bacterial infections). However, CRP does not usually increase during ICI-mediated tumor regression. Simeone et al. reported that a decrease or no change in serum levels of CRP from baseline were significantly associated with longer OS in melanoma patients treated with ipilimumab (46). Therefore, elevated CRP from baseline may indicate inflammation by tumor progression or irAE rather than an antitumor immune response from ICI treatment.

Genomic Mutations
Mutation Burden

Mutation burden, the number of mutations within a tumor genome, is different among and within the cancer types (126). Overall, multiple studies have shown that a high mutation burden was associated with a better response to ICIs (51, 52). This mechanism is not fully understood but an increased number of neoantigens (potential tumor-specific T cell targets) generated by a high mutation burden is thought to cause an enhanced response to ICIs (127). As for melanoma, our study demonstrated that acral lentiginous melanoma (ALM) and mucosal melanoma (MCM), both common types of melanoma in Asians, were less susceptible to immune checkpoint inhibitors than superficial spreading melanoma (SSM) and lentigo maligna melanoma, both major types of Caucasian melanoma (128). This may be explained, at least in part, by the lower mutation burden in ALM and MCM (129). Despite the poor ICI-mediated antitumor response in ALM patients, our retrospective study demonstrated that use of ICIs significantly improved OS in not only SSM but also ALM patients (128).

Microsatellite Instability

Mutation or silencing of mismatch repair genes, which causes deficient mismatch repair (dMMR), leads to accumulation of multiple mutations and microsatellite instability (MSI). Zhang et al. reported that the immune microenvironment in colorectal cancer differs between dMMR tumors and proficient mismatch repair (pMMR) tumors (130). The number of CD8$^+$ TIL, PD-1$^+$ TIL and IDO$^+$ tumor cells was increased in tumors with dMMR compared to those with pMMR, suggesting that dMMR is indicative of exhausted T-cell-rich environments (130). It has been reported that colon cancer with dMMR frequently shows larger tumors with poorer differentiation (131). In addition, previous studies revealed that patients with dMMR had both a poorer response to conventional chemotherapies and shorter OS than patients with pMMR in many types of cancer (132, 133). However, due to the high mutation burden, several clinical trials revealed a high response to anti-PD-1 antibodies in colorectal cancer with dMMR or high levels of MSI (MSI-H) compared to traditional treatments (53), suggesting that dMMR serves as useful indicator for choosing ICIs over other therapies. Recently, a durable response was observed in patients with dMMR or MSI-H across five clinical trials treated with pembrolizmab (KEYNOTE-016, 164, 012, 028, 158). The cancer types included colorectal, endometrial, biliary, gastric, esophageal, pancreatic and breast cancers. Based on these results, the United States Food and Drug Administration approved pembrolizumab for the treatment of any unresetable or metastatic solid tumors that display dMMR or MSI-H. A combination of nivolumab with ipilimumab was also shown to effect a promising response to dMMR/ MSI-H colorectal cancer (134).

Human Leukocyte Antigen (HLA)

HLA encodes cell surface molecules which present antigenic peptides to the T-cell receptor (TCR) on T cells. Inoue et al reported that mRNA expression of HLA-A in pre-treatment melanoma was elevated in responders to nivolumab compared to non-responders (54). There are numerous variant alleles at the HLA loci which differ in each individual and Ishida et al reported that HLA-A26, which is relatively common in Japanese but rare in Caucasians, correlated with tumor response to nivolumab in Japanese melanoma patients (55).

T Cell Receptor (TCR) Repertoire

Since the TCR determines T cell specificity with respect to tumor cells, the TCR repertoire may be predictive of the ICI-induced anti-tumor immune response. As diversity of the repertoire is increased, the likelihood of a specific immune response to tumor cells is speculated to be elevated (56). A previous study showed that both higher richness and evenness in pre-treatment peripheral blood are associated with a better response to ipilimumab in melanoma patients (56). On the other hand, Tumeh et al. showed that TILs with less diversity were significantly associated with clinical response to pembrolizumab in melanoma patients (21). It is speculated that TILs with less diversity contain a higher proportion of tumor-specific T cells, and therefore, the anti-tumor response was enhanced by ICIs. In this study, a TIL clone population expanded more than 10 times in responders than non-responders after treatment with pembrolizumab (21), revealing that both diversity and clonal expansion of T cells may predict ICI response although this indication may differ between blood and tumor tissues.

Gut Microbiome

Emergent evidence has suggested that the gut microbiome plays crucial roles for the immune response of not only intestinal diseases but also other disorders, including various type of cancers (135). Sivan et al. reported that, in mice, commensal Bifidobacterium enhanced the response to anti-PD-1 antibodies through an augmented dendritic cell function (136). Several studies have also demonstrated that distinct gut microbiota were associated with ICI response in humans. Melanoma patients whose baseline microbiota was enriched with Faecalibacterium genus and other Firmicutes showed a longer PFS and OS than those whose baseline microbiota was enriched with Bacteroides upon ipilimumab treatment (57). In addition, Gopalakrishnan et al. reported that a higher diversity of gut microbiome and relative abundance of Ruminococcaceae family bacteria before starting anti-PD-1 antibodies in melanoma patients correlated with better ORR and longer PFS (58). Moreover, Routy et al. showed that dysbiosis by administration of antibiotics inhibited ICI response in both mice and humans (59). This study also revealed a correlation between clinical responses and the relative abundance of Akkermansia muciniphilia. They also showed that transplantation of Akkermansia muciniphilia into mice enhanced the efficacy of PD-1 antibodies in an IL-12 dependent manner (59). Therefore, gut microbiota may have important implications for the immune response to ICIs.

Liquid Biopsy
Circulating Tumor DNA (ctDNA)

Tumor-derived, fragmented DNA in blood is known as ctDNA, and its precise mechanism of release remains unclear but it has been postulated that it involves a passive release from dying cells and active release from living cells (137–139). It is associated with tumor burden (140), and high levels of ctDNA are an indicator of poor prognoses in patients with various types of cancer (141). Lee et al. demonstrated that melanoma patients with a persistently elevated cDNA during the treatment of anti-PD-1 antibodies show a worse response and shorter PFS and OS (60). In addition, it has been reported that, of nine melanoma patients treated with anti-PD-1 antibodies who showed pseudoprogression (defined as a tumor size increase prior to response often seen in ICI treatment), all patients had a favorable ctDNA profile defined by undetectable ctDNA at baseline or detactable ctDNA at baseline followed by >10-fold decreases (61). In contrast, in 20 patients with true progression, all but two had an unfavorable ctDNA profile defined by detectable ctDNA at baseline that remained stable or increased. These results indicate that ctDNA is a useful marker for differentiating pseudoprogression from true progression during ICI treatment.

In addition, the mutation burden of ctDNA has been also assessed and, in line with the correlation of a high mutation burden in tumor tissues, hyper-mutated ctDNA has also been associated with improved OS in patients with diverse cancers who received ICIs (142).

Exosomes

Exosomes are microvesicles actively released from various cells, including cancer cells, and contain proteins, RNA and DNA

(63). Exosomes isolated from the plasma of cancer patients contains various immune-related proteins, including PD-1, PD-L1, and CTLA-4, with PD-L1 in exosomes showing a suppressive effect on T cell activities by signaling via PD-1 (62, 143). Similar to the correlation between circulating sPD-L1 and response to ICIs, lower baseline levels, as well as increases, in exosomal PD-L1 protein have been correlated with response to pembrolizumab in melanoma patients (62). However, opposite results were observed in the association of exosomal PD-L1 mRNA expression with response to anti-PD-1 antibodies in patients with melanoma or NSCLS (63). Baseline exosomal PD-L1 mRNA expression was higher in responders compared to non-responders and exosomal PD-L1 mRNA expression in responders was significantly decreased after treatment whereas it was stable in stabilized patients and significantly increased in progressive disease cases (63). Therefore, although the mechanism is unknown, PD-L1 proteins and transcript in the exosome may provide conflicting information on ICI response.

As for other molecules, Tucci et al. recently evaluated the circulating exosomal proteins in T cells and dendritic cells in melanoma patients treated with ipilimumab (64). They demonstrated that increased exosomal PD-1 and CD28 levels in T cells were significantly associated with longer PFS and OS while increased exosomal CD80 and CD86 in dendritic cells correlated with longer PFS (64). Such exosomal proteins may reflect potential T cell/dendritic cell activities and thus lead to predictions of ICI response.

irAE Development

Since ICIs may cause both irAEs and tumor regression through an augmented immune response, several reports have shown associations between the two events. Overall irAEs have been associated with regression of metastatic renal cell carcinoma or melanoma treated with ipilimumab (65, 144). In addition, the presence of overall irAEs was significantly associated with longer OS in melanoma patients treated with nivolumab (145). And moreover, early development of all irAEs has been associated with better ORR and longer PFS in NSCLC patients treated with nivolumab (66). However, other studies failed to show such correlations (67, 68, 146). A multivariate analysis conducted by Judo et al showed that only low grade irAEs, but not high grade irAEs, are associated with better responses to anti-PD-1 antibodies in non-melanoma patients (67). Therefore, only certain irAEs might be associated with tumor regression by ICIs. As for irAEs in each organ, several reports showed correlations between endocrine irAEs and better prognoses. Fujisawa et al. demonstrated that occurrences of endocrine irAEs were associated with longer OS in melanoma patients treated with ipilimumab after nivolumab (68). Similarly, an adjusted analysis by Kim et al. showed that development of thyroid dysfunction was significantly associated with longer PFS and OS in NSCLC patients treated with anti-PD-1 antibodies (147), suggesting that endocrine irAEs may be representative of the potential immune reaction to tumor cells. In a similar fashion, multiple studies showed that development of vitiligo correlated with better responses to ICIs in melanoma patients; this may represent a common immune response against antigens shared

by melanocytes and melanomas (69, 148). Although ICIs may cause vitiligo in patients with other cancer such as NSCLC and renal cell carcinoma (149, 150), associations with outcomes in such cases remain unclear. Several studies showed that skin irAEs, except for vitiligo, were also associated with better outcome in various types of cancer (145, 148). However, Fujisawa et al. reported conflicted findings that occurrences of skin irAEs, excluding vitiligo, correlate with a shorter OS in melanoma patients treated with ipilimumab after nivolumab (68). Since skin irAEs include various types of skin disorders, such as prurigo-like eruptions, psoriasiform dermatitis and lichenoid reactions, associations with outcomes may be different for each skin irAE.

Biomarkers of irAEs (Table 2)

The aforementioned irAEs can be induced by all ICIs. However, among the ICIs, both the frequency and the severity are highest in treatment with ipilimumab (161). Severe irAEs (grade ≥ 3) have occurred in 28–56% and 21–32% in patients treated with ipilimumab or anti-PD-1/anti-PD-L1 antibodies, respectively (10, 12, 16, 162, 163). In the combined treatment of ipilimumab plus nivolumab, much higher rates of severe irAEs are observed (16, 164). The organ most affected by irAEs is the skin followed by the gastrointestinal tract, respiratory tract and endocrine organs. A recent meta-analysis revealed that colitis, hypophysitis and rash were more frequent with anti-CTLA-4 antibodies whereas pneumonitis, hypothyroidism, arthralgia, and vitiligo were more common with anti-PD-1 antibodies (165). Most of these irAEs occur within 3–6 months from the initiation of ICI treatment (166–168). Given that most are mild and reversible if they are detected early and properly managed, biomarkers for predicting the occurrence of irAEs are essential. Compared with biomarkers for tumor response, those for irAEs have been less thoroughly investigated and some of the reported biomarkers for irAE overlap with those for tumor responses.

Body Composition Parameters

Previous reports revealed that sarcopenia was associated with poorer treatment tolerance and increased likelihood of adverse events by various chemotherapies (169, 170). In addition, low muscle attenuation (MA), which refers to increased intramuscular adipose tissue, has been associated with shorter survival in a wide variety of cancers such as melanoma and renal cell carcinoma (171, 172). Daly et al evaluated association of these body composition parameters by computer tomography with occurrences of irAEs in melanoma patients treated with ipilimumab. The multivariate analysis in this study showed that both sarcopenia and low MA were independent factors significantly associated with high-grade irAEs (151). Although the exact mechanism is unknown, many studies suggest that sarcopenia and low MA increase susceptibility to systemic inflammation (173, 174), and this may play a role in the higher frequency of severe irAEs.

Sex

Although males have been associated with a more favorable response to ICIs, a study in melanoma patients treated with ipilimumab by Valpione et al reported that females

TABLE 2 | Biomarkers for irAEs.

Biomarkers	Cancer type	Patient number	Treatment	Key data and clinical significance	References	Evidence level
Body composition parameters	Melanoma	84	Ipilimumab	Both sarcopenia and low MA were independent factors associated with high-grade irAEs.	Daly et al. (151)	2b
Sex	Melanoma	140	Ipilimumab	Females were associated with higher rates of irAEs.	Valpoine et al. (152)	2b
IL-6				IL-6 at baseline was negatively associated with irAE.		
	Melanoma	26	Ipilimumab	Lower circulating IL-6 was significantly correlated with higher incidences of colitis-related irAEs.	Chaput et al.(57)	2b
	Melanoma	15	Nivolumab	Increases in circulating IL-6 after treatment were significantly associated with development of irAEs.	Tanaka et al. (37)	4
IL-17	Melanoma	35	Ipilimumab	Circulating IL-17 levels at baseline correlated with the incidence of grade 3 irAEs of diarrhea/colitis, indicating that increased levels of circulating IL-17 may be reflective of patients with subclinical colitis.	Tarhini et al. (153)	2b
Soluble CD163, CXCL5	Melanoma	46	Nivolumab	The absolute change rate of soluble CD163 and CXCL5 after initial treatment was increased in patients with irAEs compared to those without irAEs.	Fujimura et al. (154)	2b
Blood cell counts	Melanoma, RCC, urothelial carcinom	167	Anti-PD-1 antibodies	Absolute lymphocyte and eosinophil numbers at baseline and 1 month after initial treatment were independent factors associated with a higher incidence of irAEs of grade ≥2.	Diehl et al. (155)	2b
	Melanoma	44	Anti-PD-1 antibodies	Both baseline absolute eosinophil count and relative eosinophil count at 1 month significantly correlate with the occurrence of endocrine irAEs.	Nakamura et al. (45)	2b
	Melanoma	101	Nivolumab	An increase in total WBC count and a decrease in relative lymphocyte count plus increase in relative neutrophil count on the same day of, or just prior to irAE occurrence were associated with development of lung or gastrointestinal irAEs.	Fujisawa et al. (156)	2b
autoantibodies	Melanoma, NSCLC	168	Nivolumab	TSH and TPOAb were associated with higher incidence of thyroid irAEs.	Kimbara et al. (157)	2b
	Solid cancer including melanoma, NSCLC, RCC	27	Anti-PD-1 antibodies, atezolizumab	Patients positive for type 1 diabetes antibodies at the time of presentation developed diabetes-related irAEs after fewer cycles than those without autoantibodies.	Stamatouli et al. (158)	2b
T cell repertoire	Prostate cancer	42	Ipilimumab plus granulocyte-monocyte colony-stimulating factor	An early increase in diversity and the generation of new T- cell clones correlated with the development of irAEs.	Oh et al. (159)	2b
Gut microbiome	Melanoma	26	Ipilimumab	Patients whose baseline microbiota was enriched with the Faecalibaterium genus and other Firmicutes showed a higher incidence of colitis-related irAEs.	Chaput et al. (57)	2b
	Melanoma	34	Ipilimumab	Increased representation of bacteria belonging to the Bacteroidetes phylum was associated with resistance to development of ipilimumab-induced colitis.	Dubin et al. (160)	2b

NSCLC, non-small cell lung cancer; RCC, renal cell carcinoma; irAE, immune-related adverse event; WBC, white blood cell; TPOAb, antithyroid peroxidase antibodies (TPOAb). Evidence level was evaluated based on the following criteria; 1a, systematic review/ meta-analysis of randomized controlled trials; 1b, individual randomized controlled trials; 2a, systematic review/meta-analysis of cohort studies; 2b, individual cohort study; 3a, systematic review/meta-analysis of case-control studies; 3b, individual case-control studies; 4, case series; 5, expert opinions.

were associated with higher rates of irAEs (152). Sex-specific factors, including hormones, play important roles in the immune response, and it is well-known that females are at a higher risk of several autoimmune diseases (175). Therefore, immune reactions to self-tissues mediated by female-specific factors may lead to an increased likelihood of irAEs.

Serum Factors
IL-6
Similar to the correlation with poor tumor response, it has been reported that circulating IL-6 at baseline was negatively associated with irAE occurrence in melanoma patients treated with ipilimumab (152). Another study showed that lower circulating IL-6, as well as IL-8, was significantly correlated with higher incidences of colitis-related irAEs (57). This may be explained by the immunosuppressive effects of IL-6 in certain conditions, including the induction of MDSC (176–178). In contrast, Tanaka et al. assessed the fluctuation of multiple cytokines in melanoma patients treated with nivolumab and showed that increases in circulating IL-6 after treatment were significantly associated with development of irAEs (37). These results indicate that both lower baseline IL-6 and increase after ICI treatment may serve as predictive markers for irAE occurrence.

IL-17
IL-17 is a cytokine with a variety of inflammatory effects, including the recruitment of neutrophils, and it is well-known that circulating IL-17 levels are increased in patients with inflammatory bowel disease (179). Tarhini et al. assessed candidate circulating factors which were associated with irAEs in melanoma patients treated with ipilimumab as a neoadjuvant therapy and revealed that circulating IL-17 levels at baseline significantly correlated with the incidence of grade 3 irAEs of diarrhea/colitis (153). This indicates that increased levels of circulating IL-17 may be reflective of patients with subclinical colitis, the development of which would be normally inhibited by CTLA-4.

Soluble CD163 (sCD163) and CXCL5
Circulating levels of sCD163, which is derived from macrophages, increase in various autoimmune disorders, including rheumatoid arthritis and pemphigus vulgaris, and are reflective of their activities (176, 180). CXCL5 is a chemokine which can attract CXCR2$^+$ myeloid cells and can be produced by CD163$^+$ macrophages. It is also known to be a biomarker for several autoimmune disorders (176, 181). Fujimura et al evaluated circulating sCD163 and CXCL5 levels at baseline and day 42 after initial treatment with nivolumab in melanoma patients (154), showing that the sCD163 absolute change rate was significantly increased in patients with irAEs compared to those without irAEs. Although there were no significant differences, the absolute change rate of CXCL5 also tended to be higher in patients with irAEs, suggesting that absolute changes within sCD163 and CXCL5 levels

after ICI treatment could serve as possible biomarkers for irAE development.

Blood Cells
Since both T cells and eosinophils are crucial for cellular immunity, blood cell counts of these cells may also be correlated with irAE development. A multivariate analysis conducted by Diehi et al. demonstrated that, in solid tumor patients (including melanoma, renal cell carcinoma, and urothelial carcinoma) treated with anti-PD-1 antibodies, absolute lymphocyte and eosinophil numbers at baseline and 1 month after initial treatment were independent factors that were significantly associated with a higher incidence of irAEs of grade ≥2 (155). In addition, our study demonstrated that both baseline absolute eosinophil count and relative eosinophil count at 1 month significantly correlate with the occurrence of endocrine irAEs in melanoma patients treated with anti-PD-1 antibodies (45). Therefore, circulating lymphocyte and eosinophil numbers may predict not only tumor responses but also the occurrence of ICI-mediated irAEs.

In contrast, Fujisawa et al. investigated fluctuations in blood cell count on the same day of, or just prior to irAE occurrence, in melanoma patients treated with nivolumab (156). Univariate analyses revealed that increases in total white blood cell (WBC) count and decreases in relative lymphocyte count from baseline were associated with severe irAEs of grade ≥3 although multivariate analyses failed to show independence. They also analyzed the correlation with irAEs of each organ and found that the same factors, namely an increase in total WBC count and a decrease in relative lymphocyte count plus increase in relative neutrophil count, were significantly associated with development of lung or gastrointestinal irAEs. This could be caused by neutrophil-dominant infiltration into the affected organs since DAMPs from severely damaged cells promote neutrophil recruitment (182). Indeed, active colitis in patients treated with ipilimumab saw severe neutrophil infiltration into the lamina propria (183), indicating that these factors may be useful for predicting irAEs that are currently developing or may soon develop.

Autoantibodies
Detection of autoantibodies is speculated to predict development of irAEs related to the autoantibodies (184). Kimbara et al. assessed TSH, free T3, free T4, antithyroid peroxidase antibodies (TPOAb) and antithyroglobulin antibodies at baseline in patients with solid tumors treated with nivolumab and multivariate analyses revealed that TSH and TPOAb were significantly associated with higher incidence of thyroid irAEs (157). Stamatouli et al. measured diabetes autoantibodies (glutamic and decarboxylase 65 antibodies, islet antigen 2 antibodies, and insulin autoantibodies) in solid cancer patients treated with anti-PD-1 or anti-PD-L1 antibodies, and found that patients positive for type 1 diabetes antibodies at the time of presentation developed diabetes-related irAEs after fewer cycles than those without autoantibodies (158). They also measured autoantibodies prior to treatment in three patients, and one was already positive,

indicating that autoantibodies may be useful to predict their related irAEs.

T Cell Repertoire

The T cell repertoire has been reported to correlate with irAEs as well as tumor response. Oh et al assessed the repertoire of circulating T cells in patients with metastatic castration-resistant prostate cancer treated with a combination of ipilimumab and granulocyte-monocyte colony-stimulating factor (159). They found that initial broadening in the repertoire occurred within 2 weeks of treatment, which significantly preceded irAEs onset, and an early increase in diversity and the generation of new clones were correlated with the development of irAEs. These results suggest that increased T cell diversity in response to ICI treatment could be a sign of immune response to normal tissues as well as tumor tissues.

Gut Microbiome

It is suggested that inflammatory bowel diseases (IBD) may result from a loss of tolerance to commensal bacteria and dysbiosis is a well-known factor that is significantly involved in the pathogenesis of IBD (185). Gut microbiota have been also reported as predictive of colitis-related irAEs. Melanoma patients treated with ipilimumab whose baseline microbiota was enriched with the *Faecalibaterium* genus and other Firmicutes showed a higher incidence of colitis-related irAEs although they were also associated with better outcomes (57). In contrast, this study showed no occurrences of colitis irAEs in any patients with *Bacteroidetes* (57). Similarly, Dubin et al. demonstrated that increased representation of bacteria belonging to the *Bacteroidetes phylum* was associated with resistance to development of ipilimumab-induced colitis (160).

Tumor Type

A recent meta-analysis demonstrated that the frequency of each type of irAE depends on cancer type (165). Melanoma patients had a higher frequency of skin and gastrointestinal irAEs but a lower frequency of pneumonia compared with NSCLC patients (165). In addition, dermatitis, arthritis and myalgia were more frequent in melanoma patients than in renal cell carcinoma patients whereas pneumonitis and dyspnea were found to be less common in melanoma cases (165). Although the precise mechanism remains unclear, induced immune responses to antigens of normal tissue shared with or cross-reactive with those of each cancer may be an explanation.

CONCLUSION

Although numerous predictive biomarkers for tumor response and irAEs during ICI treatment have been identified, there are no absolutely predictive biomarkers as yet. Therefore, multiple biomarkers should be taken into consideration in choosing or quitting ICI treatments. Because immune reactions induced by ICIs are quite complex and many factors are involved, identifying new biomarkers will provide mechanistic insights into the ways how ICIs modulate the anti-tumor response and irAEs in specific patients, as well as lead to the development of novel treatments to target the identified biomarkers.

AUTHOR CONTRIBUTIONS

The author confirms being the sole contributor of this work and has approved it for publication.

REFERENCES

1. Madorsky Rowdo FP, Baron A, Urrutia M, Mordoh J. Immunotherapy in cancer: a combat between tumors and the immune system; you win some, you lose some. *Front Immunol.* (2015) 6:127. doi: 10.3389/fimmu.2015.00127

2. Romano E, Kusio-Kobialka M, Foukas PG, Baumgaertner P, Meyer C, Ballabeni P, et al. Ipilimumab-dependent cell-mediated cytotoxicity of regulatory T cells *ex vivo* by nonclassical monocytes in melanoma patients. *Proc Natl Acad Sci USA.* (2015) 112:6140–5. doi: 10.1073/pnas.1417320112

3. Cho J, Ahn S, Yoo KH, Kim JH, Choi SH, Jang KT, et al. Treatment outcome of PD-1 immune checkpoint inhibitor in Asian metastatic melanoma patients: correlative analysis with PD-L1 immunohistochemistry. *Invest New Drugs.* (2016) 34:677–84. doi: 10.1007/s10637-016-0373-4

4. Robert C, Long GV, Brady B, Dutriaux C, Maio M, Mortier L, et al. Nivolumab in previously untreated melanoma without BRAF mutation. *N Engl J Med.* (2015) 372:320–30. doi: 10.1056/NEJMoa1412082

5. Robert C, Schachter J, Long GV, Arance A, Grob JJ, Mortier L, et al. Pembrolizumab versus ipilimumab in advanced melanoma. *N Engl J Med.* (2015) 372:2521–32. doi: 10.1056/NEJMoa1503093

6. Hodi FS, O'Day SJ, McDermott DF, Weber RW, Sosman JA, Haanen JB, et al. Improved survival with ipilimumab in patients with metastatic melanoma. *N Engl J Med.* (2010) 363:711–23. doi: 10.1056/NEJMoa1003466

7. Mazza C, Escudier B, Albiges L. Nivolumab in renal cell carcinoma: latest evidence and clinical potential. *Ther Adv Med Oncol.* (2017) 9:171–81. doi: 10.1177/1758834016679942

8. Kim BJ, Kim JH, Kim HS. Survival benefit of immune checkpoint inhibitors according to the histology in non-small-cell lung cancer: a meta-analysis and review. *Oncotarget.* (2017) 8:51779–85. doi: 10.18632/oncotarget.17213

9. Fehrenbacher L, Spira A, Ballinger M, Kowanetz M, Vansteenkiste J, Mazieres J, et al. Atezolizumab versus docetaxel for patients with previously treated non-small-cell lung cancer (POPLAR): a multicentre, open-label, phase 2 randomised controlled trial. *Lancet.* (2016) 387:1837–46. doi: 10.1016/s0140-6736(16) 00587-0

10. Weber J, Mandala M, Del Vecchio M, Gogas HJ, Arance AM, Cowey CL, et al. Adjuvant nivolumab versus ipilimumab in resected stage III or IV melanoma. *N Engl J Med.* (2017) 377:1824–35. doi: 10.1056/NEJMoa1709030

11. van Zeijl MC, van den Eertwegh AJ, Haanen JB, Wouters MW. (Neo) adjuvant systemic therapy for melanoma. *Eur J Surg Oncol.* (2017) 43:534–43. doi: 10.1016/j.ejso.2016.07.001

12. Eggermont AMM, Blank CU, Mandala M, Long GV, Atkinson V, Dalle S, et al. Adjuvant pembrolizumab versus placebo in resected stage III melanoma. *N Engl J Med.* (2018) 378:1789–801. doi: 10.1056/NEJMoa1802357

13. Amaria RN, Reddy SM, Tawbi HA, Davies MA, Ross MI, Glitza IC, et al. Neoadjuvant immune checkpoint blockade in high-risk resectable melanoma. *Nat Med.* (2018) 24:1649–54. doi: 10.1038/s41591-018-0197-1

14. Keung EZ, Lazar AJ, Torres KE, Wang WL, Cormier JN, Ashleigh Guadagnolo B, et al. Phase II study of neoadjuvant checkpoint blockade in patients with surgically resectable undifferentiated pleomorphic sarcoma and dedifferentiated liposarcoma. *BMC Cancer.* (2018) 18:913. doi: 10.1186/s12885-018-4829-0

15. Yeh J, Marrone KA, Forde PM. Neoadjuvant and consolidation immuno-oncology therapy in stage III non-small cell lung cancer. *J Thorac Dis.* (2018) 10:S451–S9. doi: 10.21037/jtd.2018.01.109

16. Wolchok JD, Chiarion-Sileni V, Gonzalez R, Rutkowski P, Grob JJ, Cowey CL, et al. Overall survival with combined nivolumab and ipilimumab in advanced melanoma. *N Engl J Med.* (2017) 377:1345–56. doi: 10.1056/NEJMoa1709684

17. Wu Y, Ju Q, Jia K, Yu J, Shi H, Wu H, et al. Correlation between sex and efficacy of immune checkpoint inhibitors (PD-1 and CTLA-4 inhibitors). *Int J Cancer.* (2018) 143:45–51. doi: 10.1002/ijc.31301

18. Nosrati A, Tsai KK, Goldinger SM, Tumeh P, Grimes B, Loo K, et al. Evaluation of clinicopathological factors in PD-1 response: derivation and validation of a prediction scale for response to PD-1 monotherapy. *Br J Cancer.* (2017) 116:1141–7. doi: 10.1038/bjc.2017.70

19. Nishijima TF, Muss HB, Shachar SS, Moschos SJ. Comparison of efficacy of immune checkpoint inhibitors (ICIs) between younger and older patients: a systematic review and meta-analysis. *Cancer Treat Rev.* (2016) 45:30–7. doi: 10.1016/j.ctrv.2016.02.006

20. Joseph RW, Elassaiss-Schaap J, Kefford R, Hwu WJ, Wolchok JD, Joshua AM, et al. Baseline tumor size is an independent prognostic factor for overall survival in patients with melanoma treated with pembrolizumab. *Clin Cancer Res.* (2018) 24:4960–7. doi: 10.1158/1078-0432.Ccr-17-2386

21. Tumeh PC, Harview CL, Yearley JH, Shintaku IP, Taylor EJ, Robert L, et al. PD-1 blockade induces responses by inhibiting adaptive immune resistance. *Nature.* (2014) 515:568–71. doi: 10.1038/nature13954

22. Weber JS, D'Angelo SP, Minor D, Hodi FS, Gutzmer R, Neyns B, et al. Nivolumab versus chemotherapy in patients with advanced melanoma who progressed after anti-CTLA-4 treatment (CheckMate 037): a randomised, controlled, open-label, phase 3 trial. *Lancet Oncol.* (2015) 16:375–84. doi: 10.1016/S1470-2045(15) 70076-8

23. Daud AI, Wolchok JD, Robert C, Hwu WJ, Weber JS, Ribas A, et al. Programmed death-ligand 1 expression and response to the anti-programmed death 1 antibody pembrolizumab in melanoma. *J Clin Oncol.* (2016) 34:4102–9. doi: 10.1200/JCO.2016.67.2477

24. Gandhi L, Rodriguez-Abreu D, Gadgeel S, Esteban E, Felip E, De Angelis F, et al. Pembrolizumab plus chemotherapy in metastatic non-small-cell lung cancer. *N Engl J Med.* (2018) 378:2078–92. doi: 10.1056/NEJMoa18 01005

25. Carthon BC, Wolchok JD, Yuan J, Kamat A, Ng Tang DS, Sun J, et al. Preoperative CTLA-4 blockade: tolerability and immune monitoring in the setting of a presurgical clinical trial. *Clin Cancer Res.* (2010) 16:2861–71. doi: 10.1158/1078-0432.CCR-10-0569

26. Tallerico R, Cristiani CM, Staaf E, Garofalo C, Sottile R, Capone M, et al. IL-15, TIM-3 and NK cells subsets predict responsiveness to anti-CTLA-4 treatment in melanoma patients. *Oncoimmunology.* (2017) 6:e1261242. doi: 10.1080/2162402X.2016.1261242

27. Hamid O, Schmidt H, Nissan A, Ridolfi L, Aamdal S, Hansson J, et al. A prospective phase II trial exploring the association between tumor microenvironment biomarkers and clinical activity of ipilimumab in advanced melanoma. *J Transl Med.* (2011) 9:204. doi: 10.1186/1479-5876-9-204

28. Botticelli A, Cerbelli B, Lionetto L, Zizzari I, Salati M, Pisano A, et al. Can IDO activity predict primary resistance to anti-PD-1 treatment in NSCLC? *J Transl Med.* (2018) 16:219. doi: 10.1186/s12967-018-1595-3

29. Pistillo MP, Fontana V, Morabito A, Dozin B, Laurent S, Carosio R, et al. Soluble CTLA-4 as a favorable predictive biomarker in metastatic melanoma patients treated with ipilimumab: an Italian melanoma intergroup study. *Cancer Immunol Immunother.* (2019) 68:97–107. doi: 10.1007/s00262-018-2258-1

30. Zhou J, Mahoney KM, Giobbie-Hurder A, Zhao F, Lee S, Liao X, et al. Soluble PD-L1 as a biomarker in malignant melanoma treated with checkpoint blockade. *Cancer Immunol Res.* (2017) 5:480–92. doi: 10.1158/2326-6066.CIR-16-0329

31. Okuma Y, Wakui H, Utsumi H, Sagawa Y, Hosomi Y, Kuwano K, et al. Soluble programmed cell death ligand 1 as a novel biomarker for nivolumab therapy for non-small-cell lung cancer. *Clin Lung Cancer.* (2018) 19:410-7 e1. doi: 10.1016/j.cllc.2018.04.014

32. Fujimura T, Sato Y, Tanita K, Kambayashi Y, Otsuka A, Fujisawa Y, et al. Serum level of soluble CD163 may be a predictive marker of the effectiveness of nivolumab in patients with advanced cutaneous melanoma. *Front Oncol.* (2018) 8:530. doi: 10.3389/fonc.2018.00530

33. Maccalli C, Giannarelli D, Chiarucci C, Cutaia O, Giacobini G, Hendrickx W, et al. Soluble NKG2D ligands are biomarkers associated with the clinical outcome to immune checkpoint blockade therapy of metastatic melanoma patients. *Oncoimmunology.* (2017) 6:e1323618. doi: 10.1080/2162402X.2017.13 23618

34. Ji RR, Chasalow SD, Wang L, Hamid O, Schmidt H, Cogswell J, et al. An immune-active tumor microenvironment favors clinical response to ipilimumab. *Cancer Immunol Immunother.* (2012) 61:1019–31. doi: 10.1007/s00262-011-1172-6

35. Higgs BW, Morehouse CA, Streicher K, Brohawn PZ, Pilataxi F, Gupta A, et al. Interferon gamma messenger RNA signature in tumor biopsies predicts outcomes in patients with non-small cell lung carcinoma or urothelial cancer treated with durvalumab. *Clin Cancer Res.* (2018) 24:3857–66. doi: 10.1158/1078-0432.Ccr-17-3451

36. Herbst RS, Soria JC, Kowanetz M, Fine GD, Hamid O, Gordon MS, et al. Predictive correlates of response to the anti-PD-L1 antibody MPDL3280A in cancer patients. *Nature.* (2014) 515:563–7. doi: 10.1038/nature 14011

37. Tanaka R, Okiyama N, Okune M, Ishitsuka Y, Watanabe R, Furuta J, et al. Serum level of interleukin-6 is increased in nivolumab-associated psoriasiform dermatitis and tumor necrosis factor-alpha is a biomarker of nivolumab recativity. *J Dermatol Sci.* (2017) 86:71–3. doi: 10.1016/j.jdermsci.2016.12.019

38. Martens A, Wistuba-Hamprecht K, Geukes Foppen M, Yuan J, Postow MA, Wong P, et al. Baseline peripheral blood biomarkers associated with clinical outcome of advanced melanoma patients treated with ipilimumab. *Clin Cancer Res.* (2016) 22:2908–18. doi: 10.1158/1078-0432.Ccr-15-2412

39. Wilgenhof S, Du Four S, Vandenbroucke F, Everaert H, Salmon I, Lienard D, et al. Single-center experience with ipilimumab in an expanded access program for patients with pretreated advanced melanoma. *J Immunother.* (2013) 36:215–22. doi: 10.1097/CJI.0b013e31828eed39

40. Nakamura Y, Kitano S, Takahashi A, Tsutsumida A, Namikawa K, Tanese K, et al. Nivolumab for advanced melanoma: pretreatment prognostic factors and early outcome markers during therapy. *Oncotarget.* (2016) 7:77404–15. doi: 10.18632/oncotarget.12677

41. Weide B, Martens A, Hassel JC, Berking C, Postow MA, Bisschop K, et al. Baseline biomarkers for outcome of melanoma patients treated with pembrolizumab. *Clin Cancer Res.* (2016) 22:5487–96. doi: 10.1158/1078-0432.Ccr-16-0127

42. Gebhardt C, Sevko A, Jiang H, Lichtenberger R, Reith M, Tarnanidis K, et al. Myeloid cells and related chronic inflammatory factors as novel predictive markers in melanoma treatment with ipilimumab. *Clin Cancer Res.* (2015) 21:5453–9. doi: 10.1158/1078-0432.Ccr-15-0676

43. Fujisawa Y, Yoshino K, Otsuka A, Funakoshi T, Fujimura T, Yamamoto Y, et al. Baseline neutrophil to lymphocyte ratio combined with serum lactate dehydrogenase level associated with outcome of nivolumab immunotherapy in a Japanese advanced melanoma population. *Br J Dermatol.* (2018) 179:213–5. doi: 10.1111/bjd.16427

44. Bagley SJ, Kothari S, Aggarwal C, Bauml JM, Alley EW, Evans TL, et al. Pretreatment neutrophil-to-lymphocyte ratio as a marker of outcomes in nivolumab-treated patients with advanced non-small-cell lung cancer. *Lung Cancer.* (2017) 106:1–7. doi: 10.1016/j.lungcan.2017.01.013

45. Nakamura Y, Tanaka R, Maruyama H, Ishitsuka Y, Okiyama N, Watanabe R, et al. Correlation between blood cell count and outcome of melanoma patients treated with anti-PD-1 antibodies. *Jpn J Clin Oncol.* (2019) 2019:201. doi: 10.1093/jjco/hyy201

46. Simeone E, Gentilcore G, Giannarelli D, Grimaldi AM, Caraco C, Curvietto M, et al. Immunological and biological changes during ipilimumab treatment and their potential correlation with clinical response and survival in patients with advanced melanoma. *Cancer Immunol Immunother.* (2014) 63:675–83. doi: 10.1007/s00262-014-1545-8

47. Weber J, Gibney G, Kudchadkar R, Yu B, Cheng P, Martinez AJ, et al. Phase I/II study of metastatic melanoma patients treated with nivolumab who had progressed after ipilimumab. *Cancer Immunol Res.* (2016) 4:345–53. doi: 10.1158/2326-6066.Cir-15-0193

48. Kitano S, Postow MA, Ziegler CG, Kuk D, Panageas KS, Cortez C, et al. Computational algorithm-driven evaluation of monocytic myeloid-derived suppressor cell frequency for prediction of clinical outcomes. *Cancer Immunol Res.* (2014) 2:812–21. doi: 10.1158/2326-6066.Cir-14-0013

49. Santegoets SJ, Stam AG, Lougheed SM, Gall H, Jooss K, Sacks N, et al. Myeloid derived suppressor and dendritic cell subsets are related to clinical outcome in prostate cancer patients treated with prostate GVAX and ipilimumab. *J Immunother Cancer.* (2014) 2:31. doi: 10.1186/s40425-014-0031-3

50. Delyon J, Mateus C, Lefeuvre D, Lanoy E, Zitvogel L, Chaput N, et al. Experience in daily practice with ipilimumab for the treatment of patients with metastatic melanoma: an early increase in lymphocyte and eosinophil counts is associated with improved survival. *Ann Oncol.* (2013) 24:1697–703. doi: 10.1093/annonc/mdt027

51. Snyder A, Makarov V, Merghoub T, Yuan J, Zaretsky JM, Desrichard A, et al. Genetic basis for clinical response to CTLA-4 blockade in melanoma. *N Engl J Med.* (2014) 371:2189–99. doi: 10.1056/NEJMoa1406498

52. Van Allen EM, Miao D, Schilling B, Shukla SA, Blank C, et al. Genomic correlates of response to CTLA 4 blockade in metastatic melanoma. *Science.* (2015) 350:207–11. doi: 10.1126/science.aad0095

53. Overman MJ, McDermott R, Leach JL, Lonardi S, Lenz HJ, Morse MA, et al. Nivolumab in patients with metastatic DNA mismatch repair-deficient or microsatellite instability-high colorectal cancer (CheckMate 142): an open-label, multicentre, phase 2 study. *Lancet Oncol.* (2017) 18:1182–91. doi: 10.1016/s1470-2045(17)30422-9

54. Inoue H, Park JH, Kiyotani K, Zewde M, Miyashita A, Jinnin M, et al. Intratumoral expression levels of PD-L1, GZMA, and HLA-A along with oligoclonal T cell expansion associate with response to nivolumab in metastatic melanoma. *Oncoimmunology.* (2016) 5:e1204507. doi: 10.1080/2162402x.2016.1204507

55. Ishida Y, Otsuka A, Tanaka H, Levesque MP, Dummer R, Kabashima K. HLA-A*26 is correlated with response to nivolumab in japanese melanoma patients. *J Invest Dermatol.* (2017) 137:2443–4. doi: 10.1016/j.jid.2017.06.023

56. Postow MA, Manuel M, Wong P, Yuan J, Dong Z, Liu C, et al. Peripheral T cell receptor diversity is associated with clinical outcomes following ipilimumab treatment in metastatic melanoma. *J Immunother Cancer.* (2015) 3:23. doi: 10.1186/s40425-015-0070-4

57. Chaput N, Lepage P, Coutzac C, Soularue E, Le Roux K, Monot C, et al. Baseline gut microbiota predicts clinical response and colitis in metastatic melanoma patients treated with ipilimumab. *Ann Oncol.* (2017) 28:1368–79. doi: 10.1093/annonc/mdx108

58. Gopalakrishnan V, Spencer CN, Nezi L, Reuben A, Andrews MC, Karpinets TV, et al. Gut microbiome modulates response to anti-PD-1 immunotherapy in melanoma patients. *Science.* (2018) 359:97–103. doi: 10.1126/science.aan4236

59. Routy B, Le Chatelier E, Derosa L, Duong CPM, Alou MT, Daillere R, et al. Gut microbiome influences efficacy of PD-1-based immunotherapy against epithelial tumors. *Science.* (2018) 359:91–7. doi: 10.1126/science.aan3706

60. Lee JH, Long GV, Boyd S, Lo S, Menzies AM, Tembe V, et al. Circulating tumour DNA predicts response to anti-PD1 antibodies in metastatic melanoma. *Ann Oncol.* (2017) 28:1130–6. doi: 10.1093/annonc/mdx026

61. Lee JH, Long GV, Menzies AM, Lo S, Guminski A, Whitbourne K, et al. Association between circulating tumor DNA and pseudoprogression in patients with metastatic melanoma treated with anti-programmed cell death 1 antibodies. *JAMA Oncol.* (2018) 4:717–21. doi: 10.1001/jamaoncol.2017.5332

62. Chen G, Huang AC, Zhang W, Zhang G, Wu M, Xu W, et al. Exosomal PD-L1 contributes to immunosuppression and is associated with anti-PD-1 response. *Nature.* (2018) 560:382–6. doi: 10.1038/s41586-018-0392-8

63. Del Re M, Marconcini R, Pasquini G, Rofi E, Vivaldi C, Bloise F, et al. PD-L1 mRNA expression in plasma-derived exosomes is associated with response to anti-PD-1 antibodies in melanoma and NSCLC. *Br J Cancer.* (2018) 118:820–4. doi: 10.1038/bjc.2018.9

64. Tucci M, Passarelli A, Mannavola F, Stucci LS, Ascierto PA, Capone M, et al. Serum exosomes as predictors of clinical response to ipilimumab in metastatic melanoma. *Oncoimmunology.* (2018) 7:e1387706. doi: 10.1000/2162402X.2017.1387706

65. Yang JC, Hughes M, Kammula U, Royal R, Sherry RM, Topalian SL, et al. Ipilimumab (anti-CTLA4 antibody) causes regression of metastatic renal cell cancer associated with enteritis and hypophysitis. *J Immunother.* (2007) 30:825–30. doi: 10.1097/CJI.0b013e318156e47e

66. Teraoka S, Fujimoto D, Morimoto T, Kawachi H, Ito M, Sato Y, et al. Early immune-related adverse events and association with outcome in advanced non-small cell lung cancer patients treated with nivolumab: a prospective cohort study. *J Thorac Oncol.* (2017) 12:1798–805. doi: 10.1016/j.jtho.2017.08.022

67. Judd J, Zibelman M, Handorf E, O'Neill J, Ramamurthy C, Bentota S, et al. Immune-related adverse events as a biomarker in non-melanoma patients treated with programmed cell death 1 inhibitors. *Oncologist.* (2017) 22:1232–7. doi: 10.1634/theoncologist.2017-0133

68. Fujisawa Y, Yoshino K, Otsuka A, Funakoshi T, Uchi H, Fujimura T, et al. Retrospective study of advanced melanoma patients treated with ipilimumab after nivolumab: analysis of 60 Japanese patients. *J Dermatol Sci.* (2018) 89:60–6. doi: 10.1016/j.jdermsci.2017.10.009

69. Teulings HE, Limpens J, Jansen SN, Zwinderman AH, Reitsma JB, Spuls PI, et al. Vitiligo-like depigmentation in patients with stage III-IV melanoma receiving immunotherapy and its association with survival: a systematic review and meta-analysis. *J Clin Oncol.* (2015) 33:773–81. doi: 10.1200/JCO.2014.57.4756

70. Lin PY, Sun L, Thibodeaux SR, Ludwig SM, Vadlamudi RK, Hurez VJ, et al. B7-H1-dependent sex-related differences in tumor immunity and immunotherapy responses. *J Immunol.* (2010) 185:2747–53. doi: 10.4049/jimmunol.1000496

71. Klein SL, Jedlicka A, Pekosz A. The Xs and Y of immune responses to viral vaccines. *Lancet Infect Dis.* (2010) 10:338–49. doi: 10.1016/S1473-3099(10) 70049-9

72. Kugel CH III, Douglass SM, Webster MR, Kaur A, Liu Q, Yin X, et al. Age correlates with response to anti-PD1, reflecting age-related differences in intratumoral effector and regulatory T-cell populations. *Clin Cancer Res.* (2018) 24:5347–56. doi: 10.1158/1078-0432.CCR-18-1116

73. Huang AC, Postow MA, Orlowski RJ, Mick R, Bengsch B, Manne S, et al. T-cell invigoration to tumour burden ratio associated with anti-PD-1 response. *Nature.* (2017) 545:60–5. doi: 10.1038/nature22079

74. Taylor RC, Patel A, Panageas KS, Busam KJ, Brady MS. Tumor-infiltrating lymphocytes predict sentinel lymph node positivity in patients with cutaneous melanoma. *J Clin Oncol.* (2007) 25:869–75. doi: 10.1200/JCO.2006.08.9755

75. Naito Y, Saito K, Shiiba K, Ohuchi A, Saigenji K, Nagura H, et al. CD8+ T cells infiltrated within cancer cell nests as a prognostic factor in human colorectal cancer. *Cancer Res.* (1998) 58:3491–4.

76. Diggs LP, Hsueh EC. Utility of PD-L1 immunohistochemistry assays for predicting PD-1/PD-L1 inhibitor response. *Biomark Res.* (2017) 5:12. doi: 10.1186/s40364-017-0093-8

77. Madore J, Vilain RE, Menzies AM, Kakavand H, Wilmott JS, Hyman J, et al. PD-L1 expression in melanoma shows marked heterogeneity within and between patients: implications for anti-PD-1/PD-L1 clinical trials. *Pigment Cell Melanoma Res.* (2015) 28:245–53. doi: 10.1111/pcmr.12340

78. Liakou CI, Kamat A, Tang DN, Chen H, Sun J, Troncoso P, et al. CTLA-4 blockade increases IFNgamma-producing CD4+ICOShi cells to shift the ratio of effector to regulatory T cells in cancer patients. *Proc Natl Acad Sci USA.* (2008) 105:14987–92. doi: 10.1073/pnas.0806075105

79. Koyama S, Akbay EA, Li YY, Herter-Sprie GS, Buczkowski KA, Richards WG, et al. Adaptive resistance to therapeutic PD-1 blockade is associated with upregulation of alternative immune checkpoints. *Nat Commun.* (2016) 7:10501. doi: 10.1038/ncomms10501

80. Mbongue JC, Nicholas DA, Torrez TW, Kim NS, Firek AF, Langridge WH. The role of indoleamine 2, 3-dioxygenase in immune suppression and autoimmunity. *Vaccines.* (2015) 3:703–29. doi: 10.3390/vaccines3030703

81. Fallarino F, Grohmann U, Vacca C, Orabona C, Spreca A, Fioretti MC, et al. T cell apoptosis by kynurenines. *Adv Exp Med Biol.* (2003) 527:183–90.

82. Fallarino F, Grohmann U, You S, McGrath BC, Cavener DR, Vacca C, et al. Tryptophan catabolism generates autoimmune-preventive regulatory T cells. *Transpl Immunol.* (2006) 17:58–60. doi: 10.1016/j.trim.2006.09.017

83. Rubel F, Kern JS, Technau-Hafsi K, Uhrich S, Thoma K, Hacker G, et al. Indoleamine 2,3-dioxygenase expression in primary cutaneous

melanoma correlates with breslow thickness and is of significant prognostic value for progression-free survival. *J Invest Dermatol.* (2018) 138:679–87. doi: 10.1016/j.jid.2017.09.036

84. Oaks MK, Hallett KM. Cutting edge: a soluble form of CTLA-4 in patients with autoimmune thyroid disease. *J Immunol.* (2000) 164:5015–8. doi: 10.4049/jimmunol.164.10.5015

85. Magistrelli G, Jeannin P, Herbault N, Benoit De Coignac A, Gauchat JF, Bonnefoy JY, et al. A soluble form of CTLA-4 generated by alternative splicing is expressed by nonstimulated human T cells. *Eur J Immunol.* (1999) 29:3596–602. doi: 10.1002/(SICI)1521-4141(199911)29:11<3596::AID-IMMU3596>3.0.CO;2-Y

86. Ryden A, Bolmeson C, Jonson CO, Cilio CM, Faresjo M. Low expression and secretion of circulating soluble CTLA-4 in peripheral blood mononuclear cells and sera from type 1 diabetic children. *Diabetes Metab Res Rev.* (2012) 28:84–96. doi: 10.1002/dmrr.1286

87. Sato S, Fujimoto M, Hasegawa M, Komura K, Yanaba K, Hayakawa I, et al. Serum soluble CTLA-4 levels are increased in diffuse cutaneous systemic sclerosis. *Rheumatology.* (2004) 43:1261–6. doi: 10.1093/rheumatology/keh303

88. Frigola X, Inman BA, Lohse CM, Krco CJ, Cheville JC, Thompson RH, et al. Identification of a soluble form of B7-H1 that retains immunosuppressive activity and is associated with aggressive renal cell carcinoma. *Clin Cancer Res.* (2011) 17:1915–23. doi: 10.1158/1078-0432.CCR-10-0250

89. Rossille D, Gressier M, Damotte D, Maucort-Boulch D, Pangault C, Semana G, et al. High level of soluble programmed cell death ligand 1 in blood impacts overall survival in aggressive diffuse large B-Cell lymphoma: results from a French multicenter clinical trial. *Leukemia.* (2014) 28:2367–75. doi: 10.1038/leu.2014.137

90. Wang L, Wang H, Chen H, Wang WD, Chen XQ, Geng QR, et al. Serum levels of soluble programmed death ligand 1 predict treatment response and progression free survival in multiple myeloma. *Oncotarget.* (2015) 6:41228–36. doi: 10.18632/oncotarget.5682

91. Van Gorp H, Delputte PL, Nauwynck HJ. Scavenger receptor CD163, a Jack-of-all-trades and potential target for cell-directed therapy. *Mol Immunol.* (2010) 47:1650–60. doi: 10.1016/j.molimm.2010.02.008

92. Jensen TO, Schmidt H, Moller HJ, Hoyer M, Maniecki MB, Sjoegren P, et al. Macrophage markers in serum and tumor have prognostic impact in American Joint Committee on Cancer stage I/II melanoma. *J Clin Oncol.* (2009) 27:3330–7. doi: 10.1200/jco.2008.19.9919

93. Zhang J, Basher F, Wu JD. NKG2D ligands in tumor immunity: two sides of a coin. *Front Immunol.* (2015) 6:97. doi: 10.3389/fimmu.2015.00097

94. Raulet DH. Roles of the NKG2D immunoreceptor and its ligands. *Nat Rev Immunol.* (2003) 3:781–90. doi: 10.1038/nri1199

95. Paschen A, Sucker A, Hill B, Moll I, Zapatka M, Nguyen XD, et al. Differential clinical significance of individual NKG2D ligands in melanoma: soluble ULBP2 as an indicator of poor prognosis superior to S100B. *Clin Cancer Res.* (2009) 15:5208–15. doi: 10.1158/1078-0432.CCR-09-0886

96. Chitadze G, Bhat J, Lettau M, Janssen O, Kabelitz D. Generation of soluble NKG2D ligands: proteolytic cleavage, exosome secretion and functional implications. *Scand J Immunol.* (2013) 78:120–9. doi: 10.1111/sji.12072

97. Maccalli C, Scaramuzza S, Parmiani G. TNK cells (NKG2D+ CD8+ or CD4+ T lymphocytes) in the control of human tumors. *Cancer Immunol Immunother.* (2009) 58:801–8. doi: 10.1007/s00262-008-0635-x

98. Nuckel H, Switala M, Sellmann L, Horn PA, Durig J, Duhrsen U, et al. The prognostic significance of soluble NKG2D ligands in B-cell chronic lymphocytic leukemia. *Leukemia.* (2010) 24:1152–9. doi: 10.1038/leu.2010.74

99. Groh V, Wu J, Yee C, Spies T. Tumour-derived soluble MIC ligands impair expression of NKG2D and T-cell activation. *Nature.* (2002) 419:734–8. doi: 10.1038/nature01112

100. Liu G, Lu S, Wang X, Page ST, Higano CS, Plymate SR, et al. Perturbation of NK cell peripheral homeostasis accelerates prostate carcinoma metastasis. *J Clin Invest.* (2013) 123:4410–22. doi: 10.1172/JCI69369

101. Tannenbaum CS, Hamilton TA. Immune-inflammatory mechanisms in IFNgamma-mediated anti-tumor activity. *Semin Cancer Biol.* (2000) 10:113–23. doi: 10.1006/scbi.2000.0314.

102. Bellucci R, Martin A, Bommarito D, Wang K, Hansen SH, Freeman GJ, et al. Interferon-gamma-induced activation of JAK1 and JAK2 suppresses tumor

cell susceptibility to NK cells through upregulation of PD-L1 expression. *Oncoimmunology.* (2015) 4:e1008824. doi: 10.1080/2162402x.2015.1008824

103. Balkwill F. TNF-alpha in promotion and progression of cancer. *Cancer Metastasis Rev.* (2006) 25:409–16. doi: 10.1007/s10555-006-9005-3

104. Lin WW, Karin M. A cytokine-mediated link between innate immunity, inflammation, and cancer. *J Clin Invest.* (2007) 117:1175–83. doi: 10.1172/jci31537

105. Guo Y, Xu F, Lu T, Duan Z, Zhang Z. Interleukin-6 signaling pathway in targeted therapy for cancer. *Cancer Treat Rev.* (2012) 38:904–10. doi: 10.1016/j.ctrv.2012.04.007

106. Hoejberg L, Bastholt L, Johansen JS, Christensen IJ, Gehl J, Schmidt H. Serum interleukin-6 as a prognostic biomarker in patients with metastatic melanoma. *Melanoma Res.* (2012) 22:287–93. doi: 10.1097/CMR.0b013e3283550aa5

107. Mortensen RF. C-reactive protein, inflammation, and innate immunity. *Immunol Res.* (2001) 24:163–76. doi: 10.1385/ir:24:2:163

108. Davis BP, Rothenberg ME. Eosinophils and cancer. *Cancer Immunol Res.* (2014) 2:1–8. doi: 10.1158/2326-6066.Cir-13-0196

109. Simson L, Ellyard JI, Dent LA, Matthaei KI, Rothenberg ME, Foster PS, et al. Regulation of carcinogenesis by IL-5 and CCL11: a potential role for eosinophils in tumor immune surveillance. *J Immunol.* (2007) 178:4222–9. doi: 10.4049/jimmunol.178.7.4222

110. Ishibashi S, Ohashi Y, Suzuki T, Miyazaki S, Moriya T, Satomi S, et al. Tumor-associated tissue eosinophilia in human esophageal squamous cell carcinoma. *Anticancer Res.* (2006) 26:1419–24.

111. Pretlow TP, Keith EF, Cryar AK, Bartolucci AA, Pitts AM, Pretlow TG II, et al. Eosinophil infiltration of human colonic carcinomas as a prognostic indicator. *Cancer Res.* (1983) 43:2997–3000.

112. Grivennikov SI, Greten FR, Karin M. Immunity, inflammation, and cancer. *Cell.* (2010) 140:883–99. doi: 10.1016/j.cell.2010.01.025

113. Hernandez C, Huebener P, Schwabe RF. Damage-associated molecular patterns in cancer: a double-edged sword. *Oncogene.* (2016) 35:5931–41. doi: 10.1038/onc.2016.104

114. Singel KL, Grzankowski KS, Khan A, Grimm MJ, D'Auria AC, Morrell K, et al. Mitochondrial DNA in the tumour microenvironment activates neutrophils and is associated with worse outcomes in patients with advanced epithelial ovarian cancer. *Br J Cancer.* (2019) 120:207–17. doi: 10.1038/s41416-018-0339-8

115. Lee BM, Chung SY, Chang JS, Lee KJ, Seong J. The neutrophil-lymphocyte ratio and platelet-lymphocyte ratio are prognostic factors in patients with locally advanced pancreatic cancer treated with chemoradiotherapy. *Gut Liver.* (2018) 12:342–52. doi: 10.5009/gnl17216

116. Kiriu T, Yamamoto M, Nagano T, Hazama D, Sekiya R, Katsurada M, et al. The time-series behavior of neutrophil-to-lymphocyte ratio is useful as a predictive marker in non-small cell lung cancer. *PLoS ONE.* (2018) 13:e0193018. doi: 10.1371/journal.pone.0193018

117. Tanaka A, Sakaguchi S. Regulatory T cells in cancer immunotherapy. *Cell Res.* (2017) 27:109–18. doi: 10.1038/cr.2016.151

118. Sakaguchi S, Sakaguchi N, Shimizu J, Yamazaki S, Sakihama T, Itoh M, et al. Immunologic tolerance maintained by CD25+ CD4+ regulatory T cells: their common role in controlling autoimmunity, tumor immunity, and transplantation tolerance. *Immunol Rev.* (2001) 182:18–32.

119. Onizuka S, Tawara I, Shimizu J, Sakaguchi S, Fujita T, Nakayama E. Tumor rejection by *in vivo* administration of anti-CD25 (interleukin-2 receptor alpha) monoclonal antibody. *Cancer Res.* (1999) 59:3128–33.

120. Weber R, Fleming V, Hu X, Nagibin V, Groth C, Altevogt P, et al. Myeloid-derived suppressor cells hinder the anti-cancer activity of immune checkpoint inhibitors. *Front Immunol.* (2018) 9:1310. doi: 10.3389/fimmu.2018.01310

121. Mantovani A. The growing diversity and spectrum of action of myeloid-derived suppressor cells. *Eur J Immunol.* (2010) 40:3317–20. doi: 10.1002/eji.201041170

122. Gabrilovich DI, Ostrand-Rosenberg S, Bronte V. Coordinated regulation of myeloid cells by tumours. *Nat Rev Immunol.* (2012) 12:253–68. doi: 10.1038/nri3175

123. Bedikian AY, Johnson MM, Warneke CL, Papadopoulos NE, Kim K, Hwu WJ, et al. Prognostic factors that determine the long-term survival

of patients with unresectable metastatic melanoma. *Cancer Invest.* (2008) 26:624–33. doi: 10.1080/07357900802027073

124. Kelderman S, Heemskerk B, van Tinteren H, van den Brom RR, Hospers GA, van den Eertwegh AJ, et al. Lactate dehydrogenase as a selection criterion for ipilimumab treatment in metastatic melanoma. *Cancer Immunol Immunother.* (2014) 63:449–58. doi: 10.1007/s00262-014-1528-9

125. Taniguchi Y, Tamiya A, Isa SI, Nakahama K, Okishio K, Shiroyama T, et al. Predictive factors for poor progression-free survival in patients with non-small cell lung cancer treated with nivolumab. *Anticancer Res.* (2017) 37:5857–62. doi: 10.21873/anticanres.12030

126. Alexandrov LB, Nik-Zainal S, Wedge DC, Aparicio SA, Behjati S, Biankin AV, et al. Signatures of mutational processes in human cancer. *Nature.* (2013) 500:415–21. doi: 10.1038/nature12477

127. Topalian SL, Taube JM, Anders RA, Pardoll DM. Mechanism-driven biomarkers to guide immune checkpoint blockade in cancer therapy. *Nat Rev Cancer.* (2016) 16:275–87. doi: 10.1038/nrc.2016.36

128. Nakamura Y, Fujisawa Y, Tanaka R, Maruyama H, Ishitsuka Y, Okiyama N, et al. Use of immune checkpoint inhibitors prolonged overall survival in a Japanese population of advanced malignant melanoma patients: retrospective single institutional study. *J Dermatol.* (2018) 45:1337–9. doi: 10.1111/1346-8138.14637

129. Hayward NK, Wilmott JS, Waddell N, Johansson PA, Field MA, Nones K, et al. Whole-genome landscapes of major melanoma subtypes. *Nature.* (2017) 545:175–80. doi: 10.1038/nature22071

130. Zhang Y, Sun Z, Mao X, Wu H, Luo F, Wu X, et al. Impact of mismatch-repair deficiency on the colorectal cancer immune microenvironment. *Oncotarget.* (2017) 8:85526–36. doi: 10.18632/oncotarget.20241

131. Lee V, Murphy A, Le DT, Diaz LA Jr. Mismatch repair deficiency and response to immune checkpoint blockade. *Oncologist.* (2016) 21:1200–11. doi: 10.1634/theoncologist.2016-0046

132. Goldstein J, Tran B, Ensor J, Gibbs P, Wong HL, Wong SF, et al. Multicenter retrospective analysis of metastatic colorectal cancer (CRC) with high-level microsatellite instability (MSI-H). *Ann Oncol.* (2014) 25:1032–8. doi: 10.1093/annonc/mdu100

133. Koopman M, Kortman GA, Mekenkamp L, Ligtenberg MJ, Hoogerbrugge N, Antonini NF, et al. Deficient mismatch repair system in patients with sporadic advanced colorectal cancer. *Br J Cancer.* (2009) 100:266–73. doi: 10.1038/sj.bjc.6604867

134. Overman MJ, Lonardi S, Wong KYM, Lenz HJ, Gelsomino F, Aglietta M, et al. Durable clinical benefit with nivolumab plus ipilimumab in DNA mismatch repair-deficient/microsatellite instability-high metastatic colorectal cancer. *J Clin Oncol.* (2018) 36:773–9. doi: 10.1200/jco.2017.76.9901

135. Bhatt AP, Redinbo MR, Bultman SJ. The role of the microbiome in cancer development and therapy. *CA Cancer J Clin.* (2017) 67:326–44. doi: 10.3322/caac.21398

136. Sivan A, Corrales L, Hubert N, Williams JB, Aquino-Michaels K, Earley ZM, et al. Commensal Bifidobacterium promotes antitumor immunity and facilitates anti-PD-L1 efficacy. *Science.* (2015) 350:1084–9. doi: 10.1126/science.aac4255

137. Schwarzenbach H, Hoon DS, Pantel K. Cell-free nucleic acids as biomarkers in cancer patients. *Nat Rev Cancer.* (2011) 11:426–37. doi: 10.1038/nrc3066

138. Garcia-Olmo DC, Dominguez C, Garcia-Arranz M, Anker P, Stroun M, Garcia-Verdugo JM, et al. Cell-free nucleic acids circulating in the plasma of colorectal cancer patients induce the oncogenic transformation of susceptible cultured cells. *Cancer Res.* (2010) 70:560–7. doi: 10.1158/0008-5472.Can-09-3513

139. Stroun M, Lyautey J, Lederrey C, Olson-Sand A, Anker P. About the possible origin and mechanism of circulating DNA apoptosis and active DNA release. *Clin Chim Acta.* (2001) 313:139–42.

140. Ascierto PA, Minor D, Ribas A, Lebbe C, O'Hagan A, Arya N, et al. Phase II trial (BREAK-2) of the BRAF inhibitor dabrafenib (GSK2118436) in patients with metastatic melanoma. *J Clin Oncol.* (2013) 31:3205–11. doi: 10.1200/JCO.2013.49.8691

141. Heitzer E, Ulz P, Geigl JB. Circulating tumor DNA as a liquid biopsy for cancer. *Clin Chem.* (2015) 61:112–23. doi: 10.1373/clinchem.2014.222679

142. Khagi Y, Goodman AM, Daniels GA, Patel SP, Sacco AG, Randall JM, et al. Hypermutated circulating tumor DNA: correlation with response

to checkpoint inhibitor-based immunotherapy. *Clin Cancer Res.* (2017) 23:5729–36. doi: 10.1158/1078-0432.CCR-17-1439

143. Theodoraki MN, Yerneni SS, Hoffmann TK, Gooding WE, Whiteside TL. Clinical significance of PD-L1(+) exosomes in plasma of head and neck cancer patients. *Clin Cancer Res.* (2018) 24:896–905. doi: 10.1158/1078-0432.CCR-17-2664

144. Downey SG, Klapper JA, Smith FO, Yang JC, Sherry RM, Royal RE, et al. Prognostic factors related to clinical response in patients with metastatic melanoma treated with CTL-associated antigen-4 blockade. *Clin Cancer Res.* (2007) 13:6681–8. doi: 10.1158/1078-0432.CCR-07-0187

145. Freeman-Keller M, Kim Y, Cronin H, Richards A, Gibney G, Weber JS. Nivolumab in resected and unresectable metastatic melanoma: characteristics of immune-related adverse events and association with outcomes. *Clin Cancer Res.* (2016) 22:886–94. doi: 10.1158/1078-0432.CCR-15-1136

146. Khoja L, Atenafu EG, Templeton A, Qye Y, Chappell MA, Saibil S, et al. The full blood count as a biomarker of outcome and toxicity in ipilimumab-treated cutaneous metastatic melanoma. *Cancer Med.* (2016) 5:2792–9. doi: 10.1002/cam4.878

147. Kim HI, Kim M, Lee SH, Park SY, Kim YN, Kim H, et al. Development of thyroid dysfunction is associated with clinical response to PD-1 blockade treatment in patients with advanced non-small cell lung cancer. *Oncoimmunology.* (2017) 7:e1375642. doi: 10.1080/2162402X.2017.1375642

148. Rzepecki AK, Cheng H, McLellan BN. Cutaneous toxicity as a predictive biomarker for clinical outcome in patients receiving anticancer therapy. *J Am Acad Dermatol.* (2018) 79:545–55. doi: 10.1016/j.jaad.2018.04.046

149. Kosche C, Mohindra N, Choi JN. Vitiligo in a patient undergoing nivolumab treatment for non-small cell lung cancer. *JAAD Case Rep.* (2018) 4:1042–4. doi: 10.1016/j.jdcr.2018.08.009

150. Liu RC, Consuegra G, Chou S, Fernandez Penas P. Vitiligo-like depigmentation in oncology patients treated with immunotherapies for nonmelanoma metastatic cancers. *Clin Exp Dermatol.* (2019) 2019:13867. doi: 10.1111/ced.13867

151. Daly LE, Power DG, O'Reilly A, Donnellan P, Cushen SJ, O'Sullivan K, et al. The impact of body composition parameters on ipilimumab toxicity and survival in patients with metastatic melanoma. *Br J Cancer.* (2017) 116:310–7. doi: 10.1038/bjc.2016.431

152. Valpione S, Pasquali S, Campana LG, Piccin L, Mocellin S, Pigozzo J, et al. Sex and interleukin-6 are prognostic factors for autoimmune toxicity following treatment with anti-CTLA4 blockade. *J Transl Med.* (2018) 16:94. doi: 10.1186/s12967-018-1467-x

153. Tarhini AA, Zahoor H, Lin Y, Malhotra U, Sander C, Butterfield LH, et al. Baseline circulating IL-17 predicts toxicity while TGF-beta1 and IL-10 are prognostic of relapse in ipilimumab neoadjuvant therapy of melanoma. *J Immunother Cancer.* (2015) 3:39. doi: 10.1186/s40425-015-0081-1

154. Fujimura T, Sato Y, Tanita K, Kambayashi Y, Otsuka A, Fujisawa Y, et al. Serum levels of soluble CD163 and CXCL5 may be predictive markers for immune-related adverse events in patients with advanced melanoma treated with nivolumab: a pilot study. *Oncotarget.* (2018) 9:15542–51. doi: 10.18632/oncotarget.24509

155. Diehl A, Yarchoan M, Hopkins A, Jaffee E, Grossman SA. Relationships between lymphocyte counts and treatment-related toxicities and clinical responses in patients with solid tumors treated with PD-1 checkpoint inhibitors. *Oncotarget.* (2017) 8:114268–80. doi: 10.18632/oncotarget.23217

156. Fujisawa Y, Yoshino K, Otsuka A, Funakoshi T, Fujimura T, Yamamoto Y, et al. Fluctuations in routine blood count might signal severe immune-related adverse events in melanoma patients treated with nivolumab. *J Dermatol Sci.* (2017) 88:225–31. doi: 10.1016/j.jdermsci.2017.07.007

157. Kimbara S, Fujiwara Y, Iwama S, Ohashi K, Kuchiba A, Arima H, et al. Association of antithyroglobulin antibodies with the development of thyroid dysfunction induced by nivolumab. *Cancer Sci.* (2018) 109:3583–90. doi: 10.1111/cas.13800

158. Stamatouli AM, Quandt Z, Perdigoto AL, Clark PL, Kluger H, Weiss SA, et al. Collateral damage: insulin-dependent diabetes induced with checkpoint inhibitors. *Diabetes.* (2018) 67:1471–80. doi: 10.2337/dbi18-0002

159. Oh DY, Cham J, Zhang L, Fong G, Kwek SS, Klinger M, et al. Immune toxicities elicted by CTLA-4 blockade in cancer patients are associated with

early diversification of the T-cell repertoire. *Cancer Res.* (2017) 77:1322–30. doi: 10.1158/0008-5472.Can-16-2324

160. Dubin K, Callahan MK, Ren B, Khanin R, Viale A, Ling L, et al. Intestinal microbiome analyses identify melanoma patients at risk for checkpoint-blockade-induced colitis. *Nat Commun.* (2016) 7:10391. doi: 10.1038/ncomms10391

161. De Velasco G, Je Y, Bosse D, Awad MM, Ott PA, Moreira RB, et al. Comprehensive meta-analysis of key immune-related adverse events from CTLA-4 and PD-1/PD-L1 inhibitors in cancer patients. *Cancer Immunol Res.* (2017) 5:312–8. doi: 10.1158/2326-6066.Cir-16-0237

162. Eggermont AM, Chiarion-Sileni V, Grob JJ, Dummer R, Wolchok JD, Schmidt H, et al. Adjuvant ipilimumab versus placebo after complete resection of high-risk stage III melanoma (EORTC 18071): a randomised, double-blind, phase 3 trial. *Lancet Oncol.* (2015) 16:522–30. doi: 10.1016/s1470-2045(15)70122-1

163. Perez-Gracia JL, Loriot Y, Rosenberg JE, Powles T, Necchi A, Hussain SA, et al. Atezolizumab in platinum-treated locally advanced or metastatic urothelial carcinoma: outcomes by prior number of regimens. *Eur Urol.* (2017) 2017:023. doi: 10.1016/j.eururo.2017.11.023

164. Antonia SJ, Lopez-Martin JA, Bendell J, Ott PA, Taylor M, Eder JP, et al. Nivolumab alone and nivolumab plus ipilimumab in recurrent small-cell lung cancer (CheckMate 032): a multicentre, open-label, phase 1/2 trial. *Lancet Oncol.* (2016) 17:883–95. doi: 10.1016/s1470-2045(16)30098-5

165. Khoja L, Day D, Wei-Wu Chen T, Siu LL, Hansen AR. Tumour- and class-specific patterns of immune-related adverse events of immune checkpoint inhibitors: a systematic review. *Ann Oncol.* (2017) 28:2377–85. doi: 10.1093/annonc/mdx286

166. Weber JS, Dummer R, de Pril V, Lebbe C, Hodi FS. Patterns of onset and resolution of immune-related adverse events of special interest with ipilimumab: detailed safety analysis from a phase 3 trial in patients with advanced melanoma. *Cancer.* (2013) 119:1675–82. doi: 10.1002/cncr.27969

167. Topalian SL, Sznol M, McDermott DF, Kluger HM, Carvajal RD, Sharfman WH, et al. Survival, durable tumor remission, and long-term safety in patients with advanced melanoma receiving nivolumab. *J Clin Oncol.* (2014) 32:1020–30. doi: 10.1200/jco.2013.53.0105

168. Weber JS, Hodi FS, Wolchok JD, Topalian SL, Schadendorf D, Larkin J, et al. Safety profile of nivolumab monotherapy: a pooled analysis of patients with advanced melanoma. *J Clin Oncol.* (2017) 35:785–92. doi: 10.1200/jco.2015.66.1389

169. Prado CM, Baracos VE, McCargar LJ, Reiman T, Mourtzakis M, Tonkin K, et al. Sarcopenia as a determinant of chemotherapy toxicity and time to tumor progression in metastatic breast cancer patients receiving capecitabine treatment. *Clin Cancer Res.* (2009) 15:2920–6. doi: 10.1158/1078-0432.Ccr-08-2242

170. Huillard O, Mir O, Peyromaure M, Tlemsani C, Giroux J, Boudou-Rouquette P, et al. Sarcopenia and body mass index predict sunitinib-induced early dose-limiting toxicities in renal cancer patients. *Br J Cancer.* (2013) 108:1034–41. doi: 10.1038/bjc.2013.58

171. Antoun S, Birdsell L, Sawyer MB, Venner P, Escudier B, Baracos VE. Association of skeletal muscle wasting with treatment with sorafenib in patients with advanced renal cell carcinoma: results from a placebo-controlled study. *J Clin Oncol.* (2010) 28:1054–60. doi: 10.1200/jco.2009.24.9730

172. Sabel MS, Lee J, Cai S, Englesbe MJ, Holcombe S, Wang S. Sarcopenia as a prognostic factor among patients with stage III melanoma. *Ann Surg Oncol.* (2011) 18:3579–85. doi: 10.1245/s10434-011-1976-9

173. Rollins KE, Tewari N, Ackner A, Awwad A, Madhusudan S, Macdonald IA, et al. The impact of sarcopenia and myosteatosis on outcomes of unresectable pancreatic cancer or distal cholangiocarcinoma. *Clin Nutr.* (2016) 35:1103–9. doi: 10.1016/j.clnu.2015.08.005

174. Blauwhoff-Buskermolen S, Versteeg KS, de van der Schueren MA, den Braver NR, Berkhof J, Langius JA, et al. Loss of muscle mass during chemotherapy is predictive for poor survival of patients with metastatic colorectal cancer. *J Clin Oncol.* (2016) 34:1339–44. doi: 10.1200/jco.2015.63.6043

175. Schwinge D, Schramm C. Sex-related factors in autoimmune liver diseases. *Semin Immunopathol.* (2018) 2018:715. doi: 10.1007/s00281-018-0715-8

176. Fujimura T, Mahnke K, Enk AH. Myeloid derived suppressor cells and their role in tolerance induction in cancer. *J Dermatol Sci.* (2010) 59:1–6. doi: 10.1016/j.jdermsci.2010.05.001

177. Sosa A, Lopez Cadena E, Simon Olive C, Karachaliou N, Rosell R. Clinical assessment of immune-related adverse events. *Ther Adv Med Oncol.* (2018) 10:1758835918764628. doi: 10.1177/1758835918764628

178. Patel SA, Gooderham NJ. IL6 mediates immune and colorectal cancer cell cross-talk via miR-21 and miR-29b. *Mol Cancer Res.* (2015) 13:1502–8. doi: 10.1158/1541-7786.Mcr-15-0147

179. Abraham C, Cho J. Interleukin-23/Th17 pathways and inflammatory bowel disease. *Inflamm Bowel Dis.* (2009) 15:1090–100. doi: 10.1002/ibd.20894

180. Fujimura T, Kakizaki A, Furudate S, Aiba S. A possible interaction between periostin and CD163(+) skin-resident macrophages in pemphigus vulgaris and bullous pemphigoid. *Exp Dermatol.* (2017) 26:1193–8. doi: 10.1111/exd.13157

181. Rumble JM, Huber AK, Krishnamoorthy G, Srinivasan A, Giles DA, Zhang X, et al. Neutrophil-related factors as biomarkers in EAE and MS. *J Exp Med.* (2015) 212:23–35. doi: 10.1084/jem.20141015

182. Huebener P, Pradere JP, Hernandez C, Gwak GY, Caviglia JM, Mu X, et al. The HMGB1/RAGE axis triggers neutrophil-mediated injury amplification following necrosis. *J Clin Invest.* (2015) 125:539–50. doi: 10.1172/jci76887

183. Berman D, Parker SM, Siegel J, Chasalow SD, Weber J, Galbraith S, et al. Blockade of cytotoxic T-lymphocyte antigen-4 by ipilimumab results in dysregulation of gastrointestinal immunity in patients with advanced melanoma. *Cancer Immun.* (2010) 10:11.

184. Da Gama Duarte J, Parakh S, Andrews MC, Woods K, Pasam A, Tutuka C, et al. Autoantibodies may predict immune-related toxicity: results from a phase i study of intralesional bacillus calmette-guerin followed by ipilimumab in patients with advanced metastatic melanoma. *Front Immunol.* (2018) 9:411. doi: 10.3389/fimmu.2018.00411

185. Heidarian F, Alebouyeh M, Shahrokh S, Balaii H, Zali MR. Altered fecal bacterial composition correlates with disease activity in inflammatory bowel disease and the extent of IL8 induction. *Curr Res Transl Med.* (2019) 2019:002. doi: 10.1016/j.retram.2019.01.002

14

Anti-PD-1 and Anti-CTLA-4 Therapies in Cancer: Mechanisms of Action, Efficacy and Limitations

Judith A. Seidel[1], Atsushi Otsuka[1]* and Kenji Kabashima[1,2]*

[1]Department of Dermatology, Kyoto University Graduate School of Medicine, Kyoto, Japan, [2]Singapore Immunology Network (SIgN), Institute of Medical Biology, Agency for Science, Technology and Research (A*STAR), Biopolis, Singapore, Singapore

*Correspondence:
Atsushi Otsuka
otsukamn@kuhp.kyoto-u.ac.jp;
Kenji Kabashima
kaba@kuhp.kyoto-u.ac.jp

Melanoma, a skin cancer associated with high mortality rates, is highly radio- and chemotherapy resistant but can also be very immunogenic. These circumstances have led to a recent surge in research into therapies aiming to boost anti-tumor immune responses in cancer patients. Among these immunotherapies, neutralizing antibodies targeting the immune checkpoints T-lymphocyte-associated protein 4 (CTLA-4) and programmed cell death protein 1 (PD-1) are being hailed as particularly successful. These antibodies have resulted in dramatic improvements in disease outcome and are now clinically approved in many countries. However, the majority of advanced stage melanoma patients do not respond or will relapse, and the hunt for the "magic bullet" to treat the disease continues. This review examines the mechanisms of action and the limitations of anti-PD-1/PD-L1 and anti-CTLA-4 antibodies which are the two types of checkpoint inhibitors currently available to patients and further explores the future avenues of their use in melanoma and other cancers.

Keywords: immunotherapy, cancer, melanoma, side effects, biomarkers, immune checkpoint inhibitors, mode of action

INTRODUCTION

In recent years, there has been a steep rise in the development and implementation of anti-cancer immunotherapies. The approval of anti-cytotoxic T-lymphocyte-associated protein 4 (CTLA-4) and anti-programmed cell death protein 1 (PD-1) antibodies for human use has already resulted in significant improvements in disease outcomes for various cancers, especially melanoma. Unlike radio- and chemotherapy, which aim to directly interfere with tumor cell growth and survival, immunotherapies target the tumor indirectly by boosting the anti-tumor immune responses that spontaneously arise in many patients.

Abbreviations: ctDNA, circular tumor DNA; CTLA-4, T-lymphocyte-associated protein 4; DCs, dendritic cells; IPRES, innate anti-PD-1 resistance; LDH, lactate dehydrogenase; NK, natural killer cells; PD-1, programmed cell death protein 1; IDO, indoleamine 2,3-dioxygenase; IL-12, interleukin 12; TGF-β, tumor growth factor-β; Tregs, regulatory T cells; MDSCs, myeloid-derived suppressor cells; VISTA, V-domain Ig suppressor of T cell activation; ITIM, immunoreceptor tyrosine-based inhibition motif; IFN-γ, interferon; TIM-3, T-cell immunoglobulin and mucin-domain containing-3; LAG-3, lymphocyte-activation protein 3; TIGIT, T-cell immunoreceptor with Ig and ITIM domains; TNF-α, tumor necrosis factor-α; ICOS, inducible co-stimulatory molecule; IFN-γ, interferon-γ; BTLA, B- And T-lymphocyte-associated protein; CSF-1R, colony stimulating factor-1 receptor; GM-CSF, granulocyte-macrophage colony-stimulating factor; Breg, regulatory B cell.

CANCERS EVADE AND INHIBIT IMMUNE RESPONSES

In order to understand the modes of action of immune checkpoint inhibitors, it is important to understand the dynamic interplay between cancers and the immune system during the course of the disease.

Cancer cells are genetically unstable, which contributes to their uncontrolled proliferation and the expression of antigens that can be recognized by the immune system. These antigens include normal proteins overexpressed by cancer cells and novel proteins that are generated by mutation and gene rearrangement (1). Cytotoxic CD8+ T cells are immune cells that are particularly effective at mediating anti-tumor immune responses. These cells may learn to recognize the tumor-specific antigens presented on major histocompatibility complex (MHC) class I molecules and thereby perform targeted tumor cell killing. CD8+ T cells become licensed effector cells after appropriate stimulation by antigen-presenting cells that have collected antigens at the tumor site. Apart from the antigen peptides embedded on the MHC molecules, antigen-presenting cells must provide costimulatory signals through surface receptors (such as CD28) and cytokines [such as interleukin (IL)-12] for effective T cell stimulation (2).

Tumor cells adopt a variety of mechanisms to avoid immune recognition and immunomediated destruction. Established tumors are often thought to arise through the selection of clones that are able to evade the immune system, a process known as immunoediting (3). Tumor cells may evade immune recognition directly by downregulating features that make them vulnerable such as tumor antigens or MHC class I (4–6). Alternatively, tumors may evade immune responses by taking advantage of negative feedback mechanisms that the body has evolved to prevent immunopathology. These include inhibitory cytokines such as IL-10 and tumor growth factor (TGF)-β, inhibitory cell types such as regulatory T cells (Tregs), regulatory B cells (Bregs), and myeloid-derived suppressor cells (MDSCs), metabolic modulators such as indoleamine 2,3-dioxygenase (IDO), and inhibitory receptors such as PD-1 and CTLA-4 (7, 8).

IMMUNE EXHAUSTION CONTRIBUTES TO IMMUNE DYSFUNCTION IN CANCER

Inhibitory receptors, also known as immune checkpoints, and their ligands can be found on a wide range of cell types. They are essential for central and peripheral tolerance in that they counteract simultaneous activating signaling through co-stimulatory molecules. Inhibitory receptors may act during both immune activation and ongoing immune responses. During chronic inflammation in particular, T cells are known to become exhausted and to upregulate a wide range of non-redundant inhibitory receptors that limit their effectiveness, such as PD-1, CTLA-4, T-cell immunoglobulin and mucin-domain containing-3 (TIM-3), lymphocyte-activation gene 3 (LAG-3), or T-Cell immunoreceptor with Ig And ITIM domains (TIGIT) [See **Table 1** (9–11)]. Originally described in the context of chronic viral infections, where the host fails to clear the pathogen, it is now apparent that exhausted T cells can also occur in cancer (12, 13). It is believed that, under these conditions, persistent high antigenic load leads to the T cells upregulating the inhibitory receptors, whose signaling subsequently leads to a progressive loss of proliferative potential and effector functions and in some cases to their deletion (14).

Exhaustion is therefore both a physiological mechanism designed to limit immunopathology during persistent infection and a major obstacle for anti-tumor immune responses (17). It should be noted that expression of inhibitory markers is not always a sign of immune exhaustion, because the receptors may be expressed individually during conventional immune responses (18).

THE IMMUNE CHECKPOINT RECEPTOR CTLA-4

The anti-CTLA-4 blocking antibody ipilimumab was the first immune checkpoint inhibitor to be tested and approved for the treatment of cancer patients (19, 20). CTLA-4 (CD152) is a B7/CD28 family member that inhibits T cell functions. It is constitutively expressed by Tregs but can also be upregulated by

TABLE 1 | Overview of T cell surface receptors associated with immune inhibition and dysfunction.

Receptor	Expressing cells	Ligands	Ligand-expressing cells
Programmed cell death protein 1 (PD-1) (11)	CD4 (activated/exhausted, follicular), CD8 (activated/exhausted), B cells, dendritic cells (DCs), monocytes, mast cells, Langerhans cells	PD-L1, PD-L2	Antigen-presenting cells, CD4+ T cells, non-lymphoid tissues, some tumors
T-lymphocyte-associated protein 4 (CTLA-4) (15)	CD4 (activated/exhausted, Tregs), CD8 (activated/exhausted), some tumors	CD80, CD86	Antigen-presenting cells
lymphocyte-activation protein 3 (LAG-3) (15)	CD4 (including Treg and exhausted), CD8 (including exhausted), natural killer cells (NK)	MHC class II, LSECtin	Antigen-presenting cells, liver, some tumors
T-cell immunoglobulin and mucin-domain containing-3 (TIM-3) (16)	CD4 (Th1, Th17, Treg), CD8 (including exhausted and Tc1), DC, NK, monocyte, macrophages	Galectin-9, phosphatidyl serine, high mobility group protein B1, Ceacam-1	Endothelial cells, apoptotic cells, some tumors
T-cell immunoreceptor with Ig And ITIM domains (TIGIT) (16)	CD4 (including Treg, follicular helper T cells), CD8, NK	CD155 (PVR), CD122 (PVRL2, nectin-2)	APCs, T cells, some tumors

other T cell subsets, especially CD4[+] T cells, upon activation (21). Exhausted T cells are also often characterized by the expression of CTLA-4 among other inhibitory receptors. CTLA-4 is mostly located in intracellular vesicles and is only transiently expressed upon activation in the immunological synapse before being rapidly endocytosed (22).

CTLA-4 mediates immunosuppression by indirectly diminishing signaling through the co-stimulatory receptor CD28. Although both receptors bind CD80 and CD86, CTLA-4 does so with much higher affinity, effectively outcompeting CD28 (23). CTLA-4 may also remove CD80 and CD86 (including their cytoplasmic domains) from the cell surfaces of antigen-presenting cells *via* trans-endocytosis (24), therefore reducing the availability of these stimulatory receptors to other CD28-expressing T cells. Indeed, this process is an important mechanism by which Tregs mediate immune suppression on bystander cells (25).

By limiting CD28-mediated signaling during antigen presentation, CTLA-4 increases the activation threshold of T cells, reducing immune responses to weak antigens such as self- and tumor antigens. The central role that CTLA-4 plays in immunological tolerance is exemplified by experiments in mice that lack the CTLA-4 gene globally or specifically in the Forkhead box P3 (FoxP3)[+] Treg compartment. These animals develop lymphoproliferative disorders and die at a young age (25, 26). Similarly, polymorphisms within the CTLA-4 gene are associated with autoimmune diseases in humans (27). CTLA-4 signaling has been shown to dampen immune responses against infections and tumor cells (28, 29).

THE IMMUNE CHECKPOINT RECEPTOR PD-1

The surface receptor PD-1 (CD279) was first discovered on a murine T cell hybridoma and was thought to be involved in cell death (30). It has since become clear, however, that PD-1, which is homologous to CD28, is primarily involved in inhibitory immune signaling, and is an essential regulator of adaptive immune responses (31). In both humans and mice some T cell populations constitutively express PD-1; one example is follicular helper T cells (32). Although most circulating T cells do not express the receptor, they can be induced to do so upon stimulation, through the T cell receptor (TCR) complex or exposure to cytokines such as IL-2, IL-7, IL-15, IL-21, and transforming growth factor (TGF)-β (33, 34). Other cell types, such as B cells, myeloid dendritic cells, mast cells, and Langerhans cells, can also express PD-1 which may regulate their own and bystander cell functions under pathophysiological conditions (35–38). PD-1 has two ligands: PD-L1 (B7-H1; CD274) and PD-L2 (B7-DC; CD273). Both can be found on the surface of antigen-presenting cells (such as dendritic cells, macrophages, and monocytes), but are otherwise differentially expressed on various non-lymphoid tissues (39, 40). Interferon (IFN)-γ is the main trigger known to cause PD-L1 and PD-L2 upregulation (41).

PD-1 bears an immunoreceptor tyrosine-based inhibition motif (ITIM) and an immunoreceptor tyrosine-based switch motif (ITSM) motif on its intracellular tail. The intracellular signaling events initiated upon PD-1 engagement are best described in T cells and are illustrated in **Figure 1**. In these cells, engagement of PD-1 causes tyrosine residues to become phosphorylated, starting an intracellular signaling cascade that mediates the dephosphorylation of TCR proximal signaling components (9, 42–44). Among these, CD28 has recently been found to be the primary target (45). In the presence of TCR stimulation, CD28 provides critical signals that are important for T cell activation. By interfering with early TCR/CD28 signaling and associated IL-2-dependent positive feedback, PD-1 signaling therefore results in reduced cytokine production [such as IL-2, IFN-γ, and tumor necrosis factor (TNF)-α], cell cycle progression, and pro-survival Bcl-xL gene expression, as well as reduced expression of the transcription factors involved in effector functions such as T-bet and Eomes (42, 43, 46, 47). PD-1 activity is therefore only relevant during simultaneous T cell activation, as its signal transduction can only come into effect during TCR-dependent signaling (39, 41, 48). Details about PD-1 signaling in other cell types that bear this receptor, such as B cells, remain to be elucidated.

Overall, PD-1 is crucial for the maintenance of peripheral tolerance and for containing immune responses to avoid immunopathology. Mice deficient in the receptor initially appear healthy, but develop autoimmune diseases such as lupus-like proliferative glomerulonephritis and arthritis with age and exacerbated inflammation during infections (18, 31, 49, 50). Humans with genetic polymorphisms in the PD-1 locus also have an increased likelihood of developing various autoimmune diseases (51, 52).

CTLA-4, PD-1, AND THEIR LIGANDS IN CANCER

CTLA-4 may be expressed in tumor lesions on infiltrating Tregs or exhausted conventional T cells as well as tumor cells themselves (53, 54). Despite the immunosuppressive role of CTLA-4, its association with disease prognosis is not clear; however, it should be noted that only a few studies have described the prognostic value of CTLA-4 levels in the tumor site. So far, the expression of CTLA-4 on tumors has been associated with decreased survival in nasopharyngeal carcinoma (54) and increased survival in non-small cell lung cancer (53).

PD-1 can be upregulated transiently during stimulation and constitutively during chronic immune activation (17). The inhibitory receptor has been detected on both circulating tumor-specific T cells and tumor-infiltrating lymphocytes, where it was associated with decreased T cell function in humans and mice (13, 29, 55–57). Other cell types may also upregulate PD-1 in tumor lesions. PD-1-positive dendritic cells, for example, have been identified in hepatocellular carcinoma where they exhibited a reduced ability to stimulate T cells (37). Another study identified a population of tumor-infiltrating PD-1-expressing regulatory B cells that

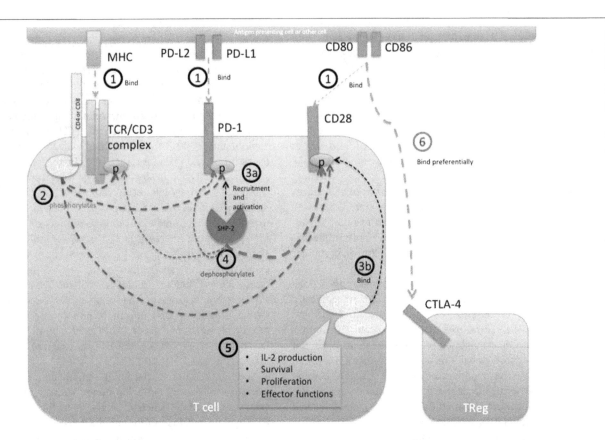

FIGURE 1 | Programmed cell death protein 1 (PD-1) mediated intracellular signaling events during T cell activation. **(1)** Upon T cell activation, the extracellular receptors PD-1, CD28, and the T cell receptor (TCR) complex (including CD4 or CD8) bind their ligands PD-L1 or PD-L2, CD80 or CD86, and major histocompatibility complex (MHC) class I or II, respectively. This brings all the receptors into close proximity with each other at the immunological synapse and allows them to interact with each other. **(2)** The Src kinase Lck (P56Lck), which is bound to the intracellular tail of CD4 and CD8, can now phosphorylate the tyrosine residues on the intracellular tails of PD-1 and CD28 as well as the CD3ζ chain of the TCR/CD3 complex. **(3a)** Phosphorylation of the immunoreceptor tyrosine-based switch motif (ITSM) motif on the intracellular tail of PD-1 allows recruitment of the Src homology region 2 domain-containing phosphatase 2 (SHP-2), resulting in the activation of SHP-2 phosphatase activity. SHP-1 may also bind PD-1 but to a lesser extent than SHP-2. **(3b)** Simultaneously, the phosphorylated tail of CD28 is now able to recruit PI-3K and Grb2 among other signaling molecules. **(4)** Through close proximity at the immunological synapse, PD-1-associated SHP-2 can dephosphorylate the cytoplasmic tail of CD28, and to a lesser extent that of the CD3ζ chain, therefore preventing the recruitment of further downstream signaling molecules associated with these molecules. SHP-2 may also dephosphorylate PD-1, causing auto-regulation of this inhibitory pathway. **(5)** CD28 provides critical signals alongside TCR stimulation, and the abrogated binding of PI3K and Grb2 to this receptor therefore leads to decreased signaling in pathways important for IL-2 production, survival, proliferation, and certain effector functions. In the absence of its ligands, PD-1 is not recruited to the immune synapse and can therefore not interfere with activation signaling. **(6)** The inhibitory receptor CTLA-4 primarily restricts CD28 signaling indirectly by reducing the availability of CD80 and CD86, to which it binds with a much higher affinity than the co-stimulatory receptor CD28. Sources (43–45).

produced IL-10; higher proportions of these cells were correlated with worse disease outcome in hepatocellular carcinoma patients (58). Tumor-associated macrophages were also recently shown to express PD-1 in both mice and humans with colorectal cancer and to impair macrophage phagocytosis (59).

Both cancer cells and tumor-infiltrating immune cells (such as macrophages) may express PD-L1 and upregulate it in response to IFN-γ (60). PD-L1 expression may therefore be indicative of active anti-tumor immune responses and may also actively contribute to local immunosuppression. The relationship between PD-1 or PD-L1 expression at the tumor site and disease outcome is thus not consistent among all tumor types and patients. High PD-1 and/or PD-L1 may correlate with poor prognosis in some cancers (including melanoma, renal cell carcinoma, esophageal, gastric, and ovarian cancers) and

with improved prognosis in others (such as angiosarcoma and gastric cancer) (55, 60–65).

EFFICACY AND MODE OF ACTION OF CHECKPOINT INHIBITORS

Both CTLA-4 and PD-1 checkpoint inhibitors have resulted in increased patient survival in a number of studies, including studies on melanoma, renal cell carcinoma, squamous cell carcinoma, and non-small cell lung cancer, when compared to conventional chemotherapies (summarized in **Table 2**). In melanoma, anti-PD-1 treatment was more effective in patients with smaller tumors (66). A direct comparison between the two checkpoint inhibitors in a Phase III clinical trial found better response (44%) and survival rates (6.9 months progression-free survival) among

TABLE-2 | Treatment outcome of clinical trials for immune checkpoint inhibitors in various cancer types.

Target	Drug	Condition	Treatment regimen	Treatment in control group	Objective response rate	Complete response rates	Overall survival (months)	Progression-free survival (months)	Grade 3-5 adverse events	Participants treated (and controls)	Reference
Programmed cell death protein -1 (PD-1) signaling	Nivolumab (IgG4a)	Melanoma (stage III/IV)	3 mg/kg/2 weeks	(vs combination therapy)	43.7%	8.9%	n/a	6.9	16.3%	316	(67)
		Renal cell carcinoma (metastatic)	3 mg/kg/2 weeks	10 mg/day Everolimus	25% (4% control)	1% (<1% control)	25.0 (19.6 control)	4.6 (4.4 control)	19% (27% control)	406 (397 control)	(68)
		Hodgkin's lymphoma (relapsed/refractory)	3 mg/kg/2 weeks	n/a	87%	17%	n/a	86% at 24 weeks	22%	23	(69)
		Squamous-cell carcinoma of the head and neck (recurrent)	3 mg/kg/2 weeks	Single-agent systemic therapy (methotrexate, docetaxel, or cetuximab)	13.3% (5.8% control)	2.5% (0.8% control)	36.0%/1 year (16.6% control)	19.7% at 6 months (9.9% control)	13.1% (35.1%)	240 (121 control)	(70)
		Non-small cell lung cancer	3 mg/kg/2 weeks	Docetaxel	19% (12% control)	1% (<1% control)	12.2 (9.4 control)	2.3 (4.2 control)	10% (54% control)	292 (290 control)	(71)
			3 mg/kg/2 weeks	Docetaxel	20% (9% control)	1% (0% control)	9.2 (6 control)	3.5 (2.8 control)	7% (55% control)	135 (137 control)	(72)
		Ovarian cancer (platinum-resistant)	1 or 3 mg/kg/2 weeks	n/a	15%	10%	20	3.5	40%	20	(62)
	Pembrolizumab (IgG4a)	Melanoma (stage III/IV)	10 mg/2 weeks or 3 weeks	(vs ipilimumab)	33.7-32.9%	5.0-6.1%	n/a	5.5-4.1	13.3-10.1%	279-277	(73)
		Merkel cell carcinoma	2 mg/kg/3 weeks	n/a	56%	16%	n/a	65% at 6 months	15%	26	(74)
		Non-small cell lung cancer	2 mg/kg/3 weeks 10 mg/kg/3 weeks 10 mg/kg/2 weeks	n/a	19.4%	n/a	12	3.7	9.5%	495	(75)
			200 mg/2 weeks (PD-L1 + patients only)	Platinum-based chemotherapy	44.8 (27.8% control)	n/a	80.2% at 6 months (72.4% control)	10.3 (6 control)	26.6% (53.3% control)	154 (154 control)	(76)
			2 or 10 mg/kg/3 weeks (PD-L1 + patients only)	Docetaxel	18/18% (9% control)	0/0% (0% control)	10.4/12.7 (8.5 control)	3.9/4.0 (4.0 control)	13/16% (35% control)	345/346 (343 control)	(77)
		Progressive metastatic colorectal cancer	10 mg/kg/every 2 weeks	n/a	40/0%	0/0%	>5 months/5	>5/2.2	41% overall	10/18	(78)
	Pidilizumab (IgG1)	B cell lymphoma (after autologous stem cell transfer)	1.5 mg/42 days	n/a	51%	34%	85% at 16 months	72% at 16 months	n/a	66	(79)

(Continued)

TABLE 2 | Continued

Target	Drug	Condition	Treatment regimen	Treatment in control group	Objective response rate	Complete response rates	Overall survival (months)	Progression-free survival (months)	Grade 3–5 adverse events	Participants treated (and controls)	Reference
		Follicular lymphoma (relapsed)	3 mg/kg/4 weeks (+ rituximab)	n/a	66%	52%	n/a	n/a	0%	29	(80)
PD-L1	Atezolizumab (IgG1)	Non-small cell lung cancer (stage III–IV)	1,200 mg/3 weeks	Docetaxel	18% (16% control)	2% (<1% control)	15.7 (10.3 control)	2.8 (4 control)	15% (43% control)	425 (425 control)	(81)
		Urothelial carcinoma (locally advanced and metastatic)	1,200 mg/3 weeks	n/a	23%	9%	15.9%	2.7	16%	119	(82)
T-lymphocyte-associated protein 4 (CTLA-4) signaling	CTLA-4 Ipilimumab (IgG1)	Melanoma (stage III/IV)	10 mg/kg plus decarbazine	Decarbazine alone	15.2% (10.3% control)	1.6% (0.8% control)	11.2 (9.1 control)	n/a	56.3% (27.5%)	250 (252 control)	(83)
			3 mg/kg/3 weeks	(vs Pembrolizumab)	11.9%	1.4%	n/a	2.8	19.9%	278 315	(73)
			3 mg/kg/3 weeks	(vs combination with nivolumab)	19%	2.2%	n/a	2.9	27.3%	311	(67)
	Tremelimumab (IgG2)	Melanoma (stage III/IV)	15 mg/kg/90 days	chemotherapy (temozolomide or dacarbazine)	10.7% (9.8% control)	3% (2% control)	12.6% (10.7 control)	20.3% at 6 months (18.1% control)	52% (37% control)	328 (327 control)	(84)
Combination therapy	Nivolumab + Ipilimumab	Melanoma (stage III/IV)	3 mg/kg/2 weeks Nivolumab 3 mg/kg/3 weeks Ipilimumab	(vs single)	57.6%	11.5%	n/a	11.5	55%	314	(67)
		Non-small cell lung cancer	Nivo + Ipi: 1 + 3 or 3 + 1 mg/ml	Nivolumab alone	23/19% (10% control)	2/0% (0%)	7.7/6 (4.4)	2.6/1.4 (1.4 control)	30/19% (13% control)	61/54 (98 control)	(85)

n/a: not available.
Where the median values for overall or progression-free survival were not reached within the time frame of a study and the percentage of patients surviving for a given time frame are shown instead.
The anti-PD-L1 antibodies avelimumab and durvalumab are currently undergoing early-stage clinical trials and therefore no data has yet been published on their efficacy.

patients treated with the anti-PD-1 antibody nivolumab than among those treated with the anti-CTLA-4 antibody ipilimumab (19% and 2.8 months). Combined administration of both nivolumab and ipilimumab resulted in even higher response rates (58%) and survival (11.5 months) (67).

Both CTLA-4 and PD-1 act independently as brakes on CD3/CD28-dependent signaling, suggesting that underlying immune responses are required for checkpoint inhibitor treatment to take effect (66). Indeed, as mentioned in the previous section, both PD-1 and CTLA-4 blockades are more effective in tumors that are infiltrated by T cells or that have high mutation rates and are therefore more immunogenic prior to treatment (86–88).

The direct immunological consequences of anti-PD-1 and anti-CTLA-4 treatments have mostly been investigated in T cells (**Figure 2**). It is thought that the blockade of CTLA-4 most likely impacts the stage of T cell activation in the draining lymph nodes when CTLA-4 expressing Tregs remove CD80/CD86 from the surface of antigen-presenting cells, thereby reducing their ability to effectively stimulate tumor-specific T cells (24). CTLA-4 blockade may also take effect at the tumor site as exhausted CTLA-4-expressing T cells and Tregs can accumulate within the tumor microenvironment (29, 53). PD-1-expressing tumor-infiltrating T cells can be disabled by PD-L1 on the surfaces of tumor cells or other infiltrating immune cells, and blocking antibodies targeting PD-1 signaling are therefore thought to mainly affect the effector stage of the immune response (13, 55–57). Since other cell types (such as dendritic cells and B cells) can also be influenced by PD-1 signaling, inhibition of the PD-1/PD-L1 pathway may also have T cell-independent effects, whose impact on immune responses during checkpoint inhibitor therapy remain to be elucidated (36, 58).

Type I immune responses, which include IFN-γ production and cytotoxic T cell functions, are important for effective anti-tumor immune responses and are associated with better responses to anti-CTLA-4 and anti-PD-1 treatments. Indeed, mouse models have shown that local IFN-γ upregulation is essential for anti-PD-1-mediated tumor regression (89). Similarly, IFN-γ and the cytotoxic granule component granzyme B were increased in regressing lesions of melanoma patients after anti-PD-1 treatment (90). Tumors in patients treated with anti-PD-1 who initially responded and then relapsed showed mutations that caused a subsequent loss in MHC class I surface expression (to avoid cytotoxic T cell recognition) or in IFN-γ response elements (6). Th9 CD4$^+$ T cells have also been suggested to play a role according to a recent study that detected a significant increase in Th9 cell frequency in patients responding to anti-PD-1 treatment (91, 92).

It may be tempting to speculate that immune checkpoint inhibitors specifically boost the function of T cells belonging to the effector memory compartment, as these cells readily express cytotoxic molecules such as perforin and granzyme B. However, these cells lack the co-stimulatory receptor CD28 through which both PD-1 and CTLA-4 inhibit T cell function (93). Two recent studies have shown that it is indeed CD28-expressing cells rather than already terminally differentiated effector cells that respond to PD-1 blockade with a proliferative burst and differentiation (94, 95).

The characteristics of a tumor itself may also influence immune checkpoint inhibitor efficacy. The mutational burden of tumor cells may increase their antigenicity but may also enhance their ability to evade treatment-induced immune responses. Indeed, a recent study identified a melanoma gene signature associated with innate anti-PD-1 resistance, which included upregulation of genes associated with angiogenesis, wound healing, mesenchymal transitioning, cell adhesion, and extracellular matrix remodeling (96).

Commensal bacteria may also play a role in influencing the efficacy of immune checkpoint inhibitors. Anti-CTLA-4 treatment was found to be ineffective in mice reared under sterile conditions and to induce a shift in the gut flora of conventionally reared mice. Further experiments showed that the presence of certain bacterial strains, in particular *Bacteroides fragilis*, promoted Th1 polarization in the animals and was associated with an improved anti-tumor immune response (97). Importantly, antibiotic treatment was also associated with reduced responses to anti-PD-1/PD-L1 treatments in cancer patients, possibly by altering the normal gut flora. Good treatment response among patients was instead associated with the presence of the commensal *Akkermansia muciniphila*, which also improved anti-PD-1 treatment responses in mice by allowing increased recruitment of CCR9 + CXCR3 + CD4 + T lymphocytes into the tumor (98).

TREATMENT-RELATED ADVERSE EVENTS AND THEIR MANAGEMENT

PD-1 and CTLA-4 prevent autoimmunity and limit immune activation to prevent bystander damage under physiological conditions. Inhibition of these receptors through therapeutic antibodies for the treatment of cancer is therefore associated with a wide range of side effects that resemble autoimmune reactions. Rates of severe side effects vary greatly by study and treatment (see **Table 2**). Clinical trials that directly compared different types of immune checkpoint inhibitors and their combination noted that more patients experienced side effects when treated with anti-CTLA-4 (27.3%) compared to anti-PD-1 (16.3%). Even more patients were affected when treated with a combination of both (55%) (67).

Almost all patients treated with immune checkpoint inhibitors experience mild side effects such as diarrhea, fatigue, pruritus, rash, nausea and decreased appetite. Severe adverse reactions include severe diarrhea, colitis, increased alanine aminotransferase levels, inflammation pneumonitis, and interstitial nephritis (67, 73, 99). There have also been reports of patients experiencing exacerbation of pre-existing autoimmune conditions such as psoriasis (91, 92, 100) or developing new ones such as type 1 diabetes mellitus (101). Particularly severe side effects may require cessation of treatment, although these patients may still respond thereafter (102). Interestingly, certain treatment-related auto-immune reactions such as rash and vitiligo have been shown to correlate with better disease prognosis (103), suggesting an overlap between auto-immune and anti-tumor immune responses.

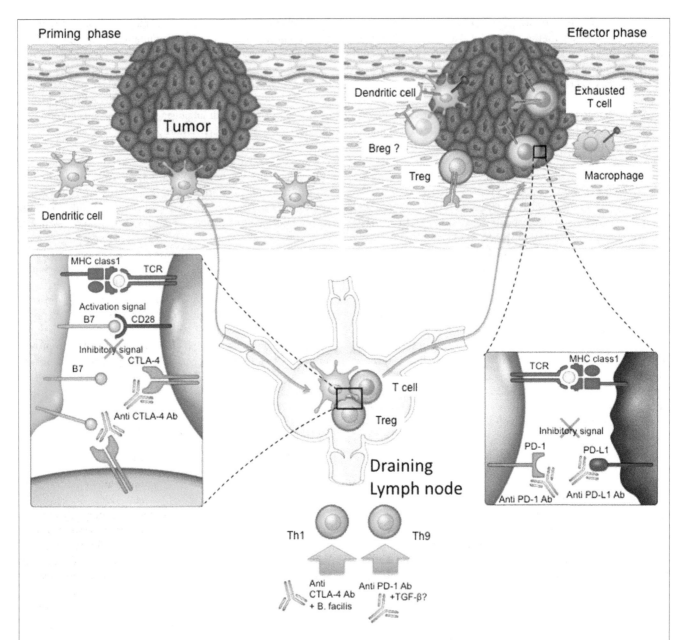

FIGURE 2 | The role of programmed cell death protein 1 (PD-1) and T-lymphocyte-associated protein 4 (CTLA-4) in the priming and effector phases of anti-tumor immune responses. For T cell priming, dendritic cells (DCs) sample antigen at the tumor site and transport it to the draining lymph nodes, where they present the antigens on their major histocompatibility complex (MHC) molecules to T cells. T cells become activated if their T cell receptors recognize and bind the antigen on MHC complexes and their CD28 costimulatory receptors bind CD80 and CD86 on DCs. CTLA-4 upregulation on T cells or bystander Tregs can interfere with the CD28 signal, as the former receptor binds CD80 and CD86 with higher affinity. Once activated, T cells migrate to the tumor site in order to kill malignant cells. Tumors or bystander cells such as macrophages may, however, upregulate PD-L1 and therefore obstruct T cell function by inducing inhibitory intracellular signaling. Anti-CTLA-4 blocking antibody may therefore restore T cell priming in the lymph nodes, and the PD-1 signaling blockade may enable T cell effector function at the tumor site. Additionally, other cell types such as Breg cells and DCs in the tumor microenvironment may express PD-1 and therefore be affected by PD-1 blockade. PD-1 and CTLA-4 blockade may also affect T helper cell profiles directly or by influencing the microbiota.

BIOMARKERS OF ANTI-PD-1/CTLA-4 TREATMENT EFFICACY

Biomarkers are needed both before and during treatment to identify the patients most or least likely to respond to immune checkpoint inhibitor treatments in order to reduce inappropriate drug exposure. Treatment response is defined as a reduction in tumor size during the course of treatment. A number of factors associated with disease prognoses in untreated patients are also linked to immune checkpoint inhibitor response rates (**Table 3**). For example, patients with smaller tumors or low serum lactate dehydrogenase (LDH) levels at baseline have a better prognosis

TABLE 3 | Biomarkers associated with favorable responses to immune checkpoint inhibitors.

	Pre-treatment	Post-treatment
Tumor	Tumor size and distribution (66) High mutation burden but no innate anti-PD-1 resistance (IPRES) gene signature (78, 86, 87, 96) PD-L1 expression on tumor cells (only confirmed by some but not all studies) (67, 108)	Reduction in tumor size
Tumor-infiltrating immune cells	Presence of CD8 + T cells inside the tumor or at the tumor margin (88) PD-L1 expression by infiltrating cells (77) Increased Th1- and CTLA-4-associated gene expression (77).	Proliferation of intratumoral CD8 + T cells (88)
Circulation	High relative lymphocyte counts (109) High relative eosinophil counts (109) High serum TGF-β levels (91, 92) Low serum LDH levels (66, 109) Low levels of ctDNA (107)	Increased levels of ICOS + T cells (110) Low neutrophil-to-lymphocyte ratio (110) High levels of Th9 cells A reduction in serum LDH levels (104) A reduction in ctDNA (107)
Host genome	Presence of HLA-A*26 allele (111)	

and are also more likely to respond to anti-PD-1 treatment (66). A reduction in LDH levels after treatment is also associated with improved response (104). Circulating tumor DNA (ctDNA), which contains melanoma-associated mutations and can be released by dead tumor cells, can be detected in the serum of some patients. CtDNA levels correlate strongly with tumor burden and progression (105, 106). A recent study in advanced stage melanoma patients treated with anti-PD-1 (alone or in combination with anti-CTLA-4) showed high treatment response rates in individuals that were ctDNA negative prior to or after treatment (107), making serum ctDNA an attractive biomarker before and during immune checkpoint treatment.

For anti-PD-1 treatments, expression of PD-L1 within the tumor microenvironment has been an obvious biomarker candidate. Although PD-L1 expression on tumor cells was correlated with treatment efficacy in melanoma patients (67, 108), it was not in patients with squamous cell carcinoma, non-small cell lung cancer and Merkel cell carcinoma (70, 72, 74). Interestingly, one study assessing the role of PD-L1 in both cancer cells and tumor-infiltrating immune cells found that only in the latter context was anti-PD-L1 treatment efficiency correlated with PD-L1 expression (77).

The presence of neoantigens on mutated tumor cells boosts anti-tumor immunogenicity and improves treatment efficacy. High genetic disparity between tumor cells and host cells is therefore an indicator of checkpoint inhibitor treatment efficacy. This was particularly noted in anti-CTLA-4-treated melanoma patients whose tumors displayed neo-antigens (87) and similarly in anti-PD-1-treated patients with colorectal cancers or non-small cell lung cancers that were mismatch-repair deficient or had high mutation rates, respectively (78, 86). Although overall mutational burden is associated with improved response to anti-PD-1 treatment, reduced responses were detected in melanoma patients whose tumors displayed the IPRES gene signature (96). Antigen presentation by the host may also play a role during anti-PD-1 treatment, as patients with the HLA-A*26 were more than twice as likely to respond than patients negative for the allele (111).

Other pre-treatment immunological factors associated with improved treatment responses include high eosinophil and lymphocyte blood counts, an abundance of CD8[+] T cells infiltrating the tumor or present at the tumor margin, and increased serum TGF-β levels in melanoma patients treated with anti-PD-1 (88, 91, 92, 109). Increased Th1 and CTLA-4 (but not FoxP3) gene expression levels were also noted in responder patients with various solid tumors (including melanoma) treated with anti-PD-L1 (77).

A number of post-treatment immunological observations have also been associated with improved immune-checkpoint inhibitor responses. For example, patients more likely to respond to anti-CTLA-4 treatment had increased numbers of inducible co-stimulatory molecule (ICOS) expressing T cells and lower neutrophil-to-lymphocyte ratios (110). An increase in CD8[+] T cell proliferation within the tumor lesion and an increased frequency of Th9 cells in the patients' circulation were also associated with treatment response (88, 91, 92).

Taken together, many of these studies indicate that immune checkpoint inhibitors are most effective in patients who already display anti-tumor immune processes prior to therapy. However, not all biomarkers listed here may be equally effective, and patients may still respond to treatment despite contrary biomarker-based predictions. Further, accessing tumor tissue may be difficult in many patients, especially after treatment, and less invasive blood-based "liquid biopsies" may therefore be more appropriate. Importantly, it has been shown that investigating several biomarkers in combination can improve treatment predictions (109). Although the recently discovered ctDNA seems to be a particularly promising biomarker candidate, more studies are needed to identify more effective biomarkers or biomarker combinations, in order to devise the most appropriate treatment strategy for each patient.

LIMITATIONS OF IMMUNE CHECKPOINT INHIBITORS

Although immune checkpoint inhibitor treatment may be effective initially, many patients will eventually relapse and develop tumor progression. A number of studies have therefore sought to understand the mechanisms by which anti-PD-1 and anti-CTLA-4 treatments lose their efficacy.

The selection pressure caused by checkpoint inhibitor treatment may give rise to tumor cells that can evade immunomediated recognition and deletion through new pathways. Tumor cells from patients refractory to anti-PD-1 treatment, for example, were recently shown to have acquired mutations making them less susceptible to T cell-mediated killing *via* loss of IFN-γ response elements or MHC class I (6).

Anti-PD-1 or anti-CTLA-4 treatment may also cause upregulation of other inhibitory receptors. For example, patients with melanoma or prostate cancer exhibited upregulation of the inhibitory receptor V-domain Ig suppressor of T cell activation (VISTA) on various tumor-infiltrating immune cells after anti-CTLA-4 treatment (112). Another study noted the upregulation of the inhibitory receptor TIM-3 (but not VISTA) on the surface of T cells in anti-PD-1-treated mice with lung cancer as well as TIM-3 upregulation on T cells in adenocarcinoma patients refractory to PD-1 treatment (113).

Most recently, a study revealed another unexpected resistance mechanism to anti-PD-1 therapy in mice whereby tumor-associated macrophages removed the therapeutic antibody from the surface of the T cells *in vivo*, thus making them once again susceptible to inhibitory signaling through the receptor. This phenomenon could be partially overcome by administration of Fc-receptor blocking agents prior to treatment (114). A better understanding of the mechanisms limiting the effectiveness of immune checkpoint inhibitors will therefore allow improvement of future treatments.

FUTURE AVENUES: EXPANDING THE IMMUNE CHECKPOINT INHIBITOR TREATMENT REPERTOIRE

PD-1 and CTLA-4 blocking agents are not effective in all patients, and even those patients who do respond initially can relapse, highlighting the need for improved or alternative treatments. Alternative inhibitory receptors have been identified that may also be targeted for anti-tumor immune therapy. These include the TIM-3, LAG-3, TIGIT, and B- And T-Lymphocyte-Associated Protein (BTLA) receptors associated with T cell exhaustion as well as VISTA, a receptor found on tumor-infiltrating myeloid cells, whose inhibition promoted anti-tumor immune responses in murine models, and CD96, which has been shown to inhibit NK cell activity in murine cancer models (115–117).

Combinations of immune checkpoint inhibitors with each other or with other treatments are also being explored. Indeed, the combination of anti-CTLA-4 with anti-PD-1 treatments showed superior efficacy compared to individual administration, but was also associated with an increase in side effects. The tryptophan-metabolizing enzyme IDO inhibits T cell function, and combining IDO-blocking agents together with immune checkpoint inhibitors has shown promising results in mice and is also currently undergoing clinical trials in humans (105, 118). Macrophages may also interfere with anti-tumor immunity or even directly restrict therapeutic antibodies (114).

Their depletion through a Colony stimulating factor-1 receptor (CSF-1R) inhibitor is therefore being explored in clinical trials together with anti-PD-1, after having shown efficacy in a glioblastoma mouse model (119). Anti-tumor T cell function induced by PD-1 blockade in mice could also be improved by a targeted increase in mitochondrial function (120).

Because immune checkpoint inhibitors work by removing brakes on the immune system rather than directly boosting immune function, patients may also benefit from combination therapies that include immunostimulatory substances. Mouse melanoma models, for example, have shown that the combination of anti-CTLA-4 with cytokines such as granulocyte-macrophage colony-stimulating factor (GM-CSF) or with agonistic antibodies targeting costimulatory receptors such as CD40, increased tumor rejection in a synergistic manner (121, 122). The genetically modified herpes simplex virus talimogene laherparepvec is designed to replicate in tumor cells and to release GM-CSF, thus attracting immune cells into the tumor environment. The virus has been tested in recent clinical trials in combination with either CTLA-4 or PD-1 in advanced-stage melanoma patients, resulting in increased treatment response rates compared to the immune checkpoint inhibitors alone (123, 124).

Even modulation of the gut microbiome may improve immune checkpoint inhibitor-based therapies. Administration of intestinal *Bifidobacteria* alone was associated with reduced tumor growth in a murine B16 melanoma model by promoting dendritic-cell mediated CD8+ T cell responses. Importantly, the administration of these bacteria also added to the therapeutic effect of anti-PD-1 treatment in these mice (125). In a similar study, administration of *B. fragilis* to sterile mice treated with anti-CTLA-4 resulted in reduced tumor growth, most likely by inducing a favorable shift toward Th1 responses (97). Studies in humans were further able to link the presence of fecal *A. muciniphila*, *Ruminococcaceae*, and *Faecalibacterium* to a favorable outcome to anti-PD-1 treatment (98, 126) Together, these findings suggest that human patients too may benefit from appropriate management of their intestinal flora while undergoing immune checkpoint inhibitor treatment.

A wide range of promising new avenues are therefore currently being explored, although their clinical efficacy remains to be confirmed by ongoing and future clinical trials.

CONCLUDING REMARKS

Although PD-1 and CTLA-4 targeting therapies have been able to increase average life expectancy for cancer patients, mortality remains high among advanced-stage patients, highlighting the need for further innovation in the field. Both anti-PD-1 and anti-CTLA-4 therapies appear to be more effective in patients with pre-existing anti-tumor immunity, suggesting that, in patients without such immunity, these drugs are unable to mediate anti-tumor immune responses *de novo*. However, as our understanding of the mechanisms of these drugs improves, avenues are being opened to improve their use not only by specifically targeting those patients who are most likely to respond through appropriate biomarker screening procedures, but also by pairing currently used immune checkpoint inhibitors with other complimentary drugs to help those patients unable to respond to the current regimens.

AUTHOR CONTRIBUTIONS

This review was drafted by JAS and AO, and critically revised by KK.

REFERENCES

1. Lawrence MS, Stojanov P, Polak P, Kryukov GV, Cibulskis K, Sivachenko A, et al. Mutational heterogeneity in cancer and the search for new cancer-associated genes. *Nature* (2013) 499(7457):214–8. doi:10.1038/nature12213

2. Pennock ND, White JT, Cross EW, Cheney EE, Tamburini BA, Kedl RM. T cell responses: naïve to memory and everything in between. *Adv Physiol Educ* (2013) 37(4):273–83. doi:10.1152/advan.00066.2013

3. Teng MW, Galon J, Fridman WH, Smyth MJ. From mice to humans: developments in cancer immunoediting. *J Clin Invest* (2015) 125(9):3338–46. doi:10.1172/JCI80004

4. Otsuka A, Dreier J, Cheng PF, Nägeli M, Lehmann H, Felderer L, et al. Hedgehog pathway inhibitors promote adaptive immune responses in basal cell carcinoma. *Clin Cancer Res* (2015) 21(6):1289–97. doi:10.1158/1078-0432.CCR-14-2110

5. Otsuka A, Levesque MP, Dummer R, Kabashima K. Hedgehog signaling in basal cell carcinoma. *J Dermatol Sci* (2015) 78(2):95–100. doi:10.1016/j.jdermsci.2015.02.007

6. Zaretsky JM, Garcia-Diaz A, Shin DS, Escuin-Ordinas H, Hugo W, Hu-Lieskovan S, et al. Mutations associated with acquired resistance to PD-1 blockade in melanoma. *N Engl J Med* (2016) 375(9):819–29. doi:10.1056/NEJMoa1604958

7. Vinay DS, Ryan EP, Pawelec G, Talib WH, Stagg J, Elkord E, et al. Immune evasion in cancer: mechanistic basis and therapeutic strategies. *Semin Cancer Biol* (2015) 35(Suppl):S185–98. doi:10.1016/j.semcancer.2015.03.004

8. Sarvaria AJ, Madrigal A, Saudemont A. B cell regulation in cancer and anti-tumor immunity. *Cell Mol Immunol* (2017) 14(8):662–74. doi:10.1038/cmi.2017.35

9. Parry RV, Chemnitz JM, Frauwirth KA, Lanfranco AR, Braunstein I, Kobayashi SV, et al. CTLA-4 and PD-1 receptors inhibit T-cell activation by distinct mechanisms. *Mol Cell Biol* (2005) 25(21):9543–53. doi:10.1128/MCB.25.21.9543-9553.2005

10. Blackburn SD, Shin H, Haining WN, Zou T, Workman CJ, Polley A, et al. Coregulation of CD8+ T cell exhaustion by multiple inhibitory receptors during chronic viral infection. *Nat Immunol* (2009) 10(1):29–37. doi:10.1038/ni.1679

11. Anderson AC, Joller N, Kuchroo VK. Lag-3, Tim-3, and TIGIT: co-inhibitory receptors with specialized functions in immune regulation. *Immunity* (2016) 44(5):989–1004. doi:10.1016/j.immuni.2016.05.001

12. Day CL, Kaufmann DE, Kiepiela P, Brown JA, Moodley ES, Reddy S, et al. PD-1 expression on HIV-specific T cells is associated with T-cell exhaustion and disease progression. *Nature* (2006) 443(7109):350–4. doi:10.1038/nature05115

13. Baitsch L, Baumgaertner P, Devêvre E, Raghav SK, Legat A, Barba L, et al. Exhaustion of tumor-specific CD8+ T cells in metastases from melanoma patients. *J Clin Invest* (2011) 121(6):2350–60. doi:10.1172/JCI46102

14. Wherry EJ. T cell exhaustion. *Nat Immunol* (2011) 12(6):492–9. doi:10.1038/ni.2035

15. Jin HT, Ahmed R, Okazaki T. Role of PD-1 in regulating T-cell immunity. *Curr Top Microbiol Immunol* (2011) 350:17–37. doi:10.1007/82_2010_116

16. Gardner D, Jeffery LE, Sansom DM. Understanding the CD28/CTLA-4 (CD152) pathway and its implications for costimulatory blockade. *Am J Transplant* (2014) 14(9):1985–91. doi:10.1111/ajt.12834

17. Speiser DE, Utzschneider DT, Oberle SG, Münz C, Romero P, Zehn D. T cell differentiation in chronic infection and cancer: functional adaptation or exhaustion? *Nat Rev Immunol* (2014) 14(11):768–74. doi:10.1038/nri3740

18. Erickson JJ, Gilchuk P, Hastings AK, Tollefson SJ, Johnson M, Downing MB, et al. Viral acute lower respiratory infections impair CD8+ T cells through PD-1. *J Clin Invest* (2012) 122(8):2967–82. doi:10.1172/JCI62860

19. Hodi FS, Mihm MC, Soiffer RJ, Haluska FG, Butler M, Seiden MV, et al. Biologic activity of cytotoxic T lymphocyte-associated antigen 4 antibody blockade in previously vaccinated metastatic melanoma and ovarian carcinoma patients. *Proc Natl Acad Sci U S A* (2003) 100(8):4712–7. doi:10.1073/pnas.0830997100

20. Phan GQ, Yang JC, Sherry RM, Hwu P, Topalian SL, Schwartzentruber DJ, et al. Cancer regression and autoimmunity induced by cytotoxic t lymphocyte-associated antigen 4 blockade in patients with metastatic melanoma. *Proc Natl Acad Sci U S A* (2003) 100(14):8372–7. doi:10.1073/pnas.1533209100

21. Chan DV, Gibson HM, Aufiero BM, Wilson AJ, Hafner MS, Mi Q-S, et al. Differential CTLA-4 expression in human CD4+ versus CD8+ T cells is associated with increased NFAT1 and inhibition of CD4+ proliferation. *Genes Immun* (2014) 15(1):25–32. doi:10.1038/gene.2013.57

22. Leung IIT, Bradshaw J, Cleaveland JS, Linsley PS. Cytotoxic T lymphocyte-associated molecule-4, a high avidity receptor for CD80 and CD86, contains an intracellular localization motif in its cytoplasmic tail. *J Biol Chem* (1995) 270(42):25107–14. doi:10.1074/jbc.270.42.25107

23. Rudd CE, Taylor A, Schneider H. CD28 and CTLA-4 coreceptor expression and signal transduction. *Immunol Rev* (2009) 229(1):12–26. doi:10.1111/j.1600-065X.2009.00770.x

24. Qureshi OS, Zheng Y, Nakamura K, Attridge K, Manzotti C, Schmidt EM, et al. Trans-endocytosis of CD80 and CD86: a molecular basis for the cell-extrinsic function of CTLA-4. *Science* (2011) 332(6029):600–3. doi:10.1126/science.1202947

25. Wing K, Onishi Y, Prieto-Martin P, Yamaguchi T, Miyara M, Fehervari Z, et al. CTLA-4 control over Foxp3+ regulatory T cell function. *Science* (2008) 322(5899):271–5. doi:10.1126/science.1160062

26. Waterhouse P, Penninger JM, Timms E, Wakeham A, Shahinian A, Lee KP, et al. Lymphoproliferative disorders with early lethality in mice deficient in Ctla-4. *Science* (1995) 270(5238):985–8. doi:10.1126/science.270.5238.985

27. Gough SC, Walker LS, Sansom DM. CTLA4 gene polymorphism and autoimmunity. *Immunol Rev* (2005) 204(1):102–15. doi:10.1111/j.0105-2896.2005.00249.x

28. Nakamoto N, Cho H, Shaked A, Olthoff K, Valiga ME, Kaminski M, et al. Synergistic reversal of intrahepatic HCV-specific CD8 T cell exhaustion by combined PD-1/CTLA-4 blockade. *PLoS Pathog* (2009) 5(2):e1000313. doi:10.1371/journal.ppat.1000313

29. Curran MA, Montalvo W, Yagita H, Allison JP. PD-1 and CTLA-4 combination blockade expands infiltrating T cells and reduces regulatory T and myeloid cells within B16 melanoma tumors. *Proc Natl Acad Sci U S A* (2010) 107(9):4275–80. doi:10.1073/pnas.0915174107

30. Ishida Y, Agata Y, Shibahara K, Honjo T. Induced expression of PD-1, a novel member of the immunoglobulin gene superfamily, upon programmed cell death. *EMBO J* (1992) 11(11):3887.

31. Nishimura H, Nose M, Hiai H, Minato N, Honjo T. Development of lupus-like autoimmune diseases by disruption of the PD-1 gene encoding an ITIM motif-carrying immunoreceptor. *Immunity* (1999) 11(2):141–51. doi:10.1016/S1074-7613(00)80089-8

32. Sage PT, Francisco LM, Carman CV, Sharpe AH. The receptor PD-1 controls follicular regulatory T cells in the lymph nodes and blood. *Nat Immunol* (2013) 14(2):152–61. doi:10.1038/ni.2496

33. Agata Y, Kawasaki A, Nishimura H, Ishida Y, Tsubat T, Yagita H, et al. Expression of the PD-1 antigen on the surface of stimulated mouse T and B lymphocytes. *Int Immunol* (1996) 8(5):765–72. doi:10.1093/intimm/8.5.765

34. Kinter AL, Godbout EJ, McNally JP, Sereti I, Roby GA, O'Shea MA, et al. The common gamma-chain cytokines IL-2, IL-7, IL-15, and IL-21 induce the expression of programmed death-1 and its ligands. *J Immunol* (2008) 181(10):6738–46. doi:10.4049/jimmunol.181.10.6738

35. Peña-Cruz V, McDonough SM, Diaz-Griffero F, Crum CP, Carrasco RD, Freeman GJ. PD-1 on immature and PD-1 ligands on migratory human Langerhans cells regulate antigen-presenting cell activity. *J Invest Dermatol* (2010) 130(9):2222–30. doi:10.1038/jid.2010.127

36. Thibult ML, Mamessier E, Gertner-Dardenne J, Pastor S, Just-Landi S, Xerri L, et al. PD-1 is a novel regulator of human B-cell activation. *Int Immunol* (2013) 25(2):129–37. doi:10.1093/intimm/dxs098

37. Lim TS, Chew V, Sieow JL, Goh S, Yeong JP, Soon AL. PD-1 expression on dendritic cells suppresses CD8+ T cell function and antitumor immunity. *Oncoimmunology* (2016) 5(3):e1085146. doi:10.1080/2162402X.2015.1085146

38. Rodrigues CP, Ferreira ACF, Pinho MP, de Moraes CJ, Bergami-Santos PC, et al. Tolerogenic IDO+ dendritic cells are induced by PD-1-expressing mast cells. *Front Immunol* (2016) 7:9. doi:10.3389/fimmu.2016.00009

39. Latchman Y, Wood CR, Chernova T, Chaudhary D, Borde M, Chernova I, et al. PD-L2 is a second ligand for PD-1 and inhibits T cell activation. *Nat Immunol* (2001) 2(3):261–8. doi:10.1038/85330

40. Freeman GJ, Wherry EJ, Ahmed R, Sharpe AH. Reinvigorating exhausted HIV-specific T cells via PD-1–PD-1 ligand blockade. *J Exp Med* (2006) 203(10):2223–7. doi:10.1084/jem.20061800

41. Brown JA, Dorfman DM, Ma FR, Sullivan EL, Munoz O, Wood CR, et al. Blockade of programmed death-1 ligands on dendritic cells enhances T cell activation and cytokine production. *J Immunol* (2003) 170(3):1257–66. doi:10.4049/jimmunol.170.3.1257

42. Patsoukis N, Brown J, Petkova V, Liu F, Li L, Boussiotis VA. Selective effects of PD-1 on Akt and Ras pathways regulate molecular components of the cell cycle and inhibit T cell proliferation. *Sci Signal* (2012) 5(230):ra46–46. doi:10.1126/scisignal.2002796

43. Chemnitz JM, Parry RV, Nichols KE, June CH, Riley JL. SHP-1 and SHP-2 associate with immunoreceptor tyrosine-based switch motif of programmed death 1 upon primary human T cell stimulation, but only receptor ligation prevents T cell activation. *J Immunol* (2004) 173(2):945–54. doi:10.4049/jimmunol.173.2.945

44. Sheppard K-A, Fitz LJ, Lee JM, Benander C, George JA, Wooters J, et al. PD-1 inhibits T-cell receptor induced phosphorylation of the ZAP70/CD3ζ signalosome and downstream signaling to PKCθ. *FEBS Lett* (2004) 574(1–3):37–41. doi:10.1016/j.febslet.2004.07.083

45. Hui E, Cheung J, Zhu J, Su X, Taylor MJ, Wallweber HA, et al. T cell costimulatory receptor CD28 is a primary target for PD-1-mediated inhibition. *Science* (2017) 355(6332):1428–33. doi:10.1126/science.aaf1292

46. Carter L, Fouser LA, Jussif J, Fitz L, Deng B, Wood CR. PD-1:PD-L inhibitory pathway affects both CD4+ and CD8+ T cells and is overcome by IL-2. *Eur J Immunol* (2002) 32(3):634–43. doi:10.1002/1521-4141(200203)32:3<634:AID-IMMU634>3.0.CO;2-9

47. Nurieva R, Thomas S, Nguyen T, Martin-Orozco N, Wang Y, Kaja MK, et al. T-cell tolerance or function is determined by combinatorial costimulatory signals. *EMBO J* (2006) 25(11):2623–33. doi:10.1038/sj.emboj.7601146

48. Freeman GJ, Long AJ, Iwai Y, Bourque K, Chernova T, Nishimura H, et al. Engagement of the Pd-1 immunoinhibitory receptor by a novel B7 family member leads to negative regulation of lymphocyte activation. *J Exp Med* (2000) 192(7):1027–34. doi:10.1084/jem.192.7.1027

49. Nishimura H, Minato N, Nakano T, Honjo T. Immunological studies on PD-1 deficient mice: implication of PD-1 as a negative regulator for B cell responses. *Int Immunol* (1998) 10(10):1563–72. doi:10.1093/intimm/10.10.1563

50. Salama AD, Chitnis T, Imitola J, Ansari MJ, Akiba H, Tushima F, et al. Critical role of the programmed death-1 (PD-1) pathway in regulation of experimental autoimmune encephalomyelitis. *J Exp Med* (2003) 198(1):71–8. doi:10.1084/jem.20022119

51. Nielsen C, Hansen D, Husby S, Jacobsen BB, Lillevang ST. Association of a putative regulatory polymorphism in the PD-1 gene with susceptibility to type 1 diabetes. *Tissue Antigens* (2003) 62(6):492–7. doi:10.1046/j.1399-0039.2003.00136.x

52. Velázquez-Cruz R, Orozco L, Espinosa-Rosales F, Carreño-Manjarrez R, Solís-Vallejo E, López-Lara ND, et al. Association of PDCD1 polymorphisms with childhood-onset systemic lupus erythematosus. *Eur J Hum Genet* (2007) 15(3):336–41. doi:10.1038/sj.ejhg.5201767

53. Salvi S, Fontana V, Boccardo S, Merlo DF, Margallo E, Laurent S, et al. Evaluation of CTLA-4 expression and relevance as a novel prognostic factor in patients with non-small cell lung cancer. *Cancer Immunol Immunother* (2012) 61(9):1463–72. doi:10.1007/s00262-012-1211-y

54. Huang PY, Guo SS, Zhang Y, Lu JB, Chen QY, Tang LQ, et al. Tumor CTLA-4 overexpression predicts poor survival in patients with nasopharyngeal carcinoma. *Oncotarget* (2016) 7(11):13060–8. doi:10.18632/oncotarget.7421

55. Ahmadzadeh M, Johnson LA, Heemskerk B, Wunderlich JR, Dudley ME, White DE, et al. Tumor antigen–specific CD8 T cells infiltrating the tumor express high levels of PD-1 and are functionally impaired. *Blood* (2009) 114(8):1537–44. doi:10.1182/blood-2008-12-195792

56. Chapon M, Randriamampita C, Maubec E, Badoual C, Fouquet S, Wang SF, et al. Progressive upregulation of PD-1 in primary and metastatic melanomas associated with blunted TCR signaling in infiltrating T lymphocytes. *J Invest Dermatol* (2011) 131(6):1300–7. doi:10.1038/jid.2011.30

57. Saito H, Kuroda H, Matsunaga T, Osaki T, Ikeguchi M. Increased PD-1 expression on CD4+ and CD8+ T cells is involved in immune evasion in gastric cancer. *J Surg Oncol* (2013) 107(5):517–22. doi:10.1002/jso.23281

58. Xiao X, Lao XM, Chen MM, Liu RX, Wei Y, Ouyang FZ, et al. PD-1hi identifies a novel regulatory b-cell population in human hepatoma that promotes disease progression. *Cancer Discov* (2016) 6(5):546–59. doi:10.1158/2159-8290.CD-15-1408

59. Gordon SR, Roy LM, Ben WD, Gregor H, Benson MG, Melissa NM, et al. PD-1 expression by tumour-associated macrophages inhibits phagocytosis and tumour immunity. *Nature* (2017) 545(7655):495–9. doi:10.1038/nature22396

60. Honda Y, Otsuka A, Ono S, Yamamoto Y, Seidel JA, Morita S, et al. Infiltration of PD-1-positive cells in combination with tumor site PD-L1 expression is a positive prognostic factor in cutaneous angiosarcoma. *Oncoimmunology* (2016) 6(1):e1253657. doi:10.1080/2162402X.2016.1253657

61. Hino R, Kabashima K, Kato Y, Yagi H, Nakamura M, Honjo T, et al. Tumor cell expression of programmed cell death-1 ligand 1 is a prognostic factor for malignant melanoma. *Cancer* (2010) 116(7):1757–66. doi:10.1002/cncr.24899

62. Hamanishi J, Mandai M, Ikeda T, Minami M, Kawaguchi A, Murayama T, et al. Safety and antitumor activity of anti–PD-1 antibody, nivolumab, in patients with platinum-resistant ovarian cancer. *J Clin Oncol* (2015) 33(34):4015–22. doi:10.1200/JCO.2015.62.3397

63. Inman BA, Sebo TJ, Frigola X, Dong H, Bergstralh EJ, Frank I. PD-L1 (B7-H1) expression by urothelial carcinoma of the bladder and BCG-induced granulomata. *Cancer* (2007) 109(8):1499–505. doi:10.1002/cncr.22588

64. Kim JW, Nam KH, Ahn SH, Park DJ, Kim HH, Kim SH, et al. Prognostic implications of immunosuppressive protein expression in tumors as well as immune cell infiltration within the tumor microenvironment in gastric cancer. *Gastric Cancer* (2016) 19(1):42–52. doi:10.1007/s10120-014-0440-5

65. Zhang Y, Kang S, Shen J, He J, Jiang L, Wang W, et al. Prognostic significance of programmed cell death 1 (PD-1) or PD-1 ligand 1 (PD-L1) expression in epithelial-originated cancer: a meta-analysis. *Medicine* (2015) 94(6):e515. doi:10.1097/MD.0000000000000515

66. Ribas A, Hamid O, Daud A, Hodi FS, Wolchok JD, Kefford R, et al. Association of pembrolizumab with tumor response and survival among patients with advanced melanoma. *JAMA* (2016) 315(15):1600–9. doi:10.1001/jama.2016.4059

67. Larkin J, Chiarion-Sileni V, Gonzalez R, Grob JJ, Cowey CL, Lao CD, et al. Combined nivolumab and ipilimumab or monotherapy in untreated melanoma. *N Engl J Med* (2015) 373(1):23–34. doi:10.1056/NEJMoa1504030

68. Motzer RJ, Escudier B, McDermott DF, George S, Hammers HJ, Srinivas S, et al. Nivolumab versus everolimus in advanced renal-cell carcinoma. *N Engl J Med* (2015) 373(19):1803–13. doi:10.1056/NEJMoa1510665

69. Ansell SM, Iwamoto FM, LaCasce A, Mukundan S, Roemer MGM, Chapuy B, et al. PD-1 blockade with nivolumab in relapsed or refractory Hodgkin's lymphoma. *N Engl J Med* (2015) 372(4):311–9. doi:10.1056/NEJMoa1411087

70. Ferris RL, Blumenschein G, Fayette J, Guigay J, Colevas AD, Licitra L, et al. Nivolumab for recurrent squamous-cell carcinoma of the head and neck. *N Engl J Med* (2016) 375(19):1856–67. doi:10.1056/NEJMoa1602252

71. Borghaei H, Paz-Ares L, Horn L, Spigel DR, Steins M, Ready NE, et al. Nivolumab versus docetaxel in advanced nonsquamous non-small-cell lung cancer. *N Engl J Med* (2015) 373(17):1627–39. doi:10.1056/NEJMoa1507643

72. Brahmer J, Reckamp KL, Baas P, Crinò L, Eberhardt WE, Poddubskaya E, et al. Nivolumab versus docetaxel in advanced squamous-cell non–small-cell lung cancer. *N Engl J Med* (2015) 373(2):123–35. doi:10.1056/NEJMoa1504627

73. Robert C, Schachter J, Long GV, Arance A, Grob JJ, Mortier L, et al. Pembrolizumab versus ipilimumab in advanced melanoma. *N Engl J Med* (2015) 372(26):2521–32. doi:10.1056/NEJMoa1503093

74. Nghiem PT, Bhatia S, Lipson EJ, Kudchadkar RR, Miller NJ, Annamalai L, et al. PD-1 Blockade with pembrolizumab in advanced Merkel-cell carcinoma. *N Engl J Med* (2016) 374(26):2542–52. doi:10.1056/NEJMoa1603702

75. Garon EB, Rizvi NA, Hui R, Leighl N, Balmanoukian AS, Eder JP, et al. Pembrolizumab for the treatment of non–small-cell lung cancer. *N Engl J Med* (2015) 372(21):2018–28. doi:10.1056/NEJMoa1501824

76. Reck M, Rodríguez-Abreu D, Robinson AG, Hui R, Csőszi T, et al. Pembrolizumab versus chemotherapy for PD-L1–positive non–small-cell lung cancer. *N Engl J Med* (2016) 375(19):1823–33. doi:10.1056/NEJMoa1606774

77. Herbst RS, Baas P, Kim DW, Felip E, Pérez-Gracia JL, Han JY, et al. Pembrolizumab versus docetaxel for previously treated, PD-L1-positive, advanced non-small-cell lung cancer (KEYNOTE-010): a randomised controlled trial. *Lancet* (2016) 387(10027):1540–50. doi:10.1016/S0140-6736(15)01281-7

78. Le DT, Uram JN, Wang H, Bartlett BR, Kemberling H, Eyring AD, et al. PD-1 blockade in tumors with mismatch-repair deficiency. *N Engl J Med* (2015) 372(26):2509–20. doi:10.1056/NEJMoa1500596

79. Armand P, Nagler A, Weller EA, Devine SM, Avigan DE, Chen YB, et al. Disabling immune tolerance by programmed death-1 blockade with pidilizumab after autologous hematopoietic stem-cell transplantation for diffuse large B-cell lymphoma: results of an international phase II trial. *J Clin Oncol* (2013) 31(33):4199–206. doi:10.1200/JCO.2012.48.3685

80. Westin JR, Chu F, Zhang M, Fayad LE, Kwak LW, Fowler N, et al. Safety and activity of PD1 blockade by pidilizumab in combination with rituximab in patients with relapsed follicular lymphoma: a single group, open-label, phase 2 trial. *Lancet Oncol* (2014) 15(1):69–77. doi:10.1016/S1470-2045(13)70551-5

81. Rittmeyer A, Barlesi F, Waterkamp D, Park K, Ciardiello F, von Pawel J, et al. Atezolizumab versus docetaxel in patients with previously treated non-small-cell lung cancer (OAK): a phase 3, open-label, multicentre randomised controlled trial. *Lancet* (2016) 389(10066):255–65. doi:10.1016/S0140-6736(16)32517-X

82. Balar AV, Galsky MD, Rosenberg JE, Powles T, Petrylak DP, Bellmunt J, et al. Atezolizumab as first-line treatment in cisplatin-ineligible patients with locally advanced and metastatic urothelial carcinoma: a single-arm, multicentre, phase 2 trial. *Lancet* (2017) 389(10064):67–76. doi:10.1016/S0140-6736(16)32455-2

83. Robert C, Thomas L, Bondarenko I, O'Day S, Weber J, Garbe C, et al. Ipilimumab plus dacarbazine for previously untreated metastatic melanoma. *N Engl J Med* (2011) 364(26):2517–26. doi:10.1056/NEJMoa1104621

84. Ribas A, Kefford R, Marshall MA, Punt CJ, Haanen JB, Marmol M, et al. Phase III randomized clinical trial comparing tremelimumab with standard-of-care chemotherapy in patients with advanced melanoma. *J Clin Oncol* (2013) 31(5):616–22. doi:10.1200/JCO.2012.44.6112

85. Antonia SJ, López-Martin JA, Bendell J, Ott PA, Taylor M, Eder JP, et al. Nivolumab alone and nivolumab plus ipilimumab in recurrent small-cell lung cancer (CheckMate 032): a multicentre, open-label, phase 1/2 trial. *Lancet Oncol* (2016) 17(7):883–95. doi:10.1016/S1470-2045(16)30098-5

86. Rizvi NA, Hellmann MD, Snyder A, Kvistborg P, Makarov V, Havel JJ, et al. Mutational landscape determines sensitivity to PD-1 blockade in non–small cell lung cancer. *Science* (2015) 348(6230):124–8. doi:10.1126/science.aaa1348

87. Snyder A, Makarov V, Merghoub T, Yuan J, Zaretsky JM, Desrichard A, et al. Genetic basis for clinical response to CTLA-4 blockade in melanoma. *N Engl J Med* (2014) 371(23):2189–99. doi:10.1056/NEJMoa1406498

88. Tumeh PC, Harview CL, Yearley JH, Shintaku IP, Taylor EJ, Robert L, et al. PD-1 blockade induces responses by inhibiting adaptive immune resistance. *Nature* (2014) 515(7528):568–71. doi:10.1038/nature13954

89. Peng W, Liu C, Xu C, Lou Y, Chen J, Yang Y, et al. PD-1 blockade enhances T-cell migration to tumors by elevating IFN-γ inducible chemokines. *Cancer Res* (2012) 72(20):5209–18. doi:10.1158/0008-5472.CAN-12-1187

90. Anegawa H, Otsuka A, Kaku Y, Nonomura Y, Fujisawa A, Endo Y, et al. Upregulation of granzyme B and interferon-γ MRNA in responding lesions by treatment with nivolumab for metastatic melanoma: a case report. *J Eur Acad Dermatol Venereol* (2016) 30(12):e231–2. doi:10.1111/jdv.13567

91. Nonomura Y, Otsuka A, Ohtsuka M, Yamamoto T, Dummer R, Kabashima K. ADAMTSL5 Is upregulated in melanoma tissues in patients with idiopathic psoriasis vulgaris induced by nivolumab. *J Eur Acad Dermatol Venereol* (2017) 31(2):e100–1. doi:10.1111/jdv.13818

92. Nonomura Y, Otsuka A, Nakashima C, Seidel JA, Kitoh A, Dainichi T, et al. Peripheral blood Th9 cells are a possible pharmacodynamic biomarker of nivolumab treatment efficacy in metastatic melanoma patients. *Oncoimmunology* (2016) 5(12):e1248327. doi:10.1080/2162402X.2016.1248327

93. Appay V, van Lier RA, Sallusto F, Roederer M. Phenotype and function of human T lymphocyte subsets: consensus and issues. *Cytometry A* (2008) 73(11):975–83. doi:10.1002/cyto.a.20643

94. Im SJ, Hashimoto M, Gerner MY, Lee J, Kissick HT, Burger MC, et al. Defining CD8+ T cells that provide the proliferative burst after PD-1 therapy. *Nature* (2016) 537(7620):417–21. doi:10.1038/nature19330

95. Kamphorst AO, Wieland A, Nasti T, Yang S, Zhang R, Barber DL, et al. Rescue of exhausted CD8 T cells by PD-1–targeted therapies Is CD28-dependent. *Science* (2017) 355(6332):1423–7. doi:10.1126/science.aaf0683

96. Hugo W, Zaretsky JM, Sun L, Song C, Moreno BH, Hu-Lieskovan S, et al. Genomic and transcriptomic features of response to anti-PD-1 therapy in metastatic melanoma. *Cell* (2017) 168(3):542. doi:10.1016/j.cell.2017.01.010

97. Vétizou M, Pitt JM, Daillère R, Lepage P, Waldschmitt N, Flament C, et al. Anticancer immunotherapy by CTLA-4 blockade relies on the gut microbiota. *Science* (2015) 350(6264):1079–84. doi:10.1126/science.aad1329

98. Routy B, Le Chatelier E, Derosa L, Duong CPM, Alou MT, Daillère R, et al. Gut microbiome influences efficacy of PD-1-based immunotherapy against epithelial tumors. *Science* (2018) 359(6371):91–7. doi:10.1126/science.aan3706

99. Abdel-Rahman O, Fouad M. A network meta-analysis of the risk of immune-related renal toxicity in cancer patients treated with immune checkpoint inhibitors. *Immunotherapy* (2016) 8(5):665–74. doi:10.2217/imt-2015-0020

100. Kato Y, Otsuka A, Miyachi Y, Kabashima K. Exacerbation of psoriasis vulgaris during nivolumab for oral mucosal melanoma. *J Eur Acad Dermatol Venereol* (2016) 30(10):e89–91. doi:10.1111/jdv.13336

101. Chae YK, Chiec L, Mohindra N, Gentzler R, Patel J, Giles F. A case of pembrolizumab-induced type-1 diabetes mellitus and discussion of immune checkpoint inhibitor-induced type 1 diabetes. *Cancer Immunol Immunother* (2016) 66(1):25–32. doi:10.1007/s00262-016-1913-7

102. Zou W, Wolchok JD, Chen L. PD-L1 (B7-H1) and PD-1 pathway blockade for cancer therapy: mechanisms, response biomarkers, and combinations. *Sci Transl Med* (2016) 8(328):328rv4. doi:10.1126/scitranslmed.aad7118

103. Freeman-Keller M, Kim Y, Cronin H, Richards A, Gibney G, Weber JS. Nivolumab in resected and unresectable metastatic melanoma: characteristics of immune-related adverse events and association with outcomes. *Clin Cancer Res* (2016) 22(4):886–94. doi:10.1158/1078-0432.CCR-15-1136

104. Diem S, Kasenda B, Spain L, Martin-Liberal J, Marconcini R, Gore M, et al. Serum lactate dehydrogenase as an early marker for outcome in patients treated with anti-PD-1 therapy in metastatic melanoma. *Br J Cancer* (2016) 114(3):256–61. doi:10.1038/bjc.2015.467

105. Sharma P, Hu-Lieskovan S, Wargo JA, Ribas A. Primary, adaptive, and acquired resistance to cancer immunotherapy. *Cell* (2017) 168(4):707–23. doi:10.1016/j.cell.2017.01.017

106. Calapre L, Warburton L, Millward M, Ziman M, Gray ES. Circulating tumour DNA (CtDNA) as a liquid biopsy for melanoma. *Cancer Lett* (2017) 404(Suppl C):62–9. doi:10.1016/j.canlet.2017.06.030

107. Lee JH, Long GV, Boyd S, Lo S, Menzies AM, Tembe V, et al. Circulating tumour DNA predicts response to anti-PD1 antibodies in metastatic melanoma. *Ann Oncol* (2017) 28(5):1130–6. doi:10.1093/annonc/mdx026

108. Topalian SL, Hodi FS, Brahmer JR, Gettinger SN, Smith DC, McDermott DF, et al. Safety, activity, and immune correlates of anti-PD-1 antibody in cancer. *N Engl J Med* (2012) 366(26):2443–54. doi:10.1056/NEJMoa1200690

109. Weide B, Martens A, Hassel JC, Berking C, Postow MA, Bisschop K, et al. Baseline biomarkers for outcome of melanoma patients treated with pembrolizumab. *Clin Cancer Res* (2016) 22(22):5487–96. doi:10.1158/1078-0432.CCR-16-0127

110. Giacomo AM, Calabrò L, Danielli R, Fonsatti E, Bertocci E, Pesce I, et al. Long-term survival and immunological parameters in metastatic melanoma patients who responded to ipilimumab 10 Mg/Kg within an expanded access programme. *Cancer Immunol Immunother* (2013) 62(6):1021–8. doi:10.1007/s00262-013-1418-6

111. Ishida Y, Otsuka A, Tanaka H, Levesque MP, Dummer R, Kabashima K. HLA-A*26 is correlated with response to nivolumab in Japanese melanoma patients. *J Invest Dermatol* (2017) 137(11):2443–4. doi:10.1016/j.jid.2017.06.023

112. Gao J, Ward JF, Pettaway CA, Shi LZ, Subudhi SK, Vence LM, et al. VISTA is an inhibitory immune checkpoint that is increased after ipilimumab therapy in patients with prostate cancer. *Nat Med* (2017) 23(5):551–5. doi:10.1038/nm.4308

113. Koyama S, Akbay EA, Li YY, Herter-Sprie GS, Buczkowski KA, Richards WG, et al. Adaptive resistance to therapeutic PD-1 blockade is associated with upregulation of alternative immune checkpoints. *Nat Commun* (2016) 7:10501. doi:10.1038/ncomms10501

114. Arlauckas SP, Garris CS, Kohler RH, Kitaoka M, Cuccarese MF, Yang KS, et al. In vivo imaging reveals a tumor-associated macrophage–mediated resistance pathway in anti–PD-1 therapy. *Sci Transl Med* (2017) 9(389):eaal3604. doi:10.1126/scitranslmed.aal3604

115. Lines JL, Sempere LF, Broughton T, Wang L, Noelle R. VISTA is a novel broad-spectrum negative checkpoint regulator for cancer immunotherapy. *Cancer Immunol Res* (2014) 2(6):510–7. doi:10.1158/2326-6066. CIR-14-0072

116. Blake SJ, Dougall WC, Miles JJ, Teng MW, Smyth MJ. Molecular pathways: targeting CD96 and TIGIT for cancer immunotherapy. *Clin Cancer Res* (2016) 22(21):5183–8. doi:10.1158/1078-0432.CCR-16-0933

117. Glen MC, Tsuyoshi F, Gabriela MW, Benjamin JB, Helen LW, Jason SR, et al. TIGIT marks exhausted T cells, correlates with disease progression, and serves as a target for immune restoration in HIV and SIV infection. *PLoS Pathog* (2016) 12(1):e1005349. doi:10.1371/journal.ppat.1005349

118. Spranger S, Koblish HK, Horton B, Scherle PA, Newton R, Gajewski TF. Mechanism of tumor rejection with doublets of CTLA-4, PD-1/PD-L1, or IDO blockade involves restored IL-2 production and proliferation of CD8(+) T cells directly within the tumor microenvironment. *J Immunother Cancer* (2014) 2:3. doi:10.1186/2051-1426-2-3

119. Antonios JP, Soto H, Everson RG, Moughon D, Orpilla JR, Shin NP, et al. Immunosuppressive tumor-infiltrating myeloid cells mediate adaptive immune resistance via a PD-1/PD-L1 mechanism in glioblastoma. *Neuro Oncol* (2017) 19(6):796–807. doi:10.1093/neuonc/now287

120. Chamoto K, Chowdhury PS, Kumar A, Sonomura K, Matsuda F, Fagarasan S, et al. Mitochondrial activation chemicals synergize with surface receptor PD-1 blockade for T cell-dependent antitumor activity. *Proc Natl Acad Sci U S A* (2017) 114(5):E761–70. doi:10.1073/pnas.1620433114

121. Quezada SA, Peggs KS, Curran MA, Allison JP. CTLA4 blockade and GM-CSF combination immunotherapy alters the intratumor balance of effector and regulatory T cells. *J Clin Invest* (2006) 116(7):1935–45. doi:10.1172/JCI27745

122. Sorensen MR, Holst PJ, Steffensen MA, Christensen JP, Thomsen AR. Adenoviral vaccination combined with CD40 stimulation and CTLA-4 blockage can lead to complete tumor regression in a murine melanoma model. *Vaccine* (2010) 28(41):6757–64. doi:10.1016/j.vaccine.2010. 07.066

123. Chesney J, Collichio F, Andtbacka RHI, Puzanov I, Glaspy J, Milhem M, et al. Interim safety and efficacy of a randomized (1:1), open-label phase 2 study of talimogene laherparepvec (T) and ipilimumab (I) vs I alone in unresected, stage IIIB-IV melanoma. *Ann Oncol* (2016) 27(suppl_6):379–400. doi:10.1093/annonc/mdw379.04

124. Ribas A, Dummer R, Puzanov I, VanderWalde A, Andtbacka RHI, Michielin O, et al. Oncolytic virotherapy promotes intratumoral T cell infiltration and improves anti-PD-1 immunotherapy. *Cell* (2017) 170(6):1109.e–19.e. doi:10.1016/j.cell.2017.08.027

125. Sivan A, Corrales L, Hubert N, Williams JB, Aquino-Michaels K, Earley ZM, et al. Commensal *Bifidobacterium* promotes antitumor immunity and facilitates anti–PD-L1 efficacy. *Science* (2015) 350(6264):1084–9. doi:10.1126/ science.aac4255

126. Gopalakrishnan V, Spencer CN, Nezi L, Reuben A, Andrews MC, Karpinets TV, et al. Gut microbiome modulates response to anti-PD-1 immunotherapy in melanoma patients. *Science* (2018) 359(6371):97–103. doi:10.1126/science. aan4236

15

Successful Treatment of Unresectable Advanced Melanoma by Administration of Nivolumab With Ipilimumab Before Primary Tumor Resection

Taku Fujimura*†, Yumi Kambayashi†, Yota Sato, Kayo Tanita, Ryo Amagai,
Akira Hashimoto, Takanori Hidaka and Setsuya Aiba

Department of Dermatology, Tohoku University Graduate School of Medicine, Sendai, Japan

*Correspondence:
Taku Fujimura
tfujimura1@mac.com

†These authors have contributed
equally to this work

Ipilimumab, in combination with nivolumab, is one of the promising drugs that enhance the anti-tumor immune response of patients with advanced melanoma. Since the co-administration of nivolumab with ipilimumab in the neoadjuvant setting expands melanoma-reactive T cells at the primary site of melanoma and has a high rate of histological complete response, the pre-surgical administration of this combination could be the optimal therapy for unresectable advanced melanoma. In this report, a case of unresectable advanced melanoma treated successfully with administration of nivolumab with ipilimumab before primary tumor resection is presented. In addition, CD8+ T cells increased among the tumor-infiltrating lymphocytes that were surrounding melanoma cells and caspase 3+ cells. The present case suggests that pre-surgical administration of nivolumab with ipilimumab could be the optimal therapy for the treatment of unresectable advanced melanoma.

Keywords: nivolumab, ipilimumab, advanced melanoma, pre-surgical administration, T cell expansion

BACKGROUND

Nivolumab, anti-PD1 antibody (Abs), monotherapy has been one of the first-line therapies for advanced melanoma, especially for BRAF mutation-negative melanoma, with a reported efficacy rate of ~30–40% (1, 2). Ipilimumab, cytotoxic T-lymphocyte antigen (CTLA-4) Abs, is another immune checkpoint inhibitor (ICI) for the treatment of advanced melanoma that activates and increases T cells, and it expands effector T cells at the site especially when given with nivolumab (3). Therefore, pre-surgical treatment with the combination of nivolumab and ipilimumab could be optimal therapy for unresectable, advanced melanoma.

CASE PRESENTATION

A 64-year-old Japanese man visited our outpatient clinic with a 3-months history of an easily bleeding, black nodule on his back. At the initial physical examination, a black nodule (8 × 7 cm) with a dark-red nodule was seen on the back (**Figure 1a**). In addition, there were numerous subcutaneous nodules on the scalp, face, trunk, and extremities. Biopsy of the primary tumor showed markedly atypical melanocytes arranged in irregular nests and solitary units

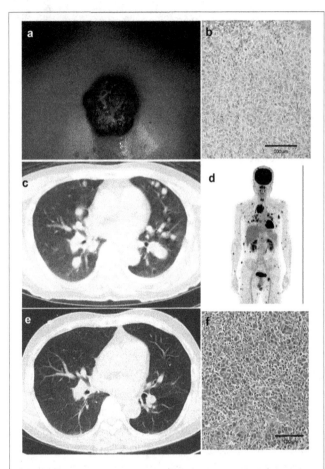

FIGURE 1 | A black nodule (8 × 7 cm) with a dark-red nodule on the back (a). Histological findings of the primary tumor before treatment: markedly atypical melanocytes arranged in irregular nests and solitary units (b). Multiple lung metastases (c), cutaneous, pharyngeal, and peritoneal nodules, lymph node metastases, and bone metastases on PET-CT (d). After treatment, multiple lung metastases are decreased (e). Histological findings of the primary tumor after single administration of nivolumab with ipilimumab showing dense infiltration of lymphocytes in the melanoma lesion (f).

(Figure 1b). The THxID kit revealed that the primary tumor possessed the BRAF^{V600E} mutation. Immunohistochemical staining showed that these melanoma cells were positive for Melan A and HMB45. PET-CT showed multiple lung (Figure 1c), cutaneous, pharyngeal, and peritoneal nodules, as well as lymph node and bone metastases (Figure 1d). Biopsy from the pharyngeal wall showed dense infiltration of markedly atypical melanocytes. In addition, serum LDH levels were elevated (336 U/l). From the above findings, the diagnosis was malignant melanoma with multiple lung, peritoneal, pharyngeal, subcutaneous, lymph node, and bone metastases [pT4bN3cM1c(1) stage IV].

TREATMENT COURSE AND OUTCOME

Since the patient had metastases in 6 organs (>3 organs) and elevated serum LDH levels, suggesting that dabrafenib

plus trametinib combined therapy might not be useful (4), nivolumab (80 mg/body/every 3 weeks) was given in combination with ipilimumab (3 mg/kg/every 3 weeks) before surgical treatment. Eighteen days after the administration of nivolumab and ipilimumab, the primary tumor was palliatively resected, and nivolumab (80 mg/body/every 3 weeks) in combination with ipilimumab (3 mg/kg/every 3 weeks) was continued for three more cycles (Supplemental Figure 1). The skin metastases regressed rapidly with scar formation, and follow-up CT 2 months after the combination therapy suggested significant regression of lung (Figure 1e), peritoneal, pharyngeal, subcutaneous, lymph node, and bone metastases. Histological findings of the resected primary tumor showed dense infiltration of lymphocytes in the melanoma lesion (Figure 1f). Four months have passed, and a grade 3 skin rash and grade 4 peripheral neuropathy, which is controlled by the intravenous administration of methylprednisolone sodium succinate at a starting dose of 2 mg/kg, were observed.

IMMUNOHISTOCHEMICAL INVESTIGATION OF TUMOR INFILTRATING LYMPHOCYTES (TILs)

Since a previous study suggested that combination therapy with nivolumab and ipilimumab significantly increased a neoantigen-specific melanoma-resident T cell clone, inducing a durable anti-immune response in melanoma patients (1), immunohistochemical staining for CD3 and CD8 was performed before and after the administration of combination therapy (Figure 2A). The ratios of CD3, CD8, PD1, and Foxp3+ cells among tumor infiltrating lymphocytes (TILs) in the primary tumor before the administration of nivolumab plus ipilimumab combination therapy and in the primary tumor 18 days after the administration of combined therapy were analyzed using the BZ-X800 (KEYENCE, Tokyo, Japan). The lymphocyte fractions, CD3+ cells, CD8+ cells, PD1+ cells, and Foxp3+ cells, were counted, and the ratios of cells staining positive on immunohistochemistry (CD3+ cells/total TILs, CD8+ cells/total TILs, PD1+ cells/total TILs, Foxp3+ cells/total TILs) were calculated in the full tumor areas of low magnification fields. These data showed a marked increase of CD8+ TILs in the post-treatment specimen (Figure 3). In addition, immunohistochemical staining for PD-L1 was performed, showing no difference between before and after the administration of combination therapy (Figure 2B). Moreover, immunofluorescence staining for caspase 3, CD8, and tyrosinase showed the induction of apoptotic cells in the melanoma lesion (Figure 2C).

Ethics Statement

The patient gave written informed consent for the publication of this case report.

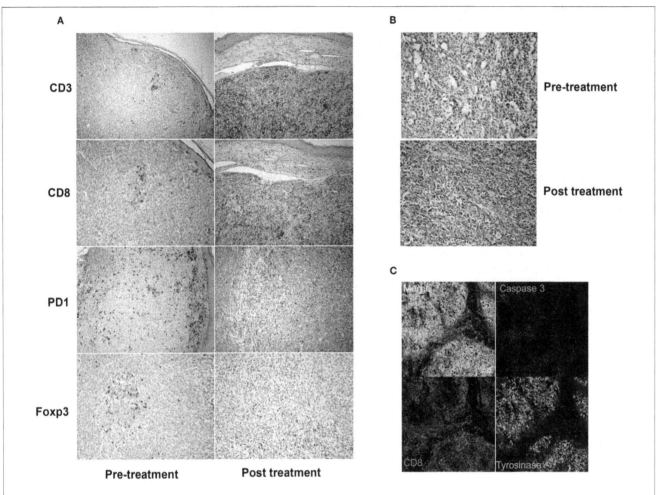

FIGURE 2 | Immunohistochemical staining for CD3, CD8, PD1, and Foxp3 before and after a single administration of nivolumab with ipilimumab **(A)**. Immunohistochemical staining for PD-L1 before and after a single administration of nivolumab with ipilimumab **(B)**. Immunofluorescence staining of CD8 (cytotoxic T cells: blue), caspase 3 (apoptotic cells: orange), and tyrosinase (melanoma cells: green) **(C)**.

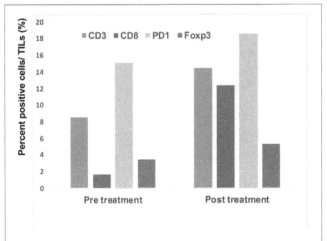

FIGURE 3 | Quantitative analysis of CD3+ T cells, CD8+ T cells, PD1-expressing cells, and Foxp3+ cells: the IHC-positive cells within the lymphocyte fraction and the percentage of IHC-positive cells per all tumor-infiltrating cells were automatically counted using a BZ-X800

DISCUSSION

Ipilimumab, in combination with nivolumab, is one of the promising drugs that enhance the anti-immune response of patients with advanced melanoma with or without BRAF gene mutation (5–7). Indeed, the response rate to this combination therapy for advanced melanoma has been reported to be 57.8% (7), and it is recommended by the NCCN guideline for cutaneous melanoma as a first-line therapy (8), despite its high toxicity. In addition, this combination therapy has a high efficacy rate even for the treatment of brain metastases of melanoma (5). Notably, Blank et al. reported that the efficacy of the combination of nivolumab and ipilimumab in the neoadjuvant setting does not parallel tumor mutation burden (TMB) and achieves a high histological complete response (CR) rate (3), suggesting that pre-surgical administration of nivolumab with ipilimumab could be the optimal treatment for unresectable advanced melanoma in real-world practice. In addition, the efficacy of a BRAF inhibitor combo, such as dabrafenib and trametinib combination therapy or encorafenib and binimetinib combination therapy, is limited in advanced melanoma with multiple organ metastases (4, 9). Although there is still insufficient evidence for the efficacy of pre-operative treatment by nivolumab plus ipilimumab, these reports suggested that pre-operative treatment by nivolumab plus ipilimumab might induce a stronger and broader tumor-specific T cell response, as in a pre-clinical study (10). In addition, Navarrete-Dechent reported one case of stage III, unresectable melanoma treated with nivolumab plus ipilimumab combined therapy, and evaluated its efficacy using reflectance confocal microscopy (11). Their report suggested that ipilimumab plus nivolumab combined immune therapy is useful for the treatment of unresectable melanoma (11).

Concerning the present case, although the patient had at least 6 organ metastases, pre-surgical administration of nivolumab with ipilimumab dramatically reduced tumor masses in all organs. Interestingly, a single administration of this combination therapy increased the ratio of CD8+ T cells among total TILs from 1.7 to 12.3% (**Figure 3**). Moreover, immunofluorescence staining showed that caspase 3+ apoptotic cells were surrounded by CD8+ T cells in the melanoma area, suggesting that increased CD8+ T cells might directly induce apoptosis of melanoma cells. Taken together, administration of nivolumab with ipilimumab before primary tumor resection increased CD8+ T cells in the primary tumor, probably a melanoma-specific T cell clone, inducing a systemic anti-melanoma immune response in advanced melanoma. To prove this hypothesis, another clinical study to evaluate nivolumab plus ipilimumab combination therapy prior to surgery is needed.

ETHICS STATEMENT

This patient gave written informed consent.

AUTHOR CONTRIBUTIONS

TF designed the research study and wrote the manuscript. TF, YK, YS, KT, and TH performed and analyze the IHC staining. TF, YK, RA, and AH treated the patients and acquired the clinical data and samples. TF and SA supervised the study.

REFERENCES

1. Yamazaki N, Kiyohara Y, Uhara H, Uehara J, Fujimoto M, Takenouchi T, et al. Efficacy and safety of nivolumab in Japanese patients with previously untreated advanced melanoma: a phase II study. *Cancer Sci.* (2017) 108:1223–30. doi: 10.1111/cas.13241
2. Larkin J, Chiarion-Sileni V, Gonzalez R, Grob JJ, Cowey CL, Lao CD, et al. Combined nivolumab and ipilimumab or monotherapy in untreated Melanoma. *N Engl J Med.* (2015) 373:23–34. doi: 10.1056/NEJMoa1504030
3. Blank CU, Rozeman EA, Fanchi LF, Sikorska K, van de Wiel B, Kvistborg P, et al. Neoadjuvant versus adjuvant ipilimumab plus nivolumab in macroscopic stage III melanoma. *Nat Med.* (2018) 24:1655–61. doi: 10.1038/s41591-018-0198-0
4. Long GV, Flaherty KT, Stroyakovskiy D, Gogas H, Levchenko E, de Braud F, et al. Dabrafenib plus trametinib versus dabrafenib monotherapy in patients with metastatic BRAF V600E/K-mutant melanoma: long-term survival and safety analysis of a phase 3 study. *Ann Oncol.* (2017) 28:1631–9. doi: 10.1093/annonc/mdx176
5. Wolchok JD, Chiarion-Sileni V, Gonzalez R, Rutkowski P, Grob JJ, Cowey CL, et al. Overall survival with combined nivolumab and ipilimumab in advanced melanoma. *N Engl J Med.* (2017) 377:1345–56. doi: 10.1056/NEJMoa1709684
6. Tawbi HA, Forsyth PA, Algazi A, Hamid O, Hodi FS, Moschos SJ, et al. Combined nivolumab and ipilimumab in melanoma metastatic to the brain. *N Engl J Med.* (2018) 379:722–30. doi: 10.1056/NEJMoa1805453
7. Hodi FS, Chiarion-Sileni V, Gonzalez R, Grob JJ, Rutkowski P, Cowey CL, et al. Nivolumab plus ipilimumab or nivolumab alone versus ipilimumab alone in advanced melanoma (CheckMate 067): 4-year outcomes of a multicentre, randomised, phase 3 trial. *Lancet Oncol.* (2018) 19:1480–92. doi: 10.1016/S1470-2045(18)30700-9
8. NCCN. *Clinical Practice Guidelines in Oncology (NCCN Guidelines®) Melanoma Version 2.* (2019). Avaliable online at: https://www.nccn.org/professionals/physician_gls/pdf/cutaneous_melanoma.pdf
9. Dummer R, Ascierto PA, Gogas HJ, Arance A, Mandala M, Liszkay G, et al. Overall survival in patients with BRAF-mutant melanoma receiving encorafenib plus binimetinib versus vemurafenib or encorafenib (COLUMBUS): a multicentre, open-label, randomised, phase 3 trial. *Lancet Oncol.* (2018) 19:1315–27. doi: 10.1016/S1470-2045(18)30497-2
10. Liu J, Blake SJ, Yong MC, Harjunpää H, Ngiow SF, Takeda K, et al. Improved efficacy of neoadjuvant compared to adjuvant immunotherapy to eradicate metastatic disease. *Cancer Discov.* (2016) 6:1382–99. doi: 10.1158/2159-8290.CD-16-0577
11. Navarrete-Dechent C, Cordova M, Postow MA, Pulitzer M, Lezcano C, Halpern AC, et al. Evaluation of the response of unresectable primary cutaneous melanoma to immunotherapy visualized with reflectance confocal microscopy: a report of 2 cases. *JAMA Dermatol.* (2019). doi: 10.1001/jamadermatol.2018.3688. [Epub ahead of print].

16

Novel Therapeutic Targets in Cutaneous Squamous Cell Carcinoma

Teruki Yanagi*, Shinya Kitamura and Hiroo Hata

Department of Dermatology, Hokkaido University Graduate School of Medicine, Sapporo, Japan

*Correspondence:
Teruki Yanagi
yanagi@med.hokudai.ac.jp

Cutaneous squamous cell carcinoma (SCC) is one of the common cancers in Caucasians, accounting for 20–30% of cutaneous malignancies. The risk of metastasis is low in most patients; however, aggressive SCC is associated with very high mortality and morbidity. Although cutaneous SCC can be treated with surgical removal, radiation and chemotherapy singly or in combination, the prognosis of patients with metastatic SCC is poor. Recently, the usage of immune checkpoint blockades has come under consideration. To develop effective therapies that are less toxic than existing ones, it is crucial to achieve a detailed characterization of the molecular mechanisms that are involved in cutaneous SCC pathogenesis and to identify new drug targets. Recent studies have identified novel molecules that are associated with SCC carcinogenesis and progression. This review focuses on recent advances in molecular studies involving SCC tumor development, as well as in new therapeutics that have become available to clinicians.

Keywords: cyclin-dependent kinase, mitochondria, Drp1, PD-1 antibody, epidermal growth factor receptor

INTRODUCTION

In light of today's demographic aging, skin cancer is becoming more prevalent. Cutaneous squamous cell carcinoma (SCC) is one of the most common cancers in Caucasian populations, and its prevalence is increasing (1). Cutaneous SCC accounts for 20–30% of cutaneous malignancies (2, 3). The risk of metastasis is low in most patients (2); however, aggressive SCC is associated with high morbidity and mortality (4). Although cutaneous SCC can be treated with surgery, radiation, and chemotherapy singly, or in combination, the prognosis of patients with metastatic SCC is almost always poor (3, 5). Today, chemotherapy with cisplatin alone or combined with 5-FU is being conducted with positive responses (6–9). However, the National Comprehensive Cancer Network Guidelines describe the evidence regarding systemic therapies for distant metastatic cutaneous SCC as limited. Recently, clinical trials on epidermal growth factor receptor (EGFR) inhibitors and immune checkpoint blockers have shown promising results as treatments for SCC (10–12). This review focuses on recent advances in molecular studies related to SCC tumor development and on new therapeutics that have become available.

RECENT PROGRESS IN CUTANEOUS SCC THERAPEUTICS

Novel Targeted Therapies

Cutaneous SCC overexpresses EGFR; thus, EGFR is a promising target for therapies. Cetuximab, an EGFR inhibitor, has been administered to cutaneous SCC patients. In some phase II studies, there have been good responses to cetuximab in patients with locally advanced or regional SCC types (10, 13–15). However, in distant metastatic diseases, it has been reported as ineffective. Also, tyrosine kinase inhibitors have been used to disrupt EGFR pathways. Case reports on gefetinib and imatinib have described slightly positive responses in cutaneous SCC patients (16, 17). Also, a single-arm phase II clinical trial has shown gefetinib to demonstrate modest antitumor activity in metastatic or locoregionally recurrent cutaneous SCC, with limited adverse events (18). Furthermore, bortezomib, a selective inhibitor of the 26S proteasome, may have antitumor effects in cutaneous SCC, although the mechanisms have not been clarified (19).

Biological Modifiers

30 years ago, isotretinoin was reported to have efficacy as a treatment for local advanced cutaneous SCC alone or in combination. Interferons have also been used for local cutaneous SCC. A phase II study on bio-chemotherapy with interferons, retinoids, and cisplatin showed a positive response in 67% of locally advanced SCC cases (20). However, the efficacy against metastatic cases remains unclear.

Cytotoxic Chemotherapy

Regrettably, recent advances in cytotoxic chemotherapy have been limited. Capecitabine, an oral prodrug of 5-FU, has been used to treat cutaneous SCC (21). In head and neck SCC cases, intra-arterial chemotherapy has been conducted as a neoadjuvant therapy (22). To date, in cutaneous SCC, no obvious evidence for positive responses has been reported, even though some cases have been described in limited detail (23).

Immune Checkpoint Inhibitors

Recently, the US FDA approved PD-1 inhibitors (immune checkpoint inhibitors) for head and neck SCCs with continued progression during or after platinum chemotherapy (24, 25). For cutaneous SCC, several case reports have shown immune checkpoint inhibitors to have promising results. Patients with advanced cutaneous SCC responded to anti-PD-1 (nivolumab and pembrolizumab), and anti-CTLA-4 (ipilimumab) agents (26–29).

Radiation With Chemotherapies or Immunotherapies

Platinum-based chemotherapy has been combined with local radiation. Cisplatin-based chemotherapy combined with concurrent radiation showed better results than cisplatin only (13, 30). Neoadjuvant chemotherapies before radiation were also reported to have promising results (31). Recently, the abscopal effect during radiation therapy after the administration of immune checkpoint inhibitors has been spotlighted. This effect is a phenomenon in which local radiotherapy is associated with the regression of metastatic cancer at a distance from the irradiated site (32). To date, abscopal effects have been observed in melanoma patients but not in cutaneous SCC. It is not clear whether these effects will occur in cutaneous SCCs; however, combined therapies of immune checkpoint inhibitors and radiation might have a synergistic effect.

Other Candidates
Human Papilloma Virus (HPV) in Cancer Cells

Until recently, the role of HPV in cutaneous SCC was not well defined. However, a meta-analysis has found evidence that HPV is associated with cutaneous SCC (33). This systematic review indicated that cutaneous SCC harbors HPV more than normal skin does. Furthermore, an increase in HPV prevalence has been observed in SCC tumors from immunosuppressive patients. A study using an animal model showed that the interaction between UVB and HPV infection strongly promotes the development of cutaneous SCC (34). Furthermore, several targeted therapies for HPV-associated head and neck SCC have been tried (35); thus, HPV might be a promising target for cutaneous SCC as well.

MicroRNAs (miRs) in Cancer Cells

MicroRNAs are short, non-coding RNAs that suppress the expression of target genes. miRs can regulate various gene targets, and they play a crucial role in biological mechanisms (36). Certain miRs are associated with the onset and progression of cancers, suggesting that miRs could be targets for cancer therapies. In cutaneous SCC, several miRs are reported to be overexpressed or downregulated (36). miR-21 and miR-31 are upregulated in cutaneous SCC. The targets of these miRs are PDCD4/GRHL3/PTEN and RhoTBT1, respectively (36, 37). To inhibit the undesirable effects of up-regulated miRs, the administration of complementary nucleic acids might be a potential cancer therapy. By contrast, miR-1, miR-34a, and miR-124 are downregulated in cutaneous SCC (36). These miRs target important molecules of cell proliferation, which tend to be activated in cancer cells. Thus, promoting the over-expression of these miRs could be an option for cancer therapies. Furthermore, various miR delivery systems have been developed. Cheng et al. reported on pHLIP-mediated miR delivery methods, in which miRs could be transported across plasma membranes under the acidic conditions found in solid tumors (38). As such, miRs are also promising targets for cutaneous SCC as well as other tumors.

Cyclin-Dependent Kinase (Cdk) 16 in Cancer Cells

Recently, Cdk4/Cdk6 inhibitor (palbociclib) showed promising results for metastatic breast cancer (39, 40). Some Cdks are overexpressed in cutaneous SCC; thus, Cdk inhibitors may become a novel therapy option. Among Cdks, we have focused on cyclin-dependent kinase 16 (Cdk16) (also known as PCTK1, PCTAIRE1) and investigated its molecular functions. Cdk16 is a member of the Cdk family (41). Molecular functions for CDK16 are reported to vesicular transport (42) and spermatogenesis (43).

To investigate the role of Cdk16 in cancerous cells, we performed gene-knockdown experiments targeting Cdk16 (44–47). In cell lines of cutaneous SCC, prostate cancer, breast cancer, cervical cancer, and melanoma, knockdown of *Cdk16* inhibited cancer cell proliferation, and induced apoptosis over time. But, no role for Cdk16 was observed in the proliferation of non-transformed cells (IMR-90 and HaCaT cells). To identify target molecules of Cdk16, we performed yeast two-hybrid screens with human Cdk16 protein as bait. We identified tumor suppressor p27 as a Cdk16 interactor and demonstrated that Cdk16 phosphorylates p27 at Ser10 by *in vitro* kinase assays (46). The knockdown of Cdk16 modulated p27 (Ser10) phosphorylation, leading to p27 accumulation in cancerous cells. In tumor xenografts of cutaneous SCC cells, the inducible conditional knockdown of Cdk16 suppressed tumor growth (47).

To evaluate the clinical importance of Cdk16, we also studied primary tumor samples In primary tumors from the patients with breast, prostate, cutaneous basal, or SCCs, Cdk16 was expressed more highly in cancer lesions than in normal tissues (46–48). In prostate cancers, a comparison of Cdk16 immunostaining with Gleason grade revealed lower expression levels in well-differentiated tumors than in less- differentiated tumors (46). In breast cancers, Cdk16 expression was elevated in *in situ* carcinomas and invasive cancers relative to the expression in normal mammary epithelium. The significantly higher levels of Cdk16 protein that are seen in invasive cancers are associated with higher histologic grades (46). Moreover, we showed that gene knockdown of *Cdk16* sensitizes cancer cells to TNF-family cytokines, such as Fas-ligand and TNF-related apoptosis-inducing ligand (49).

To advance *in vitro* results on Cdk16 silencing, we investigated the *in vivo* therapeutic potential by using siRNA encapsulated with lipid nanoparticles (LNP) (50). Therapy of Cdk16 siRNA was performed using colorectal cancer HCT116 cells and melanoma A2058 cells. Treatment with Cdk16 siRNA-LNP reduced tumor volume and weight significantly. TUNEL staining showed increased apoptosis of cancer cells treated with Cdk16 siRNA.

These findings show an expected role for Cdk16 in regulating p27 expression and tumor proliferation (**Figure 1**). We observed these functions for Cdk16 in various cancer cells (cutaneous SCCs; basal cell carcinomas; prostate, breast, and cervical cancers; and melanomas). This implies that the p27 regulation by Cdk16 is a common machinery in human cancers.

Dynamin-Related Protein 1 (Drp1) in Cancer Cells

We have also focused on the mitochondria-associated molecule Drp1 (51). Drp1 regulates mitochondrial fission. Recently, it was found to be associated with cancer cell proliferation in melanoma and lung cancer (52, 53). Disrupted mitochondrial networks induce cell cycle arrest and apoptosis (53, 54). Also, Drp1 has been reported as a prognostic factor in several malignancies, such as lung adenocarcinomas and glioblastomas (55, 56). Based on these previous studies, we investigated the role of Drp1 in cutaneous SCCs. Drp1 gene-knockdown SCC cells showed lower cell proliferation than control cells, as assessed by cell counting and clonogenic assays. DNA content Cell Cycle analysis showed Drp1 knockdown to cause G2/M phase arrest. Morphologically, the depletion of Drp1 resulted in an elongated mitochondrial network. The MEK inhibitor,

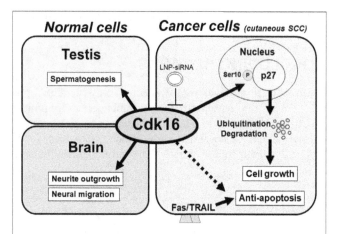

FIGURE 1 | Model of the tumorigenic role of cyclin-dependent kinase 16 (Cdk16). In normal tissue (left), Cdk16 is required for spermatogenesis and neuron differentiation. In cancer cells, including cutaneous squamous cell carcinoma (SCC) cells (right), Cdk16 phosphorylates p27 at Ser10, thereby promoting p27 ubiquitination/degradation, which leads to cell cycle progression and decreased levels of apoptosis. An unknown mechanism may also exist in the Cdk16–apoptosis pathway. Lipid nanoparticle-mediated siRNA (LNP-siRNA) therapy against Cdk16 recently succeeded in a murine xenograft model.

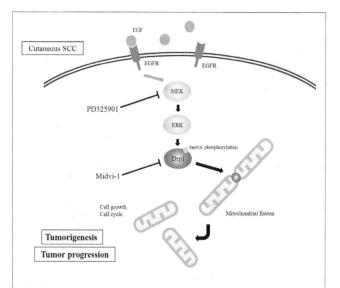

FIGURE 2 | Diagram of dynamin-related protein 1 (Drp1) function in cutaneous squamous cell carcinoma (SCC) cells. MAPK signaling activates Drp1 *via* the phosphorylation of Drp1. The overexpression of Drp1 induces mitochondrial fission, which results in cell growth and assists cell cycle.

PD325901, inhibited cell proliferation, as well as inhibiting the phosphorylation of ERK1/2 and Drp1 (Ser616). PD325901 also caused the dysregulation of the mitochondrial network. In tumor xenografts of DJM1 SCC cells, the knockdown of Drp1 suppressed tumor growth *in vivo*. Clinically, the expression levels of Drp1 were higher in cutaneous SCC specimens than in normal epidermis, and those levels correlated positively with advanced clinical stages. Our data reveal a pivotal function for Drp1 in mediating tumor growth, mitochondrial fission, and cell cycle in cutaneous SCCs (**Figure 2**), suggesting that Drp1 could be a novel target for cutaneous SCC therapies.

CONCLUDING REMARKS

In the past 10 years, novel therapeutic agents for cutaneous SCC have been developed. EGFR inhibitors and immune checkpoint inhibitors have shown particularly promising results. Furthermore, these novel treatments can be used a monotherapies or in combination with radiation; thus dermatologists and oncologists will be able to choose better treatments depending on conditions of the patient and the stage of the disease. Also, novel targeting molecules and inhibitors have been developed.

AUTHOR CONTRIBUTIONS

TY and HH designed the study. TY and SK wrote the paper. HH supervised the study.

REFERENCES

1. Burton KA, Ashack KA, Khachemoune A. Cutaneous squamous cell carcinoma: a review of high-risk and metastatic disease. *Am J Clin Dermatol* (2016) 17:491–508. doi:10.1007/s40257-016-0207-3
2. Madan V, Lear JT, Szeimies RM. Non-melanoma skin cancer. *Lancet* (2010) 375:673–85. doi:10.1016/S0140-6736(09)61196-X
3. Stratigos A, Garbe C, Lebbe C, Malvehy J, Marmol V, Pehamberger H, et al. Diagnosis and treatment of invasive squamous cell carcinoma of the skin: European consensus-based interdisciplinary guideline. *Eur J Cancer* (2015) 51:1989–2007. doi:10.1016/j.ejca.2015.06.110
4. Kopecki Z, Yang GN, Jackson JE, Melville EL, Calley MP, Murrell DF, et al. Cytoskeletal protein flightless I inhibits apoptosis, enhances tumor cell invasion and promotes cutaneous squamous cell carcinoma progression. *Oncotarget* (2015) 6:36426–40. doi:10.18632/oncotarget.5536
5. Weinberg AS, Ogle CA, Shim EK. Metastatic cutaneous squamous cell carcinoma: an update. *Dermatol Surg* (2007) 33:885–99. doi:10.1097/00042728-200708000-00001
6. Ikegawa S, Saida T, Obayashi H, Sasaki A, Esumi H, Ikeda S, et al. Cisplatin combination chemotherapy in squamous cell carcinoma and adenoid cystic carcinoma of the skin. *J Dermatol* (1989) 16:227–30. doi:10.1111/j.1346-8138.1989.tb01254.x
7. Khansur T, Kennedy A. Cisplatin and 5-fluorouracil for advanced locoregional and metastatic squamous cell carcinoma of the skin. *Cancer* (1991) 67:2030–2. doi:10.1002/1097-0142(19910415)67:8<2030::AID-CNCR2820670803>3.0.CO;2-K
8. Nakamura K, Okuyama R, Saida T, Uhara H. Platinum and anthracycline therapy for advanced cutaneous squamous cell carcinoma. *Int J Clin Oncol* (2013) 18:506–9. doi:10.1007/s10147-012-0411-y
9. Behshad R, Garcia-Zuazaga J, Bordeaux JS. Systemic treatment of locally advanced nonmetastatic cutaneous squamous cell carcinoma: a review of the literature. *Br J Dermatol* (2011) 165:1169–77. doi:10.1111/j.1365-2133.2011.10524.x
10. Lewis CM, Glisson BS, Feng L, Wan F, Tang X, Wistuba II, et al. A phase II study of gefitinib for aggressive cutaneous squamous cell carcinoma of the head and neck. *Clin Cancer Res* (2012) 18:1435–46. doi:10.1158/1078-0432.CCR-11-1951
11. Maubec E, Petrow P, Scheer-Senyarich I, Duvillard P, Lacroix L, Gelly J, et al. Phase II study of cetuximab as first-line single-drug therapy in patients with unresectable squamous cell carcinoma of the skin. *J Clin Oncol* (2011) 29:3419–26. doi:10.1200/JCO.2010.34.1735
12. Borradori L, Sutton B, Shayesteh P, Daniels GA. Rescue therapy with anti-programmed cell death protein 1 inhibitors (PD-1) of advanced cutaneous squamous cell carcinoma and basosquamous carcinoma: preliminary experience in 5 cases. *Br J Dermatol* (2016) 175:1382–6. doi:10.1111/bjd.14642
13. Fujisawa Y, Umebayashi Y, Ichikawa E, Kawachi Y, Otsuka F. Chemoradiation using low-dose cisplatin and 5-fluorouracil in locally advanced squamous cell carcinoma of the skin: a report of two cases. *J Am Acad Dermatol* (2006) 55:S81–5. doi:10.1016/j.jaad.2005.12.035
14. Reigneau M, Robert C, Routier E, Mamelle G, Moya-Plana A, Tomasic G, et al. Efficacy of neoadjuvant cetuximab alone or with platinum salt for the treatment of unresectable advanced nonmetastatic cutaneous squamous cell carcinomas. *Br J Dermatol* (2015) 173:527–34. doi:10.1111/bjd.13741
15. Preneau S, Rio E, Brocard A, Peuvrel L, Nguyen JM, Quéreux G, et al. Efficacy of cetuximab in the treatment of squamous cell carcinoma. *J Dermatolog Treat* (2014) 25:424–7. doi:10.3109/09546634.2012.751481
16. Baltaci M, Fritsch P, Weber F, Tzankov A, Sögner P, Derler AM, et al. Treatment with gefitinib (ZD1839) in a patient with advanced cutaneous squamous cell carcinoma. *Br J Dermatol* (2005) 153:234–6. doi:10.1111/j.1365-2133.2005.06709.x
17. Kawakami Y, Nakamura K, Nishibu A, Yanagihori H, Kimura H, Yamamoto T. Regression of cutaneous squamous cell carcinoma in a patient with chronic myeloid leukaemiaon imatinib mesylate treatment. *Acta Derm Venereol* (2008) 88:185–6. doi:10.2340/00015555-0368
18. William WN Jr, Feng L, Ferrarotto R, Ginsberg L, Kies M, Lippman S, et al. Gefitinib for patients with incurable cutaneous squamous cell carcinoma: a single-arm phase II clinical trial. *J Am Acad Dermatol* (2017) 77:1110–3. doi:10.1016/j.jaad.2017.07.048
19. Ramadan KM, McKenna KE, Morris TC. Clinical response of cutaneous squamous-cell carcinoma to bortezomib given for myeloma. *Lancet Oncol* (2006) 7:958–9. doi:10.1016/S1470-2045(06)70944-5
20. Shin DM, Glisson BS, Khuri FR, Clifford JL, Clayman G, Benner SE, et al. Phase II and biologic study of interferon alfa, retinoic acid, and cisplatin in advanced squamous skin cancer. *J Clin Oncol* (2002) 20:364–70. doi:10.1200/JCO.20.2.364
21. Hoff PM, Ansari R, Batist G, Cox J, Kocha W, Kuperminc M, et al. Comparison of oral capecitabine versus intravenous fluorouracil plus leucovorin as first-line treatment in 605 patients with metastatic colorectal cancer: results of a randomized phase III study. *J Clin Oncol* (2001) 19:2282–92. doi:10.1200/JCO.2001.19.8.2282
22. Robbins KT, Homma A. Intra-arterial chemotherapy for head and neck cancer: experiences from three continents. *Surg Oncol Clin N Am* (2008) 17:919–33. doi:10.1016/j.soc.2008.04.015
23. Sheen YT, Lai CS, Sheen YS, Yang SF, Sheen MC. Palmar squamous cell carcinoma successfully treated by intra-arterial infusion chemotherapy. *J Am Acad Dermatol* (2012) 67:e263–4. doi:10.1016/j.jaad.2012.03.035
24. Argiris A, Harrington KJ, Tahara M, Schulten J, Chomette P, Ferreira Castro A, et al. Evidence-based treatment options in recurrent and/or metastatic squamous cell carcinoma of the head and neck. *Front Oncol* (2017) 7:72. doi:10.3389/fonc.2017.00072
25. Bauml J, Seiwert TY, Pfister DG, Worden F, Liu SV, Gilbert J, et al. Pembrolizumab for platinum- and cetuximab-refractory head and neck cancer: results from a single-arm, phase II study. *J Clin Oncol* (2017) 35:1542–9. doi:10.1200/JCO.2016.70.1524
26. Degache E, Crochet J, Simon N, Tardieu M, Trabelsi S, Moncourier M, et al. Major response to pembrolizumab in two patients with locally advanced cutaneous squamous cell carcinoma. *J Eur Acad Dermatol Venereol* (2017). doi:10.1111/jdv.14371
27. Deinlein T, Lax SF, Schwarz T, Giuffrida R, Schmid-Zalaudek K, Zalaudek I. Rapid response of metastatic cutaneous squamous cell carcinoma to pembrolizumab in a patient with xeroderma pigmentosum: case report and review of the literature. *Eur J Cancer* (2017) 83:99–102. doi:10.1016/j.ejca.2017.06.022

28. Stevenson ML, Wang CQ, Abikhair M, Roudiani N, Felsen D, Krueger JG, et al. Expression of programmed cell death ligand in cutaneous squamous cell carcinoma and treatment of locally advanced disease with pembrolizumab. *JAMA Dermatol* (2017) 153:299–303. doi:10.1001/jamadermatol.2016.5118

29. Winkler JK, Schneiderbauer R, Bender C, Sedlaczek O, Fröhling S, Penzel R, et al. Anti-programmed cell death-1 therapy in nonmelanoma skin cancer. *Br J Dermatol* (2017) 176:498–502. doi:10.1111/bjd.14664

30. Guthrie TH Jr, Porubsky ES, Luxenberg MN, Shah KJ, Wurtz KL, Watson PR. Cisplatin-based chemotherapy in advanced basal and squamous cell carcinomas of the skin: results in 28 patients including 13 patients receiving multimodality therapy. *J Clin Oncol* (1990) 8:342–6. doi:10.1200/JCO.1990.8.2.342

31. Loeffler JS, Larson DA, Clark JR, Weichselbaum RR, Norris CM Jr, Ervin TJ. Treatment of perineural metastasis from squamous carcinoma of the skin with aggressive combination chemotherapy and irradiation. *J Surg Oncol* (1985) 29:181–3. doi:10.1002/jso.2930290310

32. Postow MA, Callahan MK, Barker CA, Yamada Y, Yuan J, Kitano S, et al. Immunologic correlates of the abscopal effect in a patient with melanoma. *N Engl J Med* (2012) 366:925–31. doi:10.1056/NEJMoa1112824

33. Wang J, Aldabagh B, Yu J, Arron ST. Role of human papillomavirus in cutaneous squamous cell carcinoma: a meta-analysis. *J Am Acad Dermatol* (2014) 70:621–9. doi:10.1016/j.jaad.2014.01.857

34. Hasche D, Stephan S, Braspenning-Wesch I, Mikulec J, Niebler M, Gröne HJ, et al. The interplay of UV and cutaneous papillomavirus infection in skin cancer development. *PLoS Pathog* (2017) 13:e1006723. doi:10.1371/journal.ppat.1006723

35. Biktasova A, Hajek M, Sewell A, Gary C, Bellinger G, Deshpande HA, et al. Demethylation therapy as a targeted treatment for human papillomavirus-associated head and neck cancer. *Clin Cancer Res* (2017) 23:7276–87. doi:10.1158/1078-0432.CCR-17-1438

36. Yu X, Li Z. The role of miRNAs in cutaneous squamous cell carcinoma. *J Cell Mol Med* (2016) 20:3–9. doi:10.1111/jcmm.12649

37. Lin N, Zhou Y, Lian X, Tu Y. MicroRNA-31 functions as an oncogenic microRNA in cutaneous squamous cell carcinoma cells by targeting RhoTBT1. *Oncol Lett* (2017) 13:1078–82. doi:10.3892/ol.2017.5554

38. Cheng CJ, Bahal R, Babar IA, Pincus Z, Barrera F, Liu C, et al. MicroRNA silencing for cancer therapy targeted to the tumour microenvironment. *Nature* (2015) 518:107–10. doi:10.1038/nature13905

39. Turner NC, Ro J, André F, Loi S, Verma S, Iwata H, et al. Palbociclib in hormone-receptor-positive advanced breast cancer. *N Engl J Med* (2015) 373:209–19. doi:10.1056/NEJMoa1505270

40. Finn RS, Martin M, Rugo HS, Jones S, Im SA, Gelmon K, et al. Palbociclib and letrozole in advanced breast cancer. *N Engl J Med* (2016) 375:1925–36. doi:10.1056/NEJMoa1607303

41. Cole AR. PCTK proteins: the forgotten brain kinases? *Neurosignals* (2009) 17:288–97. doi:10.1159/000231895

42. Ou CY, Poon VY, Maeder CI, Watanabe S, Lehrman EK, Fu AK, et al. Two cyclin-dependent kinase pathways are essential for polarized trafficking of presynaptic components. *Cell* (2010) 141:846–58. doi:10.1016/j.cell.2010.04.011

43. Mikolcevic P, Rainer J, Geley S. Orphan kinases turn eccentric: a new class of cyclin Y-activated, membrane-targeted CDKs. *Cell Cycle* (2012) 11:3758–68. doi:10.4161/cc.21592

44. Yanagi T, Matsuzawa S. PCTAIRE1/PCTK1/CDK16: a new oncotarget. *Cell Cycle* (2015) 14:463–4. doi:10.1080/15384101.2015.1006539

45. Yanagi T, Reed JC, Matsuzawa S. PCTAIRE1 regulates p27 stability, apoptosis and tumor growth in malignant melanoma. *Oncoscience* (2014) 1:624–33. doi:10.18632/oncoscience.86

46. Yanagi T, Krajewska M, Matsuzawa S, Reed JC. PCTAIRE1 phosphorylates p27 and regulates mitosis in cancer cells. *Cancer Res* (2014) 74:5795–807. doi:10.1158/0008-5472.CAN-14-0872

47. Yanagi T, Hata H, Mizuno E, Kitamura S, Imafuku K, Nakazato S, et al. PCTAIRE1/CDK16/PCTK1 is overexpressed in cutaneous squamous cell carcinoma and regulates p27 stability and cell cycle. *J Dermatol Sci* (2017) 86:149–57. doi:10.1016/j.jdermsci.2017.02.281

48. Yamaguchi Y, Yanagi T, Imafuku K, Kitamura S, Hata H, Nishihara H, et al. A case of linear basal cell carcinoma: evaluation of proliferative activity by immunohistochemical staining of PCTAIRE1 and p27. *J Eur Acad Dermatol Venereol* (2017) 31(8):e359–62. doi:10.1111/jdv.14159

49. Yanagi T, Shi R, Aza-Blanc P, Reed JC, Matsuzawa S. PCTAIRE1-knockdown sensitizes cancer cells to TNF family cytokines. *PLoS One* (2015) 10:e0119404. doi:10.1371/journal.pone.0119404

50. Yanagi T, Tachikawa K, Wilkie-Grantham R, Hishiki A, Nagai KO, Toyonaga E, et al. Lipid nanoparticle-mediated siRNA transfer against PCTAIRE1/PCTK1/Cdk16 inhibits *in vivo* cancer growth. *Mol Ther Nucleic Acids* (2016) 5:e327. doi:10.1038/mtna.2016.40

51. Kitamura S, Yanagi T, Imafuku K, Hata H, Abe R, Shimizu H. Drp1 regulates mitochondrial morphology and cell proliferation in cutaneous squamous cell carcinoma. *J Dermatol Sci* (2017) 88:298–307. doi:10.1016/j.jdermsci.2017.08.004

52. Wieder SY, Serasinghe MN, Sung JC, Choi DC, Birqe MB, Yao JL, et al. Activation of the mitochondrial fragmentation protein DRP1 correlates with BRAF(V600E) melanoma. *J Invest Dermatol* (2015) 135:2544–7. doi:10.1038/jid.2015.196

53. Qian W, Choi S, Gibson GA, Watkins SC, Bakkenist CJ, Van Houten B. Mitochondrial hyperfusion induced by loss of the fission protein Drp1 causes ATM-dependent G2/M arrest and aneuploidy through DNA replication stress. *J Cell Sci* (2012) 125:5747–57. doi:10.1242/jcs.109769

54. Zhao J, Zhang J, Yu M, Xie Y, Huang Y, Wolff DW, et al. Mitochondrial dynamics regulates migration and invasion of breast cancer cells. *Oncogene* (2013) 32:4814–24. doi:10.1038/onc.2012.494

55. Chiang YY, Chen SL, Hsiao YT, Huang CH, Lin TY, Chiang IP, et al. Nuclear expression of dynamin-related protein 1 in lung adenocarcinomas. *Mod Pathol* (2009) 22:1139–50. doi:10.1038/modpathol.2009.83

56. Xie W, Wu Q, Horbinski CM, Flavahan WA, Yang K, Zhou W, et al. Mitochondrial control by DRP1 in brain tumor initiating cells. *Nat Neurosci* (2015) 18:501–10. doi:10.1038/nn.3960

17

Dermoscopy of Melanoma and Non-melanoma Skin Cancers

Junji Kato, Kohei Horimoto, Sayuri Sato, Tomoyuki Minowa and Hisashi Uhara*

Department of Dermatology, Sapporo Medical University School of Medicine, Sapporo, Japan

Correspondence:
Hisashi Uhara
uharah@sapmed.ac.jp

Dermoscopy is a widely used non-invasive technique for diagnosing skin tumors. In melanocytic tumors, e.g., melanoma and basal cell carcinoma (BCC), the effectiveness of dermoscopic examination has been fully established over the past two decades. Moreover, dermoscopy has been used to diagnose non-melanocytic tumors. Here, we review novel findings from recent reports concerning dermoscopy of melanoma and non-melanoma skin cancers including BCC, sebaceous carcinoma, actinic keratosis, Bowen's disease, squamous cell carcinoma (SCC), Merkel cell carcinoma (MCC), extramammary Paget's disease (EMPD), and angiosarcoma.

Keywords: dermoscopy, melanoma, basal cell carcinoma, sebaceous carcinoma, actinic keratosis, Bowen's disease, squamous cell carcinoma, Merkel cell carcinoma

INTRODUCTION

Dermoscopy is a non-invasive technique for diagnosing skin lesions, which aids in the differentiation between benign and malignant alterations. Dermoscopy has been used to diagnose non-melanocytic tumors. Recently, vascular morphology has been identified as an important criteria in dermoscopic diagnosis when assessing non-melanocytic tumors. Here, we review recent reports of novel findings related to dermoscopy of melanoma and non-melanoma skin cancers.

Melanoma

Dermoscopy has been shown to improve significantly the diagnosis of melanocytic lesions in the clinical practice. Following the Consensus Net Meeting on Dermoscopy in 2000, a two-step algorithm for a method of dermoscopic diagnostic was established, especially for pigmented skin lesions (1). Marghoob and Braun subsequently devised a revised two-step algorithm including polarized dermoscopy and blood vessel morphology (2). In the second step of the revised algorithm, pattern analysis, the ABCD rule, the Menzies method (3), and the seven-point checklist are employed to diagnose melanoma. The seven-point checklist is based on seven melanoma-specific criteria; each is classified as major or minor. Major criteria consist of atypical networks, blue-whitish veils, and atypical vascular patterns while minor criteria are irregular dots/globules, irregular streaks, irregular blotches, and regression structures. A score of 2 is given to each of the major criteria, whereas a score of 1 is given to each of the minor criteria. Results yielding 3 points or more should be considered suspicious enough to justify exclusion.

Lentigo Maligna and Lentigo Maligna Melanoma

The differential diagnoses related to lentigo maligna (LM) and lentigo maligna melanoma (LMM) include a myriad of other pigmented skin lesions, including solar lentigo, seborrheic keratosis, and pigmented actinic keratosis. While the pigment network is the dermoscopic hallmark of superficial spreading melanoma (SSM) located on the trunk and extremities, a true pigment network is rarely found in LM. A pseudonetwork pattern refers to the common dermoscopic finding of melanocytic and non-melanocytic pigmented macules of the face; it is a structureless diffuse brown pigmentation interrupted by numerous, variably broad, and hypopigmented holes, which correspond to hair follicles and sweat gland openings. Based on a report by Schiffner et al., the four most important features are asymmetric pigmented follicular openings, dark rhomboidal structures, slate-gray globules, and slate-gray dots. This analysis yields a sensitivity of 89% and a specificity of 96% (4).

Nodular Melanoma

Considering that most dermoscopic features have been described in the context of SMM, the dermoscopic recognition of nodular melanoma (NM) is also challenging since the tumor often lacks the well-known melanoma-specific criteria. Therefore, several accepted dermoscopic criteria of melanoma are not detected in purely nodular tumors.

Argenziano et al. described a new predictor of NM, namely the presence of blue-black color within the lesion (5). The blue-black color is thought to reflect the combination of pigments localized in the mid-deep dermis (blue) and the epidermis (black). The authors reported that all lesion surfaces that were comprised of at least 10% blue and black areas were significantly associated with pigmented NM. Moreover, Pizzichetta et al. reported NM was related to features such as ulceration, homogeneous disorganized patterns, homogeneous blue-pigmented structureless areas, multiple (≥3) colors, the combination of polymorphous vessels and milky-red globules/areas, and symmetric shapes (6).

Acral Melanoma (Volar)

Saida et al. reported dermoscopic patterns of acral melanoma in the Japanese population (7). They found that the parallel ridge pattern (PRP) is the most specific dermoscopic finding for acral melanomas. PRP consists of a band-like pigmentation located on the ridges of the skin markings. In their report, the sensitivity and specificity of PRP for acral melanoma were 86.4 and 99%, respectively. In additional studies, Phan et al. and Ozdemir et al. reported that PRP was detectable in 53 and 60.8% of their cases (8, 9). Lallas et al. proposed the BRAAFF checklist, a score composed of four positive features, i.e., irregular blotches, PRP, asymmetry of structures, and asymmetry of colors, and two negative features such as the parallel furrow pattern (PFP) and fibrillar pattern. Based on the results of the BRAAFF checklist, they proposed a dermoscopic diagnostic algorithm that achieves 93.1% sensitivity and 86.7% specificity for acral melanoma diagnosis (10).

It is difficult to differentiate melanoma from melanocytic nevus if PRP or PFP is not observed. In melanoma on the volar skin without typical dermoscopic patterns, Mikoshiba et al. recently reported frequently observed features consisting of asymmetry, greater numbers of colors (≥3), irregular distribution of blue-white structures, dots and globules, vascular structures including milky red areas, ulcers, diffuse pigmentation, and irregular streaks (11).

Nail Apparatus (Subungual) Melanoma

Important dermoscopic features of nail apparatus (so-called subungual) melanoma include irregular lines on a brown background, micro-Hutchinson's sign triangular pigmentation on the nail plate, and a wide pigmented band (12). The width of pigmentation is an important risk factor. Ohn et al. reported the following factors to be associated with adult-onset *in situ* lesions: width of pigmentation ≥3 mm, width of pigmentation ≥6 mm (the minimum 6-mm width was more strongly associated with melanoma), multicolor pigmentation, asymmetry, border fading, and the Hutchinson sign (13). Moreover, Benati et al. reported that a width more than 2/3 of the nail plate suggested melanoma (14). They also reported that the second most important predictor of nail apparatus melanoma was the presence of gray to black color. This gray to black color was associated with 12.5% of nevus and 76% of nail apparatus melanoma.

Clinically, age is important to differentiate melanoma from melanocytic nevus. Most cases of nail apparatus melanoma are diagnosed in adults. Caution must be observed before diagnosing nail apparatus melanoma in children because irregular findings are frequently observed in the benign nevus of nails in children.

Amelanotic Melanoma

Amelanotic melanomas are a relatively rare subtype of melanomas with little or no pigment at visual inspection. Since the majority of melanoma-associated dermoscopic structures are pigmented, amelanotic melanomas remain a demanding diagnostic. The atypical vascular structures are frequently the only clue for its diagnosis (15, 16). Therefore, diagnosis and treatment are often delayed. Menzies et al. reported that the dermoscopically diagnostic accuracy of hypomelanotic or amelanotic melanomas was inferior to that of pigmented melanoma (15). In a recent study of amelanotic melanomas, Lin et al. reported polymorphous vessels as common features in 20 of 27 melanomas. However, in truly amelanotic melanomas, the vascular pattern of polymorphous vessels may not suffice as an only feature utilized to diagnose amelanotic melanoma since it is also found in other skin cancers (16).

Basal Cell Carcinoma

The value of dermoscopy of basal cell carcinoma (BCC) has been extensively demonstrated over the past few decades. Menzies et al. reported the sensitivity of diagnostic criteria for pigmented BCC was 97% (17). The dermoscopic criteria associated with BCCs include the absence of a pigment network and the presence of specific features, e.g., arborizing vessels, large blue-gray ovoid nests, multiple blue-gray globules, leaf-like areas, spoke wheel areas, and ulceration. In reports from Menzies et al. and Altamura et al., arborizing vessels (52% in Menzies et al., 48.5% in Altamura et al.), large blue-gray ovoid nests (55%, 60.8%), multiple blue-gray globules (27%, 38.5%), leaf-like areas (17%, 22.7%), spoke wheel areas (10%, 13.1%), and ulceration (27%, 34.6%) were dermoscopically observed in pigmented BCCs (17, 18). Additional features have been reported recently, specifically multiple small erosions, shiny white streaks, and concentric structures (19–23). Altamura et al. reported that multiple small erosions were seen in 14.1% of non-pigmented BCCs (18), whereas shiny white streaks have been seen only in polarized dermoscopy (22, 24). Moreover, vascular patterns such as short fine telangiectasias (SFTs), arborizing microvessels, and milky-pink backgrounds have been reported, and these patterns may be useful particularly for non-pigmented BCCs. SFTs are small vessels without branches. Micantonio et al. (20) and Emiroglu et al. (25) reported that SFTs were the second most common vascular pattern found in BCCs. These telangiectasias were significantly more common in superficial BCCs than in nodular BCCs (20). Additionally, Pan et al. reported that arborizing microvessels, short, bright red, sharply focused, fine-caliber branching vessels, were seen in 62% of superficial BCCs (26). Reports on milky-pink backgrounds indicated that they were more common in superficial BCCs (21, 25–27).

Dermoscopic characteristics for each BCC subtype have been described. Some reports differentiated between superficial BCC and other subtypes by dermoscopy (19, 24, 25). In superficial BCC, maple leaf-like areas, spoke wheel areas, SFTs, multiple small erosions, and concentric structures were frequently observed (17–19, 23). Ahnlide et al. (23) summarized dermoscopic features in the common subtype of BCC, including superficial BCC ($n = 202$), nodular BCC ($n = 76$), and infiltrated BCC ($n = 142$) (**Table 1**). Based on their reports, both in nodular and infiltrated BCCs, arborizing vessels were the most common, while ulcerations were the second most common findings. Moreover, Lallas et al. reported that blue-gray ovoid nests may be predictors for non-superficial BCCs. According to their findings, both arborizing vessels and ulcerations would exclude superficial BCC (19).

Sebaceous Carcinoma

Although the common clinical presentation of sebaceous carcinoma (SC) is a yellow or red nodule, clinical diagnosis is challenging due to the absence of criteria for dermoscopic diagnosis (28, 29). The main dermoscopic features of SC are yellowish structures, polymorphous vessels, ulcerations, and whitish-pink areas (30–36) (**Table 2**). The most common findings are yellowish structures, i.e., background, globules and yellow/yellowish areas, which were described as the heterogeneously distributing yellowish objects with varying size, shape and number in the literatures. Polymorphous vessels and ulceration are the second most common appearances. Polymorphous vessels were reported as the combination of various types of vessels, i.e., linear irregular vessels, hairpin vessels, comma-like vessels, dotted vessels, arborizing vessels, and telangiectasias. Ulcerations or crusts on the surface of the tumor suggest the possibility of malignancy, which might help distinguish SC from the benign sebaceous tumors. Whitish-pink areas were described as the homogeneous white-to-pink background (35). Dermoscopically, benign sebaceous tumors should be differentiated from SC. Benign sebaceous tumors are classified as sebaceous hyperplasia, sebaceous adenoma, and sebaceoma (31). Sebaceous hyperplasia consists of a white-yellow, umbilicated, structureless center, radially arranged yellow globules, and peripheral telangiectasias (crown vessels). The absence of polymorphous vessels and ulcerations might be helpful to differentiate from SC.

TABLE 1 | Dermoscopic features in subtype of BCC in the report of Ahnlide et al. (23).

	Nodular BCC (%)	Superficial BCC (%)	Infiltrated BCC (%)
Arborizing vessels	79.7	28.6	86.5
Blue-gray ovoid nests	28.9	21.4	18.3
Ulceration	35.3	20	58.7
Leaf-like areas/spoke wheel areas	16	37.1	50.8
Multiple small erosions	10.7	47.1	15.1
Shiny red-white, structureless areas	25.1	55.7	29.4

TABLE 2 | Dermoscopic features in sebaceous carcinoma.

References	Number of cases	Dermoscopic findings
Coates et al. (30)	2	Variably yellow background Polymorphous vessels Ulceration
Lallas et al. (31)	2	Yellowish structure White-yellowish well-circumscribed areas Polymorphous vascular pattern Ulceration
Manríquez et al. (32)	2	Yellow globules Multiple telangiectasia
Iikawa et al. (33)	1	Homogeneous yellow background Polymorphous vessels
Satomura et al. (34)	5	Yellow background Polymorphous vessels
Horimoto et al. (35)	3	Pink-whitish areas Yellow-whitish globules Polymorphous vessels Ulceration
Nair et al. (36)	1	Yellowish background with peripheral vessels Ulceration

Actinic Keratosis

A grading classification of actinic keratosis (AK) has been proposed based on clinical criteria (37). Grade I (mild) consists of slightly palpable AK, grade II (moderate) exhibits readily palpable and visible AK and grade III (severe) is characterized by very thick and hyperkeratotic AK. This clinical classification of AK corresponds to dermoscopic characteristics (38–42). In grade I, red pseudonetwork patterns and white scales are seen. In grade II, a strawberry pattern is typical. The strawberry pattern results from an erythematous background with white-to-yellow keratotic and dilated follicular openings. In addition, targetoid hair follicles are also seen in grade II (43). In grade III, either enlarged follicular plugs filled with keratotic plugs over a white to yellow background or marked hyperkeratosis are observed.

AKs cannot always be distinguished from SCC *in situ* or invasive SCC. Vascular patterns may be helpful concerning this. Casari et al. reported that the increasing atypia is usually associated with dotted vessels around follicles in severe AKs (44). Therefore, enlarging dotted vessels, forming glomerular vessels were seen *in situ* SCC. With the progression to invasive SCC, hairpin and/or linear-irregular vessels will appear.

In pigmented AK, the most typical dermoscopic structure is the superficial brown network consisting of brown, curved double lines that surround enlarged, partially confluent, keratotic follicles of various sizes. Pigmented AK may also reveal an annular-granular pattern and pseudonetwork and rhomboidal structures, which are also seen in lentigo maligna (45). The annular-granular pattern in pigmented AK tends to be more prominent and keratin may be observed in the follicular openings. Moreover, the strawberry sign, rosette pattern, and scale may help to distinguish AK from LM when making a diagnosis (43).

Bowen's Disease

The dermoscopic characteristics of Bowen's disease (BD) were first described in 2004 (46).

Based on several studies, glomerular vessels (69–97%) and scaly white-to-yellow surfaces (64–96%) were commonly observed in non-pigmented BD (26, 46–50). Brown to gray globules/dots and structureless pigmentation were observed in 21–80% and 70–78% of pigmented BD, respectively (46, 48, 50, 51). These pigmented globules/dots are often distributed at the periphery, sometimes exhibiting a streak-like or leaf-like structure. However, these are not specific to pigmented BD. Chung et al. reported that streak-like structures did not converge toward the center of the lesion, nor did they connect to a common base and therefore may be distinguished from those seen in melanocytic lesions or in BCCs (52). Recently, Yang et al. found two new dermoscopic signs by analyzing 146 lesions of BD (49). One was parallel pigmented edges at the periphery of the lesion, named the double-edge sign. The other was several aggregated large pigmented massive structures, often distributed at the periphery of the lesion, named clusters of brown structureless areas. The former was observed in 44 of 146 lesions (30.1%), and the latter was in 56 (38.4%).

In rare occasions, BD develops in the nail, periungually, in the fingers and palm, often displaying the type of pigmented BD (53–55). Nakayama et al. reported four cases of periungual pigmented BD (53). Histologically, dilated vessels in the papillary dermis corresponding to a dermoscopic finding of glomerular vessels were observed, but none of the four cases presented glomerular vessels upon dermoscopic examination. They speculated that acral skin has a thicker stratum corneum than other skin, so papillary vessels might not be detectable by dermoscopy. In addition, the PFP was found in two of four cases, while the PRP was not found in any case. Similarly, Cavicchini et al. reported a case of pigmented BD developing in the palm that showed a PFP (54). The presence of the scaly surface and the lack of the PRP may distinguish acral BD from acral melanoma. Regarding BD developed in the fingernails, several case reports described subungual BD presented longitudinal melanonychia (55–57). Additionally, Hutchinson's sign was also observed in some reports (53, 58, 59).

Squamous Cell Carcinoma

Dermoscopic criteria for squamous cell carcinoma (SCC) include the presence of keratin/scales, blood spots, white circles, white structureless areas, hairpin vessels, linear-irregular vessels perivascular white halos, and ulceration (39, 60, 61). Keratin and scales are homogeneous opaque yellow to brown structures, corresponding to hyperkeratosis and parakeratosis (60, 62). Blood spots are the multiple red to black dots in the keratin mass, corresponding to small crusts or hemangiomas (60). White circles are the bright white circles surrounding a dilated infundibulum corresponding to acanthosis and hypergranulosis of the infundibular epidermis (62). White structureless areas are the whitish areas covering large areas of tumors, corresponding to large targetoid hair follicles (39, 63). Among the criteria discussed above, keratin and white circles reached the sensitivity and specificity for SCC diagnostic at a rate of 79 and 87%, respectively (60). The presence of vessels in more than half of the tumor's surface with a diffuse distribution of vessels and bleeding significantly increased the possibility of poorly differentiated SCC. Conversely, keratin/scales are a potent predictor of well- and moderately differentiated SCC (64). However, Pyne et al. reported that moderately and poorly differentiated SCC displayed more branched and serpentine vessels than well-differentiated SCC and that moderately and poorly differentiated SCC displayed larger numbers of vessel types than well-differentiated SCC (61). Regarding lip SCC, Benati et al. recently reported that scales, white structureless areas, and white halos were observed in the majority of the cases (100, 91, and 86%, respectively) (65).

Merkel Cell Carcinoma

Several recent studies have defined useful significant dermoscopic features for Merkel cell carcinoma (MCC). The most common dermoscopic finding is the milky-red areas that are usually associated with linear irregular vessels. Jalilian et al. reported dermoscopic features of 12 MCC cases (66). All cases presented polymorphous, linear irregular vessels, and structureless areas. Milky-pink areas were observed in 11 cases. Furthermore, Harting et al. reported that milky-red areas or linear irregular vessels were most commonly observed in 10 MCC cases studies (67). Additionally, Dalle et al. observed milky-red areas in 80% of their patients. While these patterns may be observed in amelanotic melanoma, the lack of findings of pigmentation or blue-gray veils could direct diagnosis against MCC (68).

Extramammary Paget's Disease

Dermoscopic features of extramammary Paget's disease (EMPD) have not yet been established due to its rarity. Recently, Mun et al. compared the dermoscopic appearance of 35 EMPD cases and EMPD-mimicking lesions, e.g., eczematous dermatitis (ED), fungal infections (FI), and Bowen's disease (BD). In EMPD, they observed milky-red areas (32/35), dotted vessels (18/35), glomerular vessels (7/35), polymorphous vessels (6/35), surface scales (7/35), linear irregular vessels (1/35), ulcers/erosions (15/35), pigmented structures (11/35), shiny white lines (4/35), and white structureless areas (3/35) (69). Milky red areas were significantly more prevalent in EMPD than in ED, FI, or BD. Moreover, invasive EMPD correlated statistically with polymorphous vessels.

Angiosarcoma

Dermoscopic features of angiosarcoma (AS) have not yet been established due to its rarity. De Giorgi et al. described steam-like areas with a white or skin-colored central area as a characteristic dermoscopic feature of AS (70). Furthermore, Oiso et al. reported that a gradation of various colors within the lesion may be an important dermoscopic feature of AS since it is not present in common purpura or ecchymosis (71). Minagawa et al. reported that AS is characterized by the absence of well-defined vascular structures, e.g., lacunae/lagoons that are commonly found in other vascular lesions such as angioma and pyogenic granuloma. Those features might be useful toward differential diagnosis with amelanotic melanomas (72).

CONCLUSION

We summarized recent reports of novel findings related to dermoscopy of melanoma and non-melanoma skin cancers. Dermoscopy is presently thought to be effective and helpful for diagnosing melanoma and non-melanoma skin cancers. However, it is important to consider that dermoscopy is just one of several means, others being clinical history, age and gross appearance, that can be utilized in cancer diagnosis. Therefore, we should not hesitate to do a biopsy in cases in which a diagnosis cannot be reached clearly through dermoscopy.

AUTHOR CONTRIBUTIONS

JK and HU have full responsibility of this article. JK, KH, SS, TM, and HU confirmed the manuscript for submission.

REFERENCES

1. Argenziano G, Soyer HP, Chimenti S, Talamin R, Corona R, Sera F, et al. Dermoscopy of pigmented skin lesions: results of a consensus meeting via the Internet. *J Am Acad Dermatol.* (2003) 48:679–93. doi: 10.1067/mjd.2003.281

2. Marghoob AA, Braun R. Proposal for a revised 2-step algorithm for the classification of lesions of the skin using dermoscopy. *Arch Dermatol.* (2010) 146:426–28. doi: 10.1001/archdermatol.2010.41

3. Menzies SW, Ingvar C, Crotty KA, McCarthy WH. Frequency and morphologic characteristics of invasive melanomas lacking specific surface microscopic features. *Arch Dermatol.* (1996) 132:1178–82. doi: 10.1001/archderm.1996.03890340038007

4. Schiffner R, Schiffner-Rohe J, Vogt T, Landthaler M, Wlotzke U, Cognetta AB, et al. Improvement of early recognition of lentigo maligna using dermatoscopy. *J Am Acad Dermatol.* (2000) 42:25–32. doi: 10.1016/S0190-9622(00)90005-7

5. Argenziano G, Longo C, Cameron A, Cavicchini S, Gourhant JY, Lallas, et al. Blue-black rule: a simple dermoscopic clue to recognize pigmented nodular melanoma. *Br J Dermatol.* (2011) 165:1251–5. doi: 10.1111/j.1365-2133.2011.10621.x

6. Pizzichetta MA, Kittler H, Stanganelli I, Bono R, Cavicchini S, De Giorgi V, et al. Pigmented nodular melanoma: the predictive value of dermoscopic features using multivariate analysis. *Br J Dermatol.* (2015) 173:106–14. doi: 10.1111/bjd.13861

7. Saida T, Miyazaki A, Oguchi S, Ishihara Y, Yamazaki Y, Murase S, et al. Significance of dermoscopic patterns in detecting malignant melanoma on acral volar skin: results of a multicenter study in Japan. *Arch Dermatol.* (2004) 140:1233–8. doi: 10.1001/archderm.140.10.1233

8. Phan A, Dalle S, Touzet S, Ronger-Savlé S, Balme B, Thomas L. Dermoscopic features of acral lentiginous melanoma in a large series of 110 cases in a white population. *Br J Dermatol.* (2010) 162:765–71. doi: 10.1111/j.1365-2133.2009.09594.x

9. Ozdemir F, Errico MA, Yaman B, Karaarslan I. Acral lentiginous melanoma in the Turkish population and a new dermoscopic clue for the diagnosis. *Dermatol Pract Concept.* (2018) 8:140–8. doi: 10.5826/dpc.0802a14

10. Lallas A, Kyrgidis A, Koga H, Moscarella E, Tschandl P, Apalla Z, et al. The BRAAFF checklist: a new dermoscopic algorithm for diagnosing acral melanoma. *Br J Dermatol.* (2015) 173:1041–9. doi: 10.1111/bjd.14045

11. Mikoshiba Y, Minagawa A, Koga H, Yokokawa Y, Uhara H, Okuyama R. Clinical and histopathologic characteristics of melanocytic lesions on the volar skin without typical dermoscopic patterns. *JAMA Dermatol.* (2019) 155:578–84. doi: 10.1001/jamadermatol.2018.5926

12. Koga H, Saida T, Uhara H. Key point in dermoscopic differentiation between early nail apparatus melanoma and benign longitudinal melanonychia. *J Dermatol.* (2011) 38:45–52. doi: 10.1111/j.1346-8138.2010.01175.x

13. Ohn J, Jo G, Cho Y, Sheu SL, Cho KH, Mun JH. Assessment of a predictive scoring model for dermoscopy of subungual melanoma *in situ*. *JAMA Dermatol.* (2018) 154:890–96. doi: 10.1001/jamadermatol.2018.1372

14. Benati E, Ribero S, Longo C, Piana S, Puig S, Carrera C, et al. Clinical and dermoscopic clues to differentiate pigmented nail bands: an International Dermoscopy Society study. *J Eur Acad Dermatol Venereol.* (2017) 31:732–6. doi: 10.1111/jdv.13991

15. Menzies SW, Kreusch J, Byth K, Pizzichetta MA, Marghoob A, Braun R, et al. Dermoscopic evaluation of amelanotic and hypomelanotic melanoma. *Arch Dermatol.* (2008) 144:1120–7. doi: 10.1001/archderm.144.9.1120

16. Lin MJ, Xie C, Pan Y, Jalilian C, Kelly JW. Dermoscopy improves diagnostic accuracy for clinically amelanotic nodules. *Australas J Dermatol.* (2019) 60:45–9. doi: 10.1111/ajd.12902

17. Menzies SW, Westerhoff K, Rabinovitz H, Kopf AW, McCarthy WH, Katz B. Surface microscopy of pigmented basal cell carcinoma. *Arch Dermatol.* (2000) 136:1012–6. doi: 10.1001/archderm.136.8.1012

18. Altamura D, Menzies SW, Argenziano G, Zalaudek I, Soyer HP, Sera F, et al. Dermatoscopy of basal cell carcinoma: morphologic variability of global and local features and accuracy of diagnosis. *J Am Acad Dermatol.* (2010) 62:67–75. doi: 10.1016/j.jaad.2009.05.035

19. Lallas A, Apalla Z, Argenziano G, Longo C, Moscarella E, Specchio F, et al. The dermatoscopic universe of basal cell carcinoma. *Dermatol Pract Concept.* (2014) 4:11–24. doi: 10.5826/dpc.0403a02

20. Micantonio T, Gulia A, Altobelli E, Di Cesare A, Fidanza R, Riitano A, et al. Vascular patterns in basal cell carcinoma. *J Eur Acad Dermatol Venereol.* (2011) 25:358–61. doi: 10.1111/j.1468-3083.2010.03734.x

21. Giacomel J, Zalaudek I. Dermoscopy of superficial basal cell carcinoma. *Dermatol Surg.* (2005) 31:1710–3. doi: 10.1097/00042728-200512000-00014

22. Marghoob AA, Cowell L, Kopf AW, Scope A. Observation of chrysalis structures with polarized dermoscopy. *Arch Dermatol.* (2009) 145:618. doi: 10.1001/archdermatol.2009.28

23. Ahnlide I, Zalaudek I, Nilsson F, Bjellerup M, Nielsen K. Preoperative prediction of histopathological outcome in basal cell carcinoma: flat surface and multiple small erosions predict superficial basal cell carcinoma in lighter skin types. *Br J Dermatol.* (2016) 175:751–61. doi: 10.1111/bjd.14499

24. Navarrete-Dechent C, Bajaj S, Marchetti MA, Rabinovitz H, Dusza SW, Marghoob AA. Association of shiny white blotches and strands with non-pigmented basal cell carcinoma: evaluation of an additional dermoscopic diagnostic criterion. *JAMA Dermatol.* (2016) 152:546–52. doi: 10.1001/jamadermatol.2015.5731

25. Emiroglu N, Cengiz FP, Kemeriz F. The relation between dermoscopy and histopathology of basal cell carcinoma. *An Bras Dermatol.* (2015) 90:351–6. doi: 10.1590/abd1806-4841.20153446

26. Pan Y, Chamberlain AJ, Bailey M, Chong AH, Haskett M, Kelly JW. Dermatoscopy aids in the diagnosis of the solitary red scaly patch or

plaque-features distinguishing superficial basal cell carcinoma, intraepidermal carcinoma, and psoriasis. *J Am Acad Dermatol.* (2008) 59:268–74. doi: 10.1016/j.jaad.2008.05.013

27. Enache AO, Pătra?cu V, Simionescu CE, Ciurea RN, Văduva A, Stoica LE. Dermoscopy patterns and histopathological findings in nodular basal cell carcinoma-study on 68 cases. *Curr Health Sci J.* (2019) 45:116–22. doi: 10.12865/CHSJ.45.01.16

28. Nelson BR, Hamlet KR, Gillard M, Railan D, Johnson TM. Sebaceous carcinoma. *J Am Acad Dermatol.* (1995) 33:1–15. doi: 10.1016/0190-9622(95)90001-2

29. Buitrago W, Joseph AK. Sebaceous carcinoma: the great masquerader. Emerging concepts in diagnosis and treatment. *Dermatol Ther.* (2008) 21:459–66. doi: 10.1111/j.1529-8019.2008.00247.x

30. Coates D, Bowling J, Haskett M. Dermoscopic features of extraocular sebaceous carcinoma. *Australas J Dermatol.* (2011) 52:212–3. doi: 10.1111/j.1440-0960.2010.00699.x

31. Lallas A, Moscarella E, Argenziano G, Longo C, Apalla Z, Ferrara G, et al. Dermoscopy of uncommon skin tumours. *Australas J Dermatol.* (2014) 55:53–62. doi: 10.1111/ajd.12074

32. Manríquez J, Cataldo-Cerda K, Álvarez-Véliz S, Vera-Kellet C. Dermoscopy of sebaceous carcinoma: an unusual image. *G Ital Dermatol Venereol.* (2015) 150:626–8.

33. Iikawa M, Namiki T, Arima Y, Kato K, Arai M, Ueno M, et al. Extraocular sebaceous carcinoma in association with a clonal seborrheic keratosis: dermoscopic features. *J Dermatol.* (2015) 42:1105–6. doi: 10.1111/1346-8138.13043

34. Satomura H, Ogata D, Arai E, Tsuchida T. Dermoscopic features of ocular and extraocular sebaceous carcinomas. *J Dermatol.* (2017) 44:1313–6. doi: 10.1111/1346-8138.13905

35. Horimoto K, Kato J, Sumikawa Y, Hida T, Kamiya T, Sato S, et al. Dermoscopic features distinctive for extraocular sebaceous carcinoma. *J Dermatol.* (2018) 45:487–90. doi: 10.1111/1346-8138.14170

36. Nair PA, Patel T, Gandhi S. The usefulness of dermoscopy in extraocular sebaceous carcinoma. *Indian J Dermatol.* (2018) 63:440–2. doi: 10.4103/ijd.IJD_315_17

37. Rower-Huber J, Patel MJ, Forschner T, Ulrich C, Eberle J, Kerl H et al. Actinic keratosis is an early *in situ* squamous cell carcinoma: a proposal for reclassification. *Br J Dermatol.* (2007) 156:8–12. doi: 10.1111/j.1365-2133.2007.07860.x

38. Zalaudek I, Giacomel J, Argenziano G, Hofmann-Wellenhof R, Micantonio T, Di Stefani A, et al. Dermoscopy of facial nonpigmented actinic keratosis. *Br J Dermatol.* (2006) 155:951–6. doi: 10.1111/j.1365-2133.2006.07426.x

39. Zalaudek I, Giacomel J, Schmid K, Bondino S, Rosendahl C, Cavicchini S, et al. Dermatoscopy of facial actinic keratosis, intraepidermal carcinoma, and invasive squamous cell carcinoma: a progression model. *J Am Acad Dermatol.* (2012) 66:589–97. doi: 10.1016/j.jaad.2011.02.011

40. Lallas A, Argenziano G, Zendri E, Moscarella E, Longo C, Grenzi L, et al. Update on non-melanoma skin cancer and the value of dermoscopy in its diagnosis and treatment monitoring. *Expert Rev Anticancer Ther.* (2013) 13:541–58. doi: 10.1586/era.13.38

41. Russo T, Piccolo V, Lallas A, Giacomel J, Moscarella E, Alfano R, et al. Dermoscopy of malignant skin tumours: what's new? *Dermatology.* (2017) 233:64–73. doi: 10.1159/000472253

42. Deinlein T, Richtig G, Schwab C, Scarfi F, Arzberger E, Wolf I, et al. The use of dermatoscopy in diagnosis and therapy of nonmelanocytic skin cancer. *J Dtsch Dermatol Ges.* (2016) 14:144–51. doi: 10.1111/ddg.12903

43. Jaimes N, Marghoob AA. Squamous cell carcinoma, actinic keratosis and keratoacanthoma. In: Jaimes N, Marghoob AA, editors. *Pocket Guide to Dermoscopy.* Coimbatore: Jaypee Brothers Medical Publishers (P) Ltd (2017). p. 37–40.

44. Casari A, Chester J, Pellacani G. Actinic keratosis and non-invasive diagnostic techniques: an update. *Biomedicines.* (2018) 6:e8. doi: 10.3390/biomedicines6010008

45. Zalaudek I, Argenziano G. Dermoscopy of actinic keratosis, intraepidermal carcinoma and squamous cell carcinoma. *Curr Probl Dermatol.* (2015) 46:70–6. doi: 10.1159/000366539

46. Zalaudek I, Argenziano G, Leinweber B, Citarella L, Hofmann-Wellenhof R, Malvehy J, et al. Dermoscopy of Bowen's disease. *Br J Dermatol.* (2004) 150:1112–6. doi: 10.1111/j.1365-2133.2004.05924.x

47. Bugatti L, Filosa G, De Angelis R. Dermoscopic observation of Bowen's disease. *J Eur Acad Dermatol Venereol.* (2004) 18:572–4. doi: 10.1111/j.1468-3083.2004.01008.x

48. Mun JH, Kim SH, Jung DS, Ko HC, Kwon KS, Kim MB. Dermoscopic features of Bowen's disease in Asians. *J Eur Acad Dermatol Venereol.* (2010) 24:805–10. doi: 10.1111/j.1468-3083.2009.03529.x

49. Yang Y, Lin J, Fang S, Han S, Song Z. What's new in dermoscopy of Bowen's disease: two new dermoscopic signs and its differential diagnosis. *Int J Dermatol.* (2017) 56:1022–5. doi: 10.1111/ijd.13734

50. Payapvipapong K, Tanaka M. Dermoscopic classification of Bowen's disease. *Australas J Dermatol.* (2015) 56:32–5. doi: 10.1111/ajd.12200

51. Cameron A, Rosendahl C, Tschandl P, Riedl E, Kittler H. Dermatoscopy of pigmented Bowen's disease. *J Am Acad Dermatol.* (2010) 62:597–604. doi: 10.1016/j.jaad.2009.06.008

52. Chung E, Marchetti MA, Pulitzer MP, Marghoob AA. Streaks in pigmented squamous cell carcinoma *in situ.* *J Am Acad Dermatol.* (2015) 72:S64–5. doi: 10.1016/j.jaad.2014.08.044

53. Nakayama C, Hata H, Homma E, Fujita Y, Shimizu H. Dermoscopy of periungual pigmented Bowen's disease: its usefulness in differentiation from malignant melanoma. *J Eur Acad Dermatol Venereol.* (2016) 30:552–4. doi: 10.1111/jdv.12957

54. Cavicchini S, Tourlaki A, Ghislanzoni M, Alberizzi P, Alessi E. Pigmented Bowen disease of the palm: an atypical case diagnosed by dermoscopy. *J Am Acad Dermatol.* (2010) 62:356–7. doi: 10.1016/j.jaad.2009.01.035

55. Saito T, Uchi H, Moroi Y, Kiryu H, Furue M. Subungual Bowen disease revealed by longitudinal melanonychia. *J Am Acad Dermatol.* (2012) 67:e240–1. doi: 10.1016/j.jaad.2012.03.031

56. Park SW, Lee DY, Mun GH. Longitudinal melanonychia on the lateral side of the nail: a sign of Bowen disease associated with human papillomavirus. *Ann Dermatol.* (2013) 25:378–9. doi: 10.5021/ad.2013.25.3.378

57. Matsuya T, Nakamura Y, Teramoto Y, Shimizu A, Asami Y, Arai E, et al. Image gallery: Bowen's disease of a nail unit presenting with 'woodgrain appearance' - a new dermoscopic finding. *Br J Dermatol.* (2018) 178:e66. doi: 10.1111/bjd.16070

58. Baran R, Simon C. Longitudinal melanonychia: a symptom of Bowen's disease. *J Am Acad Dermatol.* (1988) 18:1359–60. doi: 10.1016/S0190-9622(88)80115-4

59. Saxena A, Kasper DA, Campanelli CD, Lee JB, Humphreys TR, Webster GF. Pigmented Bowen's disease clinically mimicking melanoma of the nail. *Dermatol Surg.* (2006) 32:1522–5. doi: 10.1111/j.1524-4725.2006.32367.x

60. Rosendahl C, Cameron A, Argenziano G, Zalaudek I, Tschandl P, Kittler H. Dermoscopy of squamous cell carcinoma and keratoacanthoma. *Arch Dermatol.* (2012) 148:1386–92. doi: 10.1001/archdermatol.2012.2974

61. Pyne J, Sapkota D, Wong JC. Squamous cell carcinoma: variation in dermatoscopic vascular features between well and non-well differentiated tumors. *Dermatol Pract Concept.* (2012) 2:204a5. doi: 10.5826/dpc.0204a05

62. Yélamos O, Braun RP, Liopyris K, Wolner ZJ, Kerl K, Gerami P, et al. Dermoscopy and dermatopathology correlates of cutaneous neoplasms. *J Am Acad Dermatol.* (2019) 80:341–63. doi: 10.1016/j.jaad.2018.07.073

63. Manfredini M, Longo C, Ferrari B, Piana S, Benati E, Casari A, et al. Dermoscopic and reflectance confocal microscopy features of cutaneous squamous cell carcinoma. *J Eur Acad Dermatol Venereol.* (2017) 31:1828–33. doi: 10.1111/jdv.14463

64. Lallas A, Pyne J, Kyrgidis A, Andreani S, Argenziano G, Cavaller A, et al. The clinical and dermoscopic features of invasive cutaneous squamous cell carcinoma depend on the histopathological grade of differentiation. *Br J Dermatol.* (2015) 172:1308–15. doi: 10.1111/bjd.13510

65. Benati E, Persechino F, Piana S, Argenziano G, Lallas A, Moscarella E, et al. Dermoscopic features of squamous cell carcinoma on the lips. *Br J Dermatol.* (2017) 177:e41–e43. doi: 10.1111/bjd.15274

66. Jalilian C, Chamberlain AJ, Haskett M, Rosendahl C, Goh M, Beck H, et al. Clinical and dermoscopic characteristics of Merkel cell carcinoma. *Br J Dermatol.* (2013) 169:294–7. doi: 10.1111/bjd.12376

67. Harting MS, Ludgate MW, Fullen DR, Johnson TM, Bichakjian CK. Dermatoscopic vascular patterns in cutaneous Merkel cell carcinoma. *J Am Acad Dermatol.* (2012) 66:923–7. doi: 10.1016/j.jaad.2011.06.020

68. Dalle S, Parmentier L, Moscarella E, Phan A, Argenziano G, Thomas L. Dermoscopy of Merkel cell carcinoma. *Dermatology.* (2012) 224:140–4. doi: 10.1159/000337411

69. Mun JH, Park SM, Kim GW, Song M, Kim HS, Ko HC, et al. Clinical and dermoscopic characteristics of extramammary Paget's disease: a study of 35 cases. *Br J Dermatol.* (2016) 174:1104–7. doi: 10.1111/bjd.14300

70. De Giorgi V, Grazzini M, Rossari S, Gori A, Verdelli A, Cervadoro E, et al. Dermoscopy pattern of cutaneous angiosarcoma. *Eur J Dermatol.* (2011) 21:113–4. doi: 10.1684/ejd.2010.1173

71. Oiso N, Matsuda H, Kawada A. Various color gradations as a dermatoscopic feature of cutaneous angiosarcoma of the scalp. *Australas J Dermatol.* (2013) 54:36–8. doi: 10.1111/j.1440-0960.2012.00885.x

72. Minagawa A, Koga H, Okuyama R. Vascular structure absence under dermoscopy in two cases of angiosarcoma on the scalp. *Int J Dermatol.* (2014) 53:350–2. doi: 10.1111/ijd.12357

18

Novel and Future Therapeutic Drugs for Advanced Mycosis Fungoides and Sézary Syndrome

Tomonori Oka and Tomomitsu Miyagaki*

Department of Dermatology, Graduate School of Medicine, The University of Tokyo, Tokyo, Japan

*Correspondence:
Tomomitsu Miyagaki
asahikari1979@gmail.com

Mycosis fungoides (MF) and Sézary syndrome (SS) are the most common subtypes of cutaneous T-cell lymphoma. The majority of MF cases present with only patches and plaques and the lesions are usually limited to the skin. On the other hand, in some cases, patients show skin tumors or erythroderma followed by lymph node involvement and rarely visceral organ involvement. SS is a rare, aggressive cutaneous T-cell lymphoma marked by exfoliative erythroderma, lymphadenopathy, and leukemic blood involvement. Because patients with relapsed or refractory MF/SS display a poor prognosis and the current treatment options are characterized by high rates of relapse, there is unmet need for the efficient treatment. This review provides a discussion of the recent and future promising therapeutic approaches in the management of advanced MF/SS. These include mogamulizumab, brentuximab vedotin, alemtuzumab, immune checkpoint inhibitors, IPH4102 (anti-KIR3DL2 antibody), histone deacetylase inhibitors (vorinostat, romidepsin, panobinostat, belinostat, and resminostat), pralatrexate, forodesine, denileukin diftitox, duvelisib, lenalidomide, and everolimus.

Keywords: mycosis fungoides, Sézary syndrome, peripheral T-cell lymphoma, clinical trial, novel therapeutic agents

INTRODUCTION

Cutaneous T-cell lymphoma (CTCL) comprises a clinically/pathologically heterogeneous group of uncommon non-Hodgkin's lymphomas that manifest primarily in the skin. Mycosis fungoides (MF) is the most common CTCL subtype that accounts for around 60% of CTCL (1). MF is generally an indolent lymphoma with slow progression over years or even decades. Typically, the initial lesions in MF are flat and erythematous skin patches, which evolve over a variable period of time into palpable plaques characterized by well-demarcated edges. In limited cases, plaques can be followed by tumors and those patients have patch, plaque, and tumor lesions simultaneously on different parts of the body. In some cases, skin lesions develop into erythroderma similar to Sézary syndrome (SS). In MF cases with tumors or erythroderma (advanced MF), lymph node or visceral involvement is sometimes observed and such cases present a poor prognosis. SS is a much rarer variant, accounting for only 3% of CTCL (1). Characteristics of SS are generalized erythroderma (defined as affecting > 80% of total body surface area), lymphadenopathy, and presence of circulating tumor cells in the blood. Progression of SS is usually more rapid compared to that of MF.

Although MF and SS are classified as distinct, separate entities, the same clinical staging system and therapeutic approaches have been used (1, 2). Patients with MF having limited T1 stage (limited patches, papules, and/or plaques covering < 10% of the skin surface) have a similar life expectancy to that of control populations (3). In addition, patients with early stage MF (stage I and IIA) have a good prognosis (a median survival: 15.8 years or more), while patients with advanced stage MF/SS (stage IIB or more) have a poor prognosis (a median survival: 4.7 years or less) (3). Current treatment consists of skin-directed therapies, such as topical corticosteroid, topical mechlorethamine, topical bexarotene, ultraviolet phototherapy, total skin electron beam therapy, and localized radiotherapy (2), for early stage disease and systemic therapies for advanced stage. For early stage MF confined to the skin, therapeutic concept is to control symptoms by skin-directed therapies with the lowest possible therapy-related side effects, as durable remissions cannot be achieved by early aggressive chemotherapy (4). For advanced stages of MF and SS, there is a variety of systemic therapies available, some of which are used from decades ago and some recently. However, currently available drug therapies are not curative treatment and the only option for curing MF/SS is stem cell transplantation (5).

As MS/SS have the chronic and recurrent nature, repeated treatment courses and maintenance regimens are necessary for disease control. Although there are available active systemic therapeutic strategies, including cytotoxic chemotherapy and biological therapy, better treatments of advanced stage and refractory MF/SS are desired by both patients and physicians. Purpose of the present paper is to review the clinical results obtained in clinical trials of novel currently used and future promising therapies for advanced MF/SS patients (**Table 1**).

MOGAMULIZUMAB

C-C chemokine receptor 4 (CCR4) is the receptor for thymus and activation-regulated chemokine and macrophage-derived chemokine and is involved in skin trafficking of type 2 helper T cells and regulatory T cells. CCR4 is also consistently expressed on the surface of tumor cells in T-cell malignancies, such as CTCL, including MF and SS, adult T-cell leukemia-lymphoma, and peripheral T-cell lymphoma (PTCL) (30–33). Mogamulizumab is a humanized IgG1 κ monoclonal antibody with a defucosylated Fc region, which selectively binds to CCR4. The antibody exerts its antitumor activity by antibody-dependent cellular cytotoxicity (34). First, mogamulizumab has been approved in Japan for relapsed or refractory CCR4+ adult

T-cell leukemia-lymphoma (2012), PTCL (2014), and CTCL (2014) (35).

Before the approval of mogamulizumab in Japan, seven patients with MF had been enrolled in a multicenter phase 2 study for patients with relapsed PTCL and CTCL in Japan (6). Intravenous infusions of 1.0 mg/kg mogamulizumab were administered to patients once per week for 8 weeks. The overall response rate (ORR) for MF patients was 28.6% [all partial response (PR) with no complete response (CR)]. A phase 1/2 study was also conducted for 38 patients with pretreated CTCL (MF and SS) in USA. Mogamulizumab was administered once weekly for 4 weeks using an escalation scheme (0.1 mg/kg and subsequent doses of 0.3 and 1.0 mg/kg) followed by 1.0 mg/kg every 2 weeks until disease progression or withdrawal. The ORR was 36.8% (CR 7.9% and PR 28.9%). Mogamulizumab was more effective for patients with SS than those with MF; ORR was 47.1% in SS ($n = 17$) and 28.6% in MF ($n = 21$). Eighteen of 19 (94.7%) patients with blood involvement had a response in blood, including 11 CRs (7). In an international, open-label, randomized, controlled phase 3 trial in patients with relapsed or refractory MF/SS (MAVORIC study), mogamulizumab (1.0 mg/kg once weekly for 4 weeks followed by every 2 weeks) significantly showed the high ORR and prolonged progression free survival (PFS) compared with 400 mg/day vorinostat (8). The ORR of mogamulizumab was 28% (21% in MF and 37% in SS), while the ORR of vorinostat was 4% (8). The median PFS was 7.7 months for the mogamulizumab group, compared with 3.1 months for vorinostat. Compartment response rates were 78/186 (42%) in skin, 83/122 (68%) in blood, 21/124 (17%) in lymph nodes, and 0/3 (0%) in viscera, suggesting that mogamulizumab is effective especially for blood involvement. In all studies, mogamulizumab showed an acceptable safety profile and common toxicities included nausea, chills, headache, fever, diarrhea, pruritus, and infusion reactions. Based on these results, mogamulizumab was approved for the treatment of patients with CTCL who have received at least 1 prior systemic therapy by the US Food and Drug Administration (FDA) and European Medicines Agency (EMA) in 2018.

BRENTUXIMAB VEDOTIN

CD30 is a cell membrane protein that belongs to the tumor necrosis factor receptor family. CD30 was originally discovered on Reed-Sternberg cells of Hodgkin's lymphoma, and its expression was subsequently demonstrated on subsets of non-Hodgkin lymphoproliferative disorders, notably systemic, and primary cutaneous anaplastic large T-cell lymphoma (ALCL) and lymphomatoid papulosis. CD30 is also expressed on tumor cells of some MF/SS cases at various levels, and cases with large cell transformation frequently show higher expression. Brentuximab vedotin (BV) is an antibody-drug conjugate composed of the cytotoxic antitubulin agent monomethyl auristatin E (MMAE) and a chimeric monoclonal anti-CD30 antibody (36). After BV binds to CD30, the antibody-drug conjugate is internalized, and the antibody is cleaved by the lysosome, leading to the intracellular release of MMAE (37). MMAE inhibits tubulin

---

Abbreviations: CTCL, cutaneous T-cell lymphoma; PTCL, peripheral T-cell lymphoma; MF, mycosis fungoides; SS, Sézary syndrome; ALCL, anaplastic large cell lymphoma; AE, adverse event; ORR, overall response rate; CR, complete response; PR, partial response; SD, stable disease; PFS, progression free survival; OS, overall survival; DOR, duration of response; CCR4, C-C chemokine receptor 4; HDAC, histone deacetylase; PNP, purine nucleoside phosphorylase; MMAE, monomethyl auristatin E; IL-2R, IL-2 receptor; PI3K, Phosphoinositide-3-kinase; FDA, Food and Drug Administration; EMA, European Medicines Agency; CTLA-4, cytotoxic T lymphocyte-associated protein 4; PD-1, programmed cell death protein 1; mTOR, mammalian target of rapamycin.

TABLE 1 | Summary of the results of clinical trials of single-agents in cutaneous T-cell lymphoma or peripheral T-cell lymphoma including a given number of mycosis fungoides or Sézary syndrome patients.

	Ref	Phase	Subtypes[†]	Number of patients[‡]	ORR, %	CRR, %	Median DOR	PFS	Approval year[§]		
									FDA	EMA	PMDA (Japan)
Mogamulizumab	(6)	2	MF/pcALCL	8(7)	37.5	0	ND	ND	2018	2018	2014
	(7)	1/2	MF/SS	38	36.8	7.9	10.4 months	50% at 11.4 months			
	(8)	3	MF/SS	186	28	3	14.1 months	50% at 7.7 months			
Brentuximab vedotin	(9)	2	MF/SS	30	70	3	ND	54% at 12 months	2017	2017	-
	(10)	3	CD30[+] MF	28	54	7	8 months	ND			
	(11)	3	CD30[+] MF	48	65	10	15.1 months	50% at 16.7 months			
Alemtuzumab	(12)	2	MF/SS	22	55	32	ND	ND	-	-	-
Nivolumab	(13)	2	MF			Ongoing			-	-	-
Pembrolizumab	(14)	2	MF/SS			Ongoing			-	-	-
IPH4102	(15)	1	MF/SS			Ongoing			-	-	-
	(16)	1	SS			Ongoing					
Vorinostat	(17)	2	MF/SS	74	29.7	0	6 months or more	ND	2007	2004 (orphan), 2009 withdrawn	2011
	(18)	2	MF/SS	33	24.2	0	3.8 months	50% at 3 months			
Romidepsin	(19)	2	MF/SS	71	33	7	13.7 months	ND	2009	2005 (orphan), 2012 refused (PTCL)	2018 (PTCL)
	(20)	2	MF/SS	96	34	6	15 months	ND			
Panobinostat	(21)	2	MF/SS	139	17.3	1.4	ND	ND	-	-	-
Belinostat	(22)	2	MF/SS/other CTCL[#]	29 (23)	13.8	10.3	3 months	ND	2014 (PTCL)	2012 (orphan, PTCL)	-
Pralatrexate	(24)	2	MF	109	58	16.7	4.4 months	50% at 5.3 months	2009 (PTCL)	2007 (orphan), 2012 refused (PTCL)	2018 (PTCL)
Forodesine	(25)	2	MF/SS	144	16	1	8.7 months	ND	-	2007 (orphan), 2012 refused (PTCL)	2018 (PTCL)
Denileukin diftitox	(26)	3	MF/SS/other CTCL[#]	100 (91)	44	10	7.8 months	50% at 26.5 months	1999	2001	-
Duvelisib	(27)	1	MF/SS/pcALCL	19 (9)	31.6	0	ND	50% at 4.5 months	-	-	-
Lenalidomide	(28)	2	MF/SS			Ongoing			-	-	-
Everolimus	(29)	2	MF			Ongoing			-	-	-

[†] When data regarding patients with MF/SS is separable in the original paper, data on MF/SS patients is shown. When inseparable, data on CTCL patients is shown.

[‡] When data regarding patients with MF/SS is inseparable in the original paper, the number of patients with MF/SS is shown in parentheses.

[§] When the drug was approved or refused not for CTCL but for PTCL, the comment "(PTCL)" is added. When the drug was approved as orphan drug from EMA, the comment "(orphan)" is added.

[#] Other CTCL includes pcALCL, peripheral T-cell lymphoma, not otherwise specified, and subcutaneous panniculitis-like T-cell lymphoma.

Ref, reference; ORR, overall response rate; CRR, complete response rate; DOR, duration of response; PFS, progression free survival; FDA, food and drug administration; EMA, European medicines agency; PMDA, pharmaceuticals and medical devices agency; MF, mycosis fungoides; pcALCL, primary cutaneous anaplastic large cell lymphoma; ND, not described; SS, Sézary syndrome; PTCL, peripheral T-cell lymphoma; CTCL, cutaneous T-cell lymphoma.

polymerization and consequently disrupts the microtubule network within the cells causing cell cycle arrest and apoptosis. In addition, a small fraction of MMAE is released from CD30[+] cells, killing neighboring cells in the tumor microenvironment in a CD30-independent manner (36, 37). BV has received regulatory approval in more than 65 countries for the treatment of relapsed or refractory Hodgkin's lymphoma and systemic ALCL (38).

The results of two phase 2 studies of BV for CD30[+] CTCL including MF/SS were reported in 2015. In one phase 2 trial of 30 evaluable patients with pretreated CD30[+] MF/SS by Kim et al, the patients received up to 16 cycles of BV (1.8 mg/kg) every 3 weeks. The ORR was observed in 21 (70%) of 30 patients (CR in one patient and PR in 20 patients), and patients with CD30 expression <5% exhibited a decreased probability of response compared with patients with CD30 expression >5%. (9). In the other trial of BV for 48 pretreated patients with primary cutaneous CD30[+] lymphoproliferative disorders, 28 patients with CD30[+] MF were included (10). BV was administered intravenously at 1.8 mg/kg every 3 weeks for a maximum of eight doses. The ORR in MF patients was 54% with CR in two cases and the response was independent of CD30 expression. Based on these promising results, the international randomized phase 3 trial (ALCANZA study) for pretreated CD30[+] CTCL (MF or primary cutaneous ALCL) had been conducted recently to compare BV against the chosen standard therapy by physicians (methotrexate or bexarotene). In this clinical trial, included cases expressed the CD30 molecule on at least 10% of the skin infiltrate BV (1.8 mg/kg every 3 weeks) and methotrexate (5–50 mg weekly) or bexarotene (300 mg/m^2 daily) were administered until disease progression or the development of major toxicity. Among the enrolled patients, 97 patients with MF were included. Forty-eight patients were treated with BV and the remaining 49 patients were treated with methotrexate or bexarotene. The ORR lasting at least 4 months was increased in the BV cohort compared with the physician's choice cohort (50 vs. 10%). Five patients achieved CR with BV, while methotrexate or bexarotene failed to achieve CR in any patient. After a median follow-up time of 17.5 months, the median PFS was 15.9 months for patients in the BV cohort and 3.5 months for patients in the methotrexate or bexarotene cohort (11). Peripheral neuropathy was the most frequent adverse event (AE) and was observed in 67% of patients undergoing treatment with BV. After a median 22.9 months of follow-up, 82% of patients with peripheral neuropathy experienced improvement or resolution. Other common side effects reported during the study included nausea, diarrhea, vomiting, alopecia, itching, fever, and loss of appetite. These data suggested that BV can be a preferable treatment option for the treatment of MF when biopsy samples have 10% or more CD30[+] malignant cells. In 2017, FDA and EMA approved BV for the treatment of adult patients with CD30[+] MF who have received prior systemic therapy.

ALEMTUZUMAB

CD52 is a small glycopeptide composed of 12 aminoacids expressed on the cell surface of several different types of leukocytes, including normal and malignant T lymphocytes. Alemtuzumab is a humanized IgG1 antibody that targets the CD52 antigen. The phase 2 study of alemtuzumab in patients with advanced MF/SS who did not respond adequately to treatment with at least PUVA, radiotherapy, or chemotherapy, showed that the ORR was 55% with 32% CR and 23% PR (12). The effect was better on erythrodermic patients (69% ORR with 38% CR) than on patients with plaques or tumors

(40% ORR with 30% CR). In that study, alemtuzumab was administered using escalating doses (5, 10, 30 mg intravenously on days 1–3) and then 30 mg/day three times a week for up to 12 weeks. Because AEs of alemtuzumab such as infusion reaction, hematologic toxicity, and infectious complications were severe, clinical trials of low-dose alemtuzumab were performed for CTCL. In 14 patients with SS treated with subcutaneous low-dose alemtuzumab (3 mg on day 1, 10 mg on day 3, then 15 mg on alternating days or 3 mg on day 1, then 10 mg on alternating days), the ORR was 85.7% with 21.4% CR and 64.3% PR (39). Infectious episodes were observed only in patients treated with 15 mg alemtuzumab. These studies suggest that low-dose alemtuzumab can be an effective treatment for erythrodermic MF/SS with acceptable safety. Consistently, a recent report on 23 patients with leukemic involvement treated with low-dose alemtuzumab (10 mg subcutaneously, three times a week) described that 13 of 17 patients presented with erythroderma showed CR and that the remaining 4 patients could be controlled by following skin-directed therapy alone. In contrast, CR was not achieved in any patient with discrete patches, plaques, or tumors (40).

IMMUNE CHECKPOINT INHIBITORS

Immune checkpoint molecules, such as cytotoxic T lymphocyte-associated protein 4 (CTLA-4) and programmed cell death protein 1 (PD-1), act as negative regulators that inhibit normal T-cell responses to avoid the emergence of pathological self-reactivity. On the other hand, cancers occasionally have the capacity to avoid anti-tumor immunity by abusing such immune checkpoint molecules. Thus, immune checkpoint inhibitors can antagonize the immunosuppressive interaction between the tumor cells and T cells and improve antitumor immune T-cell responses. In recent years, the efficacy of immune checkpoint inhibitors blocking the CTLA-4 and PD-1 pathways has been confirmed by several clinical trials in a variety of cancers. PD-1-blocking antibodies (nivolumab and pembrolizumab) and CTLA-4-blocking antibody (ipilimumab) achieved durable objective responses and improved OS in patients with solid tumors (23, 41–44) and hematologic malignancies, including Hodgkin's lymphoma (45). Concerning hematological malignancies, in 2016, nivolumab was approved for the treatment of patients with classical Hodgkin lymphoma that has relapsed or progressed after autologous hematopoietic stem cell transplantation and the following post-transplantation BV by FDA. Subsequently, FDA approved pembrolizumab for the treatment of refractory primary mediastinal large B-cell lymphoma patients in 2018.

Current data suggest that the PD-1, PD-L1/PD-L2 pathway may play a significant role in preventing immune-driven eradication of MF/SS tumor cells. Expression of PD-1 and PD-L1 has been detected in tumor cells of various morphological subsets of MF (46) as well as tumor cells circulating in the peripheral blood of SS (47). A recent phase 1b study of nivolumab in 81 patients with relapsed or refractory hematologic malignancy included 13 patients with MF. The ORR in MF patients was

15% (all PR) with 59% stable disease (SD) and the median PFS was 10 weeks (13). Khodadoust et al. presented preliminary data from a multicenter phase 2 open label study of pembrolizumab in 24 advanced and refractory CTCL patients (9 MF, 15 SS) (14). The ORR was 37.5% with 1 CR, 8 PR, and 9 SD, and the median PFS has not yet been reached. Of the 9 responding patients, 6 patients had 90% or greater decrease in modified Severity Weighted Assessment Tool score. Treatment was well-tolerated with a toxicity profile which was consistent with prior studies (48), although a notable skin flare reaction was developed in 40% of SS patients. Although it is necessary to wait for the results of several ongoing clinical trials using immune checkpoint inhibitors such as nivolumab, ipilimumab, and durvalumab (anti-PD-L1 antibody), immune checkpoint inhibition can be a novel strategy to treat advanced MF/SS.

IPH4102 (ANTI-KIR3DL2 ANTIBODY)

KIR3DL2 (CD158k), a member of the highly polymorphic killer-cell immunoglobulin-like receptor family, has the capacity to bind to MHC class I and transduce an inhibitory signal. KIR3DL2 is expressed on subsets of normal $CD8^+$ T cells and NK cells, but not on normal $CD4^+$ cells (49). On the other hand, several studies demonstrated that KIR3DL is expressed by neoplastic $CD4^+$ T cells in SS, advanced MF, and primary cutaneous ALCL (50–54). The relative specific expression of KIR3DL2 on the malignant CTCL cells makes it an ideal therapeutic target. IPH4102 is a humanized, monoclonal antibody specific toward KIR3DL2 which lacks cross-reactivity with other members of the human killer-cell immunoglobulin-like receptor family. IPH4102 selectively and efficiently can deplete $KIR3DL2^+$ cells including primary Sézary cells through antibody-dependent cell cytotoxicity and phagocytosis (55).

Preliminary results from the phase 1 study were presented at the 2017 European Organization for Research and Treatment of Cancer: Cutaneous Lymphoma Task Force in London (15). The aim of the trial is to characterize IPH4102 safety profile and identify the maximum tolerated dose and recommended phase 2 dose. A total of 25 patients, including 20 patients with SS, four patients with MF, and one patient with $CD4^+$ CTCL (neither MF nor SS), have been treated at the 10 preplanned ascending dose levels (0.0001–10 mg/kg). All patients had relapsed after or had been refractory to at least two prior systemic therapies. The ORR was 44% (1 CR and 10 PR). Two patients achieved a near CR (>90% reduction in skin involvement). The median duration of response (DOR) was 8.2 months, and the median PFS was 9.8 months. As IPH4102 was safe and well-tolerated in those dose-escalation cohorts, expansion cohorts started at the flat dose of 750 mg in 2017. Preliminary results of expansion cohorts were presented at the 60th American Society of Hematology annual meeting in 2018 (16). The study included 35 SS patients with at least two prior systemic therapies. The ORR was 42.9% (5.7% CR and 37.2% PR) with a favorable safety profile. The median DOR was 13.8 months and the median PFS was 11.7 months. Preliminary phase 1 data suggest that IPH4102 is both efficacious and well-tolerated. A global, multi-cohort, phase 2

study evaluating the potential of IPH4102 in different subtypes of T-cell lymphoma will be initiated this year (NCT03902184).

HDAC INHIBITORS

Histone deacetylase (HDAC) inhibitors have the capacity to increase acetylation of histones and other proteins, which exerts chromatin remodeling, promotion of tumor suppressor gene transcription, and apoptosis, resulting in antitumor activity. Its clinical activity is largely confined to hematologic malignancies, particularly CTCL (56). HDAC inhibitors have the prevalent AEs of fatigue, thrombocytopenia, diarrhea, and nausea in common (57).

Although vorinostat is not a novel drug, we referred to the drug in this paragraph, because it is the first approved HDAC inhibitor. Vorinostat is an oral competitive inhibitor of class I/II HDAC enzymes. In the pivotal phase 2B multicenter trial, 400 mg of vorinostat was administered daily to 74 stage IB-IVA MF/SS patients, who were previously treated with two or more prior systemic therapies, until disease progression or intolerable toxicity (17). The ORR was 29.7% (22/74) and all initial responses were confirmed PR. The other phase 2 clinical trial showed similar results (18). Eight of 33 patients (24.2%) with refractory MF/SS who had received a median of 5 prior therapies achieved PR. In 2006, FDA approved vorinostat for the treatment of CTCL patients who have progressive, persistent or recurrent disease on or following two systemic therapies. Also in Japan, the drug was approved in 2011 based on the phase 1 clinical trial conducted in Japan (58). In a recent phase 3 randomized study, vorinostat was compared with mogamulizumab in patients with stage IB-IV MF/SS (8). The ORR for the vorinostat was significantly lower than that of mogamulizumab (5 vs. 28%).

Romidepsin is a bicyclic peptide that inhibits class I HDAC selectively. Preclinical studies suggest that romidepsin is among the most potent HDAC inhibitors. Two multicenter phase 2 clinical trials of romidepsin for CTCL were conducted before 2010. In one clinical trial, 71 refractory IA-IVB MF/SS patients with a median of four prior treatments were enrolled (19). Some patients received 18 mg/m^2 romidepsin on days 1 and 5 of a 21-day cycle and to other patients romidepsin was administered at 14 mg/m^2 on days 1, 8, and 15 every 28 days. CR was observed in four patients (5.6%) and 20 patients achieved PR (28.2%). The median DOR was 13.7 months. In the other international single-arm, open-label, phase 2 study, 96 patients with IB-IVA MF/SS who had received one or more prior systemic therapies (median three), received romidepsin intravenously 14 mg/m^2 on days 1, 8, and 15 every 28 days (20). The ORR was 34% (33/96), including 6% (6/96) CRs and the median DOR was 15.0 months, which were similar to the previous study. Interestingly, in the clinical trial, romidepsin is active in subtypes of CTCL with less favorable outcomes, such as tumor stage and folliculotropic MF. The ORR was 45% (9/20) in patients with cutaneous tumors and 60% (6/10) in patients with folliculotropic disease involvement (59). Of note, Kim et al. reported that a clinically significant effect on pruritus was confirmed in a large number of patients, even in patients without any objective clinical response (60). In 2009, romidepsin was approved for the treatment of CTCL patients by FDA.

Panobinostat is an orally bioavailable pan HDAC inhibitor approved for the treatment of multiple myeloma by FDA in 2015. In a phase 2 study, 139 patients with stage IB-IVA MF/SS who had been pretreated with two or more prior systemic therapies, received 20 mg of oral panobinostat three times every week (21). The 139 patients included 79 bexarotene-exposed patients and 60 bexarotene-naïve patients. The ORR was 17.3% in all patients (15.2% in the bexarotene-exposed group and 20.0% in the bexarotene-naïve group). One CR was observed in each group. The median PFS was 4.2 months in the bexarotene-exposed group and 3.7 months in the bexarotene-naïve group. The median DOR was 5.6 months in the bexarotene-exposed group and was not reached at data cutoff in the bexarotene-naïve group.

Belinostat is an intravenous inhibitor of pan HDAC, which was approved for the treatment of relapsed or refractory PTCL by FDA in 2014. In the phase 2 clinical trial of belinostat in patients with relapsed or refractory PTCL and CTCL, 29 patients with CTCL including 17 MF patients and seven SS patients were enrolled. Patients with CTCL had received a median of four prior systemic therapies. Belinostat was administered at 1,000 mg/m^2 intravenously for consecutive 5 days of a 21-day cycle (22). The ORR was 13.8% (10.3% CR and 3.4% PR), and the median DOR was 83 days.

Resminostat is an oral drug which selectively inhibits class I, IIB, and IV HDAC enzymes. A phase 2, multicenter, double-blind, randomized, placebo-controlled trial is currently ongoing to evaluate whether resminostat can be used as maintenance treatment for MF/SS patients after disease control with other systemic therapies (NCT02953301). Patients will receive either placebo or 600 mg resminostat for consequent 5 days followed by 9 days of rest in a 14-day cycle. This clinical trial will be completed in 2020.

PRALATREXATE

Pralatrexate, an anti-neoplastic folate analog, inhibits dihydrofolate reductase, targeting DNA synthesis and resulting in tumor cell death. Pralatrexate has the improved anti-tumor activity compared to methotrexate due to higher affinity for the reduced folate carrier-1 and more selective accumulation in tumor cells.

A phase 2 study of pralatrexate in 109 patients with PTCL including 12 transformed MF patients who progressed following one or more prior systemic therapy (PROPEL study) showed that the ORR was 29% (32 of 109), including 11% CR and 18% PR, with the median DOR of 10.1 months. The median PFS and overall survival (OS) were 3.5 and 14.5 months, respectively (61). Subgroup analysis patients with transformed MF revealed that the ORR was 58% with the median DOR and PFS were 4.4 and 5.3 months, respectively per investigator assessment (24). Pralatrexate was administered at 30 mg/m^2/week for 6 weeks followed by one week of rest (7-week cycle) in this study. FDA approved pralatrexate for

the treatment of PTCL in 2009. In Japan, after phase 1/2 clinical study was conducted, pralatrexate was approved in 2018 (62).

As for CTCL, a dose de-escalation study of pralatrexate showed that the recommended regimen was identified as 15 mg/m^2/week for 3 weeks followed by 1 week of rest (4-week cycle) (63). Twenty-nine patients with refractory MF/SS and primary cutaneous ALCL with at least one prior systemic therapy received recommended dosing regimen. The ORR was 45% with 1 CR and 12 PR. In any study, the most observed toxicity is mucositis. To reduce this risk, patients received supplementation of vitamin B12 and folate, and leucovorin (folinic acid) during pralatrexate treatment. Pralatrexate can be a promising treatment with the potential to provide lasting benefit for advanced CTCL patients with the relative low toxicity. Recently, a phase 1/2 study suggested that combination therapy of 150 mg/m^2 daily bexarotene plus 15 mg/m^2/week for 3/4 weeks pralatrexate is active with high ORR (60%) and minimal toxicity for CTCL (64). A phase 1 study of pralatrexate (10 to 25 mg/m^2) and romidepsin (12 to 14 mg/m^2) on 1 of 3 schedules: every week × 3 every 28 days, every week × 2 every 21 days, and every other week every 28 days, for patients with PTCL also showed high ORR (57%) (65). These combination therapies with pralatrexate plus bexarotene or romidepsin can be an efficient and tolerated treatment option.

FORODESINE

Purine nucleoside phosphorylase (PNP) is an important enzyme for the phosphorolysis of purine nucleosides. Severe immunodeficiency syndromes are caused by congenital defects in this enzyme through selective depletion of T cells but not of B cells (66, 67). Based on increased nucleoside metabolism of malignant T cells, T-cell tumor cells can be highly sensitive to the inhibition of PNP (68). Forodesine is a potent inhibitor of PNP that causes apoptosis in both neoplastic T cells and normal T cells.

In a multicenter phase 2 open-label study, 144 patients with MF/SS who had been treated with three or more systemic therapies were enrolled. The patients received oral forodesine 200 mg daily. The drug showed limited clinical activity in this study. No CRs were observed, and only 11% of the patients achieved PR and 50% maintained SD. The median DOR was 191 days (25). Although almost all patients (96%) experienced at least one AE, most AEs were grade 1/2. Common AEs were peripheral edema, fatigue, insomnia, pruritus, diarrhea, headache, and nausea.

Forodesine was approved in Japan for the treatment of PTCL at the dose of 600 mg daily based on efficacy and safety results of the phase 1/2 clinical trial in patients with 48 relapsed PTCL including one transformed MF patient (65). In 41 evaluable patients, the ORR was 25% including 4 CRs. The most common grade 3/4 AEs were lymphopenia (96%), leukopenia (42%), and neutropenia (35%). Dose reduction and discontinuation due to AEs were uncommon. There is a possibility that such high-dose can be an effective and acceptable treatment for advanced MF/SS.

DENILEUKIN DIFTITOX

Denileukin diftitox is a genetically engineered fusion protein combining the full-length sequence of human IL-2 with the cytotoxic and membrane-translocating domains of the diphtheria toxin. After binding to the IL-2 receptor (IL-2R) on neoplastic T cells, the drug is internalized. The diphtheria toxin results in the production of a single polypeptide chain that is capable of inhibiting protein synthesis in the cells, leading to cell death (69). The human IL-2R consisted of three forms: low, intermediate, and high affinity. The high affinity IL-2R is a complex of distinct proteins of α chain (CD25), β chain (CD122), and γ chain (CD132). The intermediate one is composed of CD122 and CD132, and CD25 alone defines the low affinity one. Although denileukin diftitox can bind to all forms of the IL-2R, internalization is caused by only intermediate or

high affinity receptors (70). In addition, it is known that the baseline expression level of CD25, which is not included in the intermediate affinity IL-2R, on CTCL cell in lesional skin correlated with their clinical response to denileukin diftitox (71), suggesting that the high affinity IL-2R is the most important receptor to elicit an effect.

The largest study of denileukin diftitox was a multicenter, randomized, double-blind placebo-controlled phase 3 trial that evaluated denileukin diftitox (9 or 18 μg/kg/day) vs. placebo in 144 stage IA-III MF/SS patients who had been treated with at most three prior therapies (26). The trial excluded patients with low CD25 expression disease (defined as detectable CD25 on <20% of T cells in lesional skin). The drugs were administered for consequent 5 days every 3 weeks for up to eight cycles. The ORR for the denileukin diftitox 18 μg/kg/day group was 49.1% with 9.1% CR ($n = 55$), compared with 15.9% with

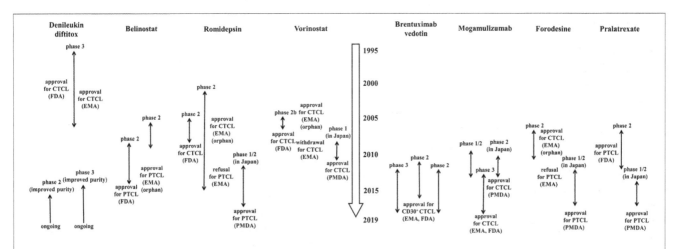

FIGURE 1 | History of clinical trials of single-agents which have been approved for cutaneous T-cell lymphoma or peripheral T-cell lymphoma by FDA, EMA, or PMDA. The data were collected on March 31, 2019. When the drug was approved as orphan drug from EMA, the comment "orphan" is added. CTCL, cutaneous T-cell lymphoma; PTCL, peripheral T-cell lymphoma; FDA, food and drug administration; EMA, European medicines agency; PMDA, pharmaceuticals and medical devices agency.

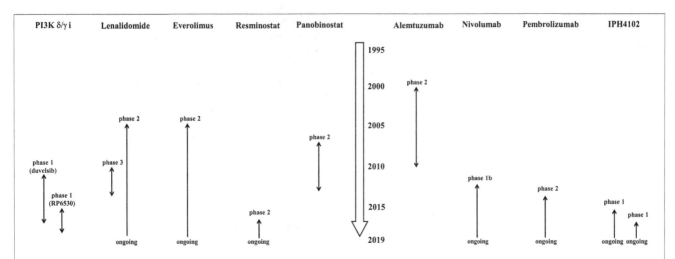

FIGURE 2 | History of clinical trials of single-agents which have not been approved for cutaneous T-cell lymphoma or peripheral T-cell lymphoma by FDA, EMA, or PMDA. The data were collected on March 31, 2019. PI3K δ/γ i, phosphoinositide-3-kinase δ/γ inhibitor.

2.3% CR for placebo ($n = 44$). For the denileukin diftitox 9 µg/kg/day group, the ORR was 37.8% ($n = 45$; 11.1% CR and 26.7% PR). The PFS was significantly prolonged for denileukin diftitox-treated patients compared to patients treated with placebo. Estimated median PFS was at least 971 days for the denileukin diftitox 18 µg/kg/day cohort, 794 days for the denileukin diftitox 9 µg/kg/day cohort, and only 124 days for placebo cohort. The drug-related severe AEs occurred in 25% of the participants receiving denileukin diftitox with premedication of acetaminophen and antihistamine. The most common drug-related severe AEs were dehydration (2%) and capillary leak syndrome (2%). To assess the denileukin diftitox effect on patients with low CD25 expression, 36 patients with MF/SS who had been excluded from the placebo-controlled trial due to low CD25 expression were enrolled in another clinical trial. In the clinical trial, patients were treated with denileukin diftitox 18 µg/kg/day for 5 consecutive days every 3 weeks for up to eight courses. The ORR was 30.6% (8.3% CR and 22.2% PR) (72). This study suggests that low CD25 expression does not necessarily preclude a meaningful clinical response to denileukin diftitox in patients with CTCL.

Denileukin diftitox had been approved by the FDA in 1999 for the treatment of patients with CTCL refractory to standard treatment options. However, denileukin diftitox is unavailable on the global market at this time. Currently, the related agent E7777 which shares an amino acid sequence with denileukin diftitox but has improved its purity and an increased percentage of active protein monomer species is being evaluated. A phase 1 study for 13 patients with PTCL conducted in Japan showed that E7777 is well-tolerated and has antitumor activity with 38% ORR (73). A phase 2 clinical trial of E7777 for relapsed or refractory PTCL and CTCL (NCT02676778) and a phase 3 clinical trial for persistent and recurrent CTCL (NCT01871727) are ongoing.

DUVELISIB

Phosphoinositide-3-kinase (PI3K) is a lipid kinase involved in intracellular signal transduction and regulates multiple cellular functions relevant to oncogenesis. The PI3K-δ and PI3K-γ isoforms, which are preferentially expressed in leukocytes, can modulate both innate and adaptive immune response (74–77). PI3K-δ and PI3K-γ mediate multiple pathways contributing to survival, proliferation, and differentiation in malignant hematopoietic cells. Moreover, PI3K signaling is involved in development of tumor microenvironment through juxta-, para-, and endocrine effects on stromal and immune cells (78–80). Additionally, PI3K-γ may also suppress antitumor immune response by inhibiting phagocytosis by tumor-associated macrophages (81). Thus, there are at least three different mechanisms via which PI3K-δ and PI3K-γ inhibitors could be effective for hematopoietic malignancies.

Duvelisib (also known as IPI-145) is an oral, dual inhibitor of PI3K-δ and PI3K-γ. In a recent phase 1 open-label trial, clinical activity of duvelisib was promising and the toxicity was acceptable in relapsed or refractory PTCL and CTCL (27). Thirty-five patients (16 PTCL, 19 CTCL) were enrolled in this study and

27 (77%) were treated at the maximum tolerated of oral duvelisib 75 mg twice daily on a 28-day cycle. The 19 patients with CTCL had received a median of six prior therapies. The CTCL population was composed of 13 patients with MF, five patients with SS, and one primary cutaneous ALCL patient. In the CTCL population, the ORR was 31.6% (all PR) and the median PFS was 4.5 months. The most common grade 3/4 AEs were increase of liver enzymes (40%), neutropenia (17%), maculopapular rash (17%), and pneumonia (17%). Thus, this study suggests that duvelisib has clinical activity with an acceptable toxicity, while further studies are needed to determine the optimal dose and identify an appropriate combination therapy. A phase 1/1b clinical trial of the other dual inhibitor of PI3K-δ and PI3K-γ, RP6530, in relapsed and refractory T-cell Lymphoma has been finished, but data analysis is incomplete (NCT02567656).

LENALIDOMIDE

Lenalidomide, a derivative of thalidomide, is an oral immunomodulatory drug with direct immune-mediated mechanism (82). Lenalidomide has been shown to induce growth arrest and apoptosis in lymphoma cell lines and FDA approved the drug for the treatment of myelodysplastic syndrome, refractory/relapsed multiple myeloma, and mantle cell lymphoma (83, 84). In addition, lenalidomide is currently being used in clinical trials to treat other various hematopoietic malignancies.

A multicenter phase 2 study of lenalidomide in 32 patients with MF/SS who progressed following a median of 4 systemic therapies was conducted between 2005 and 2010 (28). The first 19 patients received lenalidomide at a daily dose of 25 mg orally for 21 days of a 28-day cycle. The remaining 13 patients initiated treatment at a dose of 10 mg daily and the dose was then increased by 5 mg every 28 days to a maximum of 25 mg daily, based on patient safety and response. The ORR was 28% (all PR) with the median PFS of 8 months. The most frequent AEs were lower leg edema, anemia, fatigue, and transient flare reaction that mimic worsening of the patient's disease. Patients with a 25-mg starting dose showed AEs more frequently than those with a 10-mg starting dose. In a phase 3 randomized study of lenalidomide maintenance vs. observation alone after disease control with other therapies in 21 advanced CTCL patients, the median PFS was 5.3 months in the maintenance lenalidomide group ($n = 9$) and 2 months in the observation alone group ($n = 12$) (85). Because lenalidomide was used as a maintenance therapy, ORR was not evaluated. The main AEs noted in the lenalidomide arm were neutropenia, erythema multiforme, periorbital edema, hypothyroidism, and pruritus. Although statistical comparison in this study was severely underpowered, lenalidomide may be used as a maintenance therapy after debulking therapy.

EVEROLIMUS

Everolimus is an oral agent that targets the mammalian target of rapamycin (mTOR) pathway. The mTOR regulates several survival and growth pathways in a variety of cancers, which was also shown for T-cell non-Hodgkin lymphoma. In addition, an immunohistochemical study revealed that activation of mTOR pathway in MF is associated with the acquisition of a more aggressive phenotype (86). In the recent phase 2 clinical trial, 16 patients with relapsed or refractory T-cell lymphoma including 7 patients with MF were enrolled and received oral everolimus 10 mg daily. The ORR was 44% and the median PFS was 4.1 months (29). Regarding MF, three of seven patients showed PR and none reached CR. The most frequent AEs were hematologic toxicity and skin rash.

CONCLUSION

Although many patients with early CTCL have slow-progressing disease with a normal life expectancy, prognosis of patients with advanced stages of CTCL is poor. Generally speaking, CTCL is incurable without allogeneic stem cell transplantation. Current treatment outcome is characterized by high relapse rates and low durable remission rates. As treatment of advanced-stage CTCL is mostly palliative and not curable, a stage-based approach utilizing sequential therapies in an escalated manner is currently favorable. Existing clinical practice guidelines are quite heterogeneous. Consequently, therapeutic decisions should be individualized to each patient by means of a risk-proportionate approach. Although many novel therapeutic agents have been developed and clinical trials for CTCL and PTCL had or have been implemented (**Figures 1, 2**), such drugs also showed limited efficacy as reviewed in this paper. Thus, it is necessary to know which therapy is preferable for each patient with MF/SS. Creatively designed international clinical trials, such as MAVORIC study and ALCANZA study, should be encouraged.

AUTHOR CONTRIBUTIONS

TO conceived the concept and wrote the manuscript. TM co-conceived the concept, edited and improved the manuscript, and drafted the table.

REFERENCES

1. Willemze R. Cutaneous T-cell lymphoma: epidemiology, etiology, and classification. *Leuk Lymphoma*. (2003) 44 (Suppl. 3): S49–54. doi: 10.1080/10428190310001623766
2. Trautinger F, Eder J, Assaf C, Bagot M, Cozzio A, Dummer R, et al. European Organisation for Research and Treatment of Cancer consensus recommendations for the treatment of mycosis fungoides/Sézary syndrome – Update 2017. *Eur J Cancer*. (2017) 77:57–74. doi: 10.1016/j.ejca.2017.02.027
3. Agar NS, Wedgeworth E, Crichton S, Mitchell TJ, Cox M, Ferreira S, et al. Survival outcomes and prognostic factors in mycosis fungoides/sézary syndrome: validation of the revised international society for Cutaneous Lymphomas/European Organisation for research and treatment of cancer staging proposal. *J Clin Oncol*. (2010) 28:4730–9. doi: 10.1200/JCO.2009.27.7665
4. Leuchte K, Schlaak M, Stadler R, Theurich S, von Bergwelt-Baildon M. Innovative treatment concepts for cutaneous T-cell lymphoma based on microenvironment modulation. *Oncol Res Treat*. (2017) 40:262–9. doi: 10.1159/000472257
5. Virmani P, Zain J, Rosen ST, Myskowski PL, Querfeld C. Hematopoietic stem cell transplant for Mycosis fungoides and sézary syndrome. *Dermatol Clin*. (2015) 33:807–18. doi: 10.1016/j.det.2015.05.014
6. Ogura M, Ishida T, Hatake K, Taniwaki M, Ando K, Tobinai K, et al. Multicenter Phase II Study of Mogamulizumab (KW-0761), a Defucosylated Anti-CC Chemokine Receptor 4 Antibody, in Patients With Relapsed Peripheral T-Cell Lymphoma and Cutaneous T-Cell Lymphoma. *J Clin Oncol*. (2014) 32:1157–63. doi: 10.1200/JCO.2013.52.0924
7. Duvic M, Pinter-Brown LC, Foss FM, Sokol L, Jorgensen JL, Challagundla P, et al. Phase 1/2 study of mogamulizumab, a defucosylated anti-CCR4 antibody, in previously treated patients with cutaneous T-cell lymphoma. *Blood*. (2015) 125:1883–9. doi: 10.1182/blood-2014-09-600924
8. Kim YH, Bagot M, Pinter-Brown L, Rook AH, Porcu P, Horwitz SM, et al. Mogamulizumab versus vorinostat in previously treated cutaneous T-cell lymphoma (MAVORIC): an international, open-label, randomised, controlled phase 3 trial. *Lancet Oncol*. (2018) 19:1192–204. doi: 10.1016/S1470-2045(18)30379-6
9. Kim YH, Tavallaee M, Sundram U, Salva KA, Wood GS, Li S, et al. Phase II investigator-initiated study of brentuximab vedotin in mycosis fungoides and sézary syndrome with variable CD30 expression level: a multi-institution collaborative project. *J Clin Oncol*. (2015) 33:3750–8. doi: 10.1200/JCO.2014.60.3969
10. Duvic M, Tetzlaff MT, Gangar P, Clos AL, Sui D, Talpur R. Results of a phase II trial of brentuximab vedotin for CD30+ cutaneous t-cell lymphoma and lymphomatoid papulosis. *J Clin Oncol*. (2015) 33:3759–65. doi: 10.1200/JCO.2014.60.3787
11. Prince HM, Kim YH, Horwitz SM, Dummer R, Scarisbrick J, Quaglino P, et al. Brentuximab vedotin or physician's choice in CD30-positive cutaneous T-cell lymphoma (ALCANZA): an international, open-label, randomised, phase 3, multicentre trial. *Lancet*. (2017) 390:555–66. doi: 10.1016/S0140-6736(17)31266-7
12. Lundin J, Hagberg H, Repp R, Cavallin-Ståhl E, Fredén S, Juliusson G, et al. Phase 2 study of alemtuzumab (anti-CD52 monoclonal antibody) in patients with advanced mycosis fungoides/Sezary syndrome. *Blood*. (2003) 101:4267–72. doi: 10.1182/blood-2002-09-2802
13. Lesokhin AM, Ansell SM, Armand P, Scott EC, Halwani A, Gutierrez M, et al. Nivolumab in patients with relapsed or refractory hematologic malignancy: preliminary results of a phase Ib study. *J Clin Oncol*. (2016) 34:2698–704. doi: 10.1200/JCO.2015.65.9789
14. Khodadoust M, Rook AH, Porcu P, Foss FM, Moskowitz AJ, Shustov AR, et al. Pembrolizumab for treatment of relapsed/refractory mycosis fungoides and sezary syndrome: clinical efficacy in a citn multicenter phase 2 study. *Blood*. (2016) 128:181.
15. Bagot M, Porcu P, Ram-Wolff C, Khodadoust M, Basem W, Battistella M, et al. IPH4102, the first-in-class anti- KIR3DL2 mAb, is safe and clinically active in advanced cutaneous T-cell lymphoma (CTCL) patients: results from the dose-escalation part of the IPH4102–101 phase I study. In: European Organisation for Research and Treatment of Cancer: Cutaneous Lymphoma Task Force. John Wiley & Sons, Ltd (2017).
16. Bagot M, Porcu P, Basem W, Battistella M, Vermeer M, Whittaker S, et al. IPH4102; an Anti-KIR3DL2 monoclonal antibody in refractory sezary syndrome: results from a multicenter phase 1 trial. In: American Society of Hematology. John Wiley & Sons, Ltd; 2018. doi: 10.1002/hon.2437_31
17. Olsen EA, Kim YH, Kuzel TM, Pacheco TR, Foss FM, Parker S, et al. Phase IIb multicenter trial of vorinostat in patients with persistent, progressive, or treatment refractory cutaneous T-cell lymphoma. *J Clin Oncol*. (2007) 25:3109–15. doi: 10.1200/JCO.2006.10.2434

18. Duvic M, Talpur R, Ni X, Zhang C, Hazarika P, Kelly C, et al. Phase 2 trial of oral vorinostat (suberoylanilide hydroxamic acid, SAHA) for refractory cutaneous T-cell lymphoma (CTCL). *Blood.* (2007) 109:31–9. doi: 10.1182/blood-2006-06-025999

19. Piekarz RL, Frye R, Turner M, Wright JJ, Allen SL, Kirschbaum MH, et al. Phase II multi-institutional trial of the histone deacetylase inhibitor romidepsin as monotherapy for patients with cutaneous T-cell lymphoma. *J Clin Oncol.* (2009) 27:5410–7. doi: 10.1200/JCO.2008.21.6150

20. Whittaker SJ, Demierre M-F, Kim EJ, Rook AH, Lerner A, Duvic M, et al. Final results from a multicenter, international, pivotal study of romidepsin in refractory cutaneous T-cell lymphoma. *J Clin Oncol.* (2010) 28:4485–91. doi: 10.1200/JCO.2010.28.9066

21. Duvic M, Dummer R, Becker JC, Poulalhon N, Ortiz Romero P, Grazia Bernengo M, et al. Panobinostat activity in both bexarotene-exposed and -naïve patients with refractory cutaneous T-cell lymphoma: Results of a phase II trial. *Eur J Cancer.* (2013) 49:386–94. doi: 10.1016/J.EJCA.2012.08.017

22. Foss F, Advani R, Duvic M, Hymes KB, Intragumtornchai T, Lekhakula A, et al. A Phase II trial of Belinostat (PXD101) in patients with relapsed or refractory peripheral or cutaneous T-cell lymphoma. *Br J Haematol.* (2015) 168:811–9. doi: 10.1111/bjh.13222

23. Robert C, Ribas A, Wolchok JD, Hodi FS, Hamid O, Kefford R, et al. Anti-programmed-death-receptor-1 treatment with pembrolizumab in ipilimumab-refractory advanced melanoma: a randomised dose-comparison cohort of a phase 1 trial. *Lancet.* (2014) 384:1109–17. doi: 10.1016/S0140-6736(14)60958-2

24. Foss F, Horwitz SM, Coiffier B, Bartlett N, Popplewell L, Pro B, et al. Pralatrexate is an effective treatment for relapsed or refractory transformed mycosis fungoides: a subgroup efficacy analysis from the PROPEL study. *Clin Lymphoma Myeloma Leuk.* (2012) 12:238–43. doi: 10.1016/j.clml.2012.01.010

25. Dummer R, Duvic M, Scarisbrick J, Olsen EA, Rozati S, Eggmann N, et al. Final results of a multicenter phase II study of the purine nucleoside phosphorylase (PNP) inhibitor forodesine in patients with advanced cutaneous t-cell lymphomas (CTCL) (Mycosis fungoides and Sezary syndrome). *Ann Oncol.* (2014) 25:1807–12. doi: 10.1093/annonc/mdu231

26. Prince HM, Duvic M, Martin A, Sterry W, Assaf C, Sun Y, et al. Phase III placebo-controlled trial of denileukin diftitox for patients with cutaneous T-cell lymphoma. *J Clin Oncol.* (2010) 28:1870–7. doi: 10.1200/JCO.2009.26.2386

27. Horwitz SM, Koch R, Porcu P, Oki Y, Moskowitz A, Perez M, et al. Activity of the PI3K-δ,γ inhibitor duvelisib in a phase 1 trial and preclinical models of T-cell lymphoma. *Blood.* (2018) 131:888–98. doi: 10.1182/blood-2017-08-802470

28. Querfeld C, Rosen ST, Guitart J, Duvic M, Kim YH, Dusza SW, et al. Results of an open-label multicenter phase 2 trial of lenalidomide monotherapy in refractory mycosis fungoides and Sézary syndrome. *Blood.* (2014) 123:1159–66. doi: 10.1182/blood-2013-09-525915

29. Witzig TE, Reeder C, Han JJ, LaPlant B, Stenson M, Tun HW, et al. The mTORC1 inhibitor everolimus has antitumor activity *in vitro* and produces tumor responses in patients with relapsed T-cell lymphoma. *Blood.* (2015) 126:328–35. doi: 10.1182/blood-2015-02-629543

30. Ferenczi K, Fuhlbrigge RC, Kupper TS, Pinkus JL, Pinkus GS. Increased CCR4 Expression in Cutaneous T Cell Lymphoma. *J Invest Dermatol.* (2002) 119:1405–10. doi: 10.1046/J.1523-1747.2002.19610.X

31. Ishida T, Inagaki H, Utsunomiya A, Takatsuka Y, Komatsu H, Iida S, et al. CXC chemokine receptor 3 and CC chemokine receptor 4 expression in T-cell and NK-cell lymphomas with special reference to clinicopathological significance for peripheral T-cell lymphoma, unspecified. *Clin Cancer Res.* (2004) 10:5494–500. doi: 10.1158/1078-0432.CCR-04-0371

32. Ishida T, Utsunomiya A, Iida S, Inagaki H, Takatsuka Y, Kusumoto S, et al. Clinical significance of CCR4 expression in adult T-cell leukemia/lymphoma: its close association with skin involvement and unfavorable outcome. *Clin Cancer Res.* (2003) 9:3625–34.

33. Yoshie O, Fujisawa R, Nakayama T, Harasawa H, Tago H, Izawa D, et al. Frequent expression of CCR4 in adult T-cell leukemia and human T-cell leukemia virus type 1-transformed T cells. *Blood.* (2002) 99:1505–11. doi: 10.1182/blood.V99.5.1505

34. Ishii T, Ishida T, Utsunomiya A, Inagaki A, Yano H, Komatsu H, et al. Defucosylated humanized anti-CCR4 monoclonal antibody KW-0761 as a novel immunotherapeutic agent for adult T-cell leukemia/lymphoma. *Clin Cancer Res.* (2010) 16:1520–31. doi: 10.1158/1078-0432.CCR-09-2697

35. Ishida T, Jo T, Takemoto S, Suzushima H, Uozumi K, Yamamoto K, et al. Dose-intensified chemotherapy alone or in combination with mogamulizumab in newly diagnosed aggressive adult T-cell leukaemia-lymphoma: a randomized phase II study. *Br J Haematol.* (2015) 169:672–82. doi: 10.1111/bjh.13338

36. van de Donk NWCJ, Dhimolea E. Brentuximab vedotin. *MAbs.* (2012) 4:458–65. doi: 10.4161/mabs.20230

37. Deng C, Pan B, O'Connor OA. Brentuximab vedotin. *Clin Cancer Res.* (2013) 19:22–7. doi: 10.1158/1078-0432.CCR-12-0290

38. Pro B, Advani R, Brice P, Bartlett NL, Rosenblatt JD, Illidge T, et al. Brentuximab vedotin (SGN-35) in patients with relapsed or refractory systemic anaplastic large-cell lymphoma: results of a phase II study. *J Clin Oncol.* (2012) 30:2190–6. doi: 10.1200/JCO.2011.38.0402

39. Bernengo MG, Quaglino P, Comessatti A, Ortoncelli M, Novelli M, Lisa F, et al. Low-dose intermittent alemtuzumab in the treatment of Sézary syndrome: clinical and immunologic findings in 14 patients. *Haematologica.* (2007) 92:784–94. doi: 10.3324/haematol.11127

40. Watanabe R, Teague JE, Fisher DC, Kupper TS, Clark RA. Alemtuzumab therapy for leukemic cutaneous T-cell lymphoma. *JAMA Dermatol.* (2014) 150:776. doi: 10.1001/jamadermatol.2013.10099

41. Wolchok JD, Kluger H, Callahan MK, Postow MA, Rizvi NA, Lesokhin AM, et al. Nivolumab plus ipilimumab in advanced melanoma. *N Engl J Med.* (2013) 369:122–33. doi: 10.1056/NEJMoa1302369

42. Brahmer JR, Tykodi SS, Chow LQM, Hwu W-J, Topalian SL, Hwu P, et al. Safety and activity of anti-PD-L1 antibody in patients with advanced cancer. *N Engl J Med.* (2012) 366:2455–65. doi: 10.1056/NEJMoa1200694

43. Topalian SL, Hodi FS, Brahmer JR, Gettinger SN, Smith DC, McDermott DF, et al. Safety, activity, and immune correlates of anti–PD-1 antibody in cancer. *N Engl J Med.* (2012) 366:2443–54. doi: 10.1056/NEJMoa1200690

44. Eggermont AMM, Chiarion-Sileni V, Grob J-J, Dummer R, Wolchok JD, Schmidt H, et al. Prolonged survival in stage III melanoma with ipilimumab adjuvant therapy. *N Engl J Med.* (2016) 375:1845–55. doi: 10.1056/NEJMoa1611299

45. Ansell SM, Lesokhin AM, Borrello I, Halwani A, Scott EC, Gutierrez M, et al. PD-1 Blockade with nivolumab in relapsed or refractory hodgkin's lymphoma. *N Engl J Med.* (2015) 372:311–9. doi: 10.1056/NEJMoa1411087

46. Kantekure K, Yang Y, Raghunath P, Schaffer A, Woetmann A, Zhang Q, et al. Expression patterns of the immunosuppressive proteins PD-1/CD279 and PD-L1/CD274 at different stages of cutaneous T-cell lymphoma/mycosis fungoides. *Am J Dermatopathol.* (2012) 34:126–8. doi: 10.1097/DAD.0b013e31821c35cb

47. Samimi S, Benoit B, Evans K, Wherry EJ, Showe L, Wysocka M, et al. Increased Programmed Death-1 expression on CD4+ T cells in cutaneous T-cell lymphoma. *Arch Dermatol.* (2010) 146:1382. doi: 10.1001/archdermatol.2010.200

48. Herbst RS, Baas P, Kim D-W, Felip E, Pérez-Gracia JL, Han J-Y, et al. Pembrolizumab versus docetaxel for previously treated, PD-L1-positive, advanced non-small-cell lung cancer (KEYNOTE-010): a randomised controlled trial. *Lancet.* (2016) 387:1540–50. doi: 10.1016/S0140-6736(15)01281-7

49. Bagot M, Moretta A, Sivori S, Biassoni R, Cantoni C, Bottino C, et al. CD4(+) cutaneous T-cell lymphoma cells express the p140-killer cell immunoglobulin-like receptor. *Blood.* (2001) 97:1388–91. doi: 10.1182/blood.V97.5.1388

50. Wechsler J, Bagot M, Nikolova M, Parolini S, Martin-Garcia N, Boumsell L, et al. Killer cell immunoglobulin-like receptor expression delineates in situ Sézary syndrome lymphocytes. *J Pathol.* (2003) 199:77–83. doi: 10.1002/path.1251

51. Poszepczynska-Guigné E, Schiavon V, D'Incan M, Echchakir H, Musette P, Ortonne N, et al. CD158k/KIR3DL2 is a new phenotypic marker of Sezary cells: relevance for the diagnosis and follow-up of Sezary syndrome. *J Invest Dermatol.* (2004) 122:820–3. doi: 10.1111/j.0022-202X.2004.22326.x

52. Bahler DW, Hartung L, Hill S, Bowen GM, Vonderheid EC. CD158k/KIR3DL2 is a useful marker for identifying neoplastic T-cells in Sézary syndrome by flow cytometry. *Cytometry B Clin Cytom.* (2008) 74:156–62. doi: 10.1002/cyto.b.20395

53. Ortonne N, Le Gouvello S, Tabak R, Marie-Cardine A, Setiao J, Berrehar F, et al. CD158k/KIR3DL2 and NKp46 are frequently expressed

in transformed mycosis fungoides. *Exp Dermatol.* (2012) 21:461–3. doi: 10.1111/j.1600-0625.2012.01489.x

54. Moins-Teisserenc H, Daubord M, Clave E, Douay C, Félix J, Marie-Cardine A, et al. CD158k is a reliable marker for diagnosis of Sézary syndrome and reveals an unprecedented heterogeneity of circulating malignant cells. *J Invest Dermatol.* (2015) 135:247–57. doi: 10.1038/jid.2014.356

55. Marie-Cardine A, Viaud N, Thonnart N, Joly R, Chanteux S, Gauthier L, et al. IPH4102, a Humanized KIR3DL2 antibody with potent activity against cutaneous T-cell lymphoma. *Cancer Res.* (2014) 74:6060–70. doi: 10.1158/0008-5472.CAN-14-1456

56. Chun P. Histone deacetylase inhibitors in hematological malignancies and solid tumors. *Arch Pharm Res.* (2015) 38:933–49. doi: 10.1007/s12272-015-0571-1

57. Lopez AT, Bates S, Geskin L. Current Status of HDAC Inhibitors in Cutaneous T-cell Lymphoma. *Am J Clin Dermatol.* (2018) 19:805–19. doi: 10.1007/s40257-018-0380-7

58. Wada H, Tsuboi R, Kato Y, Sugaya M, Tobinai K, Hamada T, et al. Phase I and pharmacokinetic study of the oral histone deacetylase inhibitor vorinostat in Japanese patients with relapsed or refractory cutaneous T-cell lymphoma. *J Dermatol.* (2012) 39:823–8. doi: 10.1111/j.1346-8138.2012.01554.x

59. Foss F, Duvic M, Lerner A, Waksman J, Whittaker S. Clinical efficacy of romidepsin in tumor stage and folliculotropic mycosis fungoides. *Clin Lymphoma Myeloma Leuk.* (2016) 16:637–43. doi: 10.1016/j.clml.2016.08.009

60. Kim YH, Demierre M-F, Kim EJ, Lerner A, Rook AH, Duvic M, et al. Clinically meaningful reduction in pruritus in patients with cutaneous T-cell lymphoma treated with romidepsin. *Leuk Lymphoma.* (2013) 54:284–9. doi: 10.3109/10428194.2012.711829

61. O'Connor OA, Pro B, Pinter-Brown L, Bartlett N, Popplewell L, Coiffier B, et al. Pralatrexate in patients with relapsed or refractory peripheral T-cell lymphoma: results from the pivotal PROPEL study. *J Clin Oncol.* (2011) 29:1182–9. doi: 10.1200/JCO.2010.29.9024

62. Maruyama D, Nagai H, Maeda Y, Nakane T, Shimoyama T, Nakazato T, et al. Phase I/II study of pralatrexate in Japanese patients with relapsed or refractory peripheral T-cell lymphoma. *Cancer Sci.* (2017) 108:2061–8. doi: 10.1111/cas.13340

63. Horwitz SM, Kim YH, Foss F, Zain JM, Myskowski PL, Lechowicz MJ, et al. Identification of an active, well-tolerated dose of pralatrexate in patients with relapsed or refractory cutaneous T-cell lymphoma. *Blood.* (2012) 119:4115–22. doi: 10.1182/blood-2011-11-390211

64. Duvic M, Kim YH, Zinzani PL, Horwitz SM. Results from a Phase I/II open-label, dose-finding study of pralatrexate and oral bexarotene in patients with relapsed/refractory cutaneous T-cell lymphoma. *Clin Cancer Res.* (2017) 23:3552–6. doi: 10.1158/1078-0432.CCR-16-2064

65. Amengual JE, Lichtenstein R, Lue J, Sawas A, Deng C, Lichtenstein E, et al. A phase 1 study of romidepsin and pralatrexate reveals marked activity in relapsed and refractory T-cell lymphoma. *Blood.* (2018) 131:397–407. doi: 10.1182/blood-2017-09-806737

66. Bantia S, Ananth SL, Parker CD, Horn LL, Upshaw R. Mechanism of inhibition of T-acute lymphoblastic leukemia cells by PNP inhibitor—BCX-1777. *Int Immunopharmacol.* (2003) 3:879–87. doi: 10.1016/S1567-5769(03)00076-6

67. Markert ML. Purine nucleoside phosphorylase deficiency. *Immunodefic Rev.* (1991) 3:45–81.

68. Gandhi V, Kilpatrick JM, Plunkett W, Ayres M, Harman L, Du M, et al. A proof-of-principle pharmacokinetic, pharmacodynamic, and clinical study with purine nucleoside phosphorylase inhibitor immucillin-H (BCX-1777, forodesine). *Blood.* (2005) 106:4253–60. doi: 10.1182/blood-2005-03-1309

69. Bacha P, Williams DP, Waters C, Williams JM, Murphy JR, Strom TB. Interleukin 2 receptor-targeted cytotoxicity. Interleukin 2 receptor-mediated action of a diphtheria toxin-related interleukin 2 fusion protein. *J Exp Med.* (1988) 167:612–22.

70. Waters CA, Schimke PA, Snider CE, Itoh K, Smith KA, Nichols JC, et al. Interleukin 2 receptor-targeted cytotoxicity. Receptor binding requirements for entry of a diphtheria toxin-related interleukin 2 fusion protein into cells. *Eur J Immunol.* (1990) 20:785–91. doi: 10.1002/eji.1830200412

71. Talpur R, Jones DM, Alencar AJ, Apisarnthanarax N, Herne KL, Yang Y, et al. CD25 expression is correlated with histological grade and response to denileukin diftitox in cutaneous T-cell lymphoma. *J Invest Dermatol.* (2006) 126:575–83. doi: 10.1038/sj.jid.5700122

72. Prince HM, Martin AG, Olsen EA, Fivenson DP, Duvic M. Denileukin diftitox for the treatment of CD25 low-expression mycosis fungoides and Sézary syndrome. *Leuk Lymphoma.* (2013) 54:69–75. doi: 10.3109/10428194.2012.706286

73. Ohmachi K, Ando K, Ogura M, Uchida T, Tobinai K, Maruyama D, et al. E7777 in Japanese patients with relapsed/refractory peripheral and cutaneous T-cell lymphoma: a phase I study. *Cancer Sci.* (2018) 109:794–802. doi: 10.1111/cas.13513

74. Clayton E, Bardi G, Bell SE, Chantry D, Downes CP, Gray A, et al. A crucial role for the p110delta subunit of phosphatidylinositol 3-kinase in B cell development and activation. *J Exp Med.* (2002) 196:753–63. doi: 10.1084/jem.20020805

75. Okkenhaug K, Bilancio A, Farjot G, Priddle H, Sancho S, Peskett E, et al. Impaired B and T cell antigen receptor signaling in p110delta PI 3-kinase mutant mice. *Science.* (2002) 297:1031–4. doi: 10.1126/science.1073560

76. Vanhaesebroeck B, Guillermet-Guibert J, Graupera M, Bilanges B. The emerging mechanisms of isoform-specific PI3K signalling. *Nat Rev Mol Cell Biol.* (2010) 11:329–41. doi: 10.1038/nrm2882

77. Fung-Leung W-P. Phosphoinositide 3-kinase delta (PI3Kδ) in leukocyte signaling and function. *Cell Signal.* (2011) 23:603–8. doi: 10.1016/j.cellsig.2010.10.002

78. Lewis CE, Pollard JW. Distinct role of macrophages in different tumor microenvironments. *Cancer Res.* (2006) 66:605–12. doi: 10.1158/0008-5472.CAN-05-4005

79. Hanahan D, Weinberg RA. Hallmarks of cancer: the next generation. *Cell.* (2011) 144:646–74. doi: 10.1016/j.cell.2011.02.013

80. Schmid MC, Avraamides CJ, Dippold HC, Franco I, Foubert P, Ellies LG, et al. Receptor tyrosine kinases and TLR/IL1Rs unexpectedly activate myeloid cell PI3Kγ, a single convergent point promoting tumor inflammation and progression. *Cancer Cell.* (2011) 19:715–27. doi: 10.1016/j.ccr.2011.04.016

81. Kaneda MM, Messer KS, Ralainirina N, Li H, Leem CJ, Gorjestani S, et al. PI3Kγ is a molecular switch that controls immune suppression. *Nature.* (2016) 539:437–42. doi: 10.1038/nature19834

82. Gribben JG, Fowler N, Morschhauser F. Mechanisms of Action of Lenalidomide in B-Cell Non-Hodgkin Lymphoma. *J Clin Oncol.* (2015) 33:2803–11. doi: 10.1200/JCO.2014.59.5363

83. List A, Kurtin S, Roe DJ, Buresh A, Mahadevan D, Fuchs D, et al. Efficacy of lenalidomide in myelodysplastic syndromes. *N Engl J Med.* (2005) 352:549–57. doi: 10.1056/NEJMoa041668

84. Yang B, Yu R, Chi X, Lu X. Lenalidomide Treatment for multiple myeloma: systematic review and meta-analysis of randomized controlled trials. *PLoS ONE.* (2013) 8:e64354. doi: 10.1371/journal.pone.0064354

85. Bagot M, Hasan B, Whittaker S, Beylot-Barry M, Knobler R, Shah E, et al. A phase III study of lenalidomide maintenance after debulking therapy in patients with advanced cutaneous T-cell lymphoma - EORTC 21081 (NCT01098656): results and lessons learned for future trial designs. *Eur J Dermatol.* (2017) 27:286–94. doi: 10.1684/ejd.2017.3008

86. Levidou G, Siakantaris M, Papadaki T, Papadavid E, Vassilakopoulos TP, Angelopoulou MK, et al. A comprehensive immunohistochemical approach of AKT/mTOR pathway and p-STAT3 in mycosis fungoides. *J Am Acad Dermatol.* (2013) 69:375–84. doi: 10.1016/J.JAAD.2013.04.027

19

Next-Generation Sequencing Technologies for Early-Stage Cutaneous T-Cell Lymphoma

Kazuyasu Fujii and *Takuro Kanekura*

Department of Dermatology, Kagoshima University Graduate School of Medical and Dental Sciences, Kagoshima, Japan

Correspondence:
Kazuyasu Fujii
kazfujii@m2.kufm.kagoshima-u.ac.jp

The diagnosis of early stage cutaneous T-cell lymphoma is often difficult, particularly in mycosis fungoides (MF), because the clinical presentation, histological findings, and laboratory findings of MF resemble those of inflammatory skin diseases such as atopic dermatitis, psoriasis, and parapsoriasis en plaque. Furthermore, MF sometimes occurs with or after these inflammatory skin diseases. The current diagnostic criteria heavily rely on clinical impressions along with assessments of T cell clonality. To make a diagnosis of early-stage MF, the detection of a malignant clone is critical. T cell receptor (TCR) gene rearrangements have been detected by southern blotting or polymerase chain reaction for this purpose, but the results of these methods are insufficient. High-throughput TCR sequencing has provided insights into the complexities of the immune repertoire. Accordingly, his technique is more sensitive and specific than current methods, making it useful for the detection of early lesions and monitoring responses to therapy.

Keywords: mycosis fungoides, early stage, T-cell receptor, rearrangement, next-generation sequencing

INTRODUCTION

Cutaneous T cell lymphomas (CTCLs) comprise a heterogeneous class of non-Hodgkin lymphomas that are derived from skin-tropic T cells. Mycosis fungoides (MF), the most prevalent type of primary CTCL, accounts for almost half of all cases (1–3). MF is clinically characterized by erythematous patches, plaques, or skin tumors, and is can be associated with lymph node, blood, and internal organ involvement. More than two-thirds of MF patients are in early stage at first presentation (3–5). MF often starts as an unspecific erythema, similar to many inflammatory skin diseases.

Histopathologically, MF can be characterized by the epidermotropic proliferation of small- to medium-sized pleomorphic lymphocytes forming intraepidermal collections, also called Pautrier's microabscesses. This microabscess is considered the histopathological hallmark of disease, but it is only observed in <20% of early MF cases (6). These microabscesses are also usually recognized as epidermotropic atypical lymphocyte infiltration without spongiosis, although spongiotic variants of MF have been reported (7, 8). Morphologic characterization of early-stage MF might show non-specific findings (9), because skin lesions are infiltrated by large numbers of non-malignant memory T cells, often making it impossible to distinguish malignant T cell clones from activated benign infiltrating T cells based on histopathology (6). Clinical and histopathological algorithms have been developed to aid early diagnosis (10), but the specificity and sensitivity of these algorithms for early diagnosis in individual patients are by no means established. A definitive diagnosis can only be made based on careful clinicopathological correlations (9).

Early stages of MF can resemble benign inflammatory skin disorders (11, 12) like chronic dermatitis including atopic dermatitis (AD), psoriasis, and parapsoriasis en plaque (PEP), among others. AD is a common chronic inflammatory skin disorder that has a T-helper (Th) 2 type-dominant phenotype, skin-barrier dysfunction, and pruritus (13). In contrast AD is an inflammatory disorder, and its pathophysiology is similar to that of AD. Mycosis fungoides, characterized as a Th2-type disease (14, 15), is frequently linked to eosinophilia and high serum immunoglobulin E levels. Although affected skin and peripheral blood T-cells express a Th1 cytokine profile during early-stage MF (16, 17), chemokines expressed in MF lesional skin, such as CCL17, CCL11, and CCL26, are supposed to induce a Th2 milieu in MF (18).

Barrier dysfunction is also observed in MF (19). Lower levels of skin moisture, with increased transepidermal water loss, have been observed in the lesional skin of CTCL, compared to that in normal skin. CTCL lesional skin also displays decreased levels of *filaggrin* and *loricrin* mRNAs compared to those in normal skin, which has also been demonstrated for AD. Pruritus is often present in MF patients (20) and constitutes one of the most disturbing symptoms for patients (21). Therefore, it is occasionally difficult to clinically differentiate MF from AD. The coexistence of MF and AD in patients was also reported in several studies (22, 23).

Psoriasis is a common, chronic inflammatory skin disorder defined by thickened, red, scaly plaques with systemic inflammation. The relationship between MF and psoriasis is sometimes difficult to determine, as there is often significant overlap in terms of pathological and clinical observations, particularly in early stages (24). Psoriasis and MF have the abnormal function of T cells as a common symptom. Psoriasis was recognized as a Th1 disease, although recent data suggest that it might be a Th17 disease (25). MF during preliminary stages also exhibits a Th1 phenotype (26); moreover, Krejsgaard et al. (27) reported that malignant T cells from CTCL lesions produce IL-17. Therefore, many early MF cases are misdiagnosed as psoriasis, whereas another group of cases occur in which the two diseases coexist and/or psoriasis develops into MF. The prevalence of psoriasis among patients with MF was found to be higher than that estimated for the general population (24, 28) and patients with psoriasis have an elevated risk of lymphomas including CTCL (29, 30). In addition to the common symptoms, immunosuppressive agents might also promote MF development in patients with psoriasis (31).

PEP is a chronic, inflammatory skin disorder, closely resembling early-stage MF. Clinically, PEP consists of persistent, scaly, well-demarcated erythematous lesions. Pathologically, it is associated with superficial lymphocyte infiltration with various degree of epidermotropism (32). More than 30% patients with large plaque parapsoriasis develop pathologically-confirmed MF (32), and therefore, PEP is often an early manifestation of MF. However, the individual clinical course might determine the difference between early-stage MF and PEP.

Because of difficulties associated with differential diagnosis, MF often remains undiagnosed for years. Accordingly, the

average time from the appearance of lesions to a definitive diagnosis was to be estimated 3–6 years (33, 34).

T-CELL RECEPTOR CLONALITY IS AN IMPORTANT CRITERION IN MF DIAGNOSIS

Diagnosing T-cell malignancies is often hampered by difficulties in distinguishing neoplastic T cells from reactive T cells based on conventional morphological and immunopathological criteria (35). Skin lesions of MF patients are infiltrated by many non-malignant memory T cells, and thus, it is often impossible to distinguish a malignant T cell clone from activated, benign, infiltrating T cells by histopathology, particularly for early-stage lesions (10).

T-cell receptor (TCR) gene configurations are thought to be the most promising marker to identify malignant T-cell proliferation (36). TCRs are cell-surface protein heterodimers that are expressed on T cells and comprise either α and β chains or γ and δ chains. Immature T-cells rearrange their TCR genes during maturation in the thymus, then mature as either αβ or γδ lineage T-cells (37). TCRs are unique to individual T cell clones. Malignant cells in MF express αβ TCRs. The gene segments that encode variable (V), diversity (D) (β and δ chains only), joining (J), and constant (C) domains of the TCR protein exist as multiple unique sets (38). Since TCR genes are rearranged during thymic T-cell development (**Figure 1**) but not in mature T-cells, a peripheral T-cell lymphoma clone of malignant cells should only have a single TCR gene sequence. TCR genes are rearranged polyclonally in normal and reactively proliferating T cells as rearrangements are random, whereas neoplastic cells contain identically-rearranged TCR genes. Similarly, molecular analysis of such rearrangements can be useful to differentiate MF from benign skin conditions (39). Half of patients with large plaque parapsoriasis were reported to have TCR monoclonality in the lesional skin (40), and thus, the detection of monoclonality in a skin lesion generally suggests CTCL including MF, rather than inflammatory skin disorders.

CONVENTIONAL METHODS FOR DETECTING T-CELL CLONALITY

Initially, Southern blotting was used to determine TCR gene rearrangement clonality (41). This technique can detect clonal T-cell populations in most T-cell lymphomas without prior amplification, but has several disadvantages including low sensitivity and the requirement for large amounts of fresh frozen tissue. Therefore, since the effectiveness of Southern blotting in the diagnostic work-up of MF was reported (42–44) in the early 1990s, more sensitive polymerase chain reaction (PCR)-based methods have been developed. PCR amplification of rearranged TCR gamma genes using genomic DNA as the template was reported to permit the detection of clonal T cells with a sensitivity of 0.1–1% from a background population of polyclonal T-cells (45). Conventional agarose gel electrophoresis of the PCR products often fails to reliably differentiate polyclonal from

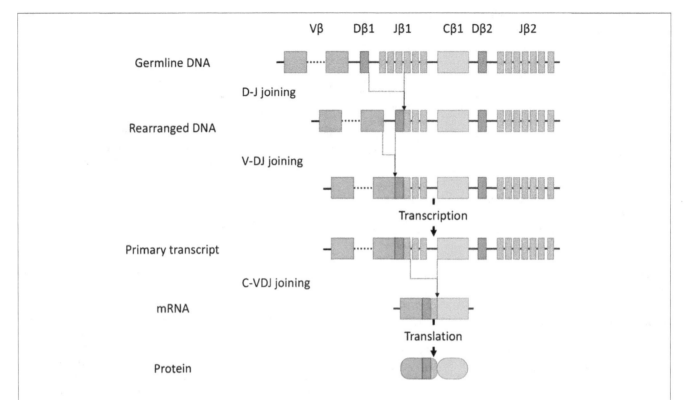

FIGURE 1 | Somatic recombination of the *TCRβ* gene. Rearrangement begins with D-J recombination followed by subsequent V-DJ recombination. The segments recombine randomly to generate TCR diversity. After transcription, intervening sequences are spliced, generating the *TCRβ* chain transcript with V, D, J, and C region segments. Finally, transcripts are translated into protein. In contrast, the *TCRα* gene lacks the D-segment, and its rearrangement starts with V-J recombination.

monoclonal TCR junctions (46), because the narrow size range of the PCR products makes multiple bands appear as single bands. Therefore, PCR amplification with subsequent denaturing gradient polyacrylamide gel electrophoresis and gel scanning (47, 48) or the Biomed GeneScan analysis of flat or capillary polyacrylamide gels (49, 50) has been used as a diagnostic assay for clonality in CTCL patients.

Despite these technical advances, current methods for TCR clonality are still sometimes insufficient for a definitive diagnosis, particularly at early stages, because early lesions often do not contain sufficient numbers of clonal T-cells (51–53). These non-quantitative tests have significant false negative and positive rates for MF (50, 54) and are particularly unreliable for early-stage MF (55).

HIGH-THROUGHPUT SEQUENCING TECHNOLOGIES FOR DIAGNOSING MF

Recent improvements in assays to assess T cell clonality have been achieved based on next-generation high-throughput sequencing (NGS) technologies. By sequencing the third complementarity-determining regions (CDR3s) of genes encoding TCRβ and TCRγ, the number of individual T cell clones present in a sample, the relative proportions of specific clones, and the CDR3 region sequences of each clone can be quantified (56, 57). Likewise, NGS represents a superior method to diagnose CTCL through

the precise identification of malignant T cell clones (58–60). This technique is more sensitive than previous techniques for the detection of clonality (59, 60). Further, NGS-based methods allow the clinician to follow specific clones when monitoring disease recurrence and progression (60). Furthermore, TCR sequencing has clarified that neoplastic cells in some MF lesions might be as few as 1% of the total population of T cells (59). These data clearly explain the difficulties encountered in the histopathological assessment of early-stage MF. In contrast, the frequencies of the most dominant T cell clones range from 1 to 10% in most cases of inflammatory skin disorders such as psoriasis and eczematous dermatitis, among others, whereas the frequency of the most dominant T cell clones adjusted by total nucleated cells could distinguish MF from inflammatory skin disorders (59). Therefore, PEP often demonstrates TCR rearrangement, and NGS-based TCR gene analysis might overcome difficulties in distinguishing PEP and early-stage MF T-cell repertoires.

Most MF cases present as early-stage, typically with a chronic, indolent clinical course. Greater than 80% of patients with early-stage disease will present with an indolent life-long course, free of disease progression, independent of the treatment modality (5). For many years, most patients will also exhibit short-term clinical response associated with recurrent disease, as well as a normal life expectancy in the majority of cases. Furthermore, the limited efficacy associated with chemotherapy has been discussed in retrospective studies (61, 62), making it clear that potentially toxic and aggressive therapies should be avoided (63, 64). However, a small number of early-stage cases will progress. Since advanced-stage patients have poor prognoses, the early identification of high-risk subpopulations is important.

Using NGS technologies, de Masson et al. (55) demonstrated that an enhanced proportion of a malignant T cell clone in the skin is strongly correlated with reductions in progression-free and overall survival for patients with CTCL, and particularly for patients with early-stage MF with a T2 distribution. Further, based on high throughput DNA sequencing of the TCRβ gene, a tumor clone frequency of >25% was found to be a strong predictor of disease progression and poor survival for MF patients with disease limited to the skin.

In summary, evidence for TCR clonality from any method is strong evidence for malignancy. However, it is not conclusive, because benign conditions have also been associated with clonal T-cell populations, such as reactive or autoimmune conditions (65, 66).

CONCLUSION

NGS can be used to assess TCR clonality with superior sensitivity compared to current methods and is useful to diagnose early stage MF. Moreover, this technique permits the tracking of specific clones across different time points or in multiple lesions for a more accurate diagnosis of MF recurrence or progression (55, 59, 60).

AUTHOR CONTRIBUTIONS

KF conceived the concept and wrote the manuscript. TK edited and improved the manuscript.

ACKNOWLEDGMENTS

We would like to thank Editage (www.editage.com) for English language editing.

REFERENCES

1. Willemze R, Jaffe ES, Burg G, Cerroni L, Berti E, Swerdlow SH, et al. WHO-EORTC classification for cutaneous lymphomas. *Blood.* (2005) 105:3768–85. doi: 10.1182/blood-2004-09-3502
2. Bradford PT, Devesa SS, Anderson WF, Toro JR. Cutaneous lymphoma incidence patterns in the United States: a population-based study of 3884 cases. *Blood.* (2009) 113:5064–73. doi: 10.1182/blood-2008-10-184168
3. Hamada T, Iwatsuki K. Cutaneous lymphoma in Japan: a nationwide study of 1733 patients. *J Dermatol.* (2014) 41:3–10. doi: 10.1111/1346-8138.12299
4. Assaf C, Gellrich S, Steinhoff M, Nashan D, Weisse F, Dippel E, et al. Cutaneous lymphomas in Germany: an analysis of the Central Cutaneous Lymphoma Registry of the German Society of Dermatology (DDG). *J Dtsch Dermatol Ges.* (2007) 5:662–8. doi: 10.1111/j.1610-0387.2007.06337.x
5. Agar NS, Wedgeworth E, Crichton S, Mitchell TJ, Cox M, Ferreira S, et al. Survival outcomes and prognostic factors in mycosis fungoides/Sezary syndrome: validation of the revised International Society for Cutaneous Lymphomas/European Organisation for Research and Treatment of Cancer staging proposal. *J Clin Oncol.* (2010) 28:4730–9. doi: 10.1200/JCO.2009.27.7665
6. Massone C, Kodama K, Kerl H, Cerroni L. Histopathologic features of early (patch) lesions of mycosis fungoides: a morphologic study on 745 biopsy specimens from 427 patients. *Am J Surg Pathol.* (2005) 29:550–60. doi: 10.1097/01.pas.0000153121.57515.c6
7. Shapiro PE, Pinto FJ. The histologic spectrum of mycosis fungoides/Sezary syndrome (cutaneous T-cell lymphoma). A review of 222 biopsies, including newly described patterns and the earliest pathologic changes. *Am J Surg Pathol.* (1994) 18:645–67. doi: 10.1097/00000478-199407000-00001
8. Shamim H, Johnson EF, Gibson LE, Comfere N. Mycosis fungoides with spongiosis: a potential diagnostic pitfall. *J Cutan Pathol.* (2019). doi: 10.1111/cup.13477. [Epub ahead of print].
9. Cerroni L. Mycosis fungoides-clinical and histopathologic features, differential diagnosis, and treatment. *Semin Cutan Med Surg.* (2018) 37:2–10. doi: 10.12788/j.sder.2018.002
10. Pimpinelli N, Olsen EA, Santucci M, Vonderheid E, Haeffner AC, Stevens S, et al. Defining early mycosis fungoides. *J Am Acad Dermatol.* (2005) 53:1053–63. doi: 10.1016/j.jaad.2005.08.057
11. Elmer KB, George RM. Cutaneous T-cell lymphoma presenting as benign dermatoses. *Am Fam Phys.* (1999) 59:2809–13.
12. Nashan D, Faulhaber D, Stander S, Luger TA, Stadler R. Mycosis fungoides: a dermatological masquerader. *Br J Dermatol.* (2007) 156:1–10. doi: 10.1111/j.1365-2133.2006.07526.x

13. Kabashima K. New concept of the pathogenesis of atopic dermatitis: interplay among the barrier, allergy, and pruritus as a trinity. *J Dermatol Sci.* (2013) 70:3–11. doi: 10.1016/j.jdermsci.2013.02.001
14. Dummer R, Kohl O, Gillessen J, Kagi M, Burg G. Peripheral blood mononuclear cells in patients with nonleukemic cutaneous T-cell lymphoma. Reduced proliferation and preferential secretion of a T helper-2-like cytokine pattern on stimulation. *Arch Dermatol.* (1993) 129:433–6. doi: 10.1001/archderm.129.4.433
15. Guenova E, Watanabe R, Teague JE, Desimone JA, Jiang Y, Dowlatshahi M, et al. TH2 cytokines from malignant cells suppress TH1 responses and enforce a global TH2 bias in leukemic cutaneous T-cell lymphoma. *Clin Cancer Res.* (2013) 19:3755–63. doi: 10.1158/1078-0432.CCR-12-3488
16. Asadullah K, Docke WD, Haeussler A, Sterry W, Volk HD. Progression of mycosis fungoides is associated with increasing cutaneous expression of interleukin-10 mRNA. *J Invest Dermatol.* (1996) 107:833–7. doi: 10.1111/1523-1747.ep12330869
17. Asadullah K, Haeussler A, Sterry W, Docke WD, Volk HD. Interferon gamma and tumor necrosis factor alpha mRNA expression in mycosis fungoides progression. *Blood.* (1996) 88:757–8.
18. Sugaya M. Chemokines and cutaneous lymphoma. *J Dermatol Sci.* (2010) 59:81–5. doi: 10.1016/j.jdermsci.2010.05.005
19. Suga H, Sugaya M, Miyagaki T, Ohmatsu H, Kawaguchi M, Takahashi N, et al. Skin barrier dysfunction and low antimicrobial peptide expression in cutaneous T-cell lymphoma. *Clin Cancer Res.* (2014) 20:4339–48. doi: 10.1158/1078-0432.CCR-14-0077
20. Beynon T, Selman L, Radcliffe E, Whittaker S, Child F, Orlowska D, et al. 'We had to change to single beds because I itch in the night': a qualitative study of the experiences, attitudes and approaches to coping of patients with cutaneous T-cell lymphoma. *Br J Dermatol.* (2015) 173:83–92. doi: 10.1111/bjd.13732
21. Sampogna F, Frontani M, Baliva G, Lombardo GA, Alvetreti G, Di Pietro C, et al. Quality of life and psychological distress in patients with cutaneous lymphoma. *Br J Dermatol.* (2009) 160:815–22. doi: 10.1111/j.1365-2133.2008.08992.x
22. Mehrany K, El-Azhary RA, Bouwhuis SA, Pittelkow MR. Cutaneous T-cell lymphoma and atopy: is there an association? *Br J Dermatol.* (2003) 149:1013–7. doi: 10.1111/j.1365-2133.2003.05551.x
23. Onsun N, Kural Y, Su O, Demirkesen C, Buyukbabani N. Hypopigmented mycosis fungoides associated with atopy in two children. *Pediatr Dermatol.* (2006) 23:493–6. doi: 10.1111/j.1525-1470.2006.00291.x
24. Nikolaou V, Marinos L, Moustou E, Papadavid E, Economidi A, Christofidou E, et al. Psoriasis in patients with mycosis fungoides: a clinicopathological study of 25 patients. *J Eur Acad Dermatol Venereol.* (2017) 31:1848–52. doi: 10.1111/jdv.14365

25. Lowes MA, Suarez-Farinas M, Krueger JG. Immunology of psoriasis. *Annu Rev Immunol.* (2014) 32:227–55. doi: 10.1146/annurev-immunol-032713-120225

26. Papadavid E, Economidou J, Psarra A, Kapsimali V, Mantzana V, Antoniou C, et al. The relevance of peripheral blood T-helper 1 and 2 cytokine pattern in the evaluation of patients with mycosis fungoides and Sezary syndrome. *Br J Dermatol.* (2003) 148:709–18. doi: 10.1046/j.1365-2133.2003.05224.x

27. Krejsgaard T, Ralfkiaer U, Clasen-Linde E, Eriksen KW, Kopp KL, Bonefeld CM, et al. Malignant cutaneous T-cell lymphoma cells express IL-17 utilizing the Jak3/Stat3 signaling pathway. *J Invest Dermatol.* (2011) 131:1331–8. doi: 10.1038/jid.2011.27

28. Donigan JM, Snowden C, Carter JB, Kimball AB. The temporal association between cutaneous T-cell lymphoma and psoriasis: implications for common biologic processes. *J Eur Acad Dermatol Venereol.* (2016) 30:e31–2. doi: 10.1111/jdv.13281

29. Morales MM, Olsen J, Johansen P, Kaerlev L, Guenel P, Arveux P, et al. Viral infection, atopy and mycosis fungoides: a European multicentre case-control study. *Eur J Cancer.* (2003) 39:511–6. doi: 10.1016/S0959-8049(02)00773-6

30. Gelfand JM, Shin DB, Neimann AL, Wang X, Margolis DJ, Troxel AB. The risk of lymphoma in patients with psoriasis. *J Invest Dermatol.* (2006) 126:2194–201. doi: 10.1038/sj.jid.5700410

31. Nikolaou V, Papadavid E, Economidi A, Marinos L, Moustou E, Karampidou K, et al. Mycosis fungoides in the era of antitumour necrosis factor-alpha treatments. *Br J Dermatol.* (2015) 173:590–3. doi: 10.1111/bjd.13705

32. Väkevä L, Sarna S, Vaalasti A, Pukkala E, Kariniemi AL, Ranki A. A retrospective study of the probability of the evolution of parapsoriasis en plaques into mycosis fungoides. *Acta Derm Venereol.* (2005) 85:318–23. doi: 10.1080/00015550510030087

33. van Doorn R, Van Haselen CW, van Voorst Vader PC, Geerts ML, Heule F, de Rie M, et al. Mycosis fungoides: disease evolution and prognosis of 309 Dutch patients. *Arch Dermatol.* (2000) 136:504–10. doi: 10.1001/archderm.136.4.504

34. Scarisbrick JJ, Quaglino P, Prince HM, Papadavid E, Hodak E, Bagot M, et al. The PROCLIPI international registry of early-stage mycosis fungoides identifies substantial diagnostic delay in most patients. *Br J Dermatol.* (2019) 181:350–7. doi: 10.1111/bjd.17258

35. Witzens M, Mohler T, Willhauck M, Scheibenbogen C, Lee KH, Keilholz U. Detection of clonally rearranged T-cell-receptor gamma chain genes from T-cell malignancies and acute inflammatory rheumatic disease using PCR amplification, PAGE, and automated analysis. *Ann Hematol.* (1997) 74:123–30. doi: 10.1007/s002770050269

36. Bertness V, Kirsch I, Hollis G, Johnson B, Bunn PA Jr. T-cell receptor gene rearrangements as clinical markers of human T-cell lymphomas. *N Engl J Med.* (1985) 313:534–8. doi: 10.1056/NEJM198508293130902

37. Robey E, Fowlkes BJ. The alpha beta versus gamma delta T-cell lineage choice. *Curr Opin Immunol.* (1998) 10:181–7. doi: 10.1016/S0952-7915(98)80247-1

38. Chitgopeker P, Sahni D. T-cell receptor gene rearrangement detection in suspected cases of cutaneous T-cell lymphoma. *J Invest Dermatol.* (2014) 134:1–5. doi: 10.1038/jid.2014.73

39. Bergman R. How useful are T-cell receptor gene rearrangement studies as an adjunct to the histopathologic diagnosis of mycosis fungoides? *Am J Dermatopathol.* (1999) 21:498–502. doi: 10.1097/00000372-199910000-00019

40. Simon M, Flaig MJ, Kind P, Sander CA, Kaudewitz P. Large plaque parapsoriasis: clinical and genotypic correlations. *J Cutan Pathol.* (2000) 27:57–60. doi: 10.1034/j.1600-0560.2000.027002057.x

41. Weiss LM, Hu E, Wood GS, Moulds C, Cleary ML, Warnke R, et al. Clonal rearrangements of T-cell receptor genes in mycosis fungoides and dermatopathic lymphadenopathy. *N Engl J Med.* (1985) 313:539–44. doi: 10.1056/NEJM198508293130903

42. Dosaka N, Tanaka T, Fujita M, Miyachi Y, Horio T, Imamura S. Southern blot analysis of clonal rearrangements of T-cell receptor gene in plaque lesion of mycosis fungoides. *J Invest Dermatol.* (1989) 93:626–9. doi: 10.1111/1523-1747.ep12319746

43. Amagai M, Hayakawa K, Amagai N, Kobayashi K, Onodera Y, Shimizu N, et al. T cell receptor gene rearrangement analysis in mycosis fungoides and disseminated lymphocytoma cutis. *Dermatologica.* (1990) 181:193–6. doi: 10.1159/000247922

44. Lynch JW Jr, Linoilla I, Sausville EA, Steinberg SM, Ghosh BC, Nguyen DT, et al. Prognostic implications of evaluation for lymph node involvement by T-cell antigen receptor gene rearrangement in mycosis fungoides. *Blood.* (1992) 79:3293–9.

45. Bourguin A, Tung R, Galili N, Sklar J. Rapid, nonradioactive detection of clonal T-cell receptor gene rearrangements in lymphoid neoplasms. *Proc Natl Acad Sci USA.* (1990) 87:8536–40. doi: 10.1073/pnas.87.21.8536

46. Kneba M, Bolz I, Linke B, Bertram J, Rothaupt D, Hiddemann W. Characterization of clone-specific rearrangement T-cell receptor gamma-chain genes in lymphomas and leukemias by the polymerase chain reaction and DNA sequencing. *Blood.* (1994) 84:574–81.

47. Wood GS, Tung RM, Haeffner AC, Crooks CF, Liao S, Orozco R, et al. Detection of clonal T-cell receptor gamma gene rearrangements in early mycosis fungoides/Sezary syndrome by polymerase chain reaction and denaturing gradient gel electrophoresis (PCR/DGGE). *J Invest Dermatol.* (1994) 103:34–41. doi: 10.1111/1523-1747.ep12389114

48. Theodorou I, Delfau-Larue MH, Bigorgne C, Lahet C, Cochet G, Bagot M, et al. Cutaneous T-cell infiltrates: analysis of T-cell receptor gamma gene rearrangement by polymerase chain reaction and denaturing gradient gel electrophoresis. *Blood.* (1995) 86:305–10.

49. Assaf C, Hummel M, Dippel E, Goerdt S, Muller HH, Anagnostopoulos I, et al. High detection rate of T-cell receptor beta chain rearrangements in T-cell lymphoproliferations by family specific polymerase chain reaction in combination with the GeneScan technique and DNA sequencing. *Blood.* (2000) 96:640–6.

50. Ponti R, Fierro MT, Quaglino P, Lisa B, Paola F, Michela O, et al. TCRgamma-chain gene rearrangement by PCR-based GeneScan: diagnostic accuracy improvement and clonal heterogeneity analysis in multiple cutaneous T-cell lymphoma samples. *J Invest Dermatol.* (2008) 128:1030–8. doi: 10.1038/sj.jid.5701109

51. Fivenson DP, Hanson CA, Nickoloff BJ. Localization of clonal T cells to the epidermis in cutaneous T-cell lymphoma. *J Am Acad Dermatol.* (1994) 31(5 Pt 1):717–23. doi: 10.1016/S0190-9622(94)70231-4

52. Ponti R, Quaglino P, Novelli M, Fierro MT, Comessatti A, Peroni A, et al. T-cell receptor gamma gene rearrangement by multiplex polymerase chain reaction/heteroduplex analysis in patients with cutaneous T-cell lymphoma (mycosis fungoides/Sezary syndrome) and benign inflammatory disease: correlation with clinical, histological and immunophenotypical findings. *Br J Dermatol.* (2005) 153:565–73. doi: 10.1111/j.1365-2133.2005.06649.x

53. Jawed SI, Myskowski PL, Horwitz S, Moskowitz A, Querfeld C. Primary cutaneous T-cell lymphoma (mycosis fungoides and Sezary syndrome): part I. Diagnosis: clinical and histopathologic features and new molecular and biologic markers. *J Am Acad Dermatol.* (2014) 70: 205 e201–216; quiz 221-202. doi: 10.1016/j.jaad.2013.07.049

54. Sandberg Y, Heule F, Lam K, Lugtenburg PJ, Wolvers-Tettero IL, van Dongen JJ, et al. Molecular immunoglobulin/T- cell receptor clonality analysis in cutaneous lymphoproliferations. Experience with the BIOMED-2 standardized polymerase chain reaction protocol. *Haematologica.* (2003) 88:659–70.

55. de Masson A, O'Malley JT, Elco CP, Garcia SS, Divito SJ, Lowry EL, et al. High-throughput sequencing of the T cell receptor beta gene identifies aggressive early-stage mycosis fungoides. *Sci Transl Med.* (2018) 10:eaar5894. doi: 10.1126/scitranslmed.aar5894

56. Weng WK, Armstrong R, Arai S, Desmarais C, Hoppe R, Kim YH. Minimal residual disease monitoring with high-throughput sequencing of T cell receptors in cutaneous T cell lymphoma. *Sci Transl Med.* (2013) 5:214ra171. doi: 10.1126/scitranslmed.3007420

57. Kirsch IR, Watanabe R, O'Malley JT, Williamson DW, Scott LL, Elco CP, et al. TCR sequencing facilitates diagnosis and identifies mature T cells as the cell of origin in CTCL. *Sci Transl Med.* (2015) 7:308ra158. doi: 10.1126/scitranslmed.aaa9122

58. Sufficool KE, Lockwood CM, Abel HJ, Hagemann IS, Schumacher JA, Kelley TW, et al. T-cell clonality assessment by next-generation sequencing improves detection sensitivity in mycosis fungoides. *J Am Acad Dermatol.* (2015) 73:228–36 e222. doi: 10.1016/j.jaad.2015.04.030

59. Hughes CF, Khot A, McCormack C, Lade S, Westerman DA, Twigger R, et al. Lack of durable disease control with chemotherapy for mycosis fungoides and Sezary syndrome: a comparative study of systemic therapy. *Blood.* (2015) 125:71–81. doi: 10.1182/blood-2014-07-588236

60. Hanel W, Briski R, Ross CW, Anderson TF, Kaminski MS, Hristov AC, et al. A retrospective comparative outcome analysis following systemic therapy in Mycosis fungoides and Sezary syndrome. *Am J Hematol.* (2016) 91:E491–5. doi: 10.1002/ajh.24564

61. Trautinger F, Knobler R, Willemze R, Peris K, Stadler R, Laroche L, et al. EORTC consensus recommendations for the treatment of mycosis fungoides/Sezary syndrome. *Eur J Cancer.* (2006) 42:1014–30. doi: 10.1016/j.ejca.2006.01.025

62. Wilcox RA. Cutaneous T-cell lymphoma: 2017 update on diagnosis, risk-stratification, and management. *Am J Hematol.* (2017) 92:1085–102. doi: 10.1002/ajh.24876

63. Plaza JA, Morrison C, Magro CM. Assessment of TCR-beta clonality in a diverse group of cutaneous T-Cell infiltrates. *J Cutan Pathol.* (2008) 35:358–65. doi: 10.1111/j.1600-0560.2007.00813.x

64. Nakasone Y, Kumagai K, Matsubara R, Shigematsu H, Kitaura K, Suzuki S, et al. Characterization of T cell receptors in a novel murine model of nickel-induced intraoral metal contact allergy. *PLoS ONE.* (2018) 13:e0209248. doi: 10.1371/journal.pone.0209248

65. Robins HS, Campregher PV, Srivastava SK, Wacher A, Turtle CJ, Kahsai O, et al. Comprehensive assessment of T-cell receptor beta-chain diversity in alphabeta T cells. *Blood.* (2009) 114:4099–107. doi: 10.1182/blood-2009-04-217604

66. Bolotin DA, Mamedov IZ, Britanova OV, Zvyagin IV, Shagin D, Ustyugova SV, et al. Next generation sequencing for TCR repertoire profiling: platform-specific features and correction algorithms. *Eur J Immunol.* (2012) 42:3073–83. doi: 10.1002/eji.201242517

20

Cutaneous Angiosarcoma: The Possibility of New Treatment Options Especially for Patients with Large Primary Tumor

Yasuhiro Fujisawa[1]*, Koji Yoshino[2], Taku Fujimura[3], Yoshiyuki Nakamura[1], Naoko Okiyama[1], Yosuke Ishitsuka[1], Rei Watanabe[1] and Manabu Fujimoto[1]

[1] Dermatology, University of Tsukuba, Tsukuba, Ibaraki, Japan, [2] Dermatology, Tokyo Metropolitan Komagome Hospital, Tokyo, Japan, [3] Dermatology, Tohoku University, Sendai, Japan

*Correspondence:
Yasuhiro Fujisawa
fujisan@md.tsukuba.ac.jp

The most widely accepted treatment for cutaneous angiosarcoma (CAS) is wide local excision and postoperative radiation to decrease the risk of recurrence. Positive surgical margins and large tumors (T2, >5 cm) are known to be associated with poor prognosis. Moreover, T2 tumors are known to be associated with positive surgical margins. According to previous reports, the majority of CAS patients in Japan had T2 tumors, whereas less than half of the patients in the studies from western countries did so. Consequently, the reported 5-year overall survival of Japanese CAS patients without distant metastasis was only 9%, lower than that for stage-IV melanoma. For patients with T2 tumors, management of subclinical metastasis should be considered when planning the initial treatment. Several attempts to control subclinical metastasis have been reported, such as using adjuvant/neoadjuvant chemotherapy in addition to conventional surgery plus radiation. Unfortunately, those attempts did not show any clinical benefit. Besides surgery, new chemotherapeutic approaches for advanced CAS have been introduced in the past couple of decades, such as paclitaxel and docetaxel. We proposed the use of chemoradiotherapy (CRT) using taxanes instead of surgery plus radiation for patients with T2 tumors without distant metastasis and showed a high response ratio with prolonged survival. However, this prolonged survival was seen only in patients who received maintenance chemotherapy after CRT, indicating that continuous chemotherapy is mandatory to control subclinical residual tumors. With the recent development of targeted drugs for cancer, many potential drugs for CAS are now available. Given that CAS expresses a high level of vascular endothelial growth factor (VEGF) receptor, drugs that target VEGF signaling pathways such as anti-VEGF monoclonal antibody and tyrosine kinase inhibitors are also promising, and several successful treatments have been reported. Besides targeted drugs, several new cytotoxic anticancer drugs such as eribulin or trabectedin have also been shown to be effective for advanced sarcoma. However, most of the clinical trials did not include a sufficient number of CAS patients. Therefore, clinical trials focusing only on CAS should be performed to evaluate the effectiveness of these new drugs.

Keywords: cutaneous angiosarcoma, concurrent chemoradiotherapy, maintenance chemotherapy, adjuvant chemotherapy, taxanes, eribulin, pazopanib, angiosarcoma of the scalp

BACKGROUND

According to the Surveillance, Epidemiology, and End Results Program database, the number of patients with sarcoma recorded between 2010 and 2014 was only 1/100 of the number of patients with carcinoma in the same period. Moreover, angiosarcoma accounts for only 1% of all sarcomas, so patients with angiosarcoma constitute only 1 in 10,000 of all patients with malignant neoplasms (1–3). Although the incidence of angiosarcoma has increased in the past couple of decades, it is around 0.5 per 1,000,000 persons, or fewer than 200 new patients, per year in the United States (3). Owing to this rarity, most previous publications have been case reports or small case series, making it difficult to interpret the results because of the selection bias and small number of patients included in those studies. Furthermore, because of this rarity, no randomized phase-3 study has been conducted, especially for angiosarcoma, and consequently, no clinical trial-proven standardized treatment has thus far been established. Although complete removal of the tumor was believed to be essential, as it is for other sarcomas (4, 5), some reports have suggested that wide-margin surgery will not deliver favorable results (6, 7). In this review, we will summarize the clinical features and current treatments of angiosarcoma and discuss the possibility of new therapeutic options for this rare disease.

CLINICAL PRESENTATION

Angiosarcoma develops in various soft tissues and organs, but the most commonly affected site is the skin [cutaneous angiosarcoma (CAS)] (8–10). According to an analysis of 434 cases of CAS, 62.1% of them developed in the head and neck, 24.4% in the trunk, 10.6% in the extremities, and 2.7% in other locations (11). CAS commonly occurs in the scalp and typically presents as an enlarging bruise-like purpura in the head and neck region and may be associated with ulceration and/or a tumor. Sometimes patients develop a thick blood crust. These head and neck CAS commonly develops in older men (12–14), whereas the secondary CAS, lymphedema-associated CAS [so-called Stewart-Treves syndrome (15)] and radiation-associated CAS (11, 16), usually develops within the lymphedema site and irradiated field >5 years after the surgery and radiation, respectively (12, 16).

Stewart-Treves syndrome was originally reported as lymphedema that developed after radical mastectomy and lymph node dissection (15), but in the past 15 years, we have never encountered Stewart-Treves syndrome that developed after the surgery for mammary carcinoma. Instead, in the same period, we experienced three cases of Stewart-Treves syndrome that developed in the lower limb after treatment for uterine carcinoma (17). This may be explained by the fact that the number of patients receiving conservative treatment for mammary carcinoma has increased, and as a consequence, the prevalence of Stewart-Treves syndrome in the upper extremity has decreased (18). On the other hand, the occurrence of radiation-induced CAS in the breast is likely to increase given that the prognosis for mammary carcinoma is gradually improving and radiation is more often used to treat (16).

While the incidence of Stewart-Treves syndrome is not well known, it has been reported to be about 1/10 to 1/20 of all CAS (19–22). Similarly, the cumulative incidence of radiation-associated CAS 15 years after radiotherapy for breast carcinoma was reported to be 0.9 per 1,000 patients (23), meaning less than 1 occurrence per 10,000 irradiated patients per year. In this review, considering its rarity and etiological difference, we will focus mainly on primary CAS, the narrow sense of CAS (24).

Distant metastasis could occur within a month of primary surgery, but typically it occurs on average after a year (4, 5). The most common site of metastasis is the lung, followed by the lymph nodes, bone, and liver (4, 5, 25). Interestingly, lung metastasis often presents as pneumothorax, which may require urgent medication (26, 27).

DIAGNOSIS AND STAGING

Patients with typical presenting symptoms can be diagnosed clinically, but the precise pathological diagnosis should be performed by an expert pathologist. The histologic features of angiosarcoma can vary between patients and even within the same patient. When the tissue specimens are taken from well-differentiated areas, the tumor cells usually form vessel-like structures and may be difficult to differentiate from normal vessels. However, the tumor vessels tend to form independent or separate networks with anastomoses (28). Other features such as cellular atypia, mitoses, and formation of multilayer endothelium can be helpful for diagnosis. On the other hand, in poorly differentiated areas, the tumor cells show sheet-like growth with hemorrhage and necrosis, which have fewer features than do vascular tumors. In such cases, positive staining for endothelial markers such as CD31, CD34, von Willbrand factor, and vascular endothelial growth factor (VEGF) are useful (29). Also, lymphatic endothelial markers such as D2-40 are positive for most superficial angiosarcomas (28).

The staging of CAS is based on the TNM staging system of the American Joint Committee on Cancer (AJCC) (**Table 1**). The tumor grade based on the pathologic features is included in the staging. In brief, localized disease is classified as stage I or II; nodal spread or T2 tumor with histologic grade 3, as stage III; and distant disease, as stage IV. However, because there is no standardized treatment algorithm for each stage, staging of CAS has little clinical benefit in the treatment decision.

PROGNOSIS AND FACTORS ASSOCIATED WITH SURVIVAL

Generally, soft-tissue sarcomas have a 50–60% survival rate (30), whereas the 5-year survival rate for angiosarcoma is <40% (12, 25, 31, 32). Several factors are reportedly associated with poor survival: older age (25, 32), worse performance status (33, 34), larger tumor size (5, 8, 20, 32, 35–40), positive margin status (31, 32, 38, 41, 42), higher histologic type or grade (32, 37, 41, 43, 44), scalp as the primary location (5, 36, 45), deeper location of the tumor (20, 31), and presence of distant metastasis (33, 38,

41, 46). On the other hand, the following factors were associated with favorable prognosis: surgery (20, 34), multimodal therapy (5, 39, 41) and postoperative radiotherapy (34, 36, 41, 43, 47, 48). The studies that included more than 50 patients with CAS only are summarized in **Table 2**. According to these five studies, tumor size seems to be a consistently poor prognostic factor; indeed, patients with tumors larger than 10 cm all died of the disease (35, 36).

A study by Sinnamon et al. (32) of 821 angiosarcomas included 211 cases of primary CAS in the head and neck. In their cohort, all cases of metastatic disease were excluded and all the patients received surgical treatment. They scored the following factors and classified the risk from low (total score 0–1), intermediate (total score 2–3), and high (total score 4–7): age > 70 as 1, black ethnicity as 1, histologic tumor grade 3 as 1, tumor size 3–7 cm as 1, tumor size larger than 7 cm as 2, microscopic residual tumor as 1, and macroscopic residual tumor as 2. By using this model, patients at high risk had a median overall survival of only 1.6 years with a hazard ratio of 5.65 when compared with patients at low risk.

This result clearly indicates that these factors strongly correlate with poor survival.

Reports from Japan and from western countries showed differences in survival. In the study from Japan of 260 cases of CAS, the 5-year overall survival among patients who could receive surgery was <20% (49) (median overall survival: < 20 months), whereas in the studies from western countries, it was 31–51% (5, 11, 25, 31, 40). CAS patients in Japan had equivalent survival to the "high risk" group reported by Sinnamon et al. (32), with a median overall survival of 1.6 years. This difference might be explained by the fact that the tumor size in Japanese patients is generally large: in the study of 260 CAS cases, 44% of the patients had tumors of at least 10 cm (originally, described as tumors larger than 100 cm^2) (49), whereas tumors larger than 5 cm (T2) constituted only 18–38% of the patients in the studies from western countries (5, 11, 25, 40). Our multicenter study, which included only Japanese patients, was also T2 dominant: only 3 of 28 patients (11%) had a T1 tumor (19). In the meta-analysis by Hwang et al., which included 128 cases from seven studies (50), the median overall survival in the T1 group was significantly longer than that in the T2 group (31.4 months and 17.3 months, respectively: $P < 0.001$). Collectively, Japanese CAS patients have larger primary tumors than do CAS patients in western countries, and consequently, the survival of Japanese CAS patients is shorter.

TREATMENT

Current Treatment Options
Surgery

Radical surgery with no residual tumor cell on the margin (R0 resection) is generally the primary goal of sarcoma treatment. In every review or set of guidelines, surgery with R0 resection is recommended as the goal of CAS treatment (28). In a systematic review by Shin et al. (51), absence of surgery was shown to correlate with poor survival; Trofymenko et al. (52) reported similar result in a study using 764 cases of CAS extracted from the National Cancer Database in the United States. Therefore, there is little doubt that surgery is one of the best choice for the management of CAS.

TABLE 1 | AJCC TNM staging system for soft tissue sarcoma.

	0	1	2	
T classification		Size<=5cm	Size>5cm	
a: superficial tumor, b: deep tumor (divided by superficial fascia)				
N classification	No nodal metastasis	Nodal metastasis		
M classification	No distant metastasis	Distant metastasis		

Stage		T	N	M	Histologic grade
I	A	1a/b			1 or not assessed
	B	2a/b			
II	A	1a/b	0	0	2 or 3
	B	2a/b			2
III		2a/b			3
		Any	1		Any
IV		Any	Any	1	

Histologic grading is defined as follows: (1) Differentiation: score from 1 to 3, (2) Mitotic count: score from 1 to 3, and (3) Tumor necrosis: score from 0 to 2.
Sum (1) to (3) and determine grade as follows.
Gx: not assessed.
G1: total score of 2 or 3.
G2: total score of 4 or 5.
G3: total score of >5.

TABLE 2 | Reported factors associated with poor survival determined by studies with >50 patients in CAS.

	N	Age	Tumor size	Pathological feature	Margin	Location	Others
Albores-Saavedra et al. (11)	434	>50	N.S.			Head and neck Deeper location	Lymph node metastasis Distant metastasis
Perez et al. (40)	88	N.S.	>5 cm		N.S.		
Holden et al. (36)	72	N.S.	>5 cm >10 cm	N.S.	N.S.		
Guadagnolo et al. (5)	70		>5 cm Satellitosis		N.S.		Surgery alone
Patel et al. (25)	55	>70	N.S.	N.S.	N.S.		Without multimodality or radiation therapy

N.S., not significant; PS, performance status.

Although no standardized treatment recommendation has been established, a margin of less than 1 cm is associated with poor survival (49). The depth of the resection has not been well discussed, but generally if the tumor does not extend into the deep fascia, a resection layer including the deep fascia is adequate. If the tumor directly invades into the deep fascia, removal of the underlying structures, e.g., the periosteum or even the outer shell of the skull, is required to obtain R0 resection.

Unfortunately, it is common to see positive microscopic (R1) or macroscopic (R2) margins even after a wide surgical margin from the visible tumor border has been obtained (4, 8, 31, 36, 41). Pawlik et al. (4) reported that in their series of 29 patients, 18 (62.1%) had an initial diagnosis of T1 (<5 cm) tumor, but 11 of those tumors turned out to be T2 (>5 cm) after surgical pathology evaluation of the resected tumor. The clinical margin of the tumor in CAS is difficult to determine because it often develops as a multifocal tumor and presents as a skip lesion. Moreover, when CAS develops near important structures such as the eye, surgical removal with an adequate margin is impossible. As a consequence, the rate of local recurrence after treatment is high reportedly ranging from 26 to 100% (5, 9, 25, 41). Lahat et al. (53) reported 32 of 44 cases of locally recurrent angiosarcoma treated with surgery, 70% of which achieved complete removal of the recurrent tumor, with a 5-year overall survival of 44%.

To reduce local recurrence, postoperative radiotherapy covering a wide area with a >50 Gy dose has been reported by several studies to be effective not only for local control but also for overall survival (4, 5). Currently, wide local excision followed by radiation is the most accepted treatment for CAS (28, 54, 55); however, despite such mutilating multimodal treatment, survival of patients, especially of those with large tumors, is still unsatisfactory (19, 32).

Other than radical surgery, palliative surgery might have role in patients with large tumors to reduce the tumor load. Some reports suggested the use of minimal surgery as part of the management of CAS (6, 56), such as for those cases with a diffuse lesion pattern involving vital structures, recurrent disease, or metastasis.

Chemotherapy

The chemotherapeutic options currently available for angiosarcoma are listed in **Table 3**. Chemotherapy using anthracyclines alone or in combination with ifosfamide have been used for unresectable and metastatic angiosarcoma (35, 57, 58). However, anthracyclines have cardiac toxicity which make it difficult to apply in older patients. Taxanes, which inhibit tubulin elongation, were introduced in the 1990s as a novel cytotoxic drug and have become accepted as standardized treatment options in various kinds of cancers such as those of the breast (59), lung (60), stomach (61), and uterus (62), because of their high efficacy. Although several clinical studies have shown that taxanes are of little benefit for sarcomas (63, 64), the angiosarcomas included in those clinical studies showed antitumor activity (64). Taxanes not only have a direct antitumor effect but also have been shown to exert an antiangiogenic effect (65, 66), which is thought to be suitable for the treatment of vascular tumors. Indeed, taxanes were shown to be effective for the treatment of Kaposi sarcoma (67, 68).

In 1999, Fata et al. (69) achieved a response ratio of 89% by using paclitaxel monotherapy for the treatment of head and neck CAS. Later, Penel et al. (70) conducted the first phase-2 trial for metastatic or locally advanced angiosarcoma, which included 30 patients treated with paclitaxel. In that clinical trial, the progression-free survival rate after 4 months was 45%, and the median overall survival was 8 months. Considering that the patients with distant metastasis consisted of 74% of the study population and 36% of them had had previous systemic chemotherapy, this result was encouraging. Italiano et al. (71) showed, albeit in a retrospective study, that paclitaxel achieved an equivalent outcome to that of anthracyclines in the treatment of advanced angiosarcoma despite the patients treated with paclitaxel being a decade older

TABLE 3 | Chemotherapy options and their effect for angiosarcoma.

Agent	Patients	N	Response/median survival (months)
Anthracyclines	Pooled analysis of 11 clinical trials for angiosarcoma from all sites Young et al. (58)	108	Response ratio: 25% for all sites PFS: 4.9, OS: 9.9
Paclitaxel	Retrospective review of angiosarcoma from all sites Italiano et al. (71)	34	Response ratio: 29.5% for all sites
		68	Response ratio: 53% for all sites Response ratio: 78% for CAS
	ANGIOTAX study: phase-2 study including angiosarcoma from all sites Penel et al. (70)	30	Response ratio: 18% for all sites Response ratio: 89% for CAS
	ANGIOTAX plus study: phase-2 study comparing paclitaxel with/without bevacizumab from all sites (showing paclitaxel arm only) Ray-Coquard et al. (74)	24	Response ratio: 45.8% for all sites PFS: 6.6, OS: 19.5
	Retrospective study for head/neck CAS Fata et al. (69)	9	Response ratio: 89% for CAS
Docetaxel	Retrospective study for CAS Nagano et al. (101)	9	Response ratio: 67% for CAS
Gemcitabine	Retrospective study with angiosarcoma from all sites Stacchiotti et al. (76)	25	Response ratio: 64% for all sites PFS: 7, OS: 17

PFS, progression-free survival; OS, overall survival; CAS, cutaneous angiosarcoma.

than those treated with anthracyclines (67.4 and 57.4 years old, respectively). Collectively, taxanes can achieve a similar level of antitumor effect to that achieved by anthracyclines, but with less toxicity, and therefore, a recent report (72) suggested using taxanes as the first-line treatment for CAS with unresectable or distant disease. Indeed, we reported (17, 73) successful treatment results using taxanes as the first-line therapy for primary CAS.

Because both taxanes have been reported to be effective, the decision about which taxane to use as the first-line might be difficult. In this review, we recommend paclitaxel as the first-line treatment since paclitaxel has been evaluated in different phase-2 studies (70, 74), whereas docetaxel has not yet been evaluated in a prospective study. However, docetaxel still has a role as a second-line therapy in patients refractory to paclitaxel (75).

Gemcitabine has been reported to be effective for sarcomas both as a single agent (76, 77) and in combination with docetaxel (78, 79). Several case series (77, 80) have been reported in which gemcitabine for the treatment of angiosarcoma was used with favorable outcomes. Moreover, albeit in a study based on a retrospective pooled analysis (76), gemcitabine showed an overall response rate of up to 68% for angiosarcoma (76). If this agent is used as monotherapy, the toxicity profile is better than that of anthracyclines but still has a significant incidence of bone marrow suppression.

Radiation

Radiation is usually delivered after surgery for better local control (28, 54, 55). However, dismal outcome have been reported when radiation was used as monotherapy (5, 38, 43). Therefore, radiation monotherapy is generally used for palliation, not for curative intent because of frequent recurrence, as high as 100% in previous studies (25, 36, 42, 43). On the other hand, Ogawa et al. (34) reported that in their cohort of 25 patients who received radiation monotherapy with curative intent, 11 of the 14 patients (79%) who received >70Gy achieved local control, whereas only 3 of the 11 patients (27%) who received <70 Gy did. A study by Scott et al. (81) of 41 patients treated with radiation recommended at least 60–65 Gy for the postoperative tumor bed and 70–75 Gy for patients who receive radiation monotherapy. Others (82) suggested that improved delivery of radiation might achieve higher efficacy. Since no prospective study has been conducted to evaluate the role of radiation as the first-line therapy, radiation monotherapy is still difficult to use as curative intent therapy for primary disease. We will discuss combination radiation and chemotherapy in the next section.

New Treatment Options
Chemoradiotherapy (CRT)

The use of chemotherapy and radiation (CRT) concurrently or concomitantly is one of the standardized treatment methods for several cancers: esophageal (83), head and neck (84), rectal (85), and cervical (86). Chemotherapeutic agents such as 5-fluorouracil (84, 85), cisplatin (87), gemcitabine (88), and taxanes (89, 90) are expected to act not only as cytotoxic but also as radiosensitizing agents. Therefore, CRT may sometimes cause higher toxicity than does monotherapy but can be justified by

its high antitumor effect, and in most cases, such side effects are manageable. Besides, although many cancer treatments introduced CRT as one of the key treatments, it was an uncommon method among cutaneous malignancies. In such a situation, we started to use cisplatin and 5-fluorouracil concurrently with radiation for the management of unresectable/metastatic cutaneous squamous cell carcinoma with the same protocol used in the head and neck and reported successful treatment results (91–93).

As described previously, a Japanese retrospective study of CAS (49) revealed that the median overall survival of patients with non-metastatic localized CAS who received surgery was less than 20 months, but this finding was not surprising because we have reported a similar dismal outcome (13.5 months) (19). We suspected that increased expression of VEGF during the wound healing process (94) caused by mutilating surgery might cause progression of residual angiosarcoma because angiosarcoma has been reported to express a VEGF receptor (95–97). As discussed in the previous section, tumor size is the most common factor for poor prognosis, which is commonly related to a positive surgical margin. Therefore, it is convincing to consider that such subclinical residual tumors could be expanded by VEGF released by surgery.

In such a situation, a retrospective study (47) of use of chemotherapy (anthracyclines) and radiation for five head and neck CAS (four scalp and one lip, three of them with high-grade tumors) was reported and achieved a median overall survival of 27.0 months, which was better than the reported median survival of face and scalp CAS (<20 months) (6, 36, 45). However, there was a concern related to use of anthracyclines for older CAS patients for whom the drug might not be tolerable. On the other hand, taxanes have a better toxicity profile, and therefore, we expected that older CAS patients could tolerate it. Moreover, taxanes are known as radiosensitizers (89, 90), and therefore, possibly an ideal agent for CRT for the treatment of CAS.

The reported cases of CAS treated with CRT are described in **Table 4**. Because the study by Mark et al. (47) did not describe the timing of the chemotherapy, we could not determine whether they used chemotherapy concurrently or concomitantly with radiation. In the study by Miki et al. (98), 5 of the 12 patients who received docetaxel, the schedule was adjusted so that the drug was administered concurrently only on the first and last weeks of radiation. Another seven patients received docetaxel for 2–6 weeks during radiation in accordance with patient status. All the patients in the other two studies received chemotherapy and radiation concurrently (19, 98, 99). Most of the arms are composed of scalp CAS, which correlated with poor survival. The response to CRT was 82% (98) and 94% (19), with a statistically higher median overall survival than that of surgery followed by radiation in both studies. Representative photographs of patients who received CRT are presented in **Figures 1A–D**.

Concurrent CRT brings severe side effects than when each treatment is delivered as monotherapy. In our study, 78% of the patients who received concurrent CRT had CTCAE grade-4 neutropenia, but the neutropenia was made manageable by use of granulocyte-colony stimulating factor and no treated-related death was observed (19). In the study by Miki et al.

TABLE 4 | Study using chemotherapy and radiation therapy for CAS.

Study	N	Patients tumor location/size	Treatment	RT dose	Response/pattern of failure	Median OS (months)
Mark et al. (47)	5	Scalp: 4 and Face: 1 Size not described	Anthracyclines	30–76.2 Gy	Response ratio: N.D. Local: 2/5 Distant: 2/5	27.0
	4	Scalp: 1 and Face: 3 Size not described	*Surgery*	50–65 Gy	Local: 1/4 Distant: 0/4	Not reached
Rhomberg et al. (99)	1	Scalp/face: 1 T2	Razoxane Vindesine	35–66 Gy	CR Alive without failure	41
Miki et al. (98)	11	Scalp: 16 and Face: 1 T1: 1 and T2: 15	Docetaxel	70 Gy	Response ratio: 82% Local: 4	33.7 ⎤
	5		*Surgery/IL-2*		Distant: 5 Both: 4	22.7 ⎦ *
Our study (19)	16	Scalp: 14, and Extremity: 2 T1: 2 and T2: 14	Docetaxel	<65Gy:12 ≥65Gy:16	Response ratio: 94% Local: 6 Distant: 7	Not reached ⎤
	12	Scalp: 10, extremity: 2 T1: 2 and T2: 10	*Surgery*		Only 1 patient still alive	15.0 ⎦ **

*P < 0.05.
**P < 0.01.
OS, overall survival; CAS, cutaneous angiosarcoma; N.D., not described; IL-2: interleukin-2.

TABLE 5 | Maintenance chemotherapy after primary therapy.

Study	N	Tumor location	Primary chemotherapy	RT dose	Maintenance chemotherapy and duration (months)		Pattern of failure	Median OS (months)
Nagano et al., 2007 (101)	9	Scalp: 6, Face: 1 Neck: 1, Leg: 1	Docetaxel	–	Docetaxel	3–22 MD: 13.5	Local: 4 Distant: 0	Not described
Rhomberg et al. 2009 (99)	5	Thyroid: 4, Scalp/face: 1	Razoxane Vindesine	35–66 Gy MD: 56 Gy	Razoxane Vindesine	6 weeks-36 MD: 12	Local or distant: 2	27.0
Our study 2014	9	Scalp: 7, Limb: 2	Docetaxel	48–80 Gy MD: 70 Gy	Docetaxel	3–50 MD: 12.5	Local/LN: 3 Distant: 2	Not reached ⎤
	7	Scalp: 7		52.5–70.4 Gy MD: 70 Gy	Not done		Local: 4 Distant: 5	21.0 ⎦ **

** P < 0.01.
RT, radiotherapy; MD, median; OS, overall survival.

(98), all the patients developed grade 1–3 dermatitis but healed uneventfully.

Taking these finding together, CRT using taxanes could achieve satisfactory antitumor activity with good tolerability and might bring better survival than does conventional surgery followed by radiation especially for CAS of the scalp. Although the use of taxanes concurrently might bring severe side effects, we suggest concurrent CRT to gain maximum antitumor effect as long as the side effects are tolerable and manageable.

Maintenance Chemotherapy

To prevent locoregional and distant failure after response to chemotherapy, some previous report continued chemotherapy to maintain the response. Gambini et al. (100) achieved complete remission of radiation-induced angiosarcoma after treatment with paclitaxel and maintained the response for 4 years by maintenance therapy with intervals of no longer than 3 weeks. Interestingly, they had local recurrence twice when the treatment was delayed, but in both instances, a new complete remission

was rapidly achieved with the same treatment and the patients remained disease-free at the time of their report. Nagano et al. (101) reported nine CAS patients treated with docetaxel, eight of whom continued docetaxel for 3–22 months (**Table 5**). None of the patients developed distant metastasis during maintenance chemotherapy. Rhomberg et al. (99) treated nine patients with angiosarcoma (five with thyroid, one with left ventricle, one with bladder, and one with scalp/face) with concurrent CRT using razoxane and vindesine. Complete remission of the tumor was obtained in six patients, five of whom received maintenance chemotherapy for 6 weeks to a year. Of those five patients, two developed recurrence but only one developed it during the maintenance chemotherapy.

In our study (19), 16 CAS patients were treated with concurrent CRT and 9 of them received maintenance chemotherapy. Locoregional relapse was seen in three of the nine patients who received maintenance chemotherapy, whereas it was seen in four of the seven patients who did not receive it. On the other hand, only two of the nine patients who received maintenance

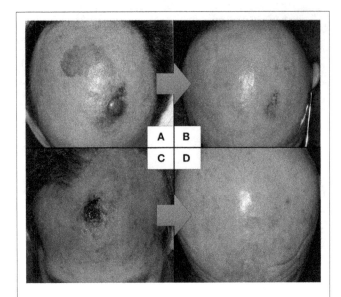

FIGURE 1 | Representative cases of CAS treated by concurrent CRT.

chemotherapy developed distant metastasis, whereas five of the seven patients who did not receive maintenance chemotherapy did develop distant metastasis ($P < 0.05$). A study by Ito et al. (75) showed that 19 patients who received maintenance chemotherapy using taxanes had significantly better survival than did 24 patients who received maintenance chemotherapy without taxanes ($P < 0.0024$) Collectively, maintenance chemotherapy after remission obtained by CRT seems to suppress tumor regrowth and development of distant metastasis. However, there is no consensus as to how long this maintenance chemotherapy should be continue. Further investigation is needed to determine the optimal length of maintenance chemotherapy.

Adjuvant/Neoadjuvant Chemotherapy
The use of adjuvant chemotherapy after complete removal of the tumor is attractive because we experience many CAS patient who develop distant metastasis even though there is no locoregional failure. However, anthracycline-based adjuvant chemotherapy did not show any survival benefit in soft tissue sarcomas (102). Indeed, we could not see any survival benefit in CAS patients by using taxanes after surgery and radiation (7). Similarly, adjuvant chemotherapy did not show a clear benefit among angiosarcoma patients treated with anthracyclines, paclitaxel, and other combinations (5, 6, 41, 44).

Some groups reported the use of chemotherapy before surgery (neoadjuvant chemotherapy) but did not show any survival benefit in face CAS (103) or in head and neck CAS (5). However, a certain percentage of patients who received neoadjuvant chemotherapy could achieve a complete response (60% in face CAS (103)) and did not require definitive surgery. Thus, the effect of neoadjuvant chemotherapy is difficult to interpret.

Since no large prospective study has been conducted to evaluate the value of adjuvant and neoadjuvant chemotherapy, those previous studies should be read with caution. However, the largest retrospective analysis of CAS including 821 patients

indicated that both adjuvant and neoadjuvant therapy after surgery did not show any survival benefit on univariate and multivariate analyses (32). Further prospective study is required to evaluate the role of adjuvant/neoadjuvant chemotherapy for CAS.

New Drugs
Anti-VEGF Drugs
Angiosarcomas express VEGFR (95, 97, 104), and overexpression of VEGF converted slow-growing vascular endothelial tumors to fast-growing malignant tumors in a mouse model and formed invasive angiosarcoma in immunodeficient mice (105). Conversely, blockade of the VEGF/VEGFR pathway inhibited tumor growth *in vitro* (106). Therefore, it is reasonable for the treatment to target the VEGF/VEGFR signaling pathway. Several studies using anti-VEGF monoclonal antibody (bevacizumab) have shown antitumor activity in angiosarcomas: 4 of 30 patients treated with bevacizumab had a partial response, with a mean time to progression of 26 weeks (107), and 2 of 2 patients treated with bevacizumab and radiation had a complete response (108).

On the basis of this background, Ray-Coquard et al. (74) conducted a non-comparative, open-label, randomized phase-2 trial to explore the activity and safety of bevacizumab and paclitaxel therapy for patients with advanced angiosarcoma. Fifty patients were randomized and assigned to two arms: (1) the paclitaxel alone or (2) the paclitaxel and bevacizumab arm. From the findings, they concluded that there is no benefit from adding bevacizumab to paclitaxel (median overall survival: 19.5 versus 15.9 months).

Other than monoclonal antibody, two small-molecule multi-tyrosine kinase inhibitors that can inhibit the VEGF/VEGFR signaling pathway have been used for the treatment of angiosarcoma patients: sorafenib (109) and pazopanib (110). A phase-2 trial including 37 patients with recurrent or metastatic angiosarcoma treated with sorafenib showed a response ratio of 14% with median progression-free survival of 3.8 months (111). No clinical trial to evaluate pazopanib activity in angiosarcoma has been conducted. In a case series using pazopanib for the treatment of taxane-resistant CAS, two of five patients achieved a partial response with median progression-free survival of 94 days (112). On the other hand, a case series of eight CAS patients treated with pazopanib did not show any benefit (113). Although we do not have enough conclusive evidence, the current first-line treatment should still be taxanes and anti-VEGF pathway therapy should be considered as the second- and third-line therapy.

Eribulin Mesylate
Eribulin mesylate suppresses microtubule polymerization and sequesters tubulin into nonfunctional aggregates, which is a mechanism distinct from those of other tubulin-targeting drugs such as taxanes (114). A phase-3 study comparing dacarbazine and eribulin in patients with advanced liposarcoma or leiomyosarcoma showed improved survival in patients treated with eribulin (115). This phase-3 study did not include angiosarcoma, and therefore, we do not have any evidence on the effect of eribulin for

angiosarcoma. However, both taxanes and eribulin target microtubule polymerization, and eribulin binds to a different site of the microtubule (116), indicating that it may be effective for patients who become resistant to taxanes. Albeit in a case report, eribulin was shown to be effective for a patient who became resistant to docetaxel (117). Currently, we are conducting a prospective, observational clinical study to evaluate eribulin in patients with CAS who became resistant to taxanes (UMIN000023331); patient enrollment for this study is expected to be completed in 2018.

Checkpoint Inhibitors

Recent development of checkpoint inhibitors in melanoma treatment dramatically improved the survival of advanced melanoma. Melanoma with higher expression of programmed death receptor ligand-1 (PD-L1) correlated with a better treatment outcome when using anti-PD-1 antibody (118). This result supports the notion of a proposed immune escape mechanism by tumor cells using their PD-L1 expression on the cell surface to bind PD-1 on cytotoxic T cells and attenuate the immune response (119). Interestingly, our study group showed that CAS with PD-1 positive cell infiltration and tumor site PD-L1 expression correlated with survival (120). This result raises the possibility of using anti-PD-1 antibody for the treatment of CAS. To the best of our knowledge, there is no on-going or planned clinical trial to use checkpoint inhibitors for advanced angiosarcoma (clinicaltrials.gov).

CURRENT RECOMMENDATION AND FUTURE PERSPECTIVE

The treatment of CAS, especially T2 tumors of the scalp, is still challenging. The surgical approach seems to be difficult because such tumors usually have an unclear border and often have skip lesions that make it difficult to determine the "true" tumor border. As patients with tumors larger than 10 cm were reported to have a catastrophic prognosis (35, 36), the current standard wide-margin resection followed by wide-field radiation might be palliative rather than curative (6). Radical surgery can reduce the tumor load; however, surgery-based treatment cannot target "subclinical" metastasis, which may have already occurred by

the time of diagnosis. Therefore, we strongly recommend starting systemic chemotherapy along with primary tumor therapy. CRT can achieve this task: systemic administration of taxanes can target subclinical metastases and also act as a radiosensitizer that will enhance the effect of radiation therapy against the primary tumor. Although neoadjuvant chemotherapy and adjuvant chemotherapy may also achieve this task, to the best of our knowledge, no study has shown the superiority of this strategy.

Collectively, we suggest considering concurrent CRT using taxanes when we encounter CAS of the scalp with a T2 tumor. We also recommend maintenance chemotherapy even if complete remission of the tumor has been achieved. On the other hand, for T1 CAS with a clear tumor border, the current standard surgery followed by radiation might be sufficient to obtain a successful result. However, these recommendations are based on a small number of retrospective studies. CRT and maintenance chemotherapy should be evaluated with prospective clinical studies to confirm the superiority of this strategy.

Moreover, we currently do not have many options for when the tumor becomes resistant to taxanes. We have already launched a clinical study to evaluate eribulin mesylate as the second-line treatment after taxane-failure. Several clinical studies are now ongoing or planned to evaluate the effect of multi-kinase inhibitors such as sorafenib or pazopanib (clinicaltrials.gov). We hope the treatment of CAS will be dramatically improved, as it has for melanoma, in the near future.

AUTHOR CONTRIBUTIONS

I have full responsibility of this article. YF wrote the part of the manuscript. KY, TF, YN, NO, RW, YI, and MF confirmed the manuscript for submission.

ACKNOWLEDGMENTS

We would like to thank F. Miyamasu of the Medical English Communication Center of the University of Tsukuba for English revision.

REFERENCES

1. Mobini N. Cutaneous epithelioid angiosarcoma: a neoplasm with potential pitfalls in diagnosis. *J Cutan Pathol* (2009) 36(3):362–9. doi:10.1111/j.1600-0560.2008.01052.x

2. Lucas DR. Angiosarcoma, radiation-associated angiosarcoma, and atypical vascular lesion. *Arch Pathol Lab Med* (2009) 133(11):1804–9. doi:10.1043/1543-2165-133.11.1804

3. Rouhani P, Fletcher CD, Devesa SS, Toro JR. Cutaneous soft tissue sarcoma incidence patterns in the U.S.: an analysis of 12,114 cases. *Cancer* (2008) 113(3):616–27. doi:10.1002/cncr.23571

4. Pawlik TM, Paulino AF, McGinn CJ, Baker LH, Cohen DS, Morris JS, et al. Cutaneous angiosarcoma of the scalp: a multidisciplinary approach. *Cancer* (2003) 98(8):1716–26. doi:10.1002/cncr.11667

5. Guadagnolo BA, Zagars GK, Araujo D, Ravi V, Shellenberger TD, Sturgis EM. Outcomes after definitive treatment for cutaneous angiosarcoma of the face and scalp. *Head Neck* (2011) 33(5):661–7. doi:10.1002/hed.21513

6. Buschmann A, Lehnhardt M, Toman N, Preiler P, Salakdeh MS, Muehlberger T. Surgical treatment of angiosarcoma of the scalp: less is more. *Ann Plast Surg* (2008) 61(4):399–403. doi:10.1097/SAP.0b013e31816b31f8

7. Fujisawa Y, Nakamura Y, Kawachi Y, Otsuka F. Comparison between taxane-based chemotherapy with conventional surgery-based therapy for cutaneous angiosarcoma: a single-center experience. *J Dermatolog Treat* (2014) 25(5):419–23. doi:10.3109/09546634.2012.754839

8. Maddox JC, Evans HL. Angiosarcoma of skin and soft tissue: a study of forty-four cases. *Cancer* (1981) 48(8):1907–21. doi:10.1002/1097-0142(19811015)48:8<1907::AID-CNCR2820480832>3.0.CO;2-T

9. Hodgkinson DJ, Soule EH, Woods JE. Cutaneous angiosarcoma of the head and neck. *Cancer* (1979) 44(3):1106–13. doi:10.1002/1097-0142(197909)44:3<1106::AID-CNCR2820440345>3.0.CO;2-C

10. Meis-Kindblom JM, Kindblom LG. Angiosarcoma of soft tissue: a study of 80 cases. *Am J Surg Pathol* (1998) 22(6):683–97. doi:10.1097/00000478-199806000-00005

11. Albores-Saavedra J, Schwartz AM, Henson DE, Kostun L, Hart A, Angeles-Albores D, et al. Cutaneous angiosarcoma. Analysis of 434 cases from the

surveillance, epidemiology, and end results program, 1973-2007. *Ann Diagn Pathol* (2011) 15(2):93–7. doi:10.1016/j.anndiagpath.2010.07.012

12. Ravi V, Patel S. Vascular sarcomas. *Curr Oncol Rep* (2013) 15(4):347–55. doi:10.1007/s11912-013-0328-2

13. Kurisetty V, Bryan BA. Aberrations in angiogenic signaling and MYC amplifications are distinguishing features of angiosarcoma. *Angiol Open Access* (2013) 1:17309. doi:10.4172/2329-9495.1000102

14. Kohen D, Dross P. Angiosarcoma of the scalp. *Del Med J* (2013) 85(9):269–72.

15. Stewart FW, Treves N. Lymphangiosarcoma in postmastectomy lymphedema; a report of six cases in elephantiasis chirurgica. *Cancer* (1948) 1(1):64–81. doi:10.1002/1097-0142(194805)1:1<64::AID-CNCR2820010105>3.0.CO;2-W

16. Depla AL, Scharloo-Karels CH, de Jong MA, Oldenborg S, Kolff MW, Oei SB, et al. Treatment and prognostic factors of radiation-associated angiosarcoma (RAAS) after primary breast cancer: a systematic review. *Eur J Cancer* (2014) 50(10):1779–88. doi:10.1016/j.ejca.2014.03.002

17. Fujisawa Y, Ito M, Mori K, Okada S, Nakamura Y, Kawachi Y, et al. Intra-arterial mitoxantrone/paclitaxel in angiosarcoma of the lower limb associated with chronic lymphedema (Stewart-Treves syndrome) in a patient with cervical cancer. *Eur J Dermatol* (2011) 21(1):119–20.

18. Sharma A, Schwartz RA. Stewart-Treves syndrome: pathogenesis and management. *J Am Acad Dermatol* (2012) 67(6):1342–8. doi:10.1016/j.jaad.2012.04.028

19. Fujisawa Y, Yoshino K, Kadono T, Miyagawa T, Nakamura Y, Fujimoto M. Chemoradiotherapy with taxane is superior to conventional surgery and radiotherapy in the management of cutaneous angiosarcoma: a multicentre, retrospective study. *Br J Dermatol* (2014) 171(6):1493–500. doi:10.1111/bjd.13110

20. Buehler D, Rice SR, Moody JS, Rush P, Hafez GR, Attia S, et al. Angiosarcoma outcomes and prognostic factors: a 25-year single institution experience. *Am J Clin Oncol* (2014) 37(5):473–9. doi:10.1097/COC.0b013e31827e4e7b

21. Lee JH, Jeong YJ, Oh DY, Kim SW, Rhie JW, Ahn ST. Clinical experience of stewart-treves syndrome in the lower leg. *Arch Plast Surg* (2013) 40(3):275–7. doi:10.5999/aps.2013.40.3.275

22. Veiga RR, Nascimento BA, Carvalho AH, Brito AC, Bittencourt MJ. Stewart-Treves Syndrome of the lower extremity. *An Bras Dermatol* (2015) 90(3 Suppl 1):232–4. doi:10.1590/abd1806-4841.20153926

23. Yap J, Chuba PJ, Thomas R, Aref A, Lucas D, Severson RK, et al. Sarcoma as a second malignancy after treatment for breast cancer. *Int J Radiat Oncol Biol Phys* (2002) 52(5):1231–7. doi:10.1016/S0360-3016(01)02799-7

24. Young RJ, Brown NJ, Reed MW, Hughes D, Woll PJ. Angiosarcoma. *Lancet Oncol* (2010) 11(10):983–91. doi:10.1016/S1470-2045(10)70023-1

25. Patel SH, Hayden RE, Hinni ML, Wong WW, Foote RL, Milani S, et al. Angiosarcoma of the scalp and face: the Mayo Clinic experience. *JAMA Otolaryngol Head Neck Surg* (2015) 141(4):335–40. doi:10.1001/jamaoto.2014.3584

26. Rosai J, Sumner HW, Kostianovsky M, Perez-Mesa C. Angiosarcoma of the skin. A clinicopathologic and fine structural study. *Hum Pathol* (1976) 7(1):83–109. doi:10.1016/S0046-8177(76)80007-X

27. Nomura M, Nakaya Y, Saito K, Miyoshi H, Kishi F, Hibino S, et al. Hemo-pneumothorax secondary to multiple cavitary metastasis in angiosarcoma of the scalp. *Respiration* (1994) 61(2):109–12. doi:10.1159/000196318

28. Vogt T, Brockmeyer N, Kutzner H, Schofer H. Brief S1 guidelines – cutaneous angiosarcoma and Kaposi sarcoma. *J Dtsch Dermatol Ges* (2013) 11(Suppl 3):2–10. doi:10.1111/ddg.12015_2

29. Ohsawa M, Naka N, Tomita Y, Kawamori D, Kanno H, Aozasa K. Use of immunohistochemical procedures in diagnosing angiosarcoma. Evaluation of 98 cases. *Cancer* (1995) 75(12):2867–74. doi:10.1002/1097-0142(19950615)75:12<2867::AID-CNCR2820751212>3.0.CO;2-8

30. Mocellin S, Rossi CR, Brandes A, Nitti D. Adult soft tissue sarcomas: conventional therapies and molecularly targeted approaches. *Cancer Treat Rev* (2006) 32(1):9–27. doi:10.1016/j.ctrv.2005.10.003

31. Fury MG, Antonescu CR, Van Zee KJ, Brennan MF, Maki RG. A 14-year retrospective review of angiosarcoma: clinical characteristics, prognostic factors, and treatment outcomes with surgery and chemotherapy. *Cancer J* (2005) 11(3):241–7. doi:10.1097/00130404-200505000-00011

32. Sinnamon AJ, Neuwirth MG, McMillan MT, Ecker BL, Bartlett EK, Zhang PJ, et al. A prognostic model for resectable soft tissue and cutaneous angiosarcoma. *J Surg Oncol* (2016) 114(5):557–63. doi:10.1002/jso.24352

33. Fayette J, Martin E, Piperno-Neumann S, Le Cesne A, Robert C, Bonvalot S, et al. Angiosarcomas, a heterogeneous group of sarcomas with specific behavior depending on primary site: a retrospective study of 161 cases. *Ann Oncol* (2007) 18(12):2030–6. doi:10.1093/annonc/mdm381

34. Ogawa K, Takahashi K, Asato Y, Yamamoto Y, Taira K, Matori S, et al. Treatment and prognosis of angiosarcoma of the scalp and face: a retrospective analysis of 48 patients. *Br J Radiol* (2012) 85(1019):e1127–33. doi:10.1259/bjr/31655219

35. Lydiatt WM, Shaha AR, Shah JP. Angiosarcoma of the head and neck. *Am J Surg* (1994) 168(5):451–4. doi:10.1016/S0002-9610(05)80097-2

36. Holden CA, Spittle MF, Jones EW. Angiosarcoma of the face and scalp, prognosis and treatment. *Cancer* (1987) 59(5):1046–57. doi:10.1002/1097-0142(19870301)59:5<1046::AID-CNCR2820590533>3.0.CO;2-6

37. Lahat G, Dhuka AR, Hallevi H, Xiao L, Zou C, Smith KD, et al. Angiosarcoma: clinical and molecular insights. *Ann Surg* (2010) 251(6):1098–106. doi:10.1097/SLA.0b013e3181dbb75a

38. Morgan MB, Swann M, Somach S, Eng W, Smoller B. Cutaneous angiosarcoma: a case series with prognostic correlation. *J Am Acad Dermatol* (2004) 50(6):867–74. doi:10.1016/j.jaad.2003.10.671

39. Naka N, Ohsawa M, Tomita Y, Kanno H, Uchida A, Myoui A, et al. Prognostic factors in angiosarcoma: a multivariate analysis of 55 cases. *J Surg Oncol* (1996) 61(3):170–6. doi:10.1002/(SICI)1096-9098(199603)61:3<170::AID-JSO2>3.0.CO;2-8

40. Perez MC, Padhya TA, Messina JL, Jackson RS, Gonzalez RJ, Bui MM, et al. Cutaneous angiosarcoma: a single-institution experience. *Ann Surg Oncol* (2013) 20(11):3391–7. doi:10.1245/s10434-013-3083-6

41. Abraham JA, Hornicek FJ, Kaufman AM, Harmon DC, Springfield DS, Raskin KA, et al. Treatment and outcome of 82 patients with angiosarcoma. *Ann Surg Oncol* (2007) 14(6):1953–67. doi:10.1245/s10434-006-9335-y

42. Sasaki R, Soejima T, Kishi K, Imajo Y, Hirota S, Kamikonya N, et al. Angiosarcoma treated with radiotherapy: impact of tumor type and size on outcome. *Int J Radiat Oncol Biol Phys* (2002) 52(4):1032–40. doi:10.1016/S0360-3016(01)02753-5

43. Mark RJ, Poen JC, Tran LM, Fu YS, Juillard GF. Angiosarcoma. A report of 67 patients and a review of the literature. *Cancer* (1996) 77(11):2400–6. doi:10.1002/(SICI)1097-0142(19960601)77:11<2400::AID-CNCR32>3.0.CO;2-Z

44. Köhler HF, Neves RI, Brechtbühl ER, Mattos Granja NV, Ikeda MK, Kowalski LP. Cutaneous angiosarcoma of the head and neck: report of 23 cases from a single institution. *Otolaryngol Head Neck Surg* (2008) 139(4):519–24. doi:10.1016/j.otohns.2008.07.022

45. Ward JR, Feigenberg SJ, Mendenhall NP, Marcus RB Jr, Mendenhall WM. Radiation therapy for angiosarcoma. *Head Neck* (2003) 25(10):873–8. doi:10.1002/hed.10276

46. Espat NJ, Lewis JJ, Woodruff JM, Antonescu C, Xia J, Leung D, et al. Confirmed angiosarcoma: prognostic factors and outcome in 50 prospectively followed patients. *Sarcoma* (2000) 4(4):173–7. doi:10.1080/13577140020025896

47. Mark RJ, Tran LM, Sercarz J, Fu YS, Calcaterra TC, Juillard GF. Angiosarcoma of the head and neck. The UCLA experience 1955 through 1990. *Arch Otolaryngol Head Neck Surg* (1993) 119(9):973–8. doi:10.1001/archotol.1993.01880210061009

48. Morrison WH, Byers RM, Garden AS, Evans HL, Ang KK, Peters LJ. Cutaneous angiosarcoma of the head and neck. A therapeutic dilemma. *Cancer* (1995) 76(2):319–27. doi:10.1002/1097-0142(19950715)76:2<319::AID-CNCR2820760224>3.0.CO;2-8

49. Mizukami S, Taguchi M, Suzuki T, Tetsuya T. Angiosarcoma: a report of 260 patients based on a study conducted by The Japanese Association of Dermatologic Surgery, and review of the literature. *Skin Cancer* (2009) 24(3):350–62. doi:10.5227/skincancer.24.350

50. Hwang K, Kim MY, Lee SH. Recommendations for therapeutic decisions of angiosarcoma of the scalp and face. *J Craniofac Surg* (2015) 26(3):e253–6. doi:10.1097/SCS.0000000000001495

51. Shin JY, Roh SG, Lee NH, Yang KM. Predisposing factors for poor prognosis of angiosarcoma of the scalp and face: systematic review and meta-analysis. *Head Neck* (2017) 39(2):380–6. doi:10.1002/hed.24554

52. Trofymenko O, Curiel-Lewandrowski C. Surgical treatment associated with improved survival in patients with cutaneous angiosarcoma. *J Eur Acad Dermatol Venereol* (2018) 32(1):e29–31. doi:10.1111/jdv.14479

53. Lahat G, Dhuka AR, Lahat S, Smith KD, Pollock RE, Hunt KK, et al. Outcome of locally recurrent and metastatic angiosarcoma. *Ann Surg Oncol* (2009) 16(9):2502–9. doi:10.1245/s10434-009-0569-3

54. Dossett LA, Harrington M, Cruse CW, Gonzalez RJ. Cutaneous angiosarcoma. *Curr Probl Cancer* (2015) 39(4):258–63. doi:10.1016/j.currproblcancer.2015.07.007

55. Shustef E, Kazlouskaya V, Prieto VG, Ivan D, Aung PP. Cutaneous angiosarcoma: a current update. *J Clin Pathol* (2017) 70(11):917–25. doi:10.1136/jclinpath-2017-204601

56. Lee BL, Chen CF, Chen PC, Lee HC, Liao WC, Perng CK, et al. Investigation of prognostic features in primary cutaneous and soft tissue angiosarcoma after surgical resection: a retrospective study. *Ann Plast Surg* (2017) 78(3 Suppl 2):S41–6. doi:10.1097/SAP.0000000000001004

57. Steward WP, Verweij J, Somers R, Blackledge G, Clavel M, Van Oosterom AT, et al. Doxorubicin plus ifosfamide with rhGM-CSF in the treatment of advanced adult soft-tissue sarcomas: preliminary results of a phase II study from the EORTC Soft-Tissue and Bone Sarcoma Group. *J Cancer Res Clin Oncol* (1991) 117(Suppl 4):S193–7. doi:10.1007/BF01613226

58. Young RJ, Natukunda A, Litière S, Woll PJ, Wardelmann E, van der Graaf WT. First-line anthracycline-based chemotherapy for angiosarcoma and other soft tissue sarcoma subtypes: pooled analysis of eleven European Organisation for Research and Treatment of Cancer Soft Tissue and Bone Sarcoma Group trials. *Eur J Cancer* (2014) 50(18):3178–86. doi:10.1016/j.ejca.2014.10.004

59. Sparano JA. Taxanes for breast cancer: an evidence-based review of randomized phase II and phase III trials. *Clin Breast Cancer* (2000) 1(1):32–40. doi:10.3816/CBC.2000.n.002

60. Novello S, Le Chevalier T. European perspectives on paclitaxel/platinum-based therapy for advanced non-small cell lung cancer. *Semin Oncol* (2001) 28(4 Suppl 14):3–9. doi:10.1053/sonc.2001.27606

61. Sakamoto J, Matsui T, Kodera Y. Paclitaxel chemotherapy for the treatment of gastric cancer. *Gastric Cancer* (2009) 12(2):69–78. doi:10.1007/s10120-009-0505-z

62. Hoskins PJ, Le N, Ellard S, Lee U, Martin LA, Swenerton KD, et al. Carboplatin plus paclitaxel for advanced or recurrent uterine malignant mixed mullerian tumors. The British Columbia Cancer Agency experience. *Gynecol Oncol* (2008) 108(1):58–62. doi:10.1016/j.ygyno.2007.08.084

63. Patel SR, Linke KA, Burgess MA, Papadopoulos NE, Plager C, Jenkins J, et al. Phase II study of paclitaxel in patients with soft tissue sarcomas. *Sarcoma* (1997) 1(2):95–7. doi:10.1080/13577149778362

64. Casper ES, Waltzman RJ, Schwartz GK, Sugarman A, Pfister D, Ilson D, et al. Phase II trial of paclitaxel in patients with soft-tissue sarcoma. *Cancer Invest* (1998) 16(7):442–6. doi:10.3109/07357909809011697

65. Belotti D, Vergani V, Drudis T, Borsotti P, Pitelli MR, Viale G, et al. The microtubule-affecting drug paclitaxel has antiangiogenic activity. *Clin Cancer Res* (1996) 2(11):1843–9.

66. Klauber N, Parangi S, Flynn E, Hamel E, D'Amato RJ. Inhibition of angiogenesis and breast cancer in mice by the microtubule inhibitors 2-methoxyestradiol and taxol. *Cancer Res* (1997) 57(1):81–6.

67. Saville MW, Lietzau J, Pluda JM, Feuerstein I, Odom J, Wilson WH, et al. Treatment of HIV-associated Kaposi's sarcoma with paclitaxel. *Lancet* (1995) 346(8966):26–8. doi:10.1016/S0140-6736(95)92654-2

68. Welles L, Saville MW, Lietzau J, Pluda JM, Wyvill KM, Feuerstein I, et al. Phase II trial with dose titration of paclitaxel for the therapy of human immunodeficiency virus-associated Kaposi's sarcoma. *J Clin Oncol* (1998) 16(3):1112–21. doi:10.1200/JCO.1998.16.3.1112

69. Fata F, O'Reilly E, Ilson D, Pfister D, Leffel D, Kelsen DP, et al. Paclitaxel in the treatment of patients with angiosarcoma of the scalp or face. *Cancer* (1999) 86(10):2034–7. doi:10.1002/(SICI)1097-0142(19991115)86:10<2034::AID-CNCR21>3.0.CO;2-P

70. Penel N, Bui BN, Bay JO, Cupissol D, Ray-Coquard I, Piperno-Neumann S, et al. Phase II trial of weekly paclitaxel for unresectable angiosarcoma: the ANGIOTAX Study. *J Clin Oncol* (2008) 26(32):5269–74. doi:10.1200/JCO.2008.17.3146

71. Italiano A, Cioffi A, Penel N, Levra MG, Delcambre C, Kalbacher E, et al. Comparison of doxorubicin and weekly paclitaxel efficacy in metastatic angiosarcomas. *Cancer* (2012) 118(13):3330–6. doi:10.1002/cncr.26599

72. Eriksson M. Histology driven chemotherapy of soft-tissue sarcoma. *Ann Oncol* (2010) 21(Suppl 7):vii270–6. doi:10.1093/annonc/mdq285

73. Nakamura Y, Hori E, Furuta J, Kawachi Y, Otsuka F. Complete long-term response of angiosarcoma of the scalp with cervical lymph node metastases treated with a combination of weekly and monthly docetaxel. *Br J Dermatol* (2010) 163(6):1357–8. doi:10.1111/j.1365-2133.2010.10000.x

74. Ray-Coquard IL, Domont J, Tresch-Bruneel E, Bompas E, Cassier PA, Mir O, et al. Paclitaxel given once per week with or without bevacizumab in patients with advanced angiosarcoma: a randomized phase II trial. *J Clin Oncol* (2015) 33(25):2797–802. doi:10.1200/JCO.2015.60.8505

75. Ito T, Uchi H, Nakahara T, Tsuji G, Oda Y, Hagihara A, et al. Cutaneous angiosarcoma of the head and face: a single-center analysis of treatment outcomes in 43 patients in Japan. *J Cancer Res Clin Oncol* (2016) 142(6):1387–94. doi:10.1007/s00432-016-2151-2

76. Stacchiotti S, Palassini E, Sanfilippo R, Vincenzi B, Arena MG, Bochicchio AM, et al. Gemcitabine in advanced angiosarcoma: a retrospective case series analysis from the Italian Rare Cancer Network. *Ann Oncol* (2012) 23(2):501–8. doi:10.1093/annonc/mdr066

77. Patel SR, Gandhi V, Jenkins J, Papadopolous N, Burgess MA, Plager C, et al. Phase II clinical investigation of gemcitabine in advanced soft tissue sarcomas and window evaluation of dose rate on gemcitabine triphosphate accumulation. *J Clin Oncol* (2001) 19(15):3483–9. doi:10.1200/JCO.2001.19.15.3483

78. Leu KM, Ostruszka LJ, Shewach D, Zalupski M, Sondak V, Biermann JS, et al. Laboratory and clinical evidence of synergistic cytotoxicity of sequential treatment with gemcitabine followed by docetaxel in the treatment of sarcoma. *J Clin Oncol* (2004) 22(9):1706–12. doi:10.1200/JCO.2004.08.043

79. Bay JO, Ray-Coquard I, Fayette J, Leyvraz S, Cherix S, Piperno-Neumann S, et al. Docetaxel and gemcitabine combination in 133 advanced soft-tissue sarcomas: a retrospective analysis. *Int J Cancer* (2006) 119(3):706–11. doi:10.1002/ijc.21867

80. Merimsky O, Meller I, Flusser G, Kollender Y, Issakov J, Weil-Ben-Arush M, et al. Gemcitabine in soft tissue or bone sarcoma resistant to standard chemotherapy: a phase II study. *Cancer Chemother Pharmacol* (2000) 45(2):177–81. doi:10.1007/s002800050027

81. Scott MT, Portnow LH, Morris CG, Marcus RB Jr, Mendenhall NP, Mendenhall WM, et al. Radiation therapy for angiosarcoma: the 35-year University of Florida experience. *Am J Clin Oncol* (2013) 36(2):174–80. doi:10.1097/COC.0b013e3182436ea3

82. Kinard JD, Zwicker RD, Schmidt-Ullrich RK, Kaufman N, Pieters R. Short communication: total craniofacial photon shell technique for radiotherapy of extensive angiosarcomas of the head. *Br J Radiol* (1996) 69(820):351–5. doi:10.1259/0007-1285-69-820-351

83. Jang R, Darling G, Wong RK. Multimodality approaches for the curative treatment of esophageal cancer. *J Natl Compr Canc Netw* (2015) 13(2):229–38. doi:10.6004/jnccn.2015.0029

84. Wee JT, Anderson BO, Corry J, D'Cruz A, Soo KC, Qian CN, et al. Management of the neck after chemoradiotherapy for head and neck cancers in Asia: consensus statement from the Asian Oncology Summit 2009. *Lancet Oncol* (2009) 10(11):1086–92. doi:10.1016/S1470-2045(09)70266-9

85. Glimelius B, Holm T, Blomqvist L. Chemotherapy in addition to preoperative radiotherapy in locally advanced rectal cancer – a systematic overview. *Rev Recent Clin Trials* (2008) 3(3):204–11. doi:10.2174/157488708785700294

86. Duenas-Gonzalez A, Campbell S. Global strategies for the treatment of early-stage and advanced cervical cancer. *Curr Opin Obstet Gynecol* (2016) 28(1):11–7. doi:10.1097/GCO.0000000000000234

87. Lagrange JL, Bondiau PY, Tessier E, Chauvel P, Renée N, Etienne MC, et al. Tumoral platinum concentrations in patients treated with repeated low-dose cisplatin as a radiosensitizer. *Int J Cancer* (1996) 68(4):452–6. doi:10.1002/(SICI)1097-0215(19961115)68:4<452::AID-IJC9>3.0.CO;2-#

88. Metro G, Fabi A, Mirri MA, Vidiri A, Pace A, Carosi M, et al. Phase II study of fixed dose rate gemcitabine as radiosensitizer for newly diagnosed glioblastoma multiforme. *Cancer Chemother Pharmacol* (2010) 65(2):391–7. doi:10.1007/s00280-009-1155-x

89. Creane M, Seymour CB, Colucci S, Mothersill C. Radiobiological effects of docetaxel (Taxotere): a potential radiation sensitizer. *Int J Radiat Biol* (1999) 75(6):731–7. doi:10.1080/095530099140078

90. Tishler RB, Schiff PB, Geard CR, Hall EJ. Taxol: a novel radiation sensitizer. *Int J Radiat Oncol Biol Phys* (1992) 22(3):613–7. doi:10.1016/0360-3016(92)90888-O

91. Shibao K, Fujisawa Y, Nakamura Y, Maruyama H, Furuta JI, Okiyama N, et al. Cutaneous squamous cell carcinoma treated with preoperative intra-arterial chemoradiation therapy. *J Dtsch Dermatol Ges* (2017) 15(7):724–6. doi:10.1111/ddg.12590

92. Fujisawa Y, Ishitsuka Y, Nakamura Y, Kawachi Y, Otsuka F, et al. Metastatic squamous cell carcinoma of the buttock treated with chemoradiation using cisplatin and 5-fluorouracil. *J Am Acad Dermatol* (2009) 60(2):355–7. doi:10.1016/j.jaad.2008.08.002

93. Fujisawa Y, Umebayashi Y, Ichikawa E, Kawachi Y, Otsuka F. Chemoradiation using low-dose cisplatin and 5-fluorouracil in locally advanced squamous cell carcinoma of the skin: a report of two cases. *J Am Acad Dermatol* (2006) 55(5 Suppl):S81–5. doi:10.1016/j.jaad.2005.12.035

94. Nissen NN, Polverini PJ, Koch AE, Volin MV, Gamelli RL, DiPietro LA. Vascular endothelial growth factor mediates angiogenic activity during the proliferative phase of wound healing. *Am J Pathol* (1998) 152(6):1445–52.

95. Itakura E, Yamamoto H, Oda Y, Tsuneyoshi M. Detection and characterization of vascular endothelial growth factors and their receptors in a series of angiosarcomas. *J Surg Oncol* (2008) 97(1):74–81. doi:10.1002/jso.20766

96. Hashimoto M, Ohsawa M, Ohnishi A, Naka N, Hirota S, Kitamura Y, et al. Expression of vascular endothelial growth factor and its receptor mRNA in angiosarcoma. *Lab Invest* (1995) 73(6):859–63.

97. McLaughlin ER, Brown LF, Weiss SW, Mulliken JB, Perez-Atayde A, Arbiser JL. VEGF and its receptors are expressed in a pediatric angiosarcoma in a patient with Aicardi's syndrome. *J Invest Dermatol* (2000) 114(6):1209–10. doi:10.1046/j.1523-1747.2000.00005-3.x

98. Miki Y, Tada T, Kamo R, Hosono MN, Tamiya H, Shimatani Y, et al. Single institutional experience of the treatment of angiosarcoma of the face and scalp. *Br J Radiol* (2013) 86(1030):20130439. doi:10.1259/bjr.20130439

99. Rhomberg W, Wink A, Pokrajac B, Eiter H, Hackl A, Pakisch B, et al. Treatment of vascular soft tissue sarcomas with razoxane. vindesine, and radiation. *Int J Radiat Oncol Biol Phys* (2009) 74(1):187–91. doi:10.1016/j.ijrobp.2008.06.1492

100. Gambini D, Visintin R, Locatelli E, Galassi B, Bareggi C, Runza L, et al. Paclitaxel-dependent prolonged and persistent complete remission four years from first recurrence of secondary breast angiosarcoma. *Tumori* (2009) 95(6):828–31.

101. Nagano T, Yamada Y, Ikeda T, Kanki H, Kamo T, Nishigori C. Docetaxel: a therapeutic option in the treatment of cutaneous angiosarcoma: report of 9 patients. *Cancer* (2007) 110(3):648–51. doi:10.1002/cncr.22822

102. Sarcoma Meta-Analysis Collaboration. Adjuvant chemotherapy for localised resectable soft tissue sarcoma in adults. *Cochrane Database Syst Rev* (2000) 4:CD001419. doi:10.1002/14651858.CD001419

103. DeMartelaere SL, Roberts D, Burgess MA, Morrison WH, Pisters PW, Sturgis EM, et al. Neoadjuvant chemotherapy-specific and overall treatment outcomes in patients with cutaneous angiosarcoma of the face with periorbital involvement. *Head Neck* (2008) 30(5):639–46. doi:10.1002/hed.20757

104. Amo Y, Masuzawa M, Hamada Y, Katsuoka K. Serum concentrations of vascular endothelial growth factor in angiosarcomas with and without p53 gene mutation. *Acta Derm Venereol* (2002) 82(5):373–4. doi:10.1080/000155502320624122

105. Arbiser JL, Larsson H, Claesson-Welsh L, Bai X, LaMontagne K, Weiss SW, et al. Overexpression of VEGF 121 in immortalized endothelial cells causes conversion to slowly growing angiosarcoma and high level expression of the VEGF receptors VEGFR-1 and VEGFR-2 in vivo. *Am J Pathol* (2000) 156(4):1469–76. doi:10.1016/S0002-9440(10)65015-8

106. Hasenstein JR, Kasmerchak K, Buehler D, Hafez GR, Cleary K, Moody JS, et al. Efficacy of Tie2 receptor antagonism in angiosarcoma. *Neoplasia* (2012) 14(2):131–40. doi:10.1593/neo.111770

107. Agulnik M, Yarber JL, Okuno SH, von Mehren M, Jovanovic BD, Brockstein BE, et al. An open-label, multicenter, phase II study of bevacizumab for the treatment of angiosarcoma and epithelioid hemangioendotheliomas. *Ann Oncol* (2013) 24(1):257–63. doi:10.1093/annonc/mds237

108. Koontz BF, Miles EF, Rubio MA, Madden JF, Fisher SR, Scher RL, et al. Preoperative radiotherapy and bevacizumab for angiosarcoma of the head and neck: two case studies. *Head Neck* (2008) 30(2):262–6. doi:10.1002/hed.20674

109. Ray-Coquard I, Italiano A, Bompas E, Le Cesne A, Robin YM, Chevreau C, et al. Sorafenib for patients with advanced angiosarcoma: a phase II Trial from the French Sarcoma Group (GSF/GETO). *Oncologist* (2012) 17(2):260–6. doi:10.1634/theoncologist.2011-0237

110. van der Graaf WT, Blay JY, Chawla SP, Kim DW, Bui-Nguyen B, Casali PG, et al. Pazopanib for metastatic soft-tissue sarcoma (PALETTE): a randomised, double-blind, placebo-controlled phase 3 trial. *Lancet* (2012) 379(9829):1879–86. doi:10.1016/S0140-6736(12)60651-5

111. Maki RG, D'Adamo DR, Keohan ML, Saulle M, Schuetze SM, Undevia SD, et al. Phase II study of sorafenib in patients with metastatic or recurrent sarcomas. *J Clin Oncol* (2009) 27(19):3133–40. doi:10.1200/JCO.2008.20.4495

112. Ogata D, Yanagisawa H, Suzuki K, Oashi K, Yamazaki N, Tsuchida T. Pazopanib treatment slows progression and stabilizes disease in patients with taxane-resistant cutaneous angiosarcoma. *Med Oncol* (2016) 33(10):116. doi:10.1007/s12032-016-0831-z

113. Kitamura S, Yanagi T, Inamura Y, Hata H, Imafuku K, Yoshino K, et al. Pazopanib does not bring remarkable improvement in patients with angiosarcoma. *J Dermatol* (2017) 44(1):64–7. doi:10.1111/1346-8138.13558

114. Jordan MA, Kamath K, Manna T, Okouneva T, Miller HP, Davis C, et al. The primary antimitotic mechanism of action of the synthetic halichondrin E7389 is suppression of microtubule growth. *Mol Cancer Ther* (2005) 4(7):1086–95. doi:10.1158/1535-7163.MCT-04-0345

115. Schöffski P, Chawla S, Maki RG, Italiano A, Gelderblom H, Choy E, et al. Eribulin versus dacarbazine in previously treated patients with advanced liposarcoma or leiomyosarcoma: a randomised, open-label, multicentre, phase 3 trial. *Lancet* (2016) 387(10028):1629–37. doi:10.1016/S0140-6736(15)01283-0

116. Jordan MA, Wilson L. Microtubules as a target for anticancer drugs. *Nat Rev Cancer* (2004) 4(4):253–65. doi:10.1038/nrc1317

117. Wada N, Uchi H, Furue M. Case of angiosarcoma of the scalp successfully controlled by eribulin. *J Dermatol* (2018) 45(1):116–7. doi:10.1111/1346-8138.13775

118. Hodi FS, Chesney J, Pavlick AC, Robert C, Grossmann KF, McDermott DF, et al. Combined nivolumab and ipilimumab versus ipilimumab alone in patients with advanced melanoma: 2-year overall survival outcomes in a multicentre, randomised, controlled, phase 2 trial. *Lancet Oncol* (2016) 17(11):1558–68. doi:10.1016/S1470-2045(16)30366-7

119. Rizvi NA, Mazières J, Planchard D, Stinchcombe TE, Dy GK, Antonia SJ, et al. Activity and safety of nivolumab, an anti-PD-1 immune checkpoint inhibitor, for patients with advanced, refractory squamous non-small-cell lung cancer (CheckMate 063): a phase 2, single-arm trial. *Lancet Oncol* (2015) 16(3):257–65. doi:10.1016/S1470-2045(15)70054-9

120. Honda Y, Otsuka A, Ono S, Yamamoto Y, Seidel JA, Morita S, et al. Infiltration of PD-1-positive cells in combination with tumor site PD-L1 expression is a positive prognostic factor in cutaneous angiosarcoma. *Oncoimmunology* (2017) 6(1):e1253657. doi:10.1080/2162402X.2016.1253657

21

The Possibility of Deep Learning-Based, Computer-Aided Skin Tumor Classifiers

Yasuhiro Fujisawa*, Sae Inoue and Yoshiyuki Nakamura

Department of Dermatology, University of Tsukuba, Tsukuba, Japan

*Correspondence:
Yasuhiro Fujisawa
fujisan@md.tsukuba.ac.jp

The incidence of skin tumors has steadily increased. Although most are benign and do not affect survival, some of the more malignant skin tumors present a lethal threat if a delay in diagnosis permits them to become advanced. Ideally, an inspection by an expert dermatologist would accurately detect malignant skin tumors in the early stage; however, it is not practical for every single patient to receive intensive screening by dermatologists. To overcome this issue, many studies are ongoing to develop dermatologist-level, computer-aided diagnostics. Whereas, many systems that can classify dermoscopic images at this dermatologist-equivalent level have been reported, a much fewer number of systems that can classify conventional clinical images have been reported thus far. Recently, the introduction of deep-learning technology, a method that automatically extracts a set of representative features for further classification has dramatically improved classification efficacy. This new technology has the potential to improve the computer classification accuracy of conventional clinical images to the level of skilled dermatologists. In this review, this new technology and present development of computer-aided skin tumor classifiers will be summarized.

Keywords: artificial intelligence, deep learning, convolutional neural network, clinical image, dermoscopy, skin tumor classifier

INTRODUCTION

The incidence of skin cancers, including melanoma and non-melanoma skin cancers (NMSC), is globally increasing. In the United States, the incidence of melanoma is reported to be 22.1 per 100,000 people, the number of new yearly melanoma patients is estimated to be more than 63,000, and melanoma is now rated as the 6th most common of all cancers (1). In spite of new therapeutic agents, such as checkpoint and BRAF inhibitors which improve survival of advanced cases, melanomas are still lethal (2–4). On the other hand, most NMSCs, which are responsible for 4.3–5.4 million new cases each year in the United States (5, 6), can be treated simply by surgical removal. Most of these (>90%) are comprised of basal cell carcinomas (BCC) and squamous cell carcinomas (SCC) (7) and skilled dermatologists can detect these by clinical appearance and a tumor magnifying dermatoscope (8). Consequently, most SCCs and BCCs are detected at an early stage and resolved by surgery alone. However, SCC can become lethal when it metastasizes, since few standardized and effective therapies for advanced SCC have been established. Although metastatic BCC is very rare, any delay in diagnosis may allow tumors to become unresectable. Therefore, early detection of all skin cancers, not limited to melanoma, is required to prevent progression of these cancers to advanced stages and reduce skin cancer-related deaths.

Skin tumor screening is one solution for the early detection of skin cancer, but it is not practical for dermatologists to check all patients for skin tumors. In most countries, primary vigilance is maintained through primary care clinics before being referred to dermatologists and, consequently, up to 20% of patients consult at primary care clinics complaining about skin-related symptoms (9–11). A study by Julian et al. reported that 16% of patients with dermatologically related diseases had benign skin tumors, 3.3% had actinic keratosis, and 3% had malignant skin tumors (10), meaning ~20% of patients who consulted a primary care doctor with skin-related complaints received a tumor diagnosis. Similar results were reported by Kerr et al. (11), showing that 11.4% of studied patients had benign skin tumors with <5% having malignant skin tumors. Although the percentage of patients with malignant skin tumors among patients who consult at primary care clinics is not so high, primary care doctors are under a heavy burden to correctly screen patients who present with

skin-related symptoms and determine which patients are to be transferred to the dermatologists. Thus, any device or service that can accurately give the probability of malignancy by analyzing a simple photograph of the tumor would be very helpful for both primary care doctors and their patients. In this context, the development of artificial intelligence (AI) that can classify skin tumor images within seconds, at a skill level similar to trained dermatologists, is an ideal solution for this problem.

MACHINE LEARNING: NECESSITY OF LABELED DATA

Artificial Intelligence (AI) is a term used to describe machine software that can mimic human cognitive functions, such as learning and problem solving (12). Machine learning achieves this via changes in the program algorithm that allow it to complete tasks more efficiently. These changes

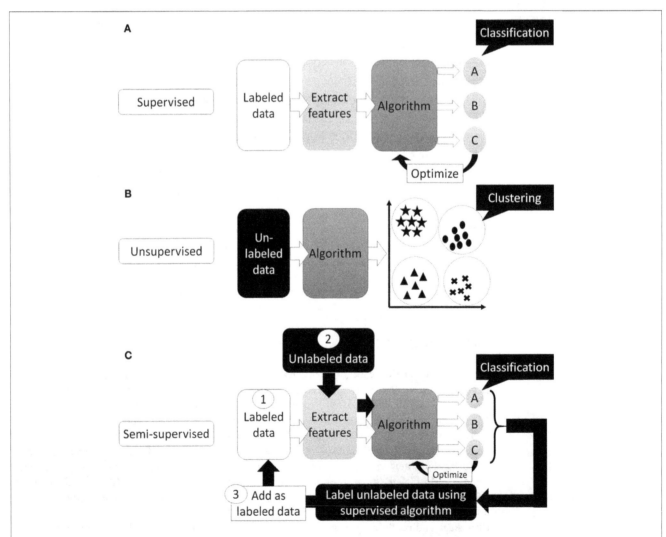

FIGURE 1 | Supervised or unsupervised training. **(A)** Supervised training which can predict classification or regression of the input data. **(B)** Unsupervised training which can cluster the data. **(C)** Semi-supervised training. First, train the algorithm by small number of labeled data. Then, use trained algorithm to "label" unlabeled data. Next, re-train algorithm using newly labeled data and originally labeled data. Finally, algorithm trained with all data and can predict classification or regression of the input data.

come from training using labeled data (supervised learning method, **Figure 1A**), data without labels (unsupervised learning method, **Figure 1B**), or both (semi-supervised learning method, **Figure 1C**) (13). For the supervised learning method, the program processes data and compares its output with the correct answer (label), adjusting its own parameters so that it can reach the correct result. This process should be repeated for as many training datasets as are available but, to achieve satisfactory efficiency, it requires a certain amount of labeled data to adjust the parameters. Thus, preparing a high enough number of datasets means that this supervised learning method could achieve a high classification efficacy (**Figure 2**). However, preparation of labeled data is often difficult, especially in the medical field. On the other hand, unsupervised learning does not require labeled data but instead uses a large amount of unlabeled data for learning. Where it differs from the supervised method is in the output of this algorithm, which clusters data instead of classifying it (**Figure 1B**). This method is useful for huge amounts of data without labels but, since this algorithm does not know the "answer," the meaning of each cluster in the output needs to be determined. The third method, semi-supervised learning, requires a small amount of labeled data with a large amount of unlabeled data. It functions on the principle that unlabeled data is classified using an algorithm trained with labeled data (**Figure 1C**). These unlabeled data are labeled with categories that were found to have high hit probability as calculated by the algorithm which was trained (supervised learning method) on the small amount of labeled data. These newly labeled data are added to the originally labeled data and supervised learning is then conducted again to re-train the algorithm. This method is useful for huge amounts of unlabeled data that would otherwise require a high cost to label. However, if a small error exists in the initial supervised learning algorithm, that error will be amplified at the end of the procedure. Collectively, the best way to train

AI algorithms is to prepare large amounts of correctly labeled data for supervised learning but this is often difficult for the medical field, since the "gold standard" pathological confirmation of lesion labels requires the excision of "all" lesions, which is not ethical for confirmed, benign lesions.

METHOD OF MACHINE LEARNING FOR IMAGE CLASSIFICATION: BEFORE THE DEEP LEARNING ERA

Developing a computer-aided diagnostic support system for skin cancer diagnosis requires many steps, as reviewed by Masood and Al-Jumaily (14) (**Figure 3**). The first step of the classification process starts by removing irrelevant structures and artifacts in the image (14, 15), such as hair, air bubbles/gel (if dermoscopy images are used), ink markings or reflectance, by using general image filters (16). These irrelevant objects or artifacts may affect the efficacy of border detection and skew the final output. Next, to analyze the internal properties for further analysis, the lesion within the objective tumor area should be separated from the surrounding skin in a procedure called segmentation. As it is not practical to manually define areas for all images, many automatic lesion segmentation systems have been reported (17–19), but this step is still a challenging task for engineers (16).

Next, the important features need to be extracted from the segmented image. Border shapes [asymmetry indices, symmetry axes, or aspect ratios (20)] or color features [average values and standard deviation of the RGB or HSV color channels (21)] are calculated and these values are used for further classification. However, there is a cost for attempting to extract more features, namely more training time, more complex algorithms, less generalization behavior, and less prediction accuracy. Thus, it is important to select only the useful feature values for classification

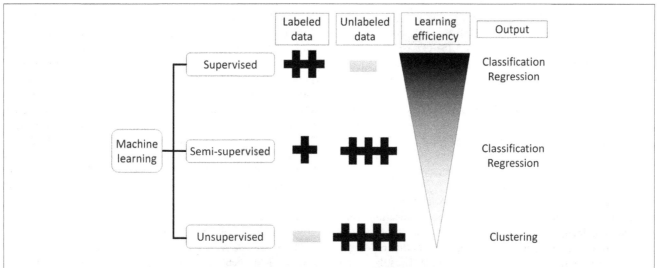

FIGURE 2 | Supervised, semi-supervised, and unsupervised training. Supervised training needs labeled data but can learn the most efficient. Unsupervised training does not need labeled data which sometimes difficult to prepare, but can only cluster the input data. Semi-supervised training can produce labeled data from unlabeled data using small number of labeled data.

while eliminating less useful ones (feature selection). There are diverse and numerous methods that have been proposed for this feature selection process (22–24).

Finally, the classification algorithm outputs the result using the selected feature values calculated in the previous phase. There are many different algorithms available for this classification task: support vector machine (25), decision tree (26), statistical [logistic regression (27)], or artificial neural network (ANN) (28). Of those, the performance of the support vector machine classifier is reported to be similar or better than other algorithms but, as it can only provide a dichotomous distinction between two classes (e.g., benign or malignant), this algorithm will not work for multi-class sorting with probabilities for each class. ANN, on the other hand, mimics the structure of biological neural networks in the human brain (**Figure 4A**) and can change connectivity between decision nodes (back propagation, **Figure 4B**) so that the network can achieve satisfactory results (28). Many ANN studies have reported on dermoscopic image analysis as (28) it has the ability to derive meaning from data which is too complex for humans to understand. The downside, however, is that ANN requires multiple repetitions of the training data to adjust network connections.

INTRODUCTION OF DEEP LEARNING TECHNOLOGY WITH CONVOLUTIONAL NEURAL NETWORKS

The image classification machine learning algorithms described above are very complex; they are based on hand-engineered features and are highly dependent on prior knowledge. For example, in some reports, more than 50 different feature values thought to be useful in the classification process, such as color, shape, or border information, were extracted from a single image for the training of the system (29, 30). In the annual ImageNet Large Scale Visual Recognition Challenge (ILSVR) computer vision competition, where 1 to 2 million images of objects are classified into 1,000 categories, a classifier using traditional machine learning had an error rate of 30% (31) compared to humans who logged an error rate of 5.1% (32). This striking gap in accuracy was dramatically reduced in the 2012 ILSVR competition; deep-learning technology using a convolutional neural network (CNN) achieved an error rate of 16.4% while other classifiers using traditional machine learning had an error rate of 26–30% (32). After the introduction of CNN, the error rates in the ILSVR competition dropped rapidly and the error rate in the 2017 competition was below 5%, indicating that CNN classified images more precisely than humans (http://image-net. org/challenges/LSVRC/2017/results).

This new CNN technology can learn and automatically determine what features are important for classification from the training image set. The extraction and selection of the features for classification was a key component of the traditional methods (33), and also the most difficult part. Thus, by using CNN, complicated image pre-processing is no longer necessary to obtain optimal feature values for the image classification. A schematic structure of CNN is shown in **Figure 5A**. In ANN,

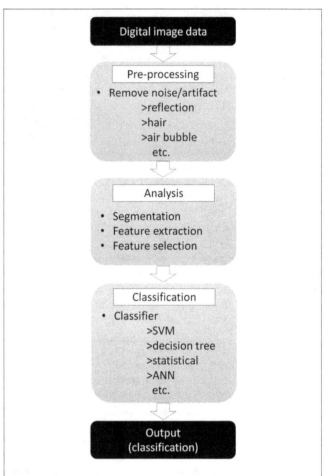

FIGURE 3 | Skin tumor classifier by "traditional" machine learning. Digital image data needs pre-processing to remove noise or artifact to improve the efficacy of the next step. Pre-processed images then analyzed to extract features required for classification step. Finally, classifier use extracted features to classify input images.

every node fully connects to the next layer (**Figure 4B**) but, in CNN, each node connects only to some nodes in the next layer (**Figure 5A**). This key feature of CNN can successfully capture the spatial and temporal dependencies in an image through the application of relevant filters (34). In this type of classifier, output values of the feature extractor usually input to a fully connected network and the softmax function finally converts input vectors to real numbers for normalization into a probability distribution (35). As an example, if the input images had 4 different classes, the final CNN layer would have 4 nodes as in **Figure 5A**. But, as the sum of the output of all 4 nodes would not be 1, it would be difficult to interpret the output. However, a softmax function that converts each node's output from 0 to 1 would allow for the components to add up to 1 and result in a final output that can be interpreted as a probability (0–100% probability).

There are many available CNN architectures used in the medical field such as LeNet (36), AlexNet (36), ZFNet (37), VGGNet (38), GoogLeNet (39, 40), ResNet (41), or SENet (42) (**Table 1**). Not only are these architectures free to use, pre-trained models are also available that are commonly trained by

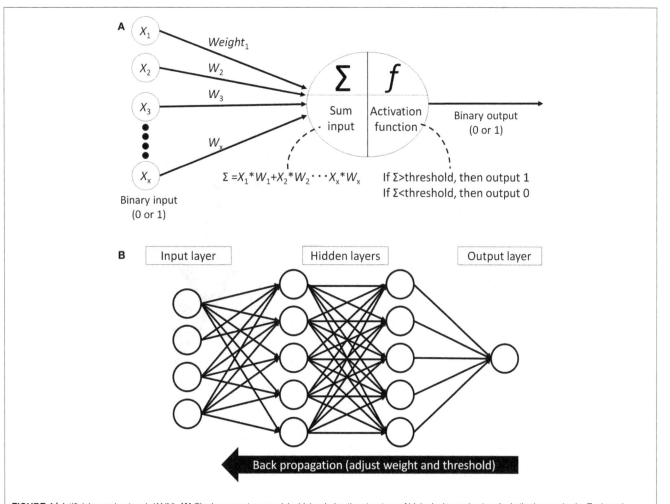

FIGURE 4 | Artificial neural network (ANN). **(A)** Single perceptron model which mimics the structure of biological neural networks in the human brain. Each node receives signal from other nodes (X1, X2... Xx). Add the multiplied values of input and weight (W) and when this sum(Σ) cross the threshold, then this node outputs signal. **(B)** An example of artificial neural network model which has hidden layer between input layer and output layer. All the nodes between the layers are fully connected and each connection has weight. Machine learning is adjusting each weights and thresholds in the network to reach the correct output (back propagation).

the previously mentioned ILSVR2012 dataset, which contains 1.2 million images within 1,000 classes (available at http://image-net.org/download-imageurls). Since the ability to extract image features by pre-trained models is very high, we can use these pre-trained models as a "feature extractor" in a technique called transfer learning (43). One example of transfer learning is shown in **Figure 5B**. Basically, the classifier part is replaced with an untrained classifier appropriate to the new task and the system is trained using a new training image dataset. This method is useful when large numbers of datasets cannot be prepared due to rarity, expense in collection/labeling, or inaccessibility (43). Therefore, transfer learning would be useful for the medical field since it is often difficult to collect images of rare diseases.

Collectively, the introduction of CNN has not only dramatically improved image classification efficacy, it has also made adoption of machine learning and image classification easier and cheaper since most of the initially needed resources are easily accessible.

SKIN TUMOR CLASSIFICATION BY USING DERMOSCOPIC IMAGES

The clinical diagnosis of melanoma is difficult since the morphological characteristics of other pigmented skin lesions may sometimes mimic it. Dermoscopy can magnify the skin and enables clinicians to better evaluate morphological features which are difficult to see with the naked eye. The introduction of dermoscopy has been reported to improve diagnostic sensitivity by 10–30% (44–46). Physicians are usually taught the ABCD-rule (47), Menzie's method (48), 7-point checklist (48), or some other pattern classification methods (49) to distinguish between melanoma and non-melanoma pigmented skin lesions. However, becoming an experienced dermoscopic reader (50, 51) who can score 90% diagnostic sensitivity (proportion of images correctly detected as malignant within all malignant images) and 59% diagnostic specificity (proportion of images correctly detected as benign within all benign images) require a significant time and training investment

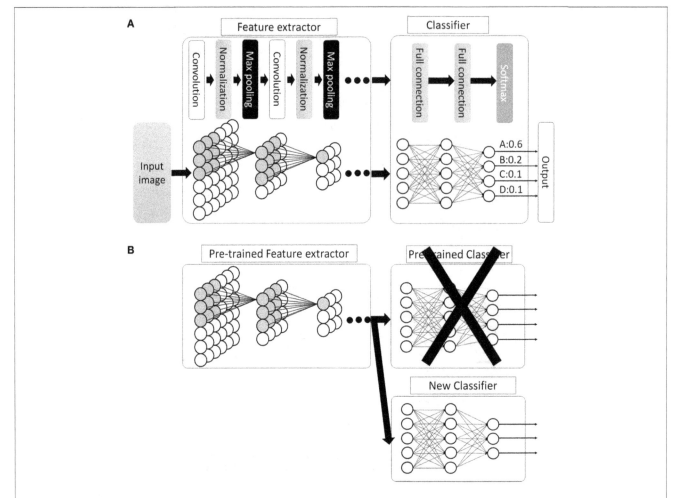

FIGURE 5 | Convolutional neural network (CNN). **(A)** Schematic image of CNN. Between the convolutional layers, each nodes connect to distinct nodes of the previous layer, which is different compared with ANN (as in **Figure 4B**, all the nodes between the layers are fully connected). By this feature, CNN can successfully capture the spatial and temporal dependencies in an image. Then, the fully connected classifier output the result as a probability distribution. **(B)** An example of transfer learning in CNN. In this example, replace classifier and use pre-trained CNN layers as feature extractor. Then, train the system to fit the new task.

(52). Moreover, even after such training, the readings are often complex and subjective.

To make readings more objective and qualitative, as well as support physicians using dermoscopy, many computer-based analyses of dermoscopic images to classify melanomas have been conducted. In a 2009 review by Rajpara et al. (53) that reviewed studies of AI classifiers (12 studies) and dermoscopy (23 studies) published between 1991 and 2002, the melanoma detection sensitivity and specificity of AI classifiers were already similar to that of physicians using dermoscopy; pooled sensitivity, and specificity for AI classifiers and physicians were 91 vs. 88% and 86 vs. 79%, respectively. In a 2013 review (14), 15 new studies on AI classifiers were included and showed sensitivities ranging from 60.7 to 98% and specificities ranging from 72 to 100%, which were similar to the previous 2009 report. Haenssle et al. reported on an AI classifier using the CNN deep learning-based algorithm and compared the classification efficiency against 58 dermatologists (54). Their CNN showed higher accuracy than most dermatologists (sensitivity 88.9 vs.

86.6% and specificity 82.5 vs. 71.3%, respectively) (54). Similar results were recently reported by Tschandl et al. (55) which compared 511 human readers, including 283 board-certified dermatologists, and 139 machine learning algorithms on a classification task consisting of 30 image batches from the test image set. When comparing 37 human experts (>10 years of experience) with the top three machine learning algorithms, the mean number of correctly classified images by humans was 18.78 images per 30 test images, whereas machine learning algorithms scored 25.43, which was statistically higher than human expert readers.

Although AI classifiers seemed to score similar marks as physicians, it is difficult to judge whether AI classifiers have already surpassed physicians or not, since most of these reports were unable to verify results by outside data and biases, such as selection bias of study training/testing data or publication bias (53). However, in spite of such possible biases, development of AI classifiers using dermoscopic images is still an attractive research area.

TABLE 1 | List of CNN architectures.

Architecture	Year	Top-5 error rate at ILSVRC*	References
LeNet	1998	NA	(36)
AlexNet	2012	15.3%	(36)
ZFNet	2013	14.8%	(37)
GoogLeNet	2014	6.67%	(39, 40)
VGG Net	2014	7.3%	(38)
ResNet-50	2015	3.6%	(41)
SENet	2017	2.3%	(42)

*ILSVRC: ImageNet Large Scale Visual Recognition Challenge.

CLASSIFICATION OF SKIN TUMOR USING CLINICAL IMAGES

As described above, many highly accurate AI classifiers focusing on melanoma detection using dermoscopic images have been developed. Although conventional machine learning algorithms that require human intervention to extract and select features have the capacity to output a binary result (benign or malignant), accurate diagnoses of multi-class skin diseases are difficult (56). Moreover, even if clinical images are cheap and easy to collect, these clinical photographs are believed to have limited morphologic information that is useful for classification (14). Collectively, outside of a binary "benign or malignant" output, AI classifiers using conventional machine learning algorithms are considered to be inferior at handling clinical images for sorting into multiple classes.

To overcome these issues, deep learning-based CNN classifiers, which surpass the general object classification capability of humans (32), became popular for use in these tasks. Several studies have been published, including from our group (39, 57, 58), since Esteva et al. (40) first reported a dermatologist-equivalent classifier of skin cancers using CNN in 2017. They used 129,450 skin lesion images for the training of a Google Inception v3 CNN architecture, which was pre-trained on the Image Net dataset consisting of 1.28 million images over 1,000 generic object classes. The CNN was fine-tuned to classify skin lesion images by the transfer learning method and was validated on its efficiency of binary classification (benign or malignant). Although the study did not reveal its overall accuracy at skin tumor classification, the CNN surpassed average-level dermatologists in the sensitivity/specificity of classifying epidermal tumors (epidermal cancers and seborrheic keratosis) and melanocytic tumors (melanoma and benign nevi). Han et al. (57) used 15,408 skin lesion images from 12 benign and malignant skin tumors to train a Microsoft ResNet-152 CNN architecture (pre-trained on the same Image Net dataset as above). Similarly, to the Esteva et al. report, they used skin tumor images to fine-tune their CNN which subsequently outperformed 16 dermatologists. They also opened their CNN to the public and it could be externally validated, which was noteworthy. In our study (39), we used only 4,800 skin lesion images from 14 benign and malignant skin tumors to train a GoogLeNet CNN architecture (pre-trained on the same Image

Net dataset as above). However, even with less images in the training set, our CNN was more accurate at image classification than 13 board-certified dermatologists and 8 dermatologist trainees (**Figure 6**), reaching a 96.3% sensitivity, and 89.5% specificity in the detection of skin cancer.

Brinker et al. (58) reported an interesting result showing that a CNN trained only with dermoscopic images could classify clinical melanoma images at a similar level to 145 dermatologists. They trained a Microsoft ResNet-50 CNN architecture (pre-trained on the same Image Net dataset as above) using 2,196 melanomas and 18,566 atypical nevi. This study is particularly interesting because this is the first report to show that dermatologist-equivalent tumor image classification was achieved by a CNN that was not trained by clinical images. This study indicates that CNN may benefit from training with dermoscopic images (that have a higher resolution than clinical images) even for low-resolution classification tasks. Another approach is to combine available data for classification as Yap et al. (59). They used 2,917 cases containing both clinical and dermoscopic images and trained a Microsoft ResNet-50 CNN architecture. They showed that a CNN trained with dermoscopic images had higher accuracy than a CNN trained with clinical images. However, when they trained their CNN on combined feature information from dermoscopic and clinical images, the accuracy outperformed single modal CNN, indicating that both clinical and dermoscopic images have distinct classification information. Collectively, the new machine learning algorithm CNN could be a "breakthrough" for developing a multi-class skin tumor classifier, which can accept clinical tumor images.

LIMITATIONS

Several issues remain for the CNN skin tumor classifier to overcome. First, there are no standardized evaluation test datasets to measure the efficacy of CNN classifiers. However, if the test dataset is known in advance, there is a risk of adapting the CNN classifier to the test dataset. Therefore, it might be better to conduct tests by a third-party organization to measure classification efficiency using closed datasets. Second, datasets used to train the CNN are comprised of regionally homogenous images, e.g., our dataset was composed of nearly 100% Asians. In a study by Han et al. (57), they tested using external tumor images (Edinburgh dataset; available from the Edinburgh Dermofit Image Library) to see if their CNN that was trained on Asian tumor images could also classify tumor images from Caucasian patients. As anticipated, both sensitivity and specificity dropped in this case. Third, although CNN requires an increased number of training datasets to improve classification efficiency, rare tumors and subtypes (such as amelanotic melanoma or pigmented basal cell carcinoma) will always mean a scarcity of available images for these diseases. Fourth, the clinical images were less standardized, with varying camera angles, orientations, multiple skin backgrounds, lighting, and even pen markings or rulers included in the photos (60). According to a study by Narla et al. (60), algorithms are more likely to classify images with rulers as malignant because images with rulers were more likely to be malignant. Fifth, the "black box" nature of CNN makes it impossible to interpret how and why CNN arrived

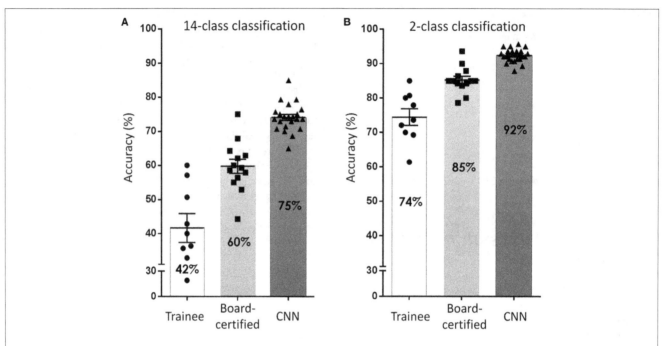

FIGURE 6 | Accuracy of skin tumor classification by our CNN classifier. **(A)** Result of 14-class classification by dermatology trainees, board-certified dermatologists, and CNN classifier. Adapted from Fujisawa et al. (39). **(B)** Result of 2-class classification (benign or malignant). In both classification level, the accuracy of CNN surpassed board-certified dermatologists.

at its output. As an example, Navarrete-Dochent et al. (61) reported that the output of their CNN was affected by the size, rotation, or color tone of images. A similar phenomenon was observed in our system; the output of our CNN was affected by changing the size parameters of the tumor (data not shown). To improve the robustness of the CNN classifier, establishment of an open-access, standardized, large skin tumor image dataset, which includes both rare tumors/subtypes and all ethnicities, is mandatory. Moreover, a robust, standardized measurement method for evaluation and comparison of systems should be established.

FUTURE PERSPECTIVE

AI classifiers for the image classification field have been dramatically improved and made more popular by the introduction of CNN. Many strategies, such as creating ensembles of multiple models (62, 63) or using additional information other than image labels, to improve the accuracy of the classifier outside of increasing the number of images for training have been reported (64). Some studies have reported that CNN algorithms have already surpassed the classification efficacy of dermatologists and, in the near future, AI classifiers may gain sufficient sensitivity and specificity to bear the screening burden for detecting malignant skin tumors. Therefore, some physicians may consider AI as a potential threat, but we believe it to be no more than a diagnostic assistance system due to many limitations detailed in previous studies and difficulty in performance comparisons within published results. Besides such limitations, AI classifiers still have important role in assisting non-dermatologist physicians, since most skin cancer patients will consult them before being transferred to dermatologists. Early detection and treatment are both still essential in the management of melanoma and, therefore, an efficient AI classifier would help to "detect" patients in the early stage of the disease. Further research is thus required to both improve classification efficacy and develop independent evaluation methodologies to accurately measure system efficacy. Moreover, integration of other medical information such as vital signs, routine blood testing, or even omics data, may give us new insights into the biology or pathology of the disease.

AUTHOR CONTRIBUTIONS

YF, SI, and YN contributed to the conception and design of the study. SI and YF wrote the first draft of the manuscript. All authors contributed to the revision of the manuscript, and read and approved the submitted version.

ACKNOWLEDGMENTS

We would like to thank Bryan J. Mathis of the Medical English Communication Center of the University of Tsukuba, for his excellent English revisions.

REFERENCES

1. *United States Cancer Statistics: Data Visualiztions.* Available online at: https://gis.cdc.gov/Cancer/USCS/DataViz.html (accessed May 28, 2019).
2. Gruber SB, Armstrong BK. Cutaneous and ocular melanoma. In: Schottenfeld D, Fraumeni JF, editors. *Cancer Epidemiology and Prevention.* New York, NY: Oxford University Press (2006). p. 1196–229. doi: 10.1093/acprof:oso/9780195149616.003.0063
3. Jemal A, Saraiya M, Patel P, Cherala SS, Barnholtz-Sloan J, Kim J, et al. Recent trends in cutaneous melanoma incidence and death rates in the United States, 1992-2006. *J Am Acad Dermatol.* (2011) 65:S17-25 e11-13. doi: 10.1016/j.jaad.2011.04.032
4. Jemal A, Simard EP, Dorell C. Annual Report to the Nation on the Status of Cancer, 1975-2009, featuring the burden and trends in human papillomavirus(HPV)-associated cancers and HPV vaccination coverage levels. *J Natl Cancer Inst.* (2013) 105:175–201. doi: 10.1093/jnci/djt083
5. Rogers HW, Weinstock MA, Feldman SR, Coldiron BM. Incidence estimate of nonmelanoma skin cancer (Keratinocyte Carcinomas) in the U.S. Population, 2012. *JAMA Dermatol.* (2015) 151:1081–6. doi: 10.1001/jamadermatol.2015.1187
6. Services UDoHaH. *The Surgeon General's Call to Action to Prevent Skin Cancer.* US Department of Health and Human Services OotSG. Washington, DC (2014).
7. Karagas MR, Weinstock MA, Nelson HH. Keratinocyte carcinomas (basal and squamous cell carcinomas of the skin. In: Schottenfeld D, Fraumeni JF, editors. *Cancer Epidemiology and Prevention.* New York, NY: Oxford University Press (2006). p. 1230–50. doi: 10.1093/acprof:oso/9780195149616.003.0064
8. Deinlein T, Richtig G, Schwab C, Scarfi F, Arzberger E, Wolf I, et al. The use of dermatoscopy in diagnosis and therapy of nonmelanocytic skin cancer. *J Dtsch Dermatol Ges.* (2016) 14:144–51. doi: 10.1111/ddg.12903
9. Verhoeven EW, Kraaimaat FW, van Weel C, van de Kerkhof PC, Duller P, van der Valk PG, et al. Skin diseases in family medicine: prevalence and health care use. *Ann Fam Med.* (2008) 6:349–54. doi: 10.1370/afm.861
10. Julian CG. Dermatology in general practice. *Br J Dermatol.* (1999) 141:518–20. doi: 10.1046/j.1365-2133.1999.03048.x
11. Kerr OA, Tidman MJ, Walker JJ, Aldridge RD, Benton EC. The profile of dermatological problems in primary care. *Clin Exp Dermatol.* (2010) 35:380–3. doi: 10.1111/j.1365-2230.2009.03586.x
12. Russell SJ, Norvig P. *Artificial Intelligence: A Modern Approach.* 3rd ed. Upper Saddle River, NJ: Prentice Hall (2009).
13. Handelman GS, Kok HK, Chandra RV, Razavi AH, Lee MJ, Asadi H. eDoctor: machine learning and the future of medicine. *J Intern Med.* (2018) 284:603–19. doi: 10.1111/joim.12822
14. Masood A, Al-Jumaily AA. Computer aided diagnostic support system for skin cancer: a review of techniques and algorithms. *Int J Biomed Imaging.* (2013) 2013:323268. doi: 10.1155/2013/323268
15. Mirzaalian H, Lee TK, Hamarneh G. Hair enhancement in dermoscopic images using dual-channel quaternion tubularness filters and MRF-based multilabel optimization. *IEEE Trans Image Process.* (2014) 23:5486–96. doi: 10.1109/TIP.2014.2362054
16. Abbas Q, Garcia IF, Emre Celebi M, Ahmad W, Mushtaq Q. Unified approach for lesion border detection based on mixture modeling and local entropy thresholding. *Skin Res Technol.* (2013) 19:314–9. doi: 10.1111/srt.12047
17. Chang WY, Huang A, Chen YC, Lin CW, Tsai J, Yang CK, et al. The feasibility of using manual segmentation in a multifeature computer-aided diagnosis system for classification of skin lesions: a retrospective comparative study. *BMJ Open.* (2015) 5:e007823. doi: 10.1136/bmjopen-2015-007823
18. Euijoon A, Lei B, Youn Hyun J, Jinman K, Changyang L, Fulham M, et al. Automated saliency-based lesion segmentation in dermoscopic images. *Conf Proc IEEE Eng Med Biol Soc.* (2015) 2015:3009–12. doi: 10.1109/EMBC.2015.7319025
19. Kasmi R, Mokrani K, Rader RK, Cole JG, Stoecker WV. Biologically inspired skin lesion segmentation using a geodesic active contour technique. *Skin Res Technol.* (2016) 22:208–22. doi: 10.1111/srt.12252
20. Aitken JF, Pfitzner J, Battistutta D, O'Rourke PK, Green AC, Martin NG. Reliability of computer image analysis of pigmented

skin lesions of Australian adolescents. *Cancer.* (1996) 78:252–7. doi: 10.1002/(SICI)1097-0142(19960715)78:2<252::AID-CNCR10>3.0.CO;2-V
21. Cascinelli N, Ferrario M, Bufalino R, Zurrida S, Galimberti V, Mascheroni L, et al. Results obtained by using a computerized image analysis system designed as an aid to diagnosis of cutaneous melanoma. *Melanoma Res.* (1992) 2:163–70. doi: 10.1097/00008390-199209000-00004
22. Marill T, Green D. On the effectiveness of receptors in recognition systems. *IEEE Trans Inform Theory.* (1963) 9:11–7. doi: 10.1109/TIT.1963.1057810
23. Whitney AW. A direct method of nonparametric measurement selection. *IEEE Trans Comput.* (1971) C-20:1100–3. doi: 10.1109/T-C.1971.223410
24. Pudil P, Novovičová J, Kittler J. Floating search methods in feature selection. *Pattern Recogn Lett.* (1994) 15:1119–25. doi: 10.1016/0167-8655(94)90127-9
25. Byvatov E, Schneider G. Support vector machine applications in bioinformatics. *Appl Bioinformatics.* (2003) 2:67–77.
26. Krzywinski M, Altman N. Classification and regression trees. *Nat Methods.* (2017) 14:757. doi: 10.1038/nmeth.4370
27. Harrell FE Jr, Lee KL, Califf RM, Pryor DB, Rosati RA. Regression modelling strategies for improved prognostic prediction. *Stat Med.* (1984) 3:143–52. doi: 10.1002/sim.4780030207
28. Ripley BD. *Pattern Recognition and Neural Networks.* Cambridge: Cambridge University Press (1996). doi: 10.1017/CBO9780511812651
29. Ferris LK, Harkes JA, Gilbert B, Winger DG, Golubets K, Akilov O, et al. Computer-aided classification of melanocytic lesions using dermoscopic images. *J Am Acad Dermatol.* (2015) 73:769–76. doi: 10.1016/j.jaad.2015.07.028
30. Chang WY, Huang A, Yang CY, Lee CH, Chen YC, Wu TY, et al. Computer-aided diagnosis of skin lesions using conventional digital photography: a reliability and feasibility study. *PLoS ONE.* (2013) 8:e76212. doi: 10.1371/journal.pone.0076212
31. Bhattacharya A, Young A, Wong A, Stalling S, Wei M, Hadley D. Precision diagnosis of melanoma and other skin lesions from digital images. *AMIA Jt Summits Transl Sci Proc.* (2017) 2017:220–6.
32. Russakovsky O, Deng J, Su H. ImageNet large scale visual recognition challenge. *Int J Comput Vision.* (2015) 115:211–52. doi: 10.1007/s11263-015-0816-y
33. Krizhevsky A, Sutskever I, Hinton G. ImageNet classification with deep convolutional neural networks. In: *25th International Conference on Neural Information Processing Systems.* New York, NY (2012). p. 1097–105. doi: 10.1145/3065386
34. Szegedy C, Liu W, Jia Y. Going deeper with convolutions. In: *IEEE Conference on Computer Vision and Pattern Recognition.* New York, NY: IEEE (2014). doi: 10.1109/CVPR.2015.7298594
35. Arribas JI, Cid-Sueiro J. A model selection algorithm for a posteriori probability estimation with neural networks. *IEEE Trans Neural Netw.* (2005) 16:799–809. doi: 10.1109/TNN.2005.849826
36. Yap MH, Pons G, Marti J, Ganau S, Sentis M, Zwiggelaar R, et al. Automated breast ultrasound lesions detection using convolutional neural networks. *IEEE J Biomed Health Inform.* (2018) 22: 1218–26. doi: 10.1109/JBHI.2017.2731873
37. Zeiler MD, Fergus R. *Visualizing and Understanding Convolutional Networks 2013.* Available online at: *arXiv[Preprint].arXiv:1311.2901* (accessed 25 July 2019).
38. Cheng PM, Malhi HS. Transfer learning with convolutional neural networks for classification of abdominal ultrasound images. *J Digit Imaging.* (2017) 30:234–43. doi: 10.1007/s10278-016-9929-2
39. Fujisawa Y, Otomo Y, Ogata Y, Nakamura Y, Fujita R, Ishitsuka Y, et al. Deep-learning-based, computer-aided classifier developed with a small dataset of clinical images surpasses board-certified dermatologists in skin tumour diagnosis. *Br J Dermatol.* (2019) 180:373–81. doi: 10.1111/bjd.16924
40. Esteva A, Kuprel B, Novoa RA, Ko J, Swetter SM, Blau HM, et al. Dermatologist-level classification of skin cancer with deep neural networks. *Nature.* (2017) 542:115–8. doi: 10.1038/nature21056
41. Baltruschat IM, Nickisch H, Grass M, Knopp T, Saalbach A. Comparison of deep learning approaches for multi-label chest X-ray classification. *Sci Rep.* (2019) 9:6381. doi: 10.1038/s41598-019-42294-8
42. Hu J, Shen L, Albanie S, Sun G, Wu E. Squeeze-and-excitation networks 2017. *arXiv[Preprint].arXiv.1709.01507.*

43. Weiss K, Khoshgoftaar TM, Wang D. A survey of transfer learning. *J Big Data*. (2016) 3:9. doi: 10.1186/s40537-016-0043-6

44. Steiner A, Pehamberger H, Wolff K. *In vivo* epiluminescence microscopy of pigmented skin lesions. II. Diagnosis of small pigmented skin lesions and early detection of malignant melanoma. *J Am Acad Dermatol*. (1987) 17:584–91. doi: 10.1016/S0190-9622(87)70240-0

45. Piccolo D, Ferrari A, Peris K, Diadone R, Ruggeri B, Chimenti S. Dermoscopic diagnosis by a trained clinician vs. a clinician with minimal dermoscopy training vs. computer-aided diagnosis of 341 pigmented skin lesions: a comparative study. *Br J Dermatol*. (2002) 147:481–6. doi: 10.1046/j.1365-2133.2002.04978.x

46. Nachbar F, Stolz W, Merkle T, Cognetta AB, Vogt T, Landthaler M, et al. The ABCD rule of dermatoscopy. High prospective value in the diagnosis of doubtful melanocytic skin lesions. *J Am Acad Dermatol*. (1994) 30:551–9. doi: 10.1016/S0190-9622(94)70061-3

47. Ahnlide I, Bjellerup M, Nilsson F, Nielsen K. Validity of ABCD rule of dermoscopy in clinical practice. *Acta Derm Venereol*. (2016) 96:367–72. doi: 10.2340/00015555-2239

48. Johr RH. Dermoscopy: alternative melanocytic algorithms-the ABCD rule of dermatoscopy, Menzies scoring method, and 7-point checklist. *Clin Dermatol*. (2002) 20:240–7. doi: 10.1016/S0738-081X(02)00236-5

49. Rao BK, Ahn CS. Dermatoscopy for melanoma and pigmented lesions. *Dermatol Clin*. (2012) 30:413–34. doi: 10.1016/j.det.2012.04.005

50. Argenziano G, Soyer HP. Dermoscopy of pigmented skin lesions–a valuable tool for early diagnosis of melanoma. *Lancet Oncol*. (2001) 2:443–9. doi: 10.1016/S1470-2045(00)00422-8

51. Kittler H, Pehamberger H, Wolff K, Binder M. Diagnostic accuracy of dermoscopy. *Lancet Oncol*. (2002) 3:159–65. doi: 10.1016/S1470-2045(02)00679-4

52. Menzies SW, Bischof L, Talbot H, Gutenev A, Avramidis M, Wong L, et al. The performance of SolarScan: an automated dermoscopy image analysis instrument for the diagnosis of primary melanoma. *Arch Dermatol*. (2005) 141:1388–96. doi: 10.1001/archderm.141.11.1388

53. Rajpara SM, Botello AP, Townend J, Ormerod AD. Systematic review of dermoscopy and digital dermoscopy/ artificial intelligence for the diagnosis of melanoma. *Br J Dermatol*. (2009) 161:591–604. doi: 10.1111/j.1365-2133.2009.09093.x

54. Haenssle HA, Fink C, Schneiderbauer R. Man against machine: diagnostic performance of a deep learning convolutional neural network for dermoscopic melanoma recognition in comparison to 58 dermatologists. *Ann Oncol*. (2018). doi: 10.1093/annonc/mdy520

55. Tschandl P, Codella N, Akay BN, Argenziano G, Braun RP, Cabo H, et al. Comparison of the accuracy of human readers versus machine-learning algorithms for pigmented skin lesion classification: an open, web-based, international, diagnostic study. *Lancet Oncol*. (2019) 20:938–47. doi: 10.1016/S1470-2045(19)30333-X

56. Han SS, Lim W, Kim MS, Park I, Park GH, Chang SE. Interpretation of the outputs of a deep learning model trained with a skin cancer dataset. *J Invest Dermatol*. (2018) 138:2275–7. doi: 10.1016/j.jid.2018.05.014

57. Han SS, Kim MS, Lim W, Park GH, Park I, Chang SE. Classification of the clinical images for benign and malignant cutaneous tumors using a deep learning algorithm. *J Invest Dermatol*. (2018) 138:1529–38. doi: 10.1016/j.jid.2018.01.028

58. Brinker TJ, Hekler A, Enk AH, Klode J, Hauschild A, Berking C, et al. A convolutional neural network trained with dermoscopic images performed on par with 145 dermatologists in a clinical melanoma image classification task. *Eur J Cancer*. (2019) 111:148–54. doi: 10.1016/j.ejca.2019.02.005

59. Yap J, Yolland W, Tschandl P. Multimodal skin lesion classification using deep learning. *Exp Dermatol*. (2018) 27:1261–7. doi: 10.1111/exd.13777

60. Narla A, Kuprel B, Sarin K, Novoa R, Ko J. Automated classification of skin lesions: from pixels to practice. *J Invest Dermatol*. (2018) 138:2108–10. doi: 10.1016/j.jid.2018.06.175

61. Navarrete-Dechent C, Dusza SW, Liopyris K, Marghoob AA, Halpern AC, Marchetti MA. Automated dermatological diagnosis: hype or reality? *J Invest Dermatol*. (2018) 138:2277–9. doi: 10.1016/j.jid.2018.04.040

62. Perez F, Avila S, Valle E. Solo or ensemble? Choosing a CNN architecture for melanoma classification. In: *The IEEE Conference on Computer Vision and Pattern Recognition (CVPR) Workshops*. Long Beach, CA: IEEE Xplore (2019).

63. Mohanraj V, Sibi Chakkaravarthy S, Vaidehi V. Ensemble of convolutional neural networks for face recognition. In: Kalita J, Balas V, Borah S, editors. *Recent Developments in Machine Learning and Data Analytics. Advances in Intelligent Systems and Computing*. Singapore: Springer (2019). doi: 10.1007/978-981-13-1280-9_43

64. Codella N, Lin C, Halpern A, Hind M, Feris R, Smith J. Collaborative human-AI (CHAI): evidence-based interpretable melanoma classification in dermoscopic images. In: *Workshop on Interpretability of Machine Intelligence in Medical Image Computing at MICCAI 2018*. (2018). doi: 10.1007/978-3-030-02628-8_11

22

Merkel Cell Carcinoma: An Update and Immunotherapy

Hiroshi Uchi*

Department of Dermatology, Graduate School of Medical Sciences, Kyushu University, Fukuoka, Japan

Correspondence:
Hiroshi Uchi
uchihir@dermatol.med.
kyushu-u.ac.jp

Merkel cell carcinoma (MCC) is a rare but aggressive skin cancer with frequent metastasis and death. MCC has a mortality rate of 30%, making it more lethal than malignant melanoma, and incidence of MCC has increased almost fourfold over the past 20 years in the USA. MCC has long been considered to be an immunogenic cancer because it occurs more frequently in immunosuppressed patients from organ transplant and HIV infection than in those with immunocompetent. Chronic UV light exposure and clonal integration of Merkel cell polyomavirus (MCPyV) are two major causative factors of MCC. Approximately 80% of MCC are associated with MCPyV, and T cells specific for MCPyV oncoproteins are present in the blood and tumors of patients. Several studies have shown that a subset of MCCs express PD-1 on tumor-infiltrating lymphocytes and express PD-L1 on tumor cells, which suggests an endogenous tumor-reactive immune response that might be unleashed by anti-PD-1 or anti-PD-L1 drugs.

Keywords: PD-1, PD-L1, Merkel cell carcinoma, Merkel cell polyomavirus, UV

BACKGROUND

Merkel cell carcinoma (MCC) is a rare but highly aggressive neuroendocrine skin cancer, which was described for the first time in 1972 as trabecular carcinoma of the skin (1). Based on the ultrastructural proof of neuroendocrine granules and the expression of CK20 and CD56 (2–4), Merkel cells were considered to be the source of MCC. However, the cells of origin of MCC remain a controversial issue. Recent studies have suggested the origin of MCC may reside in epidermal/dermal stem cells in the dermis (5) or in precursor B cells (6, 7). The incidence of MCC is rising steadily and more than one-third of patients die of MCC, making it twice as lethal as malignant melanoma (8). Risk factors for MCC include fair skin, chronic sun exposure, chronic immune suppression, and advanced age (9–12). In the USA, age-adjusted incidence increased from 0.15 to 0.44 per 100,000 from 1986 to 2004 (13). Consistent with other UV-related skin cancers, incidence rate of MCC in Queensland, Australia is higher than those in the rest of the world (age-adjusted incidence of 1.6 per 100,000) (14). The incidence of MCC in Asia is thought to be low, although no population-based data are available (15, 16). The majority of MCC is associated with Merkel cell polyomavirus (MCPyV), while the remaining is triggered by UV-mediated mutations (17, 18). MCPyV DNA integrates into the host genome of approximately up to 80% of MCCs in the northern hemisphere, whereas its presence is much lower in other geographic regions such as Australia (~30%) (17, 19). Since several lines of evidence indicate the outstanding immunogenicity of MCC, irrespective of MCPyV integration, immune modulating treatment strategies are particularly attractive. Promising results from immune checkpoint inhibitor therapy in first and second line are now available, which expands the treatment armamentarium for MCC patients.

CLINICAL AND HISTOLOGICAL FEATURES

Merkel cell carcinoma presents as a firm, painless, rapidly enlarging, red-violet cutaneous nodule with a smooth surface. The most frequently affected site is the head and neck region (50%), followed by the trunk (30%) and the limbs (10%), although MCC may arise in any body site, including the mucosae (20–22). Heath et al. developed the AEIOU acronym to define the clinical features associated with MCC: asymptomatic/lack of tenderness, expanding rapidly, immune suppression, older than age 50, and UV-exposed site on a person with fair skin. In a study of 195 patients, 89% presented with three or more of the AEIOU characteristics (23). MCC originates in the dermis and only occasionally exhibits an epidermal involvement. Histopathological characteristics of MCC include a monotonous population of tumor cells with large prominent nuclei and scant cytoplasm (24). Immunohistochemically, MCC is positive for EMA, CK20 with a perinuclear dot staining pattern, and neuroendocrine markers including synaptophysin and chromogranin (3, 25–27). Metastatic pulmonary small cell carcinoma can be excluded when the tumor cells prove negative for TTF-1 (28). Unknown primary MCC, which usually presents clinically positive nodal disease with unidentified primary tumor, are likely to have a significantly improved survival compared to those with concurrent primary tumor (29–32). Recent reports showed that unknown primary MCC had higher tumor mutational burden and lower association with MCPyV than those with known primary (33), In addition, nodal tumors from unknown primary MCC contained abundant UV-signature mutations (33), suggesting underlying immunological mechanism between regression of primary tumor and better prognosis of unknown primary MCC.

ETIOLOGY

Like Kaposi's sarcoma, immunocompromised patients with T-cell dysfunction are more likely to be affected by MCC. For example, patients with AIDS have an incidence rate that is 11–13 times greater compared with the general population (11), and solid organ transplant recipients are 5–10 times more likely to develop MCC (34, 35). Also, case reports have described spontaneous regression of MCC tumors after biopsy or an improvement in immune function, further indicating a link to the immune system (36–39). These data collectively suggested that MCC may be linked to a pathogen and in 2008, MCPyV was discovered, and it is now clear that this virus plays a key role in the majority of MCC cases (17).

Merkel cell polyomavirus is a member of the polyomavirus family comprised of non-enveloped, double-stranded circular DNA viruses. MCPyV-specific antibodies have been detected in 9% of children under 4 years of age, 35% of teenagers, and 80% of individuals 50 years or older (40), suggesting that it may be part of the cutaneous microbiome (41). Interestingly, despite this high prevalence, MCPyV has not been shown to cause any disease other than MCC (42). MCPyV-related oncogenesis requires integration of the viral genome into the host-genome and mutation of the large T (LT) antigen that is required for viral DNA replication (43). Indeed, MCPyV isolated from MCCs, in contrast with MCPyV from non-tumor sources, present mutations that are responsible for the premature truncation of the MCV LT helicase (43, 44). These mutations do not affect the Rb binding domain, but eliminate the capacity of the viral DNA to replicate. In this way, the virus loses its capability to

replicate in MCC tumor cells, but continues to express motifs that may potentially lead to uncontrolled proliferation (43, 45). Prognostic significance of tumor viral status is still controversial, but the largest cohort study so far including 282 MCC cases (281 cases with available clinical data) showed that, relative to MCPyV-positive MCC patients, MCPyV-negative MCC patients had significantly increased risk of disease progression (hazard ratio = 1.77, 95% confidence interval = 1.20–2.62) and death from MCC (hazard ratio = 1.85, 95% confidence interval = 1.19–2.89) in a multivariate analysis including age, sex, and immunosuppression (46).

Merkel cell carcinoma development is also linked to exposure to UV radiation, and primary MCC lesions preferentially develop on sun-exposed skin (20, 21). The incidence of MCC was determined to be 100-fold greater in patients who underwent PUVA treatment (47). MCPyV-negative MCC is among the most mutated of all solid tumors, including melanoma (18, 48–50). These mutations are mostly UV-signature mutations, such as p53 and Rb, commonly resulting in loss of functional protein expression (18, 49). The high mutational burden in MCC correlates to frequent amino acid changes and large numbers of UV-induced neoantigens (49). Despite significant genetic differences, both MCPyV-positive and -negative MCC exhibit nuclear accumulation of oncogenic transcription factors such as NFAT, phosphorylated CREB, and phosphorylated STAT3, indicating commonly deregulated pathogenic mechanisms (50).

TREATMENT

For patients with locoregional MCC, wide excision and/or complete lymph node dissection and/or adjuvant radiation therapy is usually recommended (51). Sentinel lymph node biopsy should be considered for patients with clinically nodal negative patients, although its impact on overall survival is still unclear (51–53).

Although cytotoxic chemotherapy (carboplatin or cisplatin plus etoposide) has been commonly used to treat patients with advanced MCC, responses are rarely durable and few studies have shown a survival benefit (54–57). Early studies showed that levels of intratumoral CD8+ T cells serve as predictors of MCC-specific survival, with 100% survival reported for patients with the highest level of CD8+ infiltrate compared to 60% survival in those with little or no CD8+ infiltration (58, 59). Then MCPyV oncoprotein-specific cells were found to be present in MCC patient blood and enriched in their tumors (60), whose frequency appears to increase with tumor burden (61). Importantly, signs of dysfunction were evident in MCPyV-specific CD8+ T cells from patients, as they expressed both PD-1 and Tim3, suggesting functional exhaustion (61). MCPyV-negative MCC is also associated with high levels of T-cell infiltrates (18). Although both MCPyV-positive and -negative tumor cells express PD-L1, the expression levels of PD-L1 in virus-positive tumors seem to be higher than those in virus-negative tumors (18, 62). These findings, therefore, provide rationale for immunotherapy targeting the PD-1 pathway in advanced MCC.

A multicenter, phase 2, non-controlled clinical trial studied pembrolizumab (anti-PD-1 Ab) 2 mg/kg every 2 weeks in

TABLE 1 | Ongoing clinical trials in MCC (http://ClinicalTrials.gov).

NCT identifier	Title	Phase	Intervention
NCT03071406	Randomized Study of Nivolumab + Ipilimumab ± SBRT for Metastatic Merkel Cell Carcinoma	2	Nivolumab Ipilimumab SBRT
NCT02643303	A Phase 1/2 Study of *In Situ* Vaccination with Tremelimumab and IV Durvalumab Plus PolyICLC in Subjects with Advanced, Measurable, Biopsy-Accessible Cancers	1/2	Durvalumab Tremelimumab Poly ICLC
NCT02488759	An Investigational Immuno-therapy Study to Investigate the Safety and Effectiveness of Nivolumab, and Nivolumab Combination Therapy in Virus-Associated Tumors (CheckMate358)	1/2	Nivolumab Ipilimumab BMS-986016 Daratumumab
NCT02584829	Localized Radiation Therapy or Recombinant Interferon Beta and Avelumab with or without Cellular Adoptive Immunotherapy in Treating Patients with Metastatic Merkel Cell Carcinoma	1/2	Avelumab Merkel cell polyomavirus TAg-specific polyclonal autologous CD8-positive T cells Interferon beta, RT
NCT03271372	Adjuvant Avelumab in Merkel Cell Cancer (ADAM)	3	Avelumab
NCT02196961	Adjuvant Therapy of Completely Resected Merkel Cell Carcinoma with Immune Checkpoint Blocking Antibodies Versus Observation (ADMEC-O)	2	Ipilimumab Nivolumab

26 patients with advanced MCC who had not received prior systemic therapy. The objective response rate (ORR) to pembrolizumab among the 25 patients with at least one evaluation during treatment was 56% including a 16% complete response (CR) rate. Of the 14 responsive patients, the response duration ranged from at least 2.2 months to at least 9.7 months. Overall, the trial had an estimated progression free survival (PFS) of 67% at 6 months. Pembrolizumab was effective in both MCPyV-positive and -negative tumors (ORR 62 and 44%, respectively, not significantly different) (63). The preliminary data from this trial led to pembrolizumab being listed as a treatment option for disseminated disease in the 2017 NCCN guidelines for MCC (64).

A multicenter, international, open-label, phase 2 clinical trial studied avelumab (anti-PD-L1 Ab) in 88 patients with distant metastatic disease who had previously received at least one line of chemotherapy. This trial found an ORR of 33% with a CR rate of 11%. At 6 months, PFS was 40% and the estimated PFS at 1 year was 30%. As with pembrolizumab, avelumab was found to be effective in both MCPyV-positive and -negative tumors (ORR 26 and 35%, respectively, not significantly different) (65). Based on these results, FDA granted an accelerated approval for avelumab as first-line treatment of patients with metastatic MCC in March 2017. In the avelumab trial, a trend toward a higher response rate was observed in patients with fewer lines of prior treatment, which along with the pembrolizumab data strongly suggest that immunotherapy targeting the PD-1 pathway should be considered for first-line treatment in patients with advanced MCC.

An international, single arm, open-label trial of nivolumab (anti-PD-1 Ab) 240 mg/body every 2 weeks included both patients who had and those who had not received prior chemotherapy (36 and 64%, respectively) is ongoing (NCT02488759;

CheckMate358). In this study, 15 of 22 patients (68%) had objective responses, and PFS at 3 months was 82%. Responses occurred in 10 of 14 treatment-naive patients including 3 CR, in 5 of 8 patients including 5 partial responses with 1–2 prior systemic therapies (63%) (**Table 1**). Based on the preliminary data from this trial, nivolumab was listed along with avelumab and pembrolizumab as a treatment option for disseminated disease in the 2018 NCCN guidelines for MCC (51).

CONCLUSION

Advanced MCC is generally considered to be sensitive to chemotherapy, but responses are transient, offering a median PFS of only 3 months (55). On the other hand, although no randomized trials compare chemotherapy with immunotherapy, data from treatment with immune checkpoint inhibitors are promising with responses both in MCPyV-positive and -negative MCC, although nearly half of patients do not derive durable benefit from these drugs. Now that avelumab has been approved for treatment of advanced MCC in the USA, EU, and Japan, the spectrum of current therapy for patients with MCC is changing. Several clinical trials of immune checkpoint inhibitors (anti-PD-1, PD-L1, and CTLA-4 Abs) administered as monotherapy or in combination with other agents or modalities are ongoing (**Table 1**) and may provide further treatment options for patients with advanced MCC in the near future.

AUTHOR CONTRIBUTIONS

The author confirms being the sole contributor of this work and approved it for publication.

REFERENCES

1. Toker C. Trabecular carcinoma of the skin. *Arch Dermatol* (1972) 105:107–10. doi:10.1001/archderm.1972.01620040075020

2. Tang CK, Toker C. Trabecular carcinoma of the skin: an ultrastructural study. *Cancer* (1978) 42:2311–21. doi:10.1002/1097-0142(197811)42:5<2311::AID-CNCR2820420531>3.0.CO;2-L

3. Moll R, Lowe A, Laufer J, Franke WW. Cytokeratin 20 in human carcinomas. A new histodiagnostic marker detected by monoclonal antibodies. *Am J Pathol* (1992) 140:427–47.

4. Gallego R, García-Caballero T, Fraga M, Beiras A, Forteza J. Neural cell adhesion molecule immunoreactivity in Merkel cells and Merkel cell tumours. *Virchows Arch* (1995) 426:317–21. doi:10.1007/BF00191370

5. Lemasson G, Coquart N, Lebonvallet N, Boulais N, Galibert MD, Marcorelles P, et al. Presence of putative stem cells in Merkel cell carcinomas. *J Eur Acad Dermatol Venereol* (2012) 26:789–95. doi:10.1111/j.1468-3083.2011.04132.x

6. Zur Hausen A, Rennspiess D, Winnepenninckx V, Speel EJ, Kurz AK. Early B-cell differentiation in Merkel cell carcinomas: clues to cellular ancestry. *Cancer Res* (2013) 73:4982–7. doi:10.1158/0008-5472.CAN-13-0616

7. Sauer CM, Haugg AM, Chteinberg E, Rennspiess D, Winnepenninckx V, Speel EJ, et al. Reviewing the current evidence supporting early B-cells as the cellular origin of Merkel cell carcinoma. *Crit Rev Oncol Hematol* (2017) 116:99–105. doi:10.1016/j.critrevonc.2017.05.009

8. Miller RW, Rabkin CS. Merkel cell carcinoma and melanoma: etiological similarities and differences. *Cancer Epidemiol Biomarkers Prev* (1999) 8:153–8.

9. Albores-Saavedra J, Batich K, Chable-Montero F, Sagy N, Schwartz AM, Henson DE. Merkel cell carcinoma demographics, morphology, and survival based on 3870 cases: a population based study. *J Cutan Pathol* (2010) 37:20–7. doi:10.1111/j.1600-0560.2009.01370.x

10. Grabowski J, Saltzstein SL, Sadler GR, Tahir Z, Blair S. A comparison of Merkel cell carcinoma and melanoma: results from the California Cancer Registry. *Clin Med Oncol* (2008) 2:327–33.

11. Engels EA, Frisch M, Goedert JJ, Biggar RJ, Miller RW. Merkel cell carcinoma and HIV infection. *Lancet* (2002) 359:497–8. doi:10.1016/S0140-6736(02)07668-7

12. Kaae J, Hansen AV, Biggar RJ, Boyd HA, Moore PS, Wohlfahrt J, et al. Merkel cell carcinoma: incidence, mortality, and risk of other cancers. *J Natl Cancer Inst* (2010) 102:793–801. doi:10.1093/jnci/djq120

13. Hodgson NC. Merkel cell carcinoma: changing incidence trends. *J Surg Oncol* (2005) 89:1–4.

14. Youlden DR, Soyer HP, Youl PH, Fritschi L, Baade PD. Incidence and survival for Merkel cell carcinoma in Queensland, Australia, 1993-2010. *JAMA Dermatol* (2014) 150:864–72. doi:10.1001/jamadermatol.2014.124

15. Chun SM, Yun SJ, Lee SC, Won YH, Lee JB. Merkel cell polyomavirus is frequently detected in Korean patients with Merkel cell carcinoma. *Ann. Dermatol* (2013) 25:203–7. doi:10.5021/ad.2013.25.2.203

16. Hattori T, Takeuchi Y, Takenouchi T, Hirofuji A, Tsuchida T, Kabumoto T, et al. The prevalence of Merkel cell polyomavirus in Japanese patients with Merkel cell carcinoma. *J Dermatol Sci* (2013) 70:99–107. doi:10.1016/j.jdermsci.2013.02.010

17. Feng H, Shuda M, Chang Y, Moore PS. Clonal integration of a polyomavirus in human Merkel cell carcinoma. *Science* (2008) 319:1096–100. doi:10.1126/science.1152586

18. Wong SQ, Waldeck K, Vergara IA, Schröder J, Madore J, Wilmott JS, et al. UV-associated mutations underlie the etiology of MCV-negative Merkel cell carcinomas. *Cancer Res* (2015) 75:5228–34. doi:10.1158/0008-5472.CAN-15-1877

19. Garneski KM, Warcola AH, Feng Q, Kiviat NB, Leonard JH, Nghiem P. Merkel cell polyomavirus is more frequently present in North American than Australian Merkel cell carcinoma tumors. *J Invest Dermatol* (2009) 129:246–8. doi:10.1038/jid.2008.229

20. Smiths VA, Camp ER, Lentsch EJ. Merkel cell carcinoma: identification of prognostic factors unique to tumors located in the head and neck based on analysis of SEER data. *Laryngoscope* (2012) 122:1283–90. doi:10.1002/lary.23222

21. Hussain SK, Sundquist J, Hemminki K. Incidence trends of squamous cell and rare skin cancers in the Swedish national cancer registry point to calendar year and age-dependent increases. *J Invest Dermatol* (2010) 130:1323–8. doi:10.1038/jid.2009.426

22. Nguyen AH, Tahseen AI, Vaudreuil AM, Caponetti GC, Huerter CJ. Clinical features and treatment of vulvar Merkel cell carcinoma: a systematic review. *Gynecol Oncol Res Pract* (2017) 4:2. doi:10.1186/s40661-017-0037-x

23. Heath M, Jaimes N, Lemos B, Mostaghimi A, Wang LC, Peñas PF, et al. Clinical characteristics of Merkel cell carcinoma at diagnosis in 195 patients: the AEIOU features. *J Am Acad Dermatol* (2008) 58:375–81. doi:10.1016/j.jaad.2007.11.020

24. Acebo E, Vidaurrazaga N, Varas C, Burgos-Bretones JJ, Díaz-Pérez JL. Merkel cell carcinoma: a clinicopathological study of 11 cases. *J Eur Acad Dermatol Venereol* (2005) 19:546–51. doi:10.1111/j.1468-3083.2005.01224.x

25. Chan JK, Suster S, Wenig BM, Tsang WY, Chan JB, Lau AL. Cytokeratin 20 immunoreactivity distinguishes Merkel cell (primary cutaneous neuroendocrine) carcinomas and salivary gland small cell carcinomas from small cell carcinomas of various sites. *Am J Surg Pathol* (1997) 21:226–34. doi:10.1097/00000478-199702000-00014

26. Visscher D, Cooper PH, Zarbo RJ, Crissman JD. Cutaneous neuroendocrine (Merkel cell) carcinoma: an immunophenotypic, clinicopathologic, and flow cytometric study. *Mod Pathol* (1989) 2:331–8.

27. Mount SL, Taatjes DJ. Neuroendocrine carcinoma of the skin (Merkel cell carcinoma). an immunoelectron-microscopic case study. *Am J Dermatopathol* (1994) 16:60–5. doi:10.1097/00000372-199402000-00012

28. Kaufmann O, Dietel M. Expression of thyroid transcription factor-1 in pulmonary and extrapulmonary small cell carcinomas and other neuroendocrine carcinomas of various primary sites. *Histopathology* (2000) 36:415–20. doi:10.1046/j.1365-2559.2000.00890.x

29. Harms KL, Healy MA, Nghiem P, Sober AJ, Johnson TM, Bichakjian CK, et al. Analysis of prognostic factors from 9387 Merkel cell carcinoma cases forms the basis for the new 8th edition AJCC staging system. *Ann Surg Oncol* (2016) 23:3564–71. doi:10.1245/s10434-016-5266-4

30. Pan Z, Chen YY, Wu X, Trisal V, Wilczynski SP, Weiss LM, et al. Merkel cell carcinoma of lymph node with unknown primary has a significantly lower association with Merkel cell polyomavirus than its cutaneous counterpart. *Mod Pathol* (2014) 27:1182–92. doi:10.1038/modpathol.2013.250

31. Chen KT, Papavasiliou P, Edwards K, Zhu F, Perlis C, Wu H, et al. A better prognosis for Merkel cell carcinoma of unknown primary origin. *Am J Surg* (2013) 206:752–7. doi:10.1016/j.amjsurg.2013.02.005

32. Foote M, Veness M, Zarate D, Poulsen M. Merkel cell carcinoma: the prognostic implications of an occult primary in stage IIIB (nodal) disease. *J Am Acad Dermatol* (2012) 67:395–9. doi:10.1016/j.jaad.2011.09.009

33. Vandeven N, Lewis CW, Makarov V, Riaz N, Paulson KG, Hippe D, et al. Merkel cell carcinoma patients presenting without a primary lesion have elevated markers of immunity, higher tumor mutation burden, and improved survival. *Clin Cancer Res* (2018) 24(4):963–71. doi:10.1158/1078-0432

34. Lanoy E, Costagliola D, Engels EA. Skin cancers associated with HIV infection and solid-organ transplantation among elderly adults. *Int J Cancer* (2010) 126:1724–31. doi:10.1002/ijc.24931

35. Clarke CA, Robbins HA, Tatalovich Z, Lynch CF, Pawlish KS, Finch JL, et al. Risk of Merkel cell carcinoma after solid organ transplantation. *J Natl Cancer Inst* (2015) 107. doi:10.1093/jnci/dju382

36. Wooff JC, Trites JR, Walsh NM, Bullock MJ. Complete spontaneous regression of metastatic Merkel cell carcinoma: a case report and review of the literature. *Am J Dermatopathol* (2010) 32:614–7. doi:10.1097/DAD.0b013e3181cd3158

37. Walsh NM. Complete spontaneous regression of Merkel cell carcinoma (1986-2016): a 30 year perspective. *J Cutan Pathol* (2016) 43:1150–4. doi:10.1111/cup.12812

38. Ahmadi Moghaddam P, Cornejo KM, Hutchinson L, Tomaszewicz K, Dresser K, Deng A, et al. Complete spontaneous regression of Merkel cell carcinoma after biopsy: a case report and review of the literature. *Am J Dermatopathol* (2016) 38:e154–8. doi:10.1097/DAD.0000000000000614

39. Burack J, Altschuler EL. Sustained remission of metastatic Merkel cell carcinoma with treatment of HIV infection. *J R Soc Med* (2003) 96:238–9. doi:10.1177/014107680309600512

40. Chang Y, Moore PS. Merkel cell carcinoma: a virus-induced human cancer. *Annu Rev Pathol* (2012) 7:123–44. doi:10.1146/annurev-pathol-011110-130227

41. Foulongne V, Kluger N, Dereure O, Mercier G, Molès JP, Guillot B, et al. Merkel cell polyomavirus in cutaneous swabs. *Emerg Infect Dis* (2013) 16:685–7. doi:10.3201/eid1604.091278

42. Spurgeon ME, Lambert PF. Merkel cell polyomavirus: a newly discovered human virus with oncogenic potential. *Virology* (2013) 435:118–30. doi:10.1016/j.virol.2012.09.029

43. Shuda M, Feng H, Kwun HJ, Rosen ST, Gjoerup O, Moore PS, et al. T antigen mutations are a human tumor-specific signature for Merkel cell polyomavirus. *Proc Natl Acad Sci U S A* (2008) 105:16272–7. doi:10.1073/pnas.0806526105

44. Duncavage EJ, Zehnbauer BA, Pfeifer JD. Prevalence of Merkel cell polyomavirus in Merkel cell carcinoma. *Mod Pathol* (2009) 22:516–21. doi:10.1038/modpathol.2009.3

45. Neumann F, Borchert S, Schmidt C, Reimer R, Hohenberg H, Fischer N, et al. Replication, gene expression and particle production by a consensus Merkel Cell Polyomavirus (MCPyV) genome. *PLoS One* (2011) 6:e29112. doi:10.1371/journal.pone.0029112

46. Moshiri AS, Doumani R, Yelistratova L, Blom A, Lachance K, Shinohara MM, et al. Polyomavirus-negative Merkel cell carcinoma: a more aggressive subtype based on analysis of 282 cases using multimodal tumor virus detection. *J Invest Dermatol* (2017) 137:819–27. doi:10.1016/j.jid.2016.10.028

47. Lunder EJ, Stern RS. Merkel-cell carcinomas in patients treated with methoxsalen and ultraviolet A radiation. *N Engl J Med* (1998) 339:1247–8. doi:10.1056/NEJM199810223391715

48. Harms PW, Vats P, Verhaegen ME, Robinson DR, Wu YM, Dhanasekaran SM, et al. The distinctive mutational spectra of polyomavirus-negative Merkel cell carcinoma. *Cancer Res* (2015) 75:3720–7. doi:10.1158/0008-5472.CAN-15-0702

49. Goh G, Walradt T, Markarov V, Blom A, Riaz N, Doumani R, et al. Mutational landscape of MCPyV-positive and MCPyV-negative Merkel cell carcinomas with implications for immunotherapy. *Oncotarget* (2016) 7:3403–15. doi:10.18632/oncotarget.6494

50. González-Vela MD, Curiel-Olmo S, Derdak S, Beltran S, Santibañez M, Martínez N, et al. Shared oncogenic pathways implicated in both virus-positive and UV-induced Merkel cell carcinomas. *J Invest Dermatol* (2017) 137:197–206. doi:10.1016/j.jid.2016.08.015

51. NCCN. *NCCN Clinical Practice Guidelines in Oncology. Merkel Cell Carcinoma. Version 1.* 2018 ed. Fort Washington, PA: National Comprehensive Cancer Network, Inc (2017).

52. Gupta SG, Wang LC, Peñas PF, Gellenthin M, Lee SJ, Nghiem P. Sentinel lymph node biopsy for evaluation and treatment of patients with Merkel cell carcinoma: the Dana-Farber experience and meta-analysis of the literature. *Arch Dermatol* (2006) 142:685–90. doi:10.1001/archderm.142.6.685

53. Fields RC, Busam KJ, Chou JF, Panageas KS, Pulitzer MP, Kraus DH, et al. Recurrence and survival in patients undergoing sentinel lymph node biopsy for Merkel cell carcinoma: analysis of 153 patients from a single institution. *Ann Surg Oncol* (2011) 18:2529–37. doi:10.1245/s10434-011-1662-y

54. Voog E, Biron P, Martin JP, Blay JY. Chemotherapy for patients with locally advanced or metastatic Merkel cell carcinoma. *Cancer* (1999) 85:2589–95. doi:10.1002/(SICI)1097-0142(19990615)85:12<2589::AID-CNCR15>3.0.CO;2-F

55. Tai PT, Yu E, Winquist E, Hammond A, Stitt L, Tonita J, et al. Chemotherapy in neuroendocrine/Merkel cell carcinoma of the skin: case series and review of 204 cases. *J Clin Oncol* (2000) 18:2493–9. doi:10.1200/JCO.2000.18.12.2493

56. Iyer JG, Blom A, Doumani R, Lewis C, Tarabadkar ES, Anderson A, et al. Response rates and durability of chemotherapy among 62 patients with metastatic Merkel cell carcinoma. *Cancer Med* (2016) 5:2294–301. doi:10.1002/cam4.815

57. Schadendorf D, Lebbé C, Zur Hausen A, Avril MF, Hariharan S, Bharmal M, et al. Merkel cell carcinoma: epidemiology, prognosis, therapy and unmet medical needs. *Eur J Cancer* (2017) 71:53–69. doi:10.1016/j.ejca.2016.10.022

58. Paulson KG, Iyer JG, Tegeder AR, Thibodeau R, Schelter J, Koba S, et al. Transcriptome-wide studies of Merkel cell carcinoma and validation of intratumoral CD8+ lymphocyte invasion as an independent predictor of survival. *J Clin Oncol* (2011) 29:1539–46. doi:10.1200/JCO.2010.30.6308

59. Paulson KG, Iyer JG, Simonson WT, Blom A, Thibodeau RM, Schmidt M, et al. CD8+ lymphocyte intratumoral infiltration as a stage-independent predictor of Merkel cell carcinoma survival: a population-based study. *Am J Clin Pathol* (2014) 142:452–8. doi:10.1309/AJCPIKDZM39CRPNC

60. Iyer JG, Afanasiev OK, McClurkan C, Paulson K, Nagase K, Jing L, et al. Merkel cell polyomavirus specific CD8(+) and CD4(+) T-cell responses identified in Merkel cell carcinomas and blood. *Clin Cancer Res* (2011) 17:6671–80. doi:10.1158/1078-0432.CCR-11-1513

61. Afanasiev OK, Yelistratova L, Miller N, Nagase K, Paulson K, Iyer JG, et al. Merkel polyomavirus specific T cells fluctuate with Merkel cell carcinoma burden and express therapeutically targetable PD-1 and Tim-3 exhaustion markers. *Clin Cancer Res* (2013) 19:5351–60. doi:10.1158/1078-0432.CCR-13-0035

62. Lipson EJ, Vincent JG, Loyo M, Kagohara LT, Luber BS, Wang H, et al. PD-L1 expression in the Merkel cell carcinoma microenvironment: association with inflammation, Merkel cell polyomavirus and overall survival. *Cancer Immunol Res* (2013) 1:54–63. doi:10.1158/2326-6066.CIR-13-0034

63. Nghiem PT, Bhatia S, Lipson EJ, Kudchadkar RR, Miller NJ, Annamalai L, et al. PD-1 blockade with pembrolizumab in advanced Merkel-cell carcinoma. *N Engl J Med* (2016) 374:2542–52. doi:10.1056/NEJMoa1603702

64. NCCN. *NCCN Clinical Practice Guidelines in Oncology. Merkel Cell Carcinoma. Version 1.* 2017 ed. Fort Washington, PA: National Comprehensive Cancer Network, Inc (2016).

65. Kaufman HL, Russell J, Hamid O, Bhatia S, Terheyden P, D'Angelo SP, et al. Avelumab in patients with chemotherapy-refractory metastatic Merkel cell carcinoma: a multicentre, single-group, open-label, phase 2 trial. *Lancet Oncol* (2016) 17:1374–85. doi:10.1016/S1470-2045(16)30364-3

23

Biomarkers for Predicting Efficacies of Anti-PD1 Antibodies

Yumi Kambayashi*, Taku Fujimura, Takanori Hidaka and Setsuya Aiba

Department of Dermatology, Tohoku University Graduate School of Medicine, Sendai, Japan

Correspondence:
Yumi Kambayashi
yumi1001@hosp.tohoku.ac.jp

Therapeutic options for treating advanced melanoma are progressing rapidly. Although anti-programmed cell death 1 (PD1) antibodies (e.g., nivolumab, pembrolizumab) have been approved as first-line and anchor drugs, respectively, for treating advanced melanoma, the efficacy appears limited as we expected, especially in Asian populations. Biomarkers to predict or evaluate the efficacy of anti-PD1 antibodies are needed to avoid subjecting patients to potentially severe adverse events associated with switching to other anti-melanoma drugs. This review focuses on the recent development of biomarkers for assessing the efficacy of anti-PD1 antibodies using routine blood tests such as the neutrophil-to-lymphocyte ratio, eosinophil ratio, serum markers such as lactate dehydrogenase, programmed cell death ligand 1 (PD-L1) expression on melanoma cells, microsatellite instability and mismatch repair deficiency assays, as well as soluble CD163, and tumor-associated macrophage-related chemokines (e.g., CXCL5, CXCL10).

Keywords: anti-PD1 antibodies, routine blood test, LDH, MSH, TMB, TAM-related factors

INTRODUCTION

Anti-programmed cell death 1 (PD-1) antibodies are in wide use for the treatment of various cancers, particularly cancers with a high tumor mutation burden (TMB) such as advanced cutaneous melanoma (1–4). Although BRAF inhibitors in combination with MEK inhibitors are useful for the treatment of BRAF^{V600}-mutant advanced melanoma, the population of BRAF^{V600}-mutant advanced melanoma is limited, particularly in the Japanese population, which contains large populations with acral lentiginous melanoma and mucosal melanoma (5, 6). Most patients with advanced melanoma are therefore administered nivolumab with or without ipilimumab, or pembrolizumab as a first-line therapy.

Ipilimumab is a fully humanized immunoglobulin (Ig)G1 monoclonal antibody that blocks cytotoxic T-lymphocyte antigen (CTLA-4) to activate and increase T cells, particularly the tumor-recognized T-cell clones that reside in primary tumors (7, 8). Combination therapy comprising nivolumab and ipilimumab or sequential administration of nivolumab and ipilimumab with a planned switch are among the most effective chemotherapies against advanced melanoma (9–11), and even increase the response rate (RR) for untreated metastasis of melanoma to the brain compared to nivolumab monotherapy (12). On the other hand, the efficacy of ipilimumab in patients with nivolumab-resistant melanoma is low after objective tumor progression compared to planned-switched patients (13). In addition, ipilimumab leads to a high frequency of immune-related adverse events (irAEs) among patients with advanced melanoma, particularly combination therapy with nivolumab (9, 11). Taken together, evaluation of the efficacy of these treatments in advance is important.

This review focuses on the recent development of biomarkers for assessing the efficacy of anti-PD1 antibodies using routine blood tests such as the neutrophil-to-lymphocyte ratio, eosinophil ratio, serum markers such as lactate dehydrogenase (LDH), PD-L1 expression on melanoma cells, microsatellite instability (MSI) and mismatch repair deficiency assays, as well as soluble CD163, and tumor-associated macrophage (TAM)-related chemokines (e.g., CXCL5, CXCL10) (**Table 1**).

SIGNIFICANCE OF ROUTINE BLOOD TESTS FOR PREDICTING THE EFFICACY OF ANTI-PD1 ANTIBODY

Leukocyte-to-Lymphocyte Ratio (LLR), Neutrophil-to-Lymphocyte Ratio (NLR), Monocyte Count, and Absolute Lymphocyte Count (ALC)

Recent reports have suggested the significance of routine blood tests, such as cell counts and cell ratios, for predicting the efficacy of anti-PD1 antibodies against advanced melanomas (14–18). Indeed, Fujisawa et al. reported that increased baseline NLR combined with serum LDH was significantly correlated with the efficacy rate of nivolumab according to multivariate analysis, and negatively correlated with efficacy of nivolumab for advanced melanoma (14). In another report, Chasseuil et al. found that increased monocyte count was significantly associated with decreased overall survival (OS) and progression-free survival (PFS) in patients with advanced melanoma according to multivariate analysis. In addition, they also reported that LLR was significantly associated with decreased OS (15). In addition, Rosner et al. reported that not only a low NLR, but also high proportion of eosinophils, high proportion of basophils, low absolute monocyte count and low LDH might be independently associated with favorable OS (16). Since several previous reports have also suggested that NLR is significantly correlated with the efficacy of ipilimumab in the treatment of melanoma patients (17, 18), baseline NLR could be one possible predictive marker for immune checkpoint inhibitor (ICI)-treated patients with advanced melanoma.

Lower ALC shows significantly less clinical benefit from anti-PD1 antibody (19), which is associated with pretreatment NLR in patients with head and neck squamous cell carcinoma. They concluded that patients with pretreatment ALC <600 cells/μl had shorter PFS than patients with pretreatment ALC ≥600 cells/μl. In another report, Soyano et al. retrospectively analyzed 157 patients with advanced non-small cell lung cancer (NSCLC) treated with anti-PD1 antibodies using logistic regression analysis, suggesting that a high baseline NLR correlated significantly with increased risks of death and disease progression (20). In addition, they also reported that a high baseline myeloid-to-lymphoid cell ratio significantly increased the risk of death, even after multivariate analysis [hazard ratio (HR) = 2.31, p = 0.002]. Indeed, a meta-analysis of 14 retrospective studies that had examined the benefits of nivolumab in patients with NSCLC suggested an association of high NLR with poor PFS and OS after nivolumab treatment (21). Moreover, they also

TABLE 1 | Highlighted papers in each chapter.

	Interest	Considerable interest
Routine blood test	14, 21, 25	23
PD-L1 expression	31	32
MSI and TMB	40, 43	3, 39
TAMs related factors	24, 50	48

reported that post-treatment NLR acted as a predictor of PFS and OS. Overall, these reports have suggested that baseline routine blood tests are important for predicting the efficacy of ICI (**Table 2**).

Clinical Use of LDH

Generally, large baseline tumor size in parallel with increased levels of LDH correlates with poor prognosis in advanced melanoma patients (25). Diem et al. first reported the benefit of measuring serum LDH in 66 patients with advanced melanoma treated using anti-PD1 antibody (22). Indeed, patients with elevated baseline LDH showed significantly shorter OS compared to patients with normal LDH. Moreover, they suggested serum LDH as a useful marker during treatment for predicting both early response of anti-PD1 antibody and progressive disease (22).

ECOG performance status (PS) and elevated LDH were reported as independent variables significantly associated with poor OS (26). More recently, Wagner et al. reported serum LDH levels and S100B among the early prognostic markers for response and OS in advanced melanoma patients treated with ICI (27). They concluded that, compared with patients showing normal LDH, increased serum LDH (>25%) was significantly associated with impaired OS when co-existing with increased serum levels of S100B (27). Increased LDH correlated with the poor prognostic factors of not only cutaneous melanoma, but also uveal melanoma, which possesses a high potential for rapid metastasis (28), and NSCLC (29). Since anti-PD1 antibody applies to various cancers, including gastric cancer, renal cell carcinoma, and Hodgkin lymphoma, measurement of LDH might offer a useful, standard marker for patients treated using ICI.

EXPRESSION LEVELS OF PD-L1

In cutaneous melanoma, both tumor cells and TAMs express PD-L1, leading to the maintenance of an immunosuppressive microenvironment at tumor sites (30, 31). Hino et al. first reported PD-L1 expression on melanoma cells as an independent prognostic factor that correlates with vertical invasion of melanoma cells (31). Accordingly, many studies have suggested that PD-L1 expression on melanoma cells can represent a biomarker for predicting the efficacy of anti-PD1 antibodies (32, 33), and even other ICIs (34). For example, PD-L1 expression on melanoma cells in pretreatment tumor biopsy samples correlated

TABLE 2 | Summary of biomarkers and their efficacy.

Treatment	Patients number	Subpopulation	Outcome	Marker	Result (95% CI) RR = 14%	p-value	References
Nivolumab	n = 90	LDH (upper normal limit)	RR	NLR > 2.2 NLR < 2.2	RR=14% RR=57%	<0.05	(14)
		LDH normal	RR	NLR > 2.2 NLR < 2.2	RR=37% RR=67%	<0.001	
Nivolumab	n = 87		OS	Monocyte count (upper normal limit)	HR = 4.31 (1.46–12.74)	0.01	(15)
			PFS	Monocyte count (upper normal limit)	HR = 3.5 (1.01–12.1)	0.04	
Nivolumab + Ipllimumab	n = 209		OS		HR = 1.95 (111–3.47)	0.02	(16)
				NLR	HR = 2.38 (1.27–4.46)	0.007	
				Eosinophils	HR = 1.86 (0.94–3.66)	0.08	
				Basophils	HR = 2.75 (1.30–5.80)	0.01	
				Absolute monocyte LDH (246<)	HR = 3.71(2.08–6.61)	<0.0001	
Lpllimumab	n = 183		OS	Baseline NLR NLR (end of treatement)	HR = 1.06 (1.01–1.10) HR = 1.06 (1.02–1.09)	0.016 <0.001	(17)
Lpllimumab	n = 720		OS PFS	ANC ANC	HR = 3.38 (2.62–4.36) HR = 2.52 (1.97–3.21)	<0.0001 <0.0001	(18)
Anti-PD1 antibody	n = 66		OS	LDH elevated LDH normal	4.3 months 15,7 months	<0.00623	(22)
Nivolumab	n = 210		RR	PD-L1 positive PD-L1 negative	52.7% (40.8–64.3) 33.1% (25.2–41.7)		(23)
Nivolumab	n = 59		RR	Increased Scd163	Sensitivity 84.6% Specificity 87.0%	<0.0030	(24)

ANC, absolute neutrophilcount; HR, hazzard ratio; NLR, neutrophilto lymphocyte ratio; OS, overall survival; PFS, progress free survival; RR, response rate; UNL, under normal limit.

with RR, PFS, and OS in advanced melanoma patients treated using anti-PD1 antibodies (33). In another report, expression of PD-L1 correlated with 24-month survival rate in patients with advanced melanoma treated with pembrolizumab (32). Indeed, median PFS in patients with PD-L1 positive melanoma cells was 6.6 months (95% confidence interval (CI), 4.2–9.7 months), while median PFS in patients with PD-L1-negative melanoma cells was 2.8 months (95%CI, 2.8-3.7 months) (32). On the other hand, Hodi et al. reported that assessment of the expression of PD-L1 alone offers a poor predictor of OS in patients treated with nivolumab or nivolumab in combination with ipilimumab (CheckMate 067) (34). Notably, even in PD-L1-negative or -intermediate expressing groups, the RR is still high (33.1%; 95%CI, 25.2-41.7%), suggesting that PD-L1 expression might represent an independent prognostic factor (35). Although those reports suggested the clinical benefits of assessing PD-L1 expression on melanoma cells in predicting the clinical outcomes of ICI treatment, the clinical utility in the real world is limited because of the low sensitivity of immunohistochemical (IHC) assays using different antibody clones, staining platforms and scoring systems in each institute (32–36). To avoid misprediction by IHC staining, more recently, Conroy et al. tried to assess the expression of PD-L1 using next-generation RNA sequencing, but the sensitivity of their system resembles that of IHC assay systems (36). In future, additional assays will be needed to improve the sensitivity of PD-L1 analysis in the prediction of clinical outcomes for ICI treatment of melanoma.

MSI AND TMB

The high RR to anti-PD1 antibodies for cancers with high frequency of MSI has been highlighted in many recent clinical studies (37, 38). Among cancer species, colorectal cancer and endometrial cancer possess a high frequency of MSI (approx. 20~33%) (38, 39), leading to the results of clinical studies that have presented significantly improved RR, PFS and OS in patients with mismatch-repair deficient colorectal cancers compared to those of mismatch repair-proficient colorectal cancers (37–39). Recent reports have also suggested that high infiltration of T-helper 1 (Th1) cells and cytotoxic T lymphocytes (CTLs) produce substantial amounts of interferon gamma (IFNγ), leading to increased expression of PD-L1 in tumors with a high frequency of MSI (37, 40). As described above, since high expression of PD-L1 can provide a biomarker for predicting the efficacy of anti-PD1 antibodies, a high frequency of MSI could correlate with RR, PFS and OS following use of anti-PD1 antibodies.

High TMB correlated with increased neoantigens in various cancers, and could provide predictors for the efficacy of ICI treatment (1, 2, 41). For example, cutaneous squamous cell carcinoma (cSCC) possesses a high TMB (50 mutations per megabase DNA pairs) (42), leading to a high RR for cemiplimab [47% (95%CI, 34–61%)] (43). In addition, since an ultraviolet (UV) damage subclass of SCC and sebaceous carcinoma harbors a high somatic mutation burden with >50 mutations per megabase, UV damage signatures in TMB in these skin cancers could be predictive biomarkers for ICI treatment (44, 45). In melanoma, Madore et al. reported that a lower non-synonymous mutation burden correlated with negative results for PD-L1 expression on melanoma cells, and significantly worse melanoma-specific survival in stage III melanoma (HR = 0.28; 95%CI, 0.12-0.66; P = 0.002) (3). In addition, significant increases in the gene expression signatures of cytotoxic T-cell (CTL) and macrophage-specific genes were seen in PD-L1-positive melanomas, correlating with better melanoma-specific survival (HR = 0.2; 95%CI, 0.05-0.87; P = 0.017). Taken together, those reports might suggest the significance of assessing TMB before the administration of ICIs, especially anti-PD1 antibodies, although further studies are needed to confirm its effectiveness.

PILOT STUDY FOR PREDICTABLE BIOMARKERS: TAM-RELATED FACTORS (SCD163, CXCL5)

TAMs are functionally reprogrammed to polarized phenotypes by exposure to various factors, leading to the maintenance of a tumor microenvironment (30). Expression of PD-L1 on TAMs is modified by both stromal factors such as regulatory T cells (Tregs) and exogenous factors including immune therapies (46). For example, in a mouse melanoma model (ret, B16 melanoma), depletion of Tregs decreased PD-L1, B7H3, and B7H4 expression on TAMs in vivo (46). In patients with esophageal carcinoma, a high density of CD163+ TAMs, which is also associated with significantly increased PD-L1 expression (47), was associated with significantly worse OS than a low density (log-rank P = 0.0025) (47). That report suggested that a high density of PD-L1-expressing CD163+ TAMs could offer a prognostic biomarker for esophageal carcinoma (47). Since PD-L1 on tumor cells could be one prognostic factor for melanoma patients treated with ICIs (as described in Chapter 3), TAM-related factors could offer biomarkers for predicting the efficacy of ICI.

TAMs in melanoma patients express not only PD-L1, but also PD-1 (48). Because PD-1 expression in TAMs is one of the key factors in M2 macrophage polarization (49), administration of an anti-PD1 antibody might repolarize TAMs, leading to TAM activation in melanoma patients. Notably, the main population of TAMs in skin cancer is CD163+ M2 macrophages, with soluble (s)CD163 as the activation marker (14). This means that CD163 activated with PD1 antibody should release sCD163, suggesting its utility as a prognostic marker for anti-PD1 antibody treatment. Indeed, serum levels of sCD163 were significantly increased in responders compared to non-responders 6 weeks after initial administration of

nivolumab for cutaneous melanoma (84.6% sensitivity, 87.0% specificity; p = 0.0030) (24). Moreover, absolute serum levels of sCD163 after 6 weeks were significantly increased in patients treated with nivolumab who developed irAEs (p = 0.0018) (49). Those reports suggested that serum sCD163 could offer a predictive marker for the efficacy and irAEs of anti-PD1 antibodies.

In addition to sCD163, TAM-related chemokines could provide another group of prognostic markers for the outcomes of anti-PD1 antibody treatment (50). For example, CXCL5 is a chemokine that can recruit neutrophils, CXCR2+ myeloid-derived suppressor cells (MDSCs) and CXCR2+ monocytes. As we previously reported, production of CXCL5 from TAMs is increased by stimulation with periostin (51), which is detected in the stroma of cutaneous melanomas (23, 49). As we previously reported, baseline serum CXCL5 is associated with the efficacy of nivolumab in advanced melanoma (50) and increased serum levels of CXCL5 correlated significantly with irAEs from nivolumab (49). Unlike CXCL5, baseline serum concentrations of CXCL10 and CCL22 have not shown any correlations with the efficacy of nivolumab against advanced melanoma (50). These data suggested that TAM-related chemokines could further improve the predictive value of sCD163 systems in the future.

Although combination therapy with nivolumab and ipilimumab is recommended by the NCCN guideline for cutaneous melanoma as a first-line therapy (52), as described above, this combination therapy leads to a high frequency of SAEs among patients with advanced melanoma (9, 11). In the future, the evaluation of serum sCD163 as well as several TAM-related chemokines will undoubtedly play an important role in avoiding the administration of ipilimumab for patients who respond to anti-PD1 antibodies.

CONCLUDING REMARKS

Although several studies have suggested useful predictive markers for the efficacy and irAEs of ICIs, exact methods to determine predictive markers remain under investigation. Further studies are needed to improve the systems for predicting the efficacy of ICI treatment.

AUTHOR CONTRIBUTIONS

YK, TF, and TH wrote manuscript. SA supervise the manuscript.

REFERENCES

1. Le DT, Durham JN, Smith KN, Wang H, Bartlett BR, Aulakh LK, et al. Mismatch repair deficiency predicts response of solid tumors to PD-1 blockade. Science. (2017) 357:409–13. doi: 10.1126/science. aan6733

2. Riaz N, Havel JJ, Makarov V, Desrichard A, Urba WJ, Sims JS, et al. Tumor and microenvironment evolution during immunotherapy with Nivolumab. Cell. (2017) 171:934–49. doi: 10.1016/j.cell.2017.09.028

3. Madore J, Strbenac D, Vilain R, Menzies AM, Yang JY, Thompson JF, et al. PD-L1 negative status is associated with lower mutation burden, differential expression of immune-related genes, and worse

survival in stage III Melanoma. *Clin Cancer Res.* (2016) 22:3915–23. doi: 10.1158/1078-0432.CCR-15-1714

4. McGranahan N, Furness AJ, Rosenthal R, Ramskov S, Lyngaa R, Saini SK, et al. Clonal neoantigens elicit T cell immunoreactivity and sensitivity to immune checkpoint blockade. *Science.* (2016) 351:1463–9. doi: 10.1126/science.aaf1490

5. Fujimura T, Hidaka T, Kambayashi Y, Aiba S. BRAF kinase inhibitors for the treatment of melanoma: developments from early stage animal studies to phase II clinical trials. *Exp Opin Invest Drugs.* (2019) 28:143–8. doi: 10.1080/13543784.2019.1558442

6. Hayward NK, Wilmott JS, Waddell N, Johansson PA, Field MA, Nones K, et al. Whole-genome landscapes of major melanoma subtypes. *Nature.* (2017) 545:175–80. doi: 10.1038/nature22071

7. Blank CU, Rozeman EA, Fanchi LF, Sikorska K, van de Wiel B, Kvistborg P, et al. Neoadjuvant versus adjuvant ipilimumab plus nivolumab in macroscopic stage III melanoma. *Nat Med.* (2018) 24:1655–61. doi: 10.1038/s41591-018-0198-0

8. Callahan MK, Wolchok JD, Allison JP. Anti-CTLA-4 antibody therapy: immune monitoring during clinical development of a novel immunotherapy. *Semin Oncol.* (2010) 37:473–84. doi: 10.1053/j.seminoncol.2010.09.001

9. Larkin J, Chiarion-Sileni V, Gonzalez R, Grob JJ, Cowey CL, Lao CD, et al. Combined nivolumab and ipilimumab or monotherapy in untreated melanoma. *N Engl J Med.* (2015) 373:23–34. doi: 10.1056/NEJMoa1504030

10. Weber JS, Gibney G, Sullivan RJ, Sosman JA, Slingluff CL Jr, Lawrence DP, et al. Sequential administration of nivolumab and ipilimumab with a planned switch in patients with advanced melanoma (CheckMate 064): an open-label, randomised, phase 2 trial. *Lancet Oncol.* (2016) 17:943–55. doi: 10.1016/S1470-2045(16)30126-7

11. Tawbi HA, Forsyth PA, Algazi A, Hamid O, Hodi FS, Moschos SJ, et al. Combined nivolumab and ipilimumab in melanoma metastatic to the brain. *N Engl J Med.* (2018) 379:722–30. doi: 10.1056/NEJMoa1805453

12. Wolchok JD, Chiarion-Sileni V, Gonzalez R, Rutkowski P, Grob JJ, Cowey CL, et al. Overall survival with combined nivolumab and ipilimumab in advanced melanoma. *N Engl J Med.* (2017) 377:1345–56. doi: 10.1056/NEJMoa1709684

13. Fujisawa Y, Yoshino K, Otsuka A, Funakoshi T, Fujimura T, Yamamoto Y, et al. Retrospective study of advanced melanoma patients treated with ipilimumab after nivolumab: analysis of 60 Japanese patients. *J Dermatol Sci.* (2018) 89:60–6. doi: 10.1016/j.jdermsci.2017.10.009

14. Fujisawa Y, Yoshino K, Otsuka A, Funakoshi T, Fujimura T, Yamamoto Y, et al. Baseline neutrophil to lymphocyte ratio combined with serum lactate dehydrogenase level associated with outcome of nivolumab immunotherapy in a Japanese advanced melanoma population. *Br J Dermatol.* (2018) 179:213–5. doi: 10.1111/bjd.16427

15. Chasseuil E, Saint-Jean M, Chasseuil H, Peuvrel L, Quéreux G, Nguyen JM, et al. Blood predictive biomarkers for nivolumab in advanced melanoma. *Acta Derm Venereol.* (2018) 98:406–10. doi: 10.2340/00015555-2872

16. Rosner S, Kwong E, Shoushtari AN, Friedman CF, Betof AS, Brady MS, et al. Peripheral blood clinical laboratory variables associated with outcomes following combination nivolumab and ipilimumab immunotherapy in melanoma. *Cancer Med.* (2018) 7:690–7. doi: 10.1002/cam4.1356

17. Khoja L, Atenafu EG, Templeton A, Qye Y, Chappell MA, Saibil S, et al. The full blood count as a biomarker of outcome and toxicity in ipilimumab-treated cutaneous metastatic melanoma. *Cancer Med.* (2016) 5:2792–9. doi: 10.1002/cam4.878

18. Ferrucci PF, Ascierto PA, Pigozzo J, Del Vecchio M, Maio M, Antonini Cappellini GC, et al. Baseline neutrophils and derived neutrophil-to-lymphocyte ratio: prognostic relevance in metastatic melanoma patients receiving ipilimumab. *Ann Oncol.* (2016) 27:732–8. doi: 10.1093/annonc/mdw016

19. Ho WJ, Yarchoan M, Hopkins A, Mehra R, Grossman S, Kang H. Association between pretreatment lymphocyte count and response to PD1 inhibitors in head and neck squamous cell carcinomas. *J Immunother Cancer.* (2018) 6:84. doi: 10.1186/s40425-018-0395-x

20. Soyano AE, Dholaria B, Marin-Acevedo JA, Diehl N, Hodge D, Luo Y, et al. Peripheral blood biomarkers correlate with outcomes in advanced non-small cell lung Cancer patients treated with anti-PD-1 antibodies. *J Immunother Cancer.* (2018) 6:129. doi: 10.1186/s40425-018-0447-2

21. Cao D, Xu H, Xu X, Guo T, Ge W. A reliable and feasible way to predict the benefits of Nivolumab in patients with non-small cell lung cancer: a pooled analysis of 14 retrospective studies. *Oncoimmunology.* (2018) 7:e1507262. doi: 10.1080/2162402X.2018.1507262

22. Diem S, Kasenda B, Spain L, Martin-Liberal J, Marconcini R, Gore M, et al. Serum lactate dehydrogenase as an early marker for outcome in patients treated with anti-PD-1 therapy in metastatic melanoma. *Br J Cancer.* (2016) 114:256–61. doi: 10.1038/bjc.2015.467

23. Fukuda K, Sugihara E, Ohta S, Izuhara K, Funakoshi T, Amagai M, et al. Periostin is a key niche component for wound metastasis of melanoma. *PLoS ONE.* (2015) 10:e0129704. doi: 10.1371/journal.pone.0129704

24. Fujimura T, Sato Y, Tanita K, Kambayashi Y, Otsuka A, Fujisawa Y, et al. Serum level of soluble CD163 may be a predictive marker of the effectiveness of nivolumab in patients with advanced cutaneous melanoma. *Front Oncol.* (2018) 8:530. doi: 10.3389/fonc.2018.00530

25. Warner AB, Postow MA. bigger is not always better: tumor size and prognosis in advanced Melanoma. *Clin Cancer Res.* (2018) 24:4915–7. doi: 10.1158/1078-0432.CCR-18-1311

26. Nakamura Y, Kitano S, Takahashi A, Tsutsumida A, Namikawa K, Tanese K, et al. Nivolumab for advanced melanoma: pretreatment prognostic factors and early outcome markers during therapy. *Oncotarget.* (2016) 7:77404–15. doi: 10.18632/oncotarget.12677

27. Wagner NB, Forschner A, Leiter U, Garbe C, Eigentler TK. S100B and LDH as early prognostic markers for response and overall survival in melanoma patients treated with anti-PD-1 or combined anti-PD-1 plus anti-CTLA-4 antibodies. *Br J Cancer.* (2018) 119:339–46. doi: 10.1038/s41416-018-0167-x

28. Heppt MV, Heinzerling L, Kähler KC, Forschner A, Kirchberger MC, Loquai C, et al. Prognostic factors and outcomes in metastatic uveal melanoma treated with programmed cell death-1 or combined PD-1/cytotoxic T-lymphocyte antigen-4 inhibition. *Eur J Cancer.* (2017) 82:56–65. doi: 10.1016/j.ejca.2017.05.038

29. Taniguchi Y, Tamiya A, Isa SI, Nakahama K, Okishio K, Shiroyama T, et al. Predictive factors for poor progression-free survival in patients with non-small cell lung cancer treated with nivolumab. *Anticancer Res.* (2017) 37:5857–62. doi: 10.21873/anticanres.12030

30. Fujimura T, Kambayashi Y, Fujisawa Y, Hidaka T, Aiba S. Tumor-associated macrophages: therapeutic targets for skin cancer. *Front Oncol.* (2018) 8:3. doi: 10.3389/fonc.2018.00003

31. Hino R, Kabashima K, Kato Y, Yagi H, Nakamura M, Honjo T, et al. Tumor cell expression of programmed cell death-1 ligand 1 is a prognostic factor for malignant melanoma. *Cancer.* (2010) 116:1757–66. doi: 10.1002/cncr.24899

32. Carlino MS, Long GV, Schadendorf D, Robert C, Ribas A, Richtig E, et al. Outcomes by line of therapy and programmed death ligand 1 expression in patients with advanced melanoma treated with pembrolizumab or ipilimumab in KEYNOTE-006: a randomised clinical trial. *Eur J Cancer.* (2018) 101:236–43. doi: 10.1016/j.ejca.2018.06.034

33. Daud AI, Wolchok JD, Robert C, Hwu WJ, Weber JS, Ribas A, et al. Programmed death-ligand 1 expression and response to the anti-programmed death 1 antibody pembrolizumab in melanoma. *J Clin Oncol.* (2016) 34:4102–9. doi: 10.1200/JCO.2016.67.2477

34. Hodi FS, Chiarion-Sileni V, Gonzalez R, Grob JJ, Rutkowski P, Cowey CL, et al. Nivolumab plus ipilimumab or nivolumab alone versus ipilimumab alone in advanced melanoma (CheckMate 067): 4-year outcomes of a multicentre, randomised, phase 3 trial. *Lancet Oncol.* (2018) 19:1480–92. doi: 10.1016/S1470-2045(18)30700-9

35. Robert C, Long GV, Brady B, Dutriaux C, Maio M, Mortier L, et al. Nivolumab in previously untreated melanoma without BRAF mutation. *N Engl J Med.* (2015) 372:320–30. doi: 10.1056/NEJMoa1412082

36. Conroy JM, Pabla S, Nesline MK, Glenn ST, Papanicolau-Sengos A, Burgher B, et al. Next generation sequencing of PD-L1 for predicting response to immune checkpoint inhibitors. *J Immunother Cancer.* (2019) 7:18. doi: 10.1186/s40425-018-0489-5

37. Dudley JC, Lin MT, Le DT, Eshleman JR. Microsatellite Instability as a Biomarker for PD-1 Blockade. *Clin Cancer Res.* (2016) 22:813–20. doi: 10.1158/1078-0432.CCR-15-1678

38. Le DT, Uram JN, Wang H, Bartlett BR, Kemberling H, Eyring AD, et al. PD-1 Blockade in tumors with mismatch-repair deficiency. *N Engl J Med.* (2015) 372:2509–20. doi: 10.1056/NEJMoa1500596

39. Zighelboim I, Goodfellow PJ, Gao F, Gibb RK, Powell MA, Rader JS, et al. Microsatellite instability and epigenetic inactivation of MLH1 and outcome of patients with endometrial carcinomas of the endometrioid type. *J Clin Oncol.* (2007) 25:2042–8. doi: 10.1200/JCO.2006.08.2107

40. Llosa NJ, Cruise M, Tam A, Wicks EC, Hechenbleikner EM, Taube JM, et al. The vigorous immune microenvironment of microsatellite instable colon cancer is balanced by multiple counter-inhibitory checkpoints. *Cancer Discov.* (2015) 5:43–51. doi: 10.1158/2159-8290.CD-14-0863

41. Samstein RM, Lee CH, Shoushtari AN, Hellmann MD, Shen R, Janjigian YY, et al. Tumor mutational load predicts survival after immunotherapy across multiple cancer types. *Nat Genet.* (2019) 51:202–6. doi: 10.1038/s41588-018-0312-8

42. Inman GJ, Wang J, Nagano A, Alexandrov LB, Purdie KJ, Taylor RG, et al. The genomic landscape of cutaneous SCC reveals drivers and a novel azathioprine associated mutational signature. *Nat Commun.* (2018) 9:3667. doi: 10.1038/s41467-018-06027-1

43. Migden MR, Rischin D, Schmults CD, Guminski A, Hauschild A, Lewis KD, et al. PD-1 blockade with cemiplimab in advanced cutaneous squamous-cell carcinoma. *N Engl J Med.* (2018) 379:341–51. doi: 10.1056/NEJMoa18 05131

44. Chan JW, Yeh I, El-Sayed IH, Algazi AP, Glastonbury CM, Ha PK, et al. Ultraviolet light-related DNA damage mutation signature distinguishes cutaneous from mucosal or other origin for head and neck squamous cell carcinoma of unknown primary site. *Head Neck.* (2019). 41, E82–5. doi: 10.1002/hed.25613

45. North JP, Golovato J, Vaske CJ, Sanborn JZ, Nguyen A, Wu W, et al. Cell of origin and mutation pattern define three clinically distinct classes of sebaceous carcinoma. *Nat Commun.* (2018) 9:1894. doi: 10.1038/s41467-018-04008-y

46. Fujimura T, Ring S, Umansky V, Mahnke K, Enk AH. Regulatory T cells (Treg) stimulate B7-H1 expression in myeloid derived suppressor cells (MDSC) in *ret* melanomas. *J Invest Dermatol.* (2012) 132:1239–46. doi: 10.1038/jid.2011.416

47. Yagi T, Baba Y, Okadome K, Kiyozumi Y, Hiyoshi Y, Ishimoto T, et al. Tumour-associated macrophages are associated with poor prognosis and programmed death ligand 1 expression in oesophageal cancer. *Eur J Cancer.* (2019) 111:38–49. doi: 10.1016/j.ejca.2019.01.018

48. Gordon SR, Maute RL, Dulken BW, Hutter G, George BM, McCracken MN, et al. PD-1 expression by tumour-associated macrophages inhibits phagocytosis and tumour immunity. *Nature.* (2017) 545:495–9. doi: 10.1038/nature22396

49. Fujimura T, Sato Y, Tanita K, Kambayashi Y, Otsuka A, Fujisawa Y, et al. Serum levels of soluble CD163 and CXCL5 may be predictive markers for immune-related adverse events in patients with advanced melanoma treated with nivolumab: a pilot study. *Oncotarget.* (2018) 9:15542–51. doi: 10.18632/oncotarget.24509

50. Fujimura T, Sato Y, Tanita K, Lyu C, Kambayash Y, Amagai R, et al. Association of baseline serum levels of CXCL5 with the efficacy of nivolumab in advanced melanoma. *Front Med.* (2019) 6:86. doi: 10.3389/fmed.2019.00086

51. Furudate S, Fujimura T, Kakizaki A, Kambayashi Y, Asano M, Watabe A, et al. The possible interaction between periostin expressed by cancer stroma and tumor-associated macrophages in developing mycosis fungoides. *Exp Dermatol.* (2016) 25:107–12. doi: 10.1111/exd.12873

52. *NCCN Clinical Practice Guidelines in Oncology (NCCN Guidelines®) Melanoma Version 2.* Available online at: https://www.nccn.org/professionals/physician_gls/pdf/cutaneous_melanoma.pdf. In. 2019 (accessed March 12, 2019).

Permissions

List of Contributors

Byung Ho Oh and Kee Yang Chung
Department of Dermatology and Cutaneous Biology Research Institute, Yonsei University College of Medicine, Seoul, South Korea

Ki Hean Kim
Department of Mechanical Engineering, Pohang University of Science and Technology, Pohang-si, South Korea

Kristian M. Hargadon
Hargadon Laboratory, Department of Biology, Hampden-Sydney College, Hampden-Sydney, VA, United States

Yasuhiro Nakamura
Department of Skin Oncology/Dermatology, Saitama Medical University International Medical Center, Saitama, Japan

Hassan Sadozai, Thomas Gruber and Mirjam Schenk
Institute of Pathology, Experimental Pathology, University of Bern, Bern, Switzerland

Robert Emil Hunger
Department of Dermatology, University Hospital Bern, Bern, Switzerland

Azusa Hiura, Koji Yoshino, Takuya Maeda, Kojiro Nagai, Satoe Oaku, Chisato Yamashita, Megumi Kato and Jiro Uehara
Department of Dermatologic Oncology, Tokyo Metropolitan Cancer and Infectious Diseases Center Komagome Hospital, Tokyo, Japan

Takayuki Nakayama and Makiko Yamashita
Department of Experimental Therapeutics, National Cancer Center Hospital, Tokyo, Japan

Shigehisa Kitano
Department of Experimental Therapeutics, National Cancer Center Hospital, Tokyo, Japan
Division of Cancer Immunotherapy, Exploratory Oncology Research and Clinical Trial Center, National Cancer Center, Tokyo, Japan

Christiane Kümpers, Mladen Jokic, Anne Offermann, Wenzel Vogel and Sven Perner
Pathology of the University Hospital Schleswig-Holstein, Luebeck and Research Center Borstel, Leibniz Lung Center, Luebeck, Germany

Ozan Haase, Victoria Grätz and Patrick Terheyden
Department of Dermatology, University of Luebeck, Luebeck, Germany

Ewan A. Langan
Department of Dermatology, University of Luebeck, Luebeck, Germany
Department of Dermatological Sciences, University of Manchester, Manchester, United Kingdom

Chunbing Lyu
Department of Dermatology, Tohoku University Graduate School of Medicine, Sendai, Japan

Yumi Nonomura
Department of Dermatology, Kyoto University Graduate School of Medicine, Kyoto, Japan

Yasuhiro Fujisawa and Ryota Tanaka
Department of Dermatology, University of Tsukuba, Tsukuba, Japan

Shigeto Matsushita
Department of Dermato-Oncology/Dermatology, National Hospital Organization Kagoshima Medical Center, Kagoshima, Japan

Hiroshi Uchi and Naoko Wada
Department of Dermatology, Kyushu University Graduate School of Medicine, Fukuoka, Japan

Yuki Yamamoto and Hisako Okuhira
Department of Dermatology, Wakayama Medical University, Wakayama, Japan

Sabrina A. Hogan, Mitchell P. Levesque and Phil F. Cheng
Department of Dermatology, UniversitätsSpital Zürich, Gloriastrasse, Zurich, Switzerland
Faculty of Medicine, Universität Zürich, Zürich, Switzerland

Judith A. Seidel and Atsushi Otsuka
Department of Dermatology, Kyoto University Graduate School of Medicine, Kyoto, Japan

Kenji Kabashima
Department of Dermatology, Kyoto University Graduate School of Medicine, Kyoto, Japan
Singapore Immunology Network (SIgN), Institute of Medical Biology, Agency for Science, Technology and Research (A*STAR), Biopolis, Singapore, Singapore

Yota Sato, Kayo Tanita, Ryo Amagai and Akira Hashimoto
Department of Dermatology, Tohoku University Graduate School of Medicine, Sendai, Japan

Teruki Yanagi, Shinya Kitamura and Hiroo Hata
Department of Dermatology, Hokkaido University Graduate School of Medicine, Sapporo, Japan

Junji Kato, Kohei Horimoto, Sayuri Sato, Tomoyuki Minowa and Hisashi Uhara
Department of Dermatology, Sapporo Medical University School of Medicine, Sapporo, Japan

Tomonori Oka and Tomomitsu Miyagaki
Department of Dermatology, Graduate School of Medicine, The University of Tokyo, Tokyo, Japan

Kazuyasu Fujii and Takuro Kanekura
Department of Dermatology, Kagoshima University Graduate School of Medical and Dental Sciences, Kagoshima, Japan

Sae Inoue, Naoko Okiyama, Yosuke Ishitsuka, Rei Watanabe and Manabu Fujimoto
Dermatology, University of Tsukuba, Tsukuba, Ibaraki, Japan

Yoshiyuki Nakamura
Department of Dermatology, Faculty of Medicine, University of Tsukuba, Tsukuba, Japan

Yumi Kambayashi, Taku Fujimura, Takanori Hidaka and Setsuya Aiba
Department of Dermatology, Tohoku University Graduate School of Medicine, Sendai, Japan

Index

Printed in the USA
CPSIA information can be obtained
at www.ICGtesting.com
JSHW050003260324
59877JS00005B/45